IGNATAVICIUS · WORKMAN

MEDICAL-SURGICAL NURSING

Patient-Centered Collaborative Care

7th

Edition

CHRIS WINKELMAN, RN, PhD, CCRN, ACNP
Associate Professor
Frances Payne Bolton School of Nursing
Case Western Reserve University;
Clinical Nurse
Trauma/Critical Care Float Pool
MetroHealth Medical Center
Cleveland, Ohio

3251 Riverport Lane
St. Louis, Missouri 63043

Clinical Companion for Medical-Surgical Nursing:
Patient-Centered Collaborative Care   ISBN: 978-1-4377-2797-5

Previous editions copyrighted 2010, 2006, 2002

International Standard Book Number: 978-1-4377-2797-5

Executive Content Strategist, Nursing: Lee Henderson
Content Coordinator: Kel McGowan
Publishing Services Manager: Deborah L. Vogel
Senior Project Manager: Jodi M. Willard
Design Direction: Jessica Williams

Printed in United States of America
Last digit is the print number: 9 8 7 6 5 4 3 2 1

Preface

Welcome to the new edition of the *Clinical Companion for Medical-Surgical Nursing: Critical Thinking for Collaborative Care!* This is a succinct reference to conditions and interventions seen in the acute care setting. It reflects the Ignatavicius and Workman text and its most recent changes.

As with the Ignatavicius and Workman text, the new feature **Nursing Safety Priority** ❗ gives cues to one of three types of situations and details essential nursing actions to promote effective care: (1) *Action Alert*—discusses an activity or intervention that promotes optimal outcomes; (2) *Critical Rescue*—signals a need for immediate attention and action to prevent a critical outcome; (3) *Drug Alert*—informs the reader about potential adverse drug reactions and strategies for administering and monitoring patient responses to drugs that have the potential to harm hospitalized patients. **National Patient Safety Goals** 🛡 are applied to assessments and interventions in congruence with The Joint Commission goals for safety in hospital settings. Genetic/genomic considerations, as well as considerations for older adults, women, and people of various cultural backgrounds have been updated to reflect the best evidence for delivery of care.

Part One, renamed *Concepts of Medical-Surgical Nursing*, provides an overview of the physiology, pathology, and collaborative management of selected common conditions in the acute care setting. This section uses the nursing process to integrate assessment, diagnostic testing, interventions, and evaluation of patient responses.

Part Two continues to feature a brief, prioritized snapshot of diseases and disorders, including new content on H1N1 influenza and sickle cell disease. Designed to be a reference for nurses in a variety of settings that deliver acute care to adults, this *Clinical Companion* stands alone. For the reader who desires more information, we recommend Ignatavicius and Workman's *Medical-Surgical Nursing: Patient-Centered Collaborative Care*, 7th edition.

The ten appendixes at the back of the text are designed to be quick capsules of concentrated knowledge. The appendixes include three common situations (head-to-toe physical assessment, normal laboratory values, discharge planning) and five less typical situations that need quick responses (electrocardiogram interpretation, care for a patient with chest tubes, caring for a patient with intubation/mechanical ventilation, environmental emergencies, chemical/biological terrorism emergencies, and vocabulary for Spanish-speaking patients).

Medical-surgical nursing is both the most and the least special-ized practice in the acute care setting. This text balances general and specialty knowledge in a format that can be carried with you in a variety of medical-surgical settings. Let us know if we left out important information you need to practice at the bedside; we are already making plans for the 8th edition.

Acknowledgments

The insight and skillful assistance of Lee Henderson, Rae Robertson, Kel McGowan, and Jodi Willard from Elsevier have improved the user-friendly format for presenting the essential information in this edition. Well done!

Students, clinicians, and my family continue to inform, inspire and sustain my enthusiasm for nursing. Thank you!

–CW

Acknowledgments

Concepts of Medical-Surgical Nursing

CANCER PATHOPHYSIOLOGY

OVERVIEW

- *Neoplasia* is any new or continued cell growth not needed for normal development or replacement of dead and damaged tissues. This new growth may be benign or cancerous.
- *Benign tumor cells* are normal cells growing in the wrong place or at the wrong time. They are not needed for normal growth and development. Although benign tumors do not invade other tissues, depending on their location, they can damage normal tissue and may need to be removed.
- *Cancer cells*, also called *malignant cells*, are abnormal, serve no useful function, and invade and destroy normal body tissues. Without treatment, cancer leads to death.
- Cancer can develop in any tissue or organ but tends to occur more commonly in tissues that continue to grow by cell division (mitosis) throughout the life span.
- All cancers start from normal cells that undergo changes at the gene level. These changes result in a loss of control over cell growth.
- *Carcinogenesis* and *oncogenesis* are additional names for cancer development.
- *Malignant transformation* is the process of changing a normal cell into a cancer cell.
- *Carcinogens* are substances that can damage normal cell DNA and change the activity of genes. Carcinogens may be chemicals, physical agents, or viruses.
- Biologic features of cancer cells and malignant tumors are:
  1. Anaplasia or loss of the specific appearance of the parent cells
  2. A large nuclear-cytoplasmic ratio or a larger-than-normal cell nucleus
  3. Loss of specific cell function
  4. Loose adherence resulting in the ability of malignant cells to migrate

   5. Rapid, persistent cell division
   6. Aneuploidy or abnormal chromosomes
   7. No response to normal cellular signals for programmed cell death (i.e., apoptosis)
- A *primary tumor* is the original tumor, identified by the normal tissue from which it arose.
- When primary tumors are located in vital organs, such as the brain or lungs, they can grow excessively and lethally damage the vital organ or crowd out healthy organ tissue and interfere with that organ's ability to perform its vital function.
- A *metastatic tumor* is one that has spread from the original site, usually through the blood or lymph, into other tissues and organs, where it can establish metastatic or secondary tumors that grow and cause more damage and dysfunction.
   1. When a metastatic tumor is in another organ, it is still a cancer from the original altered tissue.
   2. For example, when breast cancer spreads to the lung and the bone, it is breast cancer in the lung and bone, not lung cancer and not bone cancer.

CARCINOGENESIS/ONCOGENESIS

- The process of carcinogenesis or oncogenesis occurs through the steps of initiation, promotion, progression, and metastasis.
   1. *Initiation* begins the change of a normal cell into a cancer cell. Initiation is the result of expression of oncogenes (genes that cause normal cells to transform into cancerous cells) or reduced expression of suppressor genes (genes that prevent cancerous transformation of normal cells), altering cell division. If growth conditions are right, widespread metastatic disease can develop from just one cancer cell.
   2. *Promotion* is the enhancement of growth of an initiated cell. Many normal hormones and body proteins, such as insulin and estrogen, act as promoters and make initiated cells divide more often.
   3. *Progression* is the continued change of a cancer, making cells more malignant. One change is the development of a separate blood supply. Over time, changes in cell growth and function provide advantages that allow cancer cells to live and divide, no matter how the conditions around them change.
   4. *Metastasis* is the spread of a tumor into nearby or remote tissue areas by invasion.
- Cancers are classified by the type of tissue from which they arise. For example, glandular cancers are carcinomas, and connective tissue cancers are sarcomas.

- About 100 different types of cancer arise from various tissues or organs.
- Solid tumors develop from specific tissues (e.g., breast cancer and lung cancer). Hematologic cancers (e.g., leukemias and lymphomas) arise from blood cell-forming tissues and lymphatic tissues.
- Systems of cancer grading and staging are used to standardize cancer diagnosis, prognosis, and treatment.
- *Grading* of a tumor classifies cellular aspects of the cancer and ranks cancers for degree of malignancy on the basis of cancer cell appearance, growth rates, and aggressiveness compared with the normal tissues from which they arose. Low-grade cancers have fewer malignant features and are well-differentiated; high-grade cancers have more malignant features such as anaplasia.
- Tumor *ploidy* classifies tumor chromosomes as normal or abnormal. When cancer cell chromosomes are abnormal, they are called *aneuploid*. The degree of aneuploidy usually increases with the degree of malignancy.
- *Staging* determines the exact location of the cancer and its degree of metastasis at diagnosis. Staging is important, because for most cancers, the smaller the cancer is at diagnosis and the less it has spread, the greater the chances are that treatment will result in a cure. Staging also influences selection of therapy.
  1. *Clinical staging* assesses the patient's clinical manifestations and evaluates clinical signs for tumor size and possible spread.
  2. *Surgical staging* assesses the tumor size, number, sites, and spread by inspection at surgery.
  3. *Pathologic staging* is the most definitive type, determining the tumor size, number, sites, and spread by pathologic examination of tissues obtained at surgery.

CANCER ETIOLOGY AND GENETIC RISK

- Carcinogenesis takes years and depends on several tumor and patient factors.
- Three interacting factors influence cancer development: exposure to carcinogens, genetic predisposition, and immune function.
- *Oncogene activation* with overexpression is the main mechanism of carcinogenesis regardless of the specific cause. Oncogenes cause normal cells to transform into cancerous cells.
- The normal cell's suppressor genes (which control cell growth and prevent oncogene overexpression) can be damaged or mutated. As a result, the oncogenes are overexpressed.

- Both external and personal factors can activate oncogenes, damage suppressor genes, or both, leading to cancer development.
- External factors that cause cancer include:
  1. Exposure to chemical carcinogens, such as many known chemicals, tobacco, drugs, and other products used in everyday life
  2. Exposure to physical carcinogens, such as radiation and chronic irritation
  3. Infection with a carcinogenic virus, such as certain strains of the human papillomavirus (HPV)
  4. Possible dietary factors, such as low fiber intake, high intake of red meat, and high animal fat intake. Preservatives, contaminants, preparation methods, and additives (e.g., dyes, flavorings, and sweeteners) also may have cancer-promoting effects.
- Personal factors in cancer development include:
  1. Immune function, with decreased immune function increasing cancer risk
  2. Advancing age, the single most important risk factor for cancer
  3. Genetic predisposition, resulting from the inheritance of specific gene mutation(s)

Genetic/Genomic Considerations

- Genetic risk for cancer occurs in a small percentage of the population; however, people who have a genetic predisposition are at high risk for cancer development, and these predispositions can be passed from generation to generation.
- In some people, the sequence of a specific oncogene is different (has been mutated), which may allow it to be activated more easily. In other people, the oncogene is normal, but the gene controlling oncogene activity, the *suppressor gene*, is mutated and allows overexpression of one or more oncogenes, leading to a huge increase in cancer risk.
- Inherited predisposition for specific cancers, inherited conditions associated with cancer, familial clustering, and chromosomal aberrations demonstrate a pattern of genetic risk for cancer.

⊕ Cultural Awareness

- The incidence of cancer varies among races. African Americans have a higher incidence of cancer than white Americans do, and the death rate is higher for African Americans.
- Cancer sites and cancer-related mortality also vary along racial lines. One explanation for this difference is that more African Americans have less access to health care. They are more often diagnosed with later stage cancer that is more difficult to cure or control. However, this disparity in health care access does not explain all differences.

PATIENT-CENTERED COLLABORATIVE CARE

- Teach patients to use sunscreen and to wear protective clothing during sun exposure.
- Encourage patients to participate in the recommended cancer-screening activities for their age-group and cancer risk category.
- Inform all patients who smoke that tobacco use is a causative factor in 30% of all cancers. Assist anyone interested in smoking cessation to find an appropriate smoking cessation program.
- Assess the patient's knowledge about causes of cancer and his or her screening and prevention practices.
- Help patients who fear a cancer diagnosis to understand that finding cancer at an early stage increases the chances for cure.
- Ask all patients about their exposures to environmental agents that are known or suspected to increase the risk for cancer.
- Obtain a detailed family history (at least three generations) and use this information to create a pedigree to assess the patient's risk for familial or inherited cancer.
- Teach anyone, especially older adults, the "seven warning signs of cancer" (indicated by the acronym *CAUTION*):
    1. **C**hanges in bowel or bladder habits
    2. **A** sore that does not heal
    3. **U**nusual bleeding or discharge
    4. **T**hickening or lump in the breast or elsewhere
    5. **I**ndigestion or difficulty swallowing
    6. **O**bvious change in a wart or mole
    7. **N**agging cough or hoarseness

CANCER TREATMENT ISSUES

- Primary prevention of cancer involves avoiding exposure to known causes of cancer.
- Secondary prevention of cancer involves screening for early detection.
- Tertiary treatment occurs after a cancer diagnosis, and the purpose is to prolong survival time or improve quality of life.
- Therapies for cancer include surgery, radiation therapy, chemotherapy, hormonal manipulation, photodynamic therapy, immunotherapy, gene therapy, and targeted therapy.
- Various therapies may be used separately or, more commonly, in combination to kill cancer cells.
- The types and amount of therapy used depend on the specific type of cancer, whether the cancer has spread, and the health of the patient.

CANCER SURGERY

OVERVIEW

- Surgery for cancer involves the removal of diseased tissue and may be used for prophylaxis, diagnosis, cure, control, palliation, determination of therapy effectiveness, and reconstruction.
  1. *Prophylactic surgery* is the removal of at-risk tissue to prevent cancer development and is performed when a patient has an existing premalignant condition or a known family history that strongly predisposes the person to the development of a specific cancer.
  2. *Diagnostic surgery (biopsy)* is the removal of all or part of a suspected lesion for examination and testing. It provides proof of the presence of cancer.
  3. *Curative surgery* is focused on removal of all cancer tissue and alone can result in a cure rate of 27% to 30% when all visible and microscopic tumor is removed or destroyed.
  4. Cancer control, or *cytoreductive surgery,* is the removal of part of the tumor and leaving a known amount of gross tumor. It is also known as *debulking surgery,* and it does not alone result in a cure.
  5. *Palliative surgery* is focused on improving the quality of life during the survival time and is not focused on cure.
  6. *Second-look surgery* is used for a rediagnosis after treatment. The results of this surgery are used to determine whether a specific therapy should be continued or discontinued.
  7. *Reconstructive or rehabilitative surgery* increases function, enhances appearance, or both.

PATIENT-CENTERED COLLABORATIVE CARE

- The nursing care needs of the patient having surgery for cancer are similar to those related to surgery for other reasons.
- Surgery usually involves the loss of a specific body part or its function.
- The amount of function lost and how much the loss affects patients depend on the location and extent of the cancer and surgical intervention.
- Some cancer surgery results in major scarring or disfigurement.
- Two additional priority care needs are psychosocial support and assisting the patient to achieve or maintain maximum function.
  1. Assess the patient's and family's ability to cope with the uncertainty of cancer and its treatment and with the changes in body image and role.
  2. Coordinate with the health care team to provide support for the patient and family.

3. Encourage the patient and family to express their feelings and concerns.
4. Encourage the patient to look at the surgical site, touch it, and participate in any dressing changes or incisional care required.
5. Provide information about support groups, such as those sponsored by the American Cancer Society or specialty cancer organizations.
6. Discuss with the patient the idea of having a person who has coped with the same issues come for a visit.
7. Teach the patient about the importance of performing and progressing the intensity of any prescribed exercises to regain as much function as possible and prevent complications.
8. Coordinate with the physical therapist, occupational therapist, and family members to plan strategies individualized to each patient to regain or maintain optimal function.

RADIATION THERAPY

OVERVIEW

- The purpose of radiation therapy for cancer is to destroy cancer cells with minimal exposure of the normal cells to the damaging actions of radiation.
- Because the effects of radiation are seen only in the tissues in the path of the radiation beam, this type of therapy is a local treatment.
- Radiation doses vary according to the size, location, and radiation sensitivity of the tumor and surrounding normal tissues.
- Radiation therapy is classified in two categories:
  1. *Teletherapy*: The radiation source is external to the patient and remote from the tumor site. It is also called *external beam radiation*. Because the source is external, the patient is not radioactive and is not a hazard to others. This type of therapy usually is given as a series of divided doses.
  2. *Brachytherapy*: The radiation source comes into direct, continuous contact with the tumor tissues for a specific period of time. It is delivered in a solid, sealed form or unsealed within body fluids. *With all types of brachytherapy, the patient emits radiation for a period of time and is a hazard to others.*
- Side effects of radiation therapy are limited to the tissues exposed to the radiation and vary according to the site. Skin changes and hair loss are local but are likely to be permanent. Other common side effects include altered taste sensations and severe fatigue.

- Radiation damage to normal tissues during cancer therapy can start the inflammatory responses that cause tissue fibrosis and scarring. These effects may not be apparent for many years after radiation treatment.

PATIENT-CENTERED COLLABORATIVE CARE

- For teletherapy, teach patients to:
  1. Wash the irradiated area gently each day with water or with a mild soap and water.
  2. Use the hand rather than a washcloth to be gentler.
  3. Rinse soap thoroughly from the skin.
  4. Not remove any ink or dye markings that indicate exactly where the beam of radiation is to be focused.
  5. Dry the irradiated area with patting motions rather than rubbing motions; use a clean, soft towel or cloth.
  6. Powders, ointments, lotions, or creams on the skin should not be used at the radiation site unless they are prescribed by the radiologist or the radiation therapy advanced practice nurse.
  7. Wear soft clothing over the skin at the radiation site.
  8. Avoid wearing belts, buckles, straps, or any type of clothing that binds or rubs the skin at the radiation site.
  9. Avoid exposure of the irradiated area to the sun.
     a. Protect this area by wearing clothing over it but *not* by applying sunscreen agents.
     b. Avoid going outdoors between 10:00 AM and 4:00 PM to avoid the more intense sunrays.
     c. Use awnings, umbrellas, and other forms of shade when outdoors during the times when the sun's rays are most intense.
  10. Avoid heat exposure.
- For patients receiving brachytherapy:
  1. Assign the patient to a private room with a private bath.
  2. Place a "Caution: Radioactive Material" sign on the door of the patient's room.
  3. If portable lead shields are used, place them between the patient and the door.
  4. Keep the door to the patient's room closed as much as possible.
  5. Wear a dosimeter film badge at all times while caring for patients with radioactive implants. Each badge should be used only by one individual.
  6. Wear a lead apron while providing care. Always keep the front of the apron facing the source of radiation (do not turn your back toward the patient).

7. Pregnant nurses should not care for these patients; do not allow pregnant women or children younger than 16 years old to visit.

8. Limit each visitor to 30 minutes per day. Be sure visitors are at least 6 feet from the source.

9. Never touch the radioactive source with bare hands. In the rare instance that it is dislodged, use a long-handled forceps to retrieve it. Deposit the radioactive source in the lead container kept in the patient's room.

10. Save all dressings and bed linens until after the radioactive source is removed.

CHEMOTHERAPY

OVERVIEW

- *Chemotherapy* is the treatment of cancer with chemical agents. It is used to cure and to increase survival time, because it has some selectivity for killing cancer cells over normal cells.
- The tumors most sensitive to chemotherapy are those that have rapid growth.
- The effects of chemotherapy are systemic, providing the opportunity to kill metastatic cancer cells that may have escaped local treatment.
- Drugs used for chemotherapy usually are given systemically and exert their cell-damaging (cytotoxic) effects against healthy cells and cancer cells.
- The normal cells most affected by chemotherapy are those that divide rapidly, including skin, hair, intestinal tissues, spermatocytes, and blood-forming cells.
- Chemotherapy drugs are classified by the specific types of action they exert in the cancer cell and include antimetabolites, antitumor antibiotics, antimitotic agents, alkylating agents, topoisomerase inhibitors, and miscellaneous agents.
- Successful cancer chemotherapy most often involves giving more than one anticancer drug in a timed manner, known as *combination chemotherapy.*
- Drugs are selected based on known tumor sensitivity to the drugs and the degree of side effects expected.
- Dosages for most chemotherapy drugs are calculated according to the type of cancer and the patient's size, usually based on milligrams per square meter of total body surface area or on weight in kilograms.
- Although most chemotherapy drugs are given IV, they may also be given by the oral, intra-arterial, isolated limb perfusion, intracavitary, and intrathecal routes.

- Administration of IV chemotherapy is usually performed by a registered nurse who has completed an approved chemotherapy course.
- *Extravasation,* or *infiltration,* is a serious complication of IV chemotherapy administration that can lead to:
    1. Pain
    2. Infection
    3. Tissue loss
- The most important nursing intervention for extravasation is prevention by close monitoring of the access site during chemotherapy administration.
- Immediate treatment of extravasation depends on the specific drug. Coordinate with the oncologist and pharmacist to determine the type of compress and specific antidote needed for the extravasated drug.
- Perform and document the following activities for an extravasation event:
    1. Date and time when extravasation was suspected or identified
    2. Date and time when the infusion was started
    3. Time when the infusion was stopped
    4. The exact contents of the infusion fluid and the volume of fluid infused
    5. The estimated amount of fluid extravasated
    6. A diagram of the exact insertion site, and indication of whether this is a venous access device, implanted port, or a tunneled catheter
    7. The method of administration (e.g., pump, controller, rate of infusion)
    8. The needle type and size
    9. Indication on the diagram the location and number of venipuncture attempts
    10. The time between the extravasation and the last fully documented blood return.
    11. All agents administered in the previous 24 hours through this site (list agent administered, dosage and volume, and order of administration)
    12. Patient's vital signs
    13. Patient's subjective sensations and symptoms
    14. All observations of the site, including size, color, and texture
    15. A photograph of the site
    16. Administration of neutralizing or antidote agents
    17. Application of compresses and their temperature
    18. Other nursing interventions
    19. Patient's responses to nursing interventions
    20. Notification of the prescribing physician (including the time)

21. Written and oral instructions given to the patient about follow-up care
22. Any consultation request
- Sign the documentation.
- Nurses and other health care workers who prepare or give these drugs or who handle the excreta from patients within 48 hours of receiving IV chemotherapy must use extreme caution and wear personal protective equipment (PPE), including eye protection, masks, double gloves, and gown.
- Side effects of chemotherapy often include bone marrow suppression (e.g., neutropenia, anemia, thrombocytopenia), nausea and vomiting, mucositis, alopecia, changes in cognitive function, and peripheral neuropathy.

PATIENT-CENTERED COLLABORATIVE CARE
- For patients with neutropenia:
  1. Administer medications that enhance the immune system (e.g., biological response modifiers [BRMs]) as prescribed.
  2. Assess the skin and mucous membranes, lung sounds, mouth, and venous access device insertion sites every 8 hours.
  3. Urge the patient to report any indicator of infection, such as a change in skin and mucous membranes (e.g., pimple, sore, rash, open area), presence of a cough, burning on urination, pain around the venous access site, or new drainage from any location.
  4. Use good handwashing before contact with the patient.
  5. Modify the environment to protect patients who have neutropenia or thrombocytopenia.
  6. Ensure that mouth care and washing of the axillary and perianal regions are performed at least every 12 hours to reduce bioburden.
  7. Monitor for manifestations of infection.

■ NURSING SAFETY PRIORITY: Critical Rescue

The patient with neutropenia often does not develop a high fever or have purulent drainage, even when a severe infection is present. Any elevation of temperature in a patient with neutropenia is significant and is considered a sign of infection, and it should be reported to the health care provider immediately.

  8. Initiate standard protocols regarding obtaining cultures, tests, and administering antibiotics for suspected infection in neutropenic patients according to institution policy.
  9. Teach patients and family members precautions to reduce the risk for infection.

- For patients with anemia:
  1. Administer BRMs as prescribed.
  2. Assess for tachycardia and increased respiratory rate.
  3. Encourage the patient to rest.
  4. In collaboration with other members of the health care team, postpone or cancel activities that do not have a direct impact on the health of the patient.
- For patients with thrombocytopenia, provide a safe hospital environment by:
  1. Handling the patient gently
  2. Using and teaching unlicensed assistive personnel (UAP) to use a lift sheet when moving and positioning the patient in bed
  3. Avoiding IM injections and venipunctures
  4. Applying firm pressure to needle stick sites for 10 minutes
  5. Testing all urine and stool for the presence of occult blood
  6. Observing IV sites every 4 hours for bleeding
  7. Avoiding rectal temperatures, even on unconscious patients
  8. Administering prescribed suppositories carefully with liberal lubrication
  9. Instructing the patient and UAP to use an electric shaver rather than a razor
  10. When providing mouth care or supervising others in providing mouth care, instruct about:
      a. Using a soft-bristled toothbrush or tooth sponges
      b. Not using floss
      c. Checking to ensure that dentures fit and do not rub
- For patients with chemotherapy-induced nausea and vomiting (CINV):
  1. Administer prescribed antiemetics on a scheduled, rather than PRN, basis.
  2. Ensure that premedication with antiemetics occurs before each session of IV chemotherapy.
  3. Assess patients for dehydration and electrolyte imbalances.
  4. Teach patients to continue the therapy as prescribed, even when the nausea and vomiting appear controlled.

Considerations for Older Adults

- Sometimes, older patients have received lower doses of chemotherapy drugs to avoid debilitating adverse effects of chemotherapeutic agents such as the side effects of severe nausea and vomiting, cardiac or renal injury, or metabolic derangements leading to the need for hospitalization or the outcome of dysfunction. Monitor older adults closely for both early-onset and extended adverse effects from all cancer treatments.

- The older adult can become dehydrated more quickly if CINV is not adequately controlled. Teach older adult patients to be pro-active with taking their prescribed antiemetics and to contact their health care provider if the CINV does not resolve within 12 hours or becomes worse.

- For patients with mucositis:
  1. Examine the patient's mouth, including the roof, under the tongue, and between the teeth and cheek, every 4 hours.
  2. Document the location, size, and character of fissures, blisters, sores, or drainage.
  3. Brush the teeth and tongue with a soft-bristled brush or sponges every 8 hours.
  4. Rinse the mouth with a solution of 50% peroxide and 50% half-normal saline every 12 hours. (Rinsing with lukewarm water can be done as often as the patient desires.)
  5. Avoid the use of alcohol or glycerin-based mouthwashes.
  6. Encourage the patient to drink 3 or more liters of water per day, as long as another health problem does not require limiting fluid intake.
  7. Administer antimicrobial and topical analgesic drugs as prescribed.
  8. Assist the patient in using artificial saliva as needed, if prescribed.
  9. Urge the patient to avoid using tobacco or drinking alcoholic beverages.
  10. Assist the patient in menu choices to avoid spicy, salty, acidic, dry, rough, or hard food.
  11. Suggest that dentures be worn only during meals.
  12. Offer complete mouth care before and after every meal.
- For patients with alopecia:
  1. Reassure patients that hair loss is temporary and that hair regrowth usually begins about 1 month after completion of chemotherapy.
  2. Inform the patient that the new hair may differ from the original hair in color, texture, and thickness.
  3. Teach the patient to protect the scalp from injury by avoiding direct sunlight on the scalp through the use of hats or other head coverings.
  4. Teach the patient to wear some head covering underneath helmets, headphones, headsets, and other items that rub the head.
  5. Assist patients in selecting a type of head covering (e.g., wigs, scarves, turbans, caps, hats) that suits their income and lifestyle.

- For patients with changes in cognitive function:
  1. Support the patient who reports this side effect. Listen to the patient's concerns and tell him or her that other patients have also reported such problems.
  2. Warn patients against participating in other behaviors that could alter cognitive functioning, such as excessive alcohol intake, recreational drug use, and taking part in activities that increase the risk for head injury.
- For patients with chemotherapy-induced peripheral neuropathy, teach patients to prevent injury by:
  1. Not walking around in bare feet or stocking feet
  2. Always wearing shoes with a protective sole
  3. Making sure shoes are long enough and wide enough to prevent creating sores or blisters (avoid pointed-toe shoes and high heels)
  4. Providing a long break-in period for new shoes; not wearing new shoes for longer than 2 hours at a time
  5. Inspecting feet daily (with a mirror) for open areas or redness
  6. Avoiding extremes of temperature; wearing warm clothing in the winter, especially over hands, feet, and ears
  7. Testing water temperature with a thermometer when washing dishes or bathing and using warm water rather than hot water (less than 110° F [43.3° C])
  8. Setting hot water heater temperature at or below 110° F (43.3° C)
  9. Using potholders when cooking
  10. Using gloves when washing dishes or gardening
  11. Not eating foods that are steaming hot
  12. Getting up from a lying or sitting position slowly
  13. Looking at the feet and the floor or ground when walking to assess how the ground, floor, or step changes
  14. Not using area rugs, especially those that slide easily
  15. Using handrails when going up or down steps

HORMONAL MANIPULATION

- Hormonal manipulation can help control some types of cancer by decreasing the amount of hormones reaching hormone-sensitive tumors.
- Some drugs are hormone antagonists that compete with natural hormones at the tumor's receptor sites, preventing a needed hormone from binding to the receptor.
- Hormone inhibitors suppress the production of specific hormones in the normal hormone-producing organs.

- Androgens and the antiestrogen receptor drugs cause masculinizing effects in women, with increased chest and facial hair, interruption of the menstrual period, and shrinkage of breast tissue.
- Other effects for men and women receiving androgens include acne, fluid retention, hypercalcemia, deep vein thrombosis, and liver dysfunction (with prolonged therapy).
- Feminine manifestations often appear in men who take estrogens, progestins, or antiandrogen receptor drugs, including thinning facial hair, smoother skin, and gynecomastia. Testicular and penile atrophy also occur to some degree.

PHOTODYNAMIC THERAPY

OVERVIEW

- *Photodynamic therapy (PDT)* is the selective destruction of cancer cells through a chemical reaction triggered by different types of laser light.
- It is most commonly used for nonmelanoma skin cancers, ocular tumors, GI tumors, and lung cancers located in the airways.
- An agent that sensitizes cells to light is injected IV along with a dye. These drugs enter all cells but leave normal cells more rapidly than cancer cells. Usually within 48 to 72 hours, most of the drug has collected in high concentrations in cancer cells. At this time, a laser light is focused on the tumor. The light activates a chemical reaction within those cells, retaining the sensitizing drug that induces irreversible cell damage.

PATIENT-CENTERED COLLABORATIVE CARE

- The patient has increased sensitivity to light for up to 12 weeks after the photosensitizing drug is injected, with the most sensitivity in the immediate 48 hours after a treatment.
- The most intense period of light sensitivity is after injection and before the laser treatment. During this time, the patient is at high risk for sunburn and eye pain.
- Before photosensitizing therapy, teach the patient to:
  1. Bring protective clothing (e.g., shirts with long sleeves and high collars, long pants or skirt, gloves, socks, and a wide-brimmed hat) and UV-protective sunglasses when he or she comes to be injected with the photosensitizing agent.
  2. Have someone else drive the patient home if possible, so that he or she can be covered with a sheet or light blanket.
  3. Plan to avoid exposure to sunlight for 1 to 3 months.
  4. Cover all windows with light-blocking shades or heavy drapes or curtains.

5. Replace high-wattage light bulbs with lower wattage ones, and use as few as possible.

- After photosensitizing therapy, teach the patient to:
  1. Continue to wear all protective clothing and to avoid sunlight and high-wattage indoor lights.
  2. Drink plenty of water to prevent becoming dehydrated.
  3. Refrain from taking any newly prescribed or over-the-counter (OTC) drugs without contacting the physician who performed the PDT. Some drugs make the light sensitivity even worse; other drugs interact with the photosensitizing drug.
  4. Start re-exposure to sunlight and other bright lights slowly. Start by exposing only about 1 inch of skin to sunlight at a time. Start with 10 minutes, and increase the time by about 5 minutes each day.
  5. Remember that sunscreen cannot prevent severe sunburn during this time.
  6. If pain or blistering occurs, notify the PDT health care team.
  7. Continue to wear dark glasses, even indoors, until eye pain no longer occurs when in a normally lighted environment.
  8. After 3 months, see an ophthalmologist to check for retinal damage.

IMMUNOTHERAPY: BIOLOGICAL RESPONSE MODIFIERS

OVERVIEW

- BRMs modify the patient's biologic responses to tumor cells. Many of those in use for cancer therapy affect *cytokines* or *growth factors.* Cytokines are small proteins made by white blood cells (WBCs).
- Cytokines for cancer therapy generally enhance the immune system and can:
  1. Stimulate the immune system to recognize cancer cells and take actions to eliminate or destroy them
  2. Serve a supporting role by stimulating faster recovery of bone marrow function after treatment-induced suppression
- Two common types of BRMs used as cancer therapy are:
  1. *Interleukins (ILs),* which help different immune system cells recognize and destroy abnormal body cells. In particular, IL-1, -2, and -6 appear to "charge up" the immune system and enhance attacks on cancer cells by macrophages, natural killer (NK) cells, and tumor-infiltrating lymphocytes.

2. *Interferons (IFNs)*, which can:
   a. Slow tumor cell division.
   b. Stimulate the growth and activation of NK cells.
   c. Induce cancer cells to resume a more normal appearance and function.
   d. Inhibit the expression of oncogenes.

PATIENT-CENTERED COLLABORATIVE CARE

- Side effects of ILs include manifestations of inflammatory reactions:
  1. Widespread edema
  2. Chills, fever
  3. Rigors (severe shaking with chills)
  4. Flu-like general malaise
  5. Skin reactions
  6. Peripheral neuropathy (later, with high doses)
- Management includes:
  1. Giving meperidine (Demerol) for rigors
  2. Giving acetaminophen for fever
  3. Advising patients to apply moisturizers (perfume-free) to the skin and to use mild soap to clean the skin
  4. Teaching patients to protect involved skin areas from the sun with clothing or the use of sunscreen agents, to avoid swimming, and to refrain from using topical steroid creams on affected areas

TARGETED THERAPY

- Targeted therapies take advantage of one or more differences in cancer cell growth or metabolism that are not present or only slightly present in normal cells.
- Agents used as targeted therapies often are antibodies that work to disrupt cancer cell division by:
  1. Targeting and blocking growth factor receptors, especially the epithelial growth factor receptors (EGFRs) or the vascular endothelial growth factor receptors (VEGFRs). When a cancer cell's growth depends on having the growth factors bind to their specific receptors, blocking the receptor slows or eliminates the cancer cell's growth.
     NOTE: For therapies that bind to the EGFR and VEGFR receptors, normal cells in the skin, GI tract, and mucous membranes also express these receptors and may develop open sores, rashes, and acne-type lesions.
  2. Blocking signal transduction pathways in cancer cells so that the signals for turning on cell genes for division and function

does not occur. These drugs include tyrosine kinase inhibitors (TKIs), multikinase inhibitors (MKIs) and proteasome inhibitors.

3. Blocking the growth of blood vessels so that nutrients cannot be delivered to tumors (angiogenesis inhibitors)

4. Using monoclonal antibodies that bind to cancer cell receptors or cytosol proteins needed for cancer cell function or division

   NOTE: Allergic reactions can occur in patients receiving monoclonal antibodies as a result of the expression of animal proteins from the original development model.

- Targeted therapies work only on cancer cells that overexpress the actual target substance. Each person's cancer cells are evaluated to determine whether the cells have enough of a target to be affected by targeted therapy.

ONCOLOGIC EMERGENCIES

- Oncologic emergencies are acute complications associated with cancer and its treatment that often require immediate intervention to avoid life-threatening situations. These complications include sepsis and disseminated intravascular coagulation (DIC), syndrome of inappropriate antidiuretic hormone (SIADH), spinal cord compression (SCC), hypercalcemia, and tumor lysis syndrome (TLS).

- Sepsis and DIC

  1. Microorganisms enter the bloodstream and grow unchecked, because the patient often has low a WBC count and impaired immune function. This problem can lead to septic shock and death.

  2. DIC is a clotting problem triggered by sepsis, by the release of clotting factors from cancer cells, or by blood transfusions. Extensive abnormal clotting occurs throughout the small blood vessels, using up the existing clotting factors and platelets. This process is then followed by extensive bleeding that can range from minimal to fatal hemorrhage.

  3. Management focuses on prevention, early detection, and prompt aggressive treatment.

  4. For prevention:

     a. Identify those patients at greatest risk for sepsis and DIC.

     b. Use aseptic technique during care for open skin areas, nonintact mucosa, or any invasive procedure.

     c. Teach patients and family members the early manifestations of infection and sepsis and when to seek medical assistance.

5. For treatment:
   a. Administer timely IV antibiotic therapy.
   b. With DIC, anticipate IV administration of clotting factors.
   c. With severe sepsis, anticipate administration of activated protein C (drotrecogin alpha [Xigris]).

- SIADH
  1. Certain cancers secrete or stimulate the secretion of antidiuretic hormone (ADH) when it is not needed by the body for fluid and electrolyte balance. The result is retention of pure water and dilution of electrolytes. In addition to lung and other cancers, SIADH can be caused by morphine and cyclophosphamide.
  2. Assess for:
     a. Weight gain daily
     b. Decreased urine output
     c. Weakness and fatigue
     d. Muscle cramps
     e. Low serum sodium levels of 115 to 120 mEq/L (normal range is 135 to 145 mEq/L)
     f. Decreased and altered mentation and seizures when sodium levels are less than 110 mEq/L; this is a medical emergency.
  3. Management includes:
     a. Free water restriction
     b. Increased sodium intake
     c. Drug therapy, most often with demeclocycline
     d. Immediate cancer therapy to cause tumor regression
  4. Monitor for indications of fluid overload and pulmonary edema:
     a. Increased pulse quality
     b. Increasing neck vein distension
     c. Presence of crackles in lungs
     d. Increasing peripheral edema
- SCC
  1. SCC and damage occur when a tumor directly enters the spinal cord or when the vertebrae collapse from tumor degradation of the bone. It most commonly occurs with lung, prostate, breast, and colon cancers.
  2. Manifestations include:
     a. Back pain
     b. Numbness or tingling
     c. Reduced motor and sensory function
     d. Paralysis (which may be permanent)

❗NURSING SAFETY PRIORITY: Action Alert

Early recognition and treatment of spinal cord compression are key to a good outcome. Assess any cancer patient with new-onset back pain, muscle weakness or a sensation of "heaviness" in the arms or legs, numbness or tingling in the hands or feet, loss of ability to distinguish hot and cold, or an unsteady gait, and report these findings to the oncologist immediately.

3. Teach patients and families the manifestations of early SCC and instruct them to seek help as soon as problems are apparent.
4. Management is often palliative and may include:
   a. High-dose corticosteroids to reduce swelling around the spinal cord
   b. High-dose radiation to the site
   c. Intense chemotherapy to reduce tumor size
   d. Surgery to remove the tumor from the area (less common)
   e. External back or neck braces to reduce pressure on the spinal cord or spinal nerves
- Hypercalcemia
   1. Hypercalcemia (high serum calcium level) occurs most often in patients with bone metastasis. Tumors can also secrete parathyroid hormone, causing bone to release calcium. Decreased mobility and dehydration worsen hypercalcemia.
   2. Early manifestations of hypercalcemia include:
      a. Fatigue
      b. Loss of appetite
      c. Nausea and vomiting
      d. Constipation
      e. Polyuria (increased urine output)
   3. Later manifestations include:
      a. Severe muscle weakness
      b. Loss of deep tendon reflexes
      c. Paralytic ileus
      d. Dehydration
      e. Abnormalities of the electrocardiogram (ECG)
   4. Management includes:
      a. Oral hydration
      b. Parenteral hydration with normal saline
      c. Drug therapy to reduce calcium levels *temporarily*:
         (1) Oral glucocorticoids
         (2) Calcitonin

        (3) Bisphosphonates

        (4) Diphosphonate

        (5) Mithramycin

     d. Dialysis (if renal impairment is present)

- Superior vena cava (SVC) syndrome
  1. SVC syndrome occurs when the SVC is compressed or obstructed by tumor growth or by the formation of clots in the vessel. It is most common in patients with lymphomas, lung cancer, and cancers of the breast, esophagus, colon, and testes.
  2. Manifestations result from blockage of blood flow from the head, neck, and upper trunk. Early manifestations include:
     a. Facial edema, especially around the eyes, on arising
     b. Tightness of the shirt or blouse collar (Stokes' sign)
  3. Later manifestations include:
     a. Edema in the arms and hands
     b. Dyspnea
     c. Erythema of the upper body
     d. Epistaxis (nosebleeds)
  4. Late manifestations include:
     a. Hemorrhage
     b. Cyanosis
     c. Mental status changes
     d. Decreased cardiac output and hypotension
  5. Management includes:
     a. High-dose radiation therapy to the mediastinal area
     b. Stenting of the vena cava
     c. Surgery (rarely)
- TLS
  1. TLS occurs when large numbers of tumor cells are destroyed rapidly and their intracellular contents, including potassium and purines (DNA components), are released into the bloodstream faster than the body can eliminate them. The purines are converted to uric acid. Untreated TLS can cause renal failure and death by hyperkalemia and cardiac arrest.
  2. TLS is most often seen in patients receiving radiation or chemotherapy for cancers that are very sensitive to these therapies, including leukemia, lymphoma, small cell lung cancer, and multiple myeloma.
  3. Prevention through hydration is the best management for TLS.
     a. Instruct at-risk patients to drink at least 3000 mL (5000 mL is more desirable) of fluid the day before, the day of, and for 3 days after treatment.

    b. Stress the importance of adhering to the antiemetic reg-
        imen so that oral hydration can be accomplished.
    c. Instruct patients to contact the cancer clinic immediately
        if nausea and vomiting prevent adequate fluid intake, so
        IV fluids can be started.
    d. Management of actual TLS includes:
       (1) Aggressive fluid resuscitation
       (2) Osmotic diuretics
       (3) Drug therapy to increase the excretion of purines
           such as allopurinol (Aloprim, Zyloprim); rasburi-
           case (Elitek), or febuxostat (Uloric)
       (4) Drug therapy to reduce serum potassium levels
         i. Sodium polystyrene sulfonate
         ii. IV infusions of glucose and insulin
       (5) Dialysis (for severe hyperkalemia and hyperuricemia)

END-OF-LIFE CARE

OVERVIEW

- Although dying is part of the normal life cycle, it is often feared
  as a time of pain and suffering.
- *Death* is the lack of integrated tissue and organ function, manifested by cessation of heartbeat, absence of spontaneous respirations, or irreversible brain dysfunction.
- A *good death* is one that is free from avoidable distress and suffering for patients, families, and caregivers, in agreement with
  patients' and families' wishes, and consistent with clinical practice standards.
- A *bad death* is one that is associated with pain, not having one's
  wishes followed at the end of one's life, isolation, abandonment,
  and agonizing about losses.
- *Advance directives* are legal documents that detail preferences for
  health care, including care at the end of life. Advance directives
  can be instructional (e.g., medical directives, living wills) or
  establish proxy decision makers (i.e., durable power of attorney
  for health care). The Patient Self-Determination Act of 1990
  requires that all patients admitted to any health care agency
  be provided information about establishing advance directives
  if they do not already have them.
- The desired outcomes for a patient near the end of life are:
  1. Needs and preferences met
  2. Control of symptoms of distress
  3. Meaningful interactions between the patient and family
  4. A peaceful death

- Hospice care philosophy uses a coordinated, interdisciplinary approach to focus on quality of life among patients at the end of life and their family. This approach neither hastens nor postpones death; hospice staff provides interventions to meet the needs of a dying patient.

PATIENT-CENTERED COLLABORATIVE CARE
Assessment
- Obtain patient information to identify the risks for and symptoms of distress:
  1. Diagnosis
  2. Past medical history
  3. Recent state of health
- Assess any symptom of distress in terms of intensity, frequency, duration, quality, and exacerbating (worsening) and relieving factors.
- Use a consistent method for rating the intensity of symptoms to facilitate ongoing assessments and evaluate treatment response.
- Assess and document the effects of an intervention on distress and comfort.
- Assess the patient for:
  1. Physical manifestations of approaching death
     a. Symptoms of distress needing management: pain, breathlessness and weakness, inability to manage self-care
     b. Cold, mottled, discolored extremities
     c. Increased sleeping
     d. Food and fluid decrease
     e. Incontinence
     f. Congestion and gurgling
     g. Breathing pattern change
     h. Disorientation
     i. Restlessness
  2. Emotional manifestations of approaching death
     a. Withdrawal
     b. Vision-like experiences
     c. Letting go
     d. Saying goodbye

■ NURSING SAFETY PRIORITY: Action Alert
Do not deny or argue with what the dying person claims about talking to people you cannot see or hear and seeing objects and places not visible to you.

  3. Family's perception of patient's symptoms
  4. Vital signs: anticipate hypotension, slow, fast, or irregular heartbeat, and fast, shallow, or irregular respiratory rate

5. Psychosocial issues that may have an influence on the dying experience, control of symptoms, and family bereavement
   a. Cultural considerations, values, and religious beliefs of patient and family
   b. Fear, anxiety
   c. Knowledge deficits regarding the process of dying
   d. Coping problems
6. Signs that death has occurred
   a. Breathing stops
   b. Heart stops beating
   c. Pupils become fixed and dilated
   d. Body color becomes pale and waxen
   e. Body temperature drops
   f. Muscles and sphincters relax
   g. Urine and stool may be released
   h. Eyes may remain open and there is no blinking
   i. Jaw may fall open
   j. Trickling of fluids internally may be heard

⊕ Cultural Awareness

- Death-related beliefs and practices vary by ethnicity, religion, and race.
  1. Christianity
     a. Eternal life (Heaven) is a gift that is granted to all who accept salvation through Jesus Christ.
     b. Jesus Christ is believed to be the Son of God, both human and divine, and a mediator between God and sinful human beings.
     c. There are many Christian denominations that have variations in beliefs regarding medical care near the end of life.
     d. Funerals tend to be highly involved ceremonies with defined rituals; family, friends, and acquaintances of the deceased make an effort to attend.
     e. Roman Catholics are encouraged to receive sacrament of Anointing of the Sick, administered by a priest at any point during an illness.
     f. Roman Catholic moral tradition acknowledges that, in some situations, forgoing of treatment would be morally permissible (Supportive Care Coalition, 2008)
  2. Judaism
     a. There is a strong belief in the sacredness of life, one God, and the importance of community (i.e., belonging to a group). God and humans are bound together by a covenant.

    b. There is variation in religious beliefs. Not all Jewish believers accept all tenets of the Torah (the Five Books of Moses).

    c. If an individual is suffering pain, there is an obligation to alleviate it, even if it contradicts achieving the maximum life-span for this person.

    d. Torah law sanctions avoiding invasive procedures that do not offer hope of a cure, including giving high (although not fatal) doses of analgesics.

    e. There is a belief that the soul does not completely leave this world until after burial.

    f. The body, which was the vessel and vehicle to the soul, deserves reverence and respect.

    g. The body should not be left unattended until the funeral, which should take place as soon as possible (preferably within 24 hours).

    h. Autopsies should not be performed, except under special circumstances.

    i. The body should not be embalmed, displayed, or cremated.

    j. A 7-day mourning period, called *Shivah*, follows the person's death for the immediate next of kin.

3. Islam (Muslim)

    a. The religion is based on belief in one God (Allah) and his prophet Muhammad. The Qur'an is the scripture of Islam, composed of Muhammad's revelations of the Word of God (Allah).

    b. Life is meant to be a test for the preparation of everlasting life in the hereafter.

    c. God has prescribed an appointed time of death for everyone.

    d. The Qur'an encourages humans to seek treatment and not to refuse treatment. The belief is that only Allah cures, but that Allah cures through the work of humans.

    e. A dying person of Muslim faith may wish to lie facing Mecca.

    f. Upon death, the eyelids are to be closed and the body should be covered. Before moving and handling the body, contact someone from the person's mosque to perform rituals of bathing and wrapping the body in cloth.

    g. Preparation for burial takes place as soon as possible after death.

    h. Death is seen as the transition to the other side, with Islam being the vehicle that will take one there.

Interventions

- Weakness management: patients commonly experience weakness and fatigue as death nears, which may impair the ability to swallow.
    1. After the patient is unable to swallow, oral intake should stop to prevent aspiration.
    2. Educate families about the risk for aspiration, reinforce that anorexia is a part of the dying process, and that giving fluids can actually *increase* discomfort.
    3. Apply emollient to the lips, and moisten the mouth and lips with ice chips or swabs.
    4. In collaboration with a pharmacist experienced in palliative care, identify alternative routes and/or alternative drugs to maintain control of symptoms, choosing the least invasive route, such as oral, buccal mucosa, transdermal, or rectal.

∎ NURSING SAFETY PRIORITY: Action Alert

Avoid the subcutaneous or IV routes for drug delivery, because these methods are invasive and painful, and they can cause infection.

- Pain management: pain is the symptom that dying patients fear the most.
    1. Patients who have had their pain controlled with long-acting opioids should continue their scheduled doses of opioids to prevent pain recurrence.
    2. For unrelieved pain, provide morphine solution (20 mg/1 mL solution), 0.25 to 0.5 mL orally or sublingually every 2 to 3 hours as needed.
    3. Depending on the brand of long-acting opioid, oral capsules may be given rectally, sublingually, or through the buccal mucosa when swallowing is impaired.
    4. Nonpharmacologic pain management strategies can be incorporated with pharmacologic therapy and include:
        a. Massage
        b. Music therapy
        c. Therapeutic touch
        d. Aromatherapy
- Breathlessness and dyspnea management: dyspnea is a subjective experience in which the patient has an uncomfortable feeling of breathlessness, described as terrifying.
    1. Treatment is based on physical assessment and the underlying condition. *Pharmacologic interventions should begin early in the course of dyspnea, near death.* Nonpharmacologic interventions can be used in conjunction with, but not in place of, drug therapy.

2. Morphine is the standard treatment for dyspnea near death. Patients who have not been receiving opioids are given starting doses of 10 to 30 mg orally. Those who have taken morphine or other opioids for pain may need much higher doses of morphine (up to 50% more than their usual dose) for relief of dyspnea. For unrelieved dyspnea, morphine solution can be given orally or sublingually as needed and as frequently as every 2 hours.

3. Fear and anxiety may accompany breathlessness, and benzodiazepines can work with morphine to control dyspnea.

4. Bronchodilators may be used for bronchospasms, and corticosteroids may be used for inflammatory problems.

5. Diuretics may be given for vascular overload with pulmonary edema caused by heart failure.

6. Antibiotics may be indicated for dyspnea from a respiratory infection.

7. Administer anticholinergic medications to reduce secretions, such as atropine (packaged as ophthalmic drops but given sublingually) or hyoscyamine. Scopolamine, 1 to 3 transdermal patches every 72 hours, can also be used.

8. Administer 2 to 6 L of oxygen via nasal cannula and monitor patient responses; continue this therapy if dyspnea is relieved.

9. Use nonpharmacologic interventions to relieve dyspnea, including:
   a. Circulating cool air (e.g., with an air conditioner and fan)
   b. Applying wet cloths on the patient's face
   c. Positioning the patient (head of bed elevation) to facilitate chest expansion
   d. Positioning patient on the side to drain oral secretions and minimize gurgling
   e. Encouraging imagery and deep breathing

- Nausea and vomiting management. In addition to the dying process, both reversible causes (i.e., pain, urinary retention, and constipation) and medications can contribute to nausea and vomiting.
   1. When constipation is the cause of nausea and vomiting, administer a biphosphate enema for immediate fecal release.
   2. Determine whether opioids, benzodiazepines, or anticholinergics (new drugs or new doses) are contributing to nausea and/or vomiting, and consider stopping or decreasing the drug.
   3. Administer prescribed antiemetic drugs.
   4. Remove sources of odors and keep the room temperature at a level that the patient desires.
   5. For some patients, aromatherapy with peppermint or rosewood may relieve nausea.

- Restlessness and agitation management: agitation at the end of life is common and may be caused by pain, urinary retention, constipation, or another reversible cause.
  1. Determine whether the patient is in pain; treat accordingly.
  2. Determine whether the patient is experiencing urinary retention; insert a straight or Foley catheter. (See previous bullet for treatment of constipation.)
  3. For severe restlessness, administer medications. First line: haloperidol, 0.5 to 1 mg orally or sublingually every 4 hours. Alternative: lorazepam, 0.5 to 1 mg as an elixir or tablet dissolved in 0.5 mL water, administered against buccal mucosa every 4 hours to keep the patient comfortable. If the patient becomes more agitated after lorazepam, discontinue and contact hospice.
  4. Music therapy or aromatherapy may produce relaxation; consider patient preferences for music or lavender, peppermint, or other soothing aromas.
- Seizure management: seizures may occur with brain tumors, advanced AIDS, and pre-existing seizure disorders.
  1. If the patient has been taking antiepileptic drugs, give drugs around-the-clock to maintain a high seizure threshold.
  2. Drug therapy may include benzodiazepines or barbiturates given by the oral or rectal routes.
- Management of the refractory symptoms of distress: a few patients experience symptoms of distress that do not respond to typical interventions used at the end of life.
  1. Use established protocols for drug dosages with the intention of alleviating suffering, not hastening death.
  2. Palliative sedation, although controversial, may be used to alleviate distressing symptoms.

! NURSING SAFETY PRIORITY: Action Alert

The ethical responsibility of the nurse in caring for patients near death is to follow guidelines for drug use to manage symptoms and to facilitate prompt and effective symptom management.

- Psychosocial management: the personal experience of dying or of losing a loved one through death can be extremely difficult. Sudden, unexpected deaths of younger people tend to be more traumatic for families than deaths after longer terminal illnesses; however, grief, bereavement, and mourning are usually experienced regardless of the circumstances of death.
  1. Offer physical and emotional support by "being with" the patient.
  2. Respect cultural preferences.

3. Be realistic.
4. Encourage reminiscence.
5. Promote spirituality.
6. Foster hope by listening and caring.
7. Avoid explanations of the loss.
8. Communicate with the patient and involve the patient and family in decisions.
9. Provide referrals to bereavement specialists.
10. Teach about the physical signs of death (described in previous sections).
11. Ensure that the patient is receiving palliative care to manage symptoms.

■ NURSING SAFETY PRIORITY: Action Alert

Do not try to explain the loss in philosophic or religious terms. Statements such as "Everything happens for the best," or "God sends us only as much as we can bear," are not helpful when the bereaved person has yet to express feelings of anguish or anger.

- Provide for the care of the patient after death.
  1. Provide all care with respect to communicate that the person was important and valued.
  2. Notify mortality services and LifeBank of death if this step is hospital or agency policy.
  3. Ask the family or significant others if they wish to help wash the patient, comb his or her hair, or otherwise prepare the body.
     a. If no autopsy is planned, remove or cut all tubes and lines according to agency policy.
     b. Determine whether any organs will be donated after death (e.g., bone, corneas, or body for research or education).
     c. Close the patient's eyes.
     d. Insert dentures if the patient wore them.
     e. Straighten the patient, and lower the bed to a flat position.
     f. Place a pillow under the patient's head.
     g. Place waterproof pads under the patient's hips and around the perineum to absorb any excrement.
  4. Clean the patient's room or unit.
  5. Allow the family or significant others to see the patient in private and to perform any religious or cultural customs they wish (e.g., prayer).
  6. Assess that all who need to see the patient have done so before transferring the patient to the funeral home or morgue.

7. Notify the hospital chaplain or appropriate religious leader if requested by the family or significant others.
8. Ensure that the nurse or physician has completed and signed the death certificate.
9. Prepare the patient for transfer to either a morgue or funeral home; wrap the patient in a shroud and attach identification tags per agency policy.

INFLAMMATION AND IMMUNITY

OVERVIEW

- Inflammation and immunity are provided through the actions and products of white blood cells (WBCs), also called *leukocytes.*
- There are several types of WBCs, and these cell types are the basis of the differential of the WBC count. The differential can be used to determine the patient's risk for infection, the presence or absence of infection, the presence or absence of an allergic reaction, and whether an infection is bacterial or viral.
- WBCs provide protection through many defensive actions, including:
  1. Recognition of self versus non-self. Self-tolerance is the special ability of WBCs to recognize healthy self cells using proteins in cell membranes. WBCs are the only body cells able to recognize non-self cells and to attack them. One example of membrane proteins that provide self-identification are human leukocyte antigens (HLAs) found specifically in tissues; HLAs are inherited from parents.
  2. Destruction of foreign invaders, cellular debris, and unhealthy or abnormal self cells
  3. Production of antibodies directed against invaders
  4. Complement activation
  5. Production of cytokines that stimulate increased formation of leukocytes in bone marrow and increase specific leukocyte activity
- Immunocompetence requires that inflammation, antibody-mediated, and cell-mediated responses all have optimal functioning. Inflammation is a general, nonspecific protective response.
  1. Inflammation
     a. The five cardinal manifestations of inflammation are redness, warmth, swelling, pain, and loss of function. Inflammation and infection are not the same thing. Infection almost always is accompanied by inflammation, but inflammation often occurs without infection.
     b. The tissue responses to inflammation are helpful if they are confined to the area of invasion or infection and do

not extend beyond the acute phase. Chronic inflammation can damage tissues and reduce function.

 c. Inflammation cannot be transferred from one person to another.

2. Antibody-mediated immunity (AMI), also known as *humoral immunity*

 a. Antigen-antibody interactions neutralize, eliminate, or destroy foreign proteins.

 b. Antibodies are produced by sensitized B-lymphocytes (B-cells).

 c. AMI can be transferred from one person or animal to another.

 d. Antibodies transferred from one person into another person have a short-term effect.

 e. Natural active immunity is the most beneficial and long-lasting type of immunity.

 f. Vaccinations cause artificial active immunity and require "boosting" for best long-term effects.

3. Cell-mediated immunity (CMI)

 a. Controls and coordinates the entire inflammatory and immune response

- Immune function peaks between 20 and 40 years of age; the older adult is at an increased risk for infection and cancer development.
- Patients who take immunosuppressive drugs for any reason have an increased risk for infection and cancer development.
- Transplant rejection is a normal response of the immune system that can damage or destroy the transplanted organ. Patients who receive transplanted organs (unless they are from an identical sibling) need to take immunosuppressive drugs daily to prevent transplant rejection.

ORGANIZATION OF THE IMMUNE SYSTEM

- The immune system is not located in any one organ or body area, but most immune system cells come from the bone marrow. Some cells mature in the bone marrow; others leave the bone marrow and mature in different body sites.
- When mature, many immune system cells are released into the blood, where they circulate to most body areas and have specific effects.
- Each WBC has a specific function. The cells of the immune system and their functions are as follows:
  1. *Neutrophils* nonspecifically ingest and phagocytize microorganisms and foreign protein.

2. *Macrophages* nonspecifically recognize foreign proteins and microorganisms, ingesting and phagocytizing these invaders.
3. *Monocytes* destroy bacteria and cellular debris; they also mature into macrophages.
4. *Eosinophils* have weak phagocytic action and release vasoactive amines during allergic reactions.
5. *Basophils* release histamine and heparin in areas of tissue damage.
6. *Lymphocytes,* which have two categories of specialized cells, each with subtypes.
    a. B-lymphocytes are essential to AMI. They sense foreign cells and proteins and exist as either *plasma cells* or *memory cells,* secreting immunoglobulins in response to the presence of a specific antigen.
    b. T-lymphocytes are essential to CMI and are further characterized as *helper or inducer T-cells* (enhance immune activity through secretion of various factors, cytokines, and lymphokines), *suppressor T-cells* (regulate immune activity by preventing hypersensitivity); *cytotoxic or cytolytic T-cells* (selectively attack and destroy non-self cells, including virally infected cells, grafts, and transplanted organs), or *natural killer (NK) cells* (nonselectively attack non-self cells, especially body cells that have undergone mutation and become malignant; also attack grafts and transplanted organs).

- *Phagocytosis* is the engulfing and destruction of invaders. This action also rids the body of debris after tissue injury. Neutrophils and macrophages are most efficient at phagocytosis. Phagocytosis involves seven steps:
    1. *Exposure and invasion:* for phagocytosis to start, leukocytes must first be exposed to organisms, foreign proteins, or debris from damaged tissues.
    2. *Attraction:* to ensure the WBC comes into direct contact with the target (antigen, invader, or foreign protein), damaged tissues and blood vessels secrete chemotaxins (chemical attractants) that can combine with the surface of invading foreign proteins to improve attraction.
    3. *Adherence:* this process allows the phagocytic cell to bind to the surface of the target.
    4. *Recognition:* this process occurs when the phagocytic cell sticks to the surface of the target cell and recognizes it as non-self. This action ensures that phagocytosis occurs only against non-self or unhealthy self cells.
    5. *Cellular ingestion:* phagocytosis (engulfment) into the phagocyte is needed, because the destruction of the target cell occurs inside the phagocytic cell.

6. *Phagosome formation:* this occurs when the phagocyte's granules are inside the vacuole and fuse to the invader.
7. *Degradation:* the phagosome enzymes digest the engulfed target, which is the final step.

INFLAMMATION

- Inflammation, also called *natural immunity*, provides immediate protection against the effects of tissue injury and invading foreign proteins.
- The purpose of inflammation is to start blood vessel and tissue reactions to rid the body of harmful microorganisms and other invaders.
- Inflammation differs from immunity in two important ways:
  1. Inflammatory protection is immediate but short term against injury or invading organisms. It does not provide true immunity on repeated exposure to the same organism and cannot be transferred to another person.
  2. Inflammation is a nonspecific body defense to invasion or injury and can be started by almost any event, regardless of where it occurs or what causes it.
- The classic manifestations of inflammation are:
  1. Warmth
  2. Redness
  3. Swelling
  4. Pain
  5. Decreased function
- Symptoms of inflammation can be local or widespread, depending on the intensity, severity, and duration of exposure to the initiating injury or invasion.
- Inflammation occurs in response to tissue injury and to invasion by organisms. Infection is usually accompanied by inflammation; however, inflammation can occur without infection.
  1. Examples of inflammation without infection include sprain injuries to joints, myocardial infarction, sterile surgical incisions, blister formation, and thrombophlebitis.
  2. Examples of inflammation caused by noninfectious invasion by foreign proteins include allergic rhinitis, contact dermatitis, and other allergic reactions.
  3. Examples of inflammation caused by infection include otitis media, appendicitis, peritonitis, and viral hepatitis.
- Four types of WBCs (leukocytes) are involved in inflammation:
  1. Neutrophils
  2. Macrophages
  3. Eosinophils
  4. Basophils

SEQUENCE OF INFLAMMATORY RESPONSES

- Inflammatory responses occur in a predictable sequence of three stages. The sequence is the same regardless of the triggering event, and the timing may overlap.
  1. *Stage I* is the vascular part of the inflammatory response. Injured tissues and the leukocytes in this area secrete histamine, serotonin, and kinins that constrict the small veins and dilate the arterioles in the area of injury. These blood vessel changes cause redness and warmth of the tissues. This increased blood flow increases delivery of nutrients to injured tissues, causing redness, swelling, and pain. The duration of these responses depends on the severity of the initiating event, but they usually subside within 24 to 72 hours.
     a. Macrophages, or monocytes that are tissue-specific, are filled with vesicles that secrete the chemical messengers to alter vessel diameter and blood flow.
     b. Cytokines, such as colony-stimulating factors (CSFs), are secreted by activated WBCs and damaged tissue to trigger the bone marrow to increase the rate of WBC production from 14 days to a matter of hours.
  2. *Stage II* is the cellular exudate part of the response in which neutrophilia (increased number of circulating neutrophils) occurs. Exudate in the form of pus occurs, containing dead WBCs, necrotic tissue, and fluids that escape from damaged cells.
     a. The most active cell in this stage is the neutrophil, which can increase in count up to five times within 12 hours after the onset of inflammation as a result of cytokine stimulation.
     b. Neutrophils attack and destroy organisms and remove dead tissue through phagocytosis.
     c. The arachidonic acid (AA) cascade starts to increase the inflammatory response by converting fatty acids in plasma membranes into AA. Enzymes (including cyclooxygenase) then convert AA into many chemicals that are further processed into the substances that continue the inflammatory response in the tissues. Some of these substances include histamine, leukotrienes, prostaglandins, serotonin, and kinins.
  3. *Stage III* features tissue repair and replacement. Although this stage is completed last, it begins at the time of injury and is critical to the final function of the inflamed area.
     a. Some of the WBCs involved in inflammation start the replacement of lost tissues or repair of damaged tissues by inducing the remaining healthy cells to divide.

b. In tissues that are unable to divide, WBCs trigger new blood vessel growth (angiogenesis) and scar tissue formation. Because scar tissue does not behave like normal tissue, loss of function occurs wherever damaged tissues are replaced with scar tissue.

CONSEQUENCES OF INFLAMMATION

- When inflammation occurs in response to invasion by infectious microorganisms, its actions can eliminate or destroy the invaders and prevent the person from becoming ill.
- Inflammation is needed to trigger both AMI and CMI.
- When inflammatory responses are prolonged or occur at inappropriate times or in inappropriate places, they can cause tissue damage with extensive fibrosis, scarring, and loss of healthy tissue function.

IMMUNITY

ANTIBODY-MEDIATED IMMUNITY

- AMI, also known as *humoral immunity*, involves antigen-antibody interactions to neutralize, eliminate, or destroy foreign proteins. Antibodies are produced by B-lymphocytes (B-cells).
- B-cells become sensitized to a specific foreign protein (antigen) and produce antibodies directed specifically against that protein. The expressed antibody (rather than the B-cell) causes one of several actions to neutralize, eliminate, or destroy that antigen.
- B-cells start as lymphocytes in the bone marrow, the primary lymphoid tissue, and migrate into many secondary lymphoid tissues, where maturation is completed. The secondary lymphoid tissues for B-cell maturation are the spleen, parts of lymph nodes, tonsils, and the mucosa of the intestinal tract.
- The body learns to make enough of any specific antibody to provide long-lasting immunity and protection against specific organisms or toxins.
- Seven steps are needed to produce a specific antibody directed against a specific antigen whenever the person is exposed to that antigen:
  1. *Exposure or invasion* is needed, because antibody actions occur inside the body or on a few body surfaces. Without exposure, an antibody cannot be made.
  2. *Antigen recognition* is the recognition of the invader by an unsensitized B-cell. This process involves macrophages and helper-inducer T-cells.

3. *Lymphocyte sensitization* occurs when the B-cell recognizes the antigen as non-self and becomes sensitized to this antigen. A single naive B-cell can become sensitized only once.
4. *Antibody production and release* occurs at a rate as high as 300 molecules of antibody per second by each sensitized B-lymphocyte. These antibody molecules are released and can bind to their specific antigen. *Circulating antibodies can be transferred from one person to another to provide the receiving person with immediate immunity of short duration.*
5. *Antibody-antigen binding* occurs when the tips of the Y-shaped antibody recognize the specific antigen and bind to it. The binding stimulates reactions to neutralize, eliminate, or destroy the antigen.
6. *Antibody-binding actions* include agglutination, lysis, complement fixation, precipitation, and inactivation or neutralization, all of which can neutralize, eliminate, or destroy the antigen.
7. *Sustained immunity (memory)* is critical in providing long-lasting immunity to a specific antigen. It results from memory B-cells made during the lymphocyte sensitization stage. These memory cells remain sensitized to the specific antigen to which they were originally exposed. On re-exposure to the same antigen, the memory cells rapidly respond, and each new cell can rapidly make large amounts of the antibody specific for the sensitizing antigen. This ability of the memory cells to respond on re-exposure to the same antigen that originally sensitized the B-cell allows a rapid and large immune (anamnestic) response to the antigen. Such large quantities of antibody are made that the invading organisms usually are removed completely, and the person does not become ill. Because of this process, most people do not become ill with chickenpox or other infectious diseases more than once, even though they are exposed many times to the causative organism. Without the action of memory, people would remain susceptible to specific diseases on subsequent exposure to the organisms, and no sustained immunity would be generated.

- All antibodies are immunoglobulins (Ig), also called *gamma globulins,* because they are globular proteins that confer immunity.
- There are five antibody types:
  1. IgA is the secretory antibody found on body surfaces and secretions to prevent antigen entry.
  2. IgM is the antibody type a sensitized B-cell makes on first exposure to an antigen. Because it is large and is a complex, it has

10 binding sites to efficiently bind antigen, even though it is produced in small amounts. This antibody ensures that an initial infectious illness, such as chickenpox, lasts only 5 to 10 days.

3. IgG is the most common antibody found in the blood. On re-exposure to the same antigen, the already sensitized B-cell makes large amounts of the IgG type of antibody against that antigen. The enormous numbers produced make IgG antibodies efficient at clearing the antigen and protecting the person from again becoming ill with the disease.

4. IgE is the antibody type that is responsible for many allergic reactions.

5. IgD activates B-cells and modifies the activity of IgM.

ACQUIRING ANTIBODY-MEDIATED IMMUNITY

- *Adaptive immunity* is the immunity that a person's body learns to make (or can receive) as an adaptive response to invasion by organisms or foreign proteins. AMI is an acquired immunity, is active or passive, and is acquired naturally or artificially.

  1. *Active immunity* occurs when antigens enter the body and the body responds by actively making specific antibodies against the antigen.

     a. Natural active immunity occurs when an antigen enters the body without human assistance and the body responds by actively making antibodies against that antigen (e.g., chickenpox virus). *This type of immunity is the most effective and the longest lasting.*

     b. Artificial active immunity is the protection developed by vaccination or immunization. Small amounts of specific antigens are placed as a vaccination into a person and the immune system responds by actively making antibodies against the antigen.

  2. *Passive immunity* occurs when antibodies against an antigen are in a person's body but were transferred to the person's body after being made in the body of another person or animal. It provides only immediate short-term protection against a specific antigen.

     a. Natural passive immunity occurs when antibodies are passed from the mother to the fetus through the placenta or to the infant through colostrum and breast milk.

     b. Artificial passive immunity involves injecting a person with antibodies that were produced in another person or animal.

- AMI works with inflammation to protect against infection. However, AMI can provide the most effective, long-lasting immunity only when its actions are combined with those of CMI.

CELL-MEDIATED IMMUNITY

- CMI, or cellular immunity, involves many WBC actions and interactions. This type of immunity is provided by lymphocyte stem cells that mature in the secondary lymphoid tissues of the thymus and pericortical areas of lymph nodes. These cells are known as *T-lymphocytes (T-cells)*.
- Certain CMI responses influence and regulate the activities of AMI and inflammation by producing and releasing cytokines. For total immunocompetence, CMI must function optimally.
- Cytokines are small protein hormones produced by the many WBCs. One cell produces a cytokine, which exerts its effects on other cells of the immune system and on other body cells.
  1. The cells responding to the cytokine may be located close to or remote from the cytokine-secreting cell.
  2. Cytokines act like *messengers* that tell specific cells how and when to respond.
  3. Cytokines include the interleukins, interferons, colony-stimulating factors, and tumor necrosis factor.
- Four T-lymphocyte subsets that are critically important for the development and continuation of CMI are:
  1. *Helper-inducer T-cells* (T4 cells, T_H cells, CD4+ cells) that easily recognize self cells versus non-self cells. In response to the recognition of non-self (antigen), helper-inducer T-cells secrete cytokines that can enhance the activity of other WBCs.
  2. *Suppressor T-cells* (T8 cells, CD8+ cells, T_S cells) regulate CMI by preventing hypersensitivity (continuous overreactions) when a person is exposed to non-self cells or proteins. These cells secrete cytokines that inhibit immune-system cell action and work in opposition to helper-inducer T-cells. Immune function is well balanced when T4+ cells outnumber T8+ cells by a 2:1 ratio.
  3. *Cytotoxic or cytolytic T-cells* are a subset of suppressor cells that destroys cells containing a processed antigen's major histocompatibility complex (MHC). This activity is most effective against self cells infected by parasites, such as viruses or protozoa.
  4. *NK cells* (CD16 cells) have direct cytotoxic effects on some non-self cells that are independent of the interactions of other WBCs. NK cells conduct "seek and destroy" missions in the body to eliminate non-self cells. NK cells are most effective in destroying unhealthy or abnormal self cells, such as cancer cells and virally infected body cells.
- CMI helps protect the body through the ability to differentiate self from non-self.

- The non-self cells most easily recognized by CMI are cancer cells and the self cells infected by organisms that live within host cells.
- CMI watches for and rids the body of self cells that might potentially harm the body.
- It is important in preventing the development of cancer and metastasis.

INFECTION

OVERVIEW

- An infection is the invasion of a body tissue by microorganisms that allows replication of the microorganism and results in tissue damage.
- A *pathogen* is any microorganism, also called an *agent*, capable of producing disease.
- *Virulence* is the degree to which a pathogen can invade the body and cause disease after infection.
- Normal *flora* are microorganisms that live in or on the human host without causing disease. Some microbes are beneficial, but when these flora move to another body area, they can be pathogenic.
- *Colonization* is the process of having pathogenic organisms living and growing in or on a body area without causing disease or damage.
- *Toxins* are protein molecules released by bacteria to affect host cells at a distant site.
  1. Exotoxins are released by the bacteria into the host's body.
  2. Endotoxins remain within the bacterial cell walls and are released when the bacterium is attacked.
- *Microorganisms* are parasites that live at the host's expense.
- Infectious diseases can be communicable (transmitted from person to person, such as influenza) or not communicable (e.g., peritonitis).
- Transmission of infection requires these factors:
  1. Reservoir (or source) of infectious agents
     a. Animate reservoirs include people, animals, and insects
     b. Inanimate reservoirs include soil, water, other environmental sources, or medical equipment
  2. Susceptible host with a portal of entry
  3. Mode of transmission
  4. Portal of exit (exit of the microbe from the host often occurs through the portal of entry but can exit by other routes)
- Prevention of infection transmission involves disrupting the three factors or breaking the chain of infection at any point.

- Host factors that increase the susceptibility to infection are:
  1. Congenital or acquired immune deficiencies
  2. Alteration of normal flora by antibiotic therapy
  3. Advancing age
  4. Hormonal changes (e.g., pregnancy, diabetes, corticosteroid therapy, or adrenal insufficiency)
  5. Defective phagocytosis
  6. Breaks in skin or mucous membranes
  7. Interference with flow of urine, tears, or saliva
  8. Impaired cough reflex or ciliary action
  9. Malnutrition or dehydration
  10. Smoking, alcohol consumption, inhalation of toxic chemicals
  11. Invasive therapy, chemotherapy, radiation therapy, steroid therapy, surgery
- Common modes of infection transmission are:
  1. Contact transmission (most common)
     a. Direct (person-to-person) contact, in which the source and host have physical contact and microorganisms are transferred directly (e.g., common cold)
     b. Indirect contact, in which the transfer of microorganisms occurs from a source to a host by passive transfer from a contaminated object (e.g., staphylococcal organisms)
  2. Droplet transmission from contact with infected secretions or droplets (e.g., influenza)
  3. Airborne transmission from small airborne particles containing pathogens that leave the infected source, are suspended in the air, and enter a susceptible host (e.g., *Mycobacterium tuberculosis* or the varicella zoster virus)
  4. Vector transmission, in which insects carry pathogens between two or more hosts, such as the deer tick that causes Lyme disease
- Human physiologic defenses against infection include:
  1. Intact skin and mucous membranes
  2. Normal flora
  3. Secretions and natural movements of the respiratory, GI, and genitourinary tracts
  4. Inflammation and phagocytosis (natural immunity)
  5. Antibody-mediated immunity (AMI) and cell-mediated immunity (CMI)
- A hospital-acquired infection (HAI) is an infection acquired while the patient was in an inpatient setting. It occurs while the patient is receiving health care. Old terms for this include *nosocomial* and *iatrogenic.*

- HAIs can be prevented or controlled in at least five major ways:
  1. Hand hygiene
     a. Handwashing (wetting, soaping, lathering, applying friction under running water for at least 15 seconds, rinsing, and adequate drying)
     b. Alcohol-based hand rubs (ABHRs)
  2. Use of personal protective equipment (PPE), also called *barriers*
  3. Adequate staffing
  4. Disinfection or sterilization
  5. Patient placement and transport

◾NURSING SAFETY PRIORITY: Drug Alert

Do not use an ABHR before inserting eyedrops, ointments, or contact lenses. Alcohol can irritate the patient's eyes, causing burning and redness.

- Centers for Disease Control and Prevention (CDC) Transmission-Based Guidelines include:
  1. *Standard Precautions* assume that all body excretions, secretions, and moist membranes and tissues, excluding perspiration, are potentially infectious; the precautions should be used in the care of all patients.
     a. Respiratory Hygiene and Cough Etiquette (RH/CE) for respiratory illnesses
        (1) Patient, staff, and visitor education
        (2) Posted signs
        (3) Hand hygiene
        (4) Covering the nose and mouth with a tissue and prompt tissue disposal or using surgical masks
        (5) Separation from the person with respiratory infection by more than 3 feet (1 m)
     b. Safe injection practices, using a sterile, single-use disposable needle and syringe for each injection, prevention of contamination of injection equipment and drug, and use of retractable needles
  2. Transmission-Based Precautions
     a. *Airborne Precautions* for patients known or suspected to have infections transmitted by the airborne transmission route (e.g., tuberculosis, measles [rubeola], and chickenpox [varicella])
        (1) Negative airflow rooms
        (2) Enclosed booths with high-efficiency particulate air (HEPA) filtration or ultraviolet light

b. *Droplet Precautions* for patients known or suspected to have infections transmitted by the droplet transmission route (e.g., influenza, mumps, pertussis, meningitis)
c. *Contact Precautions* for patients known or suspected to have infections transmitted by direct contact or contact with items in the environment (e.g., significant multidrug-resistant organism [MDRO] infection or colonization, pediculosis, scabies, respiratory syncytial virus [RSV], and *Clostridium difficile*)

🔳 NURSING SAFETY PRIORITY: Critical Rescue

The CDC recommends that private rooms be used for patients in Airborne or Protective Environment Precautions. It is acceptable for patients with similar multidrug resistant diagnoses to share a room.

- A number of microorganisms have become resistant to certain antibiotics, and once useful drugs no longer control these infectious agents (MDROs):
  1. Methicillin-resistant *Staphylococcus aureus* (MRSA)
  2. Community-associated MRSA (CA-MRSA)
  3. Vancomycin-resistant *Enterococcus* (VRE)
  4. Vancomycin-intermediate *S. aureus* (VISA)
  5. Vancomycin-resistant *S. aureus* (VRSA)

🔳 NURSING SAFETY PRIORITY: Drug Alert

Help prevent the development of drug resistance by teaching patients to complete their prescribed antibiotic therapy and not stop the drug when they are feeling better.

- Complications from infection are relapse, cellulitis, pneumonia, abscess formation, sepsis, septic shock, disseminated intravascular coagulation (DIC), multi-system organ failure, and death.

PATIENT-CENTERED COLLABORATIVE CARE
Assessment
- Obtain patient information about:
  1. Age
  2. History of tobacco or alcohol use
  3. Current illness or disease (e.g., diabetes)
  4. Past and current drug use (e.g., prescribed, over-the-counter [OTC], recreational, injection)
  5. Nutritional status
  6. Previous vaccinations or immunizations
  7. Exposure to infectious agents
  8. Contact with animals, including pets

9. Insect bites
10. Travel history
11. Sexual history
12. Transfusion history
13. Previous infection history
14. Onset order of symptoms

- Assess for and document:
  1. Skin manifestations
     a. Redness
     b. Warmth
     c. Swelling
     d. Drainage or pus
     e. Pain
  2. Generalized manifestations
     a. Fever (usually a temperature above 101° F [38° C] or 99° F [37° C] for older adults)
     b. Chills
     c. Malaise and fatigue
     d. Lymphadenopathy
     e. Joint pain
     f. Muscle aches
     g. Photophobia
  3. GI tract manifestations
     a. Nausea and vomiting
     b. Diarrhea
  4. Genitourinary manifestations
     a. Dysuria
     b. Frequency
     c. Urgency
     d. Hematuria
     e. Purulent drainage
     f. Pelvic or flank pain
  5. Respiratory tract manifestations
     a. Cough
     b. Congestion
     c. Rhinorrhea
     d. Sore throat
     e. Chest pain
  6. Psychosocial dysfunction
     a. Anxiety and frustration
     b. Lack of knowledge
     c. Social isolation
  7. Abnormal laboratory findings
     a. Positive culture
     b. Positive serologic results

     c. High or low WBC count

     d. Elevated erythrocyte sedimentation rate (ESR)

  8. Abnormal imaging findings

     a. Chest x-ray, sinus or joint films, GI studies

     b. Computed tomography (CT)

     c. Magnetic resonance imaging (MRI)

     d. Ultrasonography

  9. Biopsy

Planning and Implementation

- Interventions to reduce fever include:
  1. Antimicrobials
  2. Antipyretics
  3. External cooling

■ NURSING SAFETY PRIORITY: Action Alert

Avoid making the patient shiver during any form of external cooling. Shivering may indicate that the patient is being cooled too quickly.

  4. Fluid administration

- Effective anti-infective therapy requires:
  1. Agent appropriate for the known organism
  2. Sufficient dosage and duration of treatment
  3. Timely administration (avoid delays or skipped doses)

- Nursing interventions include:
  1. Obtaining and reviewing an allergy history before giving antibiotics
  2. Monitoring the patient for side effects of antibiotics, such as nausea, vomiting, or rash
  3. Using best practices to reduce fever, which can vary by age, underlying pathology, or institutional policy.
  4. Monitoring for manifestations of dehydration
     a. Thirst
     b. Decreased skin turgor
     c. Dry skin and mucous membranes
  5. Encouraging fluid intake
  6. Measuring intake and output
  7. Monitoring vital signs and oxygen saturation
  8. Monitoring skin intactness, color and temperature

☑ NATIONAL PATIENT SAFETY GOAL

Fever may contribute to skin moistness or increase the potential for pressure ulcer formation. Monitor the patient more often and provide pressure-relieving interventions for vulnerable patients.

9. Assessing level of consciousness and for seizure activity
10. Monitoring laboratory values
11. Providing or assisting with oral hygiene
12. Teaching the patient and family about the mode of transmission of infection and mechanisms that prevent spread to others

Community-Based Care

- Urge immunization against respiratory infections for adults older than 50 years, anyone with a chronic illness, and anyone who lives with an older adult or a person with a chronic illness.
- Remove indwelling urinary catheters as soon as possible to prevent urinary tract infections.
- Emphasize the importance of a clean home environment, especially for the patient who continues to be immunocompromised or who is uniquely susceptible to superinfection.
- Demonstrate proper handwashing with patient and family and ask for a return demonstration to assess learning.
- Teach the patient and family about:
  1. What is causing the illness
  2. Whether the infection can be spread to others
  3. Modes of transmission
  4. Specific precautions for transmission prevention, including:
     a. Whether any special household cleaning is necessary and if so, what those special steps include
     b. How to dispose of any used needles and syringes safely and legally
     c. Cleaning clothing soiled with blood or other body fluids by washing them with bleach or disinfectant (e.g., Lysol)
     d. Cleaning measures to be based on actual available equipment and facilities
  5. The importance of adhering to the prescribed antibiotic therapy regimen, including:
     a. Timing of doses
     b. Number of days
     c. Any specific drug administration instructions (e.g., before meals, with meals, without other agents) and the possible side effects
     d. Allergic manifestations and the need to notify a health care provider if an adverse reaction occurs
     e. What to do if a drug dose is missed (e.g., doubling the dosage or waiting until the next dose time)
  6. Managing IV drug therapy
- Refer to home health care agencies as needed.

PAIN

OVERVIEW

- *Pain* is an unpleasant sensory and emotional experience associated with actual or potential tissue damage.
- It is the most common reason for a patient to seek medical care and the number one reason for a person to take medication.
- Self-report is always the most reliable indication of pain.
- The nurse's primary role in pain management is to advocate for the patient by believing reports of pain.
- The Joint Commission standards of care require that patients in all health care settings, including home care, have a right to effective pain management.
- There are two main types of pain:
  1. *Acute pain* results from sudden accidental trauma or surgery. It is usually temporary, has a sudden onset, and is localized. Features include:
     a. Physiologic responses
        (1) Increased heart rate
        (2) Increased blood pressure
        (3) Increased respiratory rate
        (4) Dilated pupils
        (5) Sweating
     b. Common behavioral responses
        (1) Restlessness
        (2) Inability to concentrate
        (3) Apprehension
        (4) Overall distress
  2. *Chronic pain* or *persistent pain* persists for longer than 3 months, is often poorly localized, and is hard to describe. It may not be associated with sympathetic nervous system responses of tachycardia or hypertension. It is often associated with depression, interference with personal relationships, and inability to maintain activities of daily living. Chronic pain is further divided into two subtypes, cancer and non-cancer pain:
     a. Chronic cancer pain is associated with:
        (1) The cancer itself
        (2) Nerve compression
        (3) Invasion of tissue
        (4) Bone metastasis
        (5) Cancer treatments (e.g. chemotherapy, radiation therapy)
     b. Chronic non-cancer pain is the more common type and is associated with tissue injury that has healed or a chronic non-cancer diagnosis such as arthritis or back pain.

   c. Chronic pain is also categorized as:
     (1) Nociceptive or visceral-somatic, with normal processing of pain signals
     (2) Neuropathic, originally the result of nerve injury, the abnormal processing of pain signals. Processing abnormalities may be generated either in the peripheral or central nervous systems.

⬛ NURSING SAFETY PRIORITY: Action Alert

Although many characteristics of chronic pain are similar in different patients, be aware that each situation is unique and requires a highly specialized plan of care.

- The attitudes of health care professionals toward pain influence the way they perceive and interact with patients in pain.
- Factors such as age, gender, sociocultural background, and genetics influence the patient's ability to process and react to pain. For example, men have more cluster headaches, back pain, gout, peripheral vascular disease, and postherpetic neuralgia.
- Many patients are reluctant to report pain. When they do, they may underreport its severity.
- Some patients, especially older adults, are reluctant to take pain medications, especially opioid analgesics, because they fear becoming addicted to or used to the drug.
- Although pain is familiar to everyone, it is so complex that there is no single universal treatment.

Considerations for Older Adults

- Age can influence how pain is perceived, assessed, and treated. The incidence of pain in older adults is high, as is the risk for undertreatment.

Women's Health Considerations

- Certain chronic painful conditions are more common in women. Women have more migraine headaches, tension headaches, rheumatoid arthritis and osteoarthritis, fibromyalgia, and multiple sclerosis.

- Definitions important to pain management:
  1. *Addiction* is a primary, chronic neurobiologic disease with one or more of the following: impaired control over drug use, compulsive use, continued use despite harm, and craving.
  2. *Pseudoaddiction* is a health care-induced syndrome created by the undertreatment of pain. Features include patient behaviors such as anger and escalating demands for more or different medications, and results in suspicion and avoidance by staff.

3. *Tolerance* is a state of adaptation in which exposure to a drug induces changes that result in a decrease in one or more of the drug's effects over time.

4. *Physical dependence* is adaptation manifested by a drug class-specific withdrawal syndrome that can be produced by abrupt cessation, rapid dose reduction, decreasing blood level of the drug, or administration of an antagonist. It occurs in everyone who takes opioids over a period of time.

5. *Withdrawal* or *abstinence syndrome* results when a patient who is physically dependent on opioids abruptly ceases using them.

6. *Placebo* is any medical treatment or nursing care that produces an effect in a patient because of its therapeutic intent and not because of its actual physical or chemical properties.

■ NURSING SAFETY PRIORITY: Drug Alert

Carefully explain the difference between physical dependence and addiction when a patient starts on opioid therapy. NOTE: tolerance, physical dependence, and addiction can co-exist.

■ NURSING SAFETY PRIORITY: Action Alert

Because of the deception involved and the need for informed consent, *never* administer a placebo to your patient.

PATIENT-CENTERED COLLABORATIVE CARE
Assessment

- Assess and record pain history information:
  1. Pain experience, including the sequence of events (precipitating and relieving factors, localization, character and quality of pain, and duration of pain)
  2. Nature of adjustments, if any, in life or in the family
  3. Beliefs about the cause of the pain and what should be done about it (patient's expectations).
- Assess for physical and clinical manifestations:
  1. Patient's statement of pain
  2. Tachycardia and increased or decreased blood pressure (heart rate and blood pressure less likely to be altered with chronic pain)
  3. Altered movement, such as splinting or listlessness
  4. Functional status impairment
  5. Location of pain
     a. Localized (pain is confined to the site of origin)
     b. Projected (pain occurs along a specific nerve or nerves)

      c. Radiating (diffuse pain occurs around the site of origin that is not well localized)

      d. Referred (pain is perceived in an area distant from the site of painful stimuli)

  6. Intensity and quality of pain

      a. Pain intensity (e.g., number rating scale of 0 to 10, with 10 being the worst possible pain)

      b. Verbal descriptions to convey the quality of pain or descriptive scales, such as "none" to "moderate" to "severe"

      c. Faces Pain Rating scale of smile to frown

- To assess pain in cognitively impaired or nonverbal patients:
  1. Use self-report (when possible).
  2. Search for potential causes of pain.
  3. Observe patient behaviors, such as facial expressions, slowed movements, or rubbing a site.
  4. Use surrogate reporting (e.g., family member).
  5. Attempt an analgesic trial.

Considerations for Older Adults

- Six common pain indicators among older adults are:
  1. Facial expression (e.g., grimacing, crying)
  2. Verbalizations or vocalizations (e.g., screaming)
  3. Body movements (e.g., restlessness)
  4. Changes in interpersonal interactions
  5. Changes in activity patterns or routines
  6. Mental status changes (e.g., confusion, increased confusion)

Interventions
Nonsurgical Management

- Drug therapy: selection of drugs is based on level of pain, drug effects and adverse effects, and knowledge of the advantages and disadvantages for each route of administration.
  1. The non-opioid analgesics are the first-line therapy for mild to moderate pain. They are typically available without a prescription and administered orally, rectally, or topically.
  2. Examples of non-opioid analgesics:
     a. Few anti-inflammatory effects: acetaminophen (Tylenol)

■NURSING SAFETY PRIORITY: Drug Alert

Teach patients to take no more the 3600 mg daily (2400 mg for older adults) of acetaminophen and for no longer than 4 weeks without informing their health care provider about the amount of acetaminophen they take each day. Remind them to have liver and renal function laboratory tests done on a regular basis as prescribed to monitor for early indicators of adverse drug events.

   b. Nonsteroidal anti-inflammatory drugs (NSAIDs) such as:
      (1) Aspirin
      (2) Ketorolac (Toradol)
      (3) Ibuprofen (Motrin, Advil, other names)
      (4) Naproxen (Naprosyn)
      (5) Ketoprofen (Orudis)
      (6) Celecoxib (Celebrex)

◾NURSING SAFETY PRIORITY: Drug Alert

Aspirin and other NSAIDs can cause GI disturbances, interfere with renal function, and reduce the ability of platelets to aggregate and stop bleeding. Therefore observe the patient for gastric discomfort, edema, hypernatremia, and bleeding or bruising. Teach the patient and family to report these problems to the health care provider immediately if they occur.

3. Opioid analgesics are used to manage moderate to severe pain. They can be administered by any route. Examples include:
   a. Hydromorphone (Dilaudid)
   b. Morphine (Roxanol, Avinza, Kadian)
   c. Fentanyl (Sublimaze)
   d. Codeine
   e. Hydrocodone
   f. Oxycodone
   g. Methadone (Dolophine)
   h. Oxymorphone (Opana, Numorphan)
   i. Meperidine (Demerol)

◾NURSING SAFETY PRIORITY: Critical Rescue

The key to assessing opioid-induced adverse effects is to monitor for sedation. After the first dose of an opioid, determine how easily the patient is aroused. *Stop the medication if the patient is difficult to arouse!* Be sure to assess the patient's level of consciousness with subsequent doses. Monitor respiratory rate and depth, especially while sleeping, and reduce the dose or stop the drug if respiratory compromise occurs during initial dosing.

◾NURSING SAFETY PRIORITY: Drug Alert

The maximum dose of meperidine is 15 mg/kg/day. The administration of meperidine is often restricted to 2 consecutive days because of the accumulation of the toxic metabolite normeperidine. Adverse central nervous system (CNS) symptoms may occur with use of this drug, particularly in older adults or others with renal insufficiency. Typical CNS adverse effects are tremors, nervousness, delirium (acute confusion), seizures, and psychosis. Do not give meperidine to older adults in any form. Oral and continuous infusions of the drug should not be administered to any patient.

The drug also blocks the reuptake of both serotonin and norepinephrine by the neurons and can cause serotonin syndrome. This is a potentially fatal condition that is seen in patients taking meperidine with selective serotonin reuptake inhibitors (SSRIs), tricyclic antidepressants, triptan migraine drugs, or monoamine oxidase inhibitors (MAOIs). The early manifestations of this combination are CNS abnormalities such as muscle rigidity and delirium, but the condition can progress to life-threatening cardiac dysrhythmias, hyperthermia, and disseminated intravascular coagulation (DIC).

- Nursing care issues related to opioid therapy:
  1. Consider onset and duration of drug before administration.
  2. Monitor and prevent complications from side effects. Side effects, in order of seriousness, can include respiratory depression, sedation, constipation, nausea and vomiting, urinary retention, and pruritus (itching).
     a. Monitor respiratory rate and depth, especially when the patient is sleeping.
     b. Sedation occurs before opioid-induced respiratory depression, so nurse-monitored sedation levels are recommended by use of a sedation scale for opioid-naive (not currently on an opioid) patients or those receiving opioids IV or epidurally. The key to assessing sedation is determining how easily the patient is aroused.
     c. Whenever a patient is started on regular doses of opioids, intervene to prevent constipation or to treat it early with a stool softener.

❗ NURSING SAFETY PRIORITY: Drug Alert

Respiratory depression is managed with an opioid antagonist, naloxone (Narcan). It is a fast-acting drug given IV to reverse the opioid effect. The respiratory-depressant effect of the opioid is usually longer acting than naloxone. Continue to monitor the patient after giving the drug, because respiratory depression can recur, necessitating additional naloxone.

- Nursing care issues with patient-controlled analgesia (PCA):
  1. PCA delivers a set amount of drug through IV access, allowing the patient to control the dosage of opioid received, improving pain relief and increasing patient satisfaction.

2. Morphine, fentanyl, and hydromorphone are the most commonly used drugs for PCA.
3. Drug security is achieved through a locked syringe pump system or locked drug reservoir system.
4. When the patient presses the button or pendant (on ambulatory pumps), the appropriate bolus or demand dose is delivered. A basal rate may also be continuously administered.
5. Teach patients how to use PCA and to report side effects, such as dizziness, nausea and vomiting, and inability to void.
6. Monitor the patient's vital signs, particularly respirations, and check his or her sedation level at least every 2 hours initially or per agency protocol.
7. Do not allow a proxy or staff to administer a bolus or push the button. If the patient is unable to use the PCA device effectively, discontinue PCA and use another mode of drug delivery.

- Nursing care issues for epidural analgesia are:
  1. Epidural analgesia is the instillation of a pain-blocking agent, usually an opioid analgesic alone or in combination with a local anesthetic, such as bupivacaine, into the epidural space.
  2. Epidural analgesia is most commonly used for the management of acute pain.
  3. Morphine (preservative-free), hydromorphone (Dilaudid), and fentanyl (Sublimaze) are the most commonly used opioids for epidural administration.
  4. Pruritus (itching), nausea, and vomiting are common side effects of epidural opioids.
  5. A temporary, externalized epidural catheter is used for acute pain control. This device is not sutured to the skin and is easily dislodged. Be sure to tape the catheter in two places to anchor it properly.
  6. Complications that occur with epidural analgesia are directly related to catheter placement, catheter maintenance, and the type of analgesic.
  7. Infection is rare but can occur as a result of failure to maintain aseptic technique during catheter placement, through direct drug instillation, during infusion of solution and tubing changes, and from a failure to maintain aseptic conditions for indwelling catheters at the site of insertion or at the site of tube junctions.

◼ NURSING SAFETY PRIORITY: Action Alert

To prevent infections, ensure that all catheter line connections are secure and that an occlusive sterile dressing is maintained over the catheter site.

8. There is a risk for respiratory depression resulting from high plasma or cerebrospinal fluid concentrations of the instilled drug. Monitor the patient's respirations and sedation level at frequent intervals during and after the administration of epidural opioids and immediately report any concerns to the health care provider.

9. Urinary retention is a common problem associated with epidural analgesia and is more likely to occur in men than in woman.

10. Lower motor weakness is common when an epidural local anesthetic is used in combination with an opioid. Assist patients who get out of bed for the first time to determine the degree of leg weakness.

❗NURSING SAFETY PRIORITY: Action Alert

Do not delegate this activity and assessment to unlicensed assistive personnel.

- Adjuvant analgesics may be used to relieve pain alone or in combination with other analgesics by potentiating or enhancing the effectiveness of the analgesic.
  1. Antiepileptic drugs (AEDs or anticonvulsants)
     a. Gabapentin (Neurontin)
     b. Pregabalin (Lyrica)
     c. Topiramate (Topamax)
  2. Tricyclic antidepressants
     a. Amitriptyline (Elavil)
     b. Nortriptyline (Pamelor)
     c. Imipramine (Tofranil)
  3. Other antidepressants
     a. Trazodone (Desyrel)
     b. Paroxetine (Paxil)
     c. Sertraline (Zoloft)
  4. Antianxiety drugs
     a. Alprazolam (Xanax)
     b. Lorazepam (Ativan)
     c. Oxazepam (Serax, Zapex)
     d. Clonazepam (Klonopin)
  5. Local anesthetics may be given orally (systemic effects), topically, and via epidural routes. Examples include:
     a. Epidural bupivacaine
     b. Oral mexiletine
     c. Xylocaine
     d. Lidocaine patch (Lidoderm patch)
     e. Lidocaine and prilocaine (EMLA cream)
     f. Lidocaine (ELA-Max cream)

      6. Multimodal (balanced) analgesia for epidural pain management is a combination of opioids, non-opioids, and/or local anesthetics to relieve acute pain, usually postoperative pain.

      7. Local short-acting gels and creams for cryotherapy. Examples include:

        a. Biofreeze

        b. Bengay

- Nonpharmacologic interventions
  1. Physical measures
     a. Cutaneous (skin) stimulation strategies
        (1) Application of heat, cold, and pressure
        (2) Therapeutic touch
        (3) Massage
        (4) Vibration
     b. Physical and occupational therapy
        (1) Exercise to strengthen muscles or to provide alternative approaches to avoid painful maneuvers
        (2) Massage or manipulation
        (3) Splinting of joints
     c. Transcutaneous electrical nerve stimulation (TENS)
  2. Cognitive-behavioral measures
     a. Distraction
     b. Imagery
     c. Relaxation (may be combined with music therapy)
     d. Hypnosis
  3. Complementary and alternative therapies
     a. Music therapy
     b. Acupuncture and acupressure
     c. Prayer and meditation
     d. Magnet therapy
     e. Herbal supplements
- Invasive techniques for chronic pain
  1. Nerve blocks
  2. Spinal cord stimulation

Community-Based Care

- Pain can be managed in any setting, including the home; some patients require parenteral pain medications at home; therefore provide health teaching to ensure continuity of care.
- Refer patients whose pain is difficult to manage to pain specialists and/or pain centers.
- Communicate and coordinate the plan of care for pain management as the patient transfers between health care agencies and home.

- Make appropriate referrals for physical therapy, a clinical nurse specialist in pain management, a social worker, and hospice or palliative care.
- Plan a home care nurse referral for patients who will require assistance or supervision with the patient's pain relief regimen at home.
- Home agency practices and professional support at home are required if patients leave the hospital with infusion therapy for pain management.
- Ensure that the patient, especially one who is on opioids, has enough pain medication to last at least until the first follow-up visit.
- Teach the patient and family about analgesic regimens, including any technical skills needed to administer or deliver the analgesic, the purpose and action of various drugs, their side effects or adverse reactions, and the importance of dosage intervals.
- If the patient is on a flexible analgesic schedule, teach the patient and family how to safely increase and decrease the drug within the prescribed dosing guidelines.

PERIOPERATIVE CARE
PREOPERATIVE ISSUES
OVERVIEW
- The preoperative period begins when the patient is scheduled for surgery and ends at the time of transfer to the surgical suite.
- The primary roles of the nurse are educator, patient advocate, and promoter of health.
- *Inpatient* refers to a patient who is admitted to a hospital the day before or the day of surgery and requires hospitalization after surgery.
- *Outpatient* and *ambulatory* refer to a patient who goes to the surgical area the day of the surgery and returns home on the same day (same-day surgery [SDS]).
- The primary reasons for surgery are:
  1. Diagnostic
  2. Curative
  3. Restorative
  4. Palliative
  5. Cosmetic
- The urgency of surgery may be:
  1. Elective
  2. Urgent
  3. Emergency

- The risk of surgery may be:
  1. Minor
  2. Major
- The extent of surgery can be:
  1. Simple
  2. Radical
  3. Minimally invasive surgery (MIS)

Considerations for Older Adults

- The older adult may have a variety of health-related issues that can have an impact on the planning of care and outcome of surgery, including:
  1. Multiple comorbidities
  2. Malnutrition
  3. Endocrine dysfunction with reduced stress response
  4. Increased risk for cardiopulmonary complications after surgery
  5. Increased risk for delirium (e.g., related to unfamiliar surroundings, change in routine, drugs given, and other factors)
  6. Increased risk of a fall and resultant injury
  7. Dysfunction or impaired self-care abilities
  8. Inadequate support systems

PATIENT-CENTERED COLLABORATIVE CARE
Assessment
- Obtain a focused assessment.
- Take and record vital signs and report:
  1. Hypotension or hypertension
  2. Heart rate less than 60 or more than 120 beats/min
  3. Irregular heart rate
  4. Chest pain
  5. Shortness of breath or dyspnea
  6. Tachypnea
  7. Pulse oximetry reading of less than 94%
- Assess for and report any signs or symptoms of infection, including:
  1. Fever
  2. Purulent sputum
  3. Dysuria or cloudy, foul-smelling urine
  4. Any red, swollen, draining IV or wound site
  5. Increased white blood cell count
- Assess for and report signs or symptoms that could contraindicate surgery, including:
  1. Increased prothrombin time (PT), international normalized ratio (INR), or activated partial thromboplastin time (aPTT)

    2. Hypokalemia or hyperkalemia
    3. Patient report of possible pregnancy or positive pregnancy test
- Assess for and report other clinical conditions that may need to be evaluated by a physician or advanced nurse practitioner before proceeding with the surgical plans, including:
    1. Change in mental status
    2. Vomiting
    3. Rash
    4. Recent administration of an anticoagulant drug
    5. Family or personal history of malignant hyperthermia with anesthesia
- Use a standardized list so that the following items are available before the start of the procedure:
    1. History and physical
    2. Signed, dated, and witnessed procedure consent form
    3. Nursing assessment
    4. Preanesthesia assessment
    5. Labeled diagnostic and radiology test results including chest x-ray, electrocardiogram, and tests specific to the condition or surgical procedure (e.g., computed tomography scan, magnetic resonance imaging scans, abdominal films, or orthopedic films)
    6. Any required blood products, implants, devices and/or special equipment for the procedure

✓ NATIONAL PATIENT SAFETY GOAL

Implement the Universal Protocol for preventing wrong site, wrong procedure, and wrong person surgery:
1. Conduct a preprocedure verification process to verify the correct procedure, correct patient, and correct site, involving the patient if possible. A checklist is required.
2. Mark the procedure site. If possible, involve the patient.

⬛ NURSING SAFETY PRIORITY: Critical Rescue

Document any abnormal findings and communicate with the surgeon and the anesthesia provider immediately. Some abnormalities must be corrected before surgery.

Planning and Implementation

- Explore the patient's level of knowledge and understanding, and then provide information about informed consent, dietary restrictions, specific preparation for surgery (bowel and skin preparations), exercises after surgery, and plans for pain management.
- Ensure informed consent is obtained from the patient (or legal designee) by the surgeon before sedation is given and before

surgery is performed. *Consent* implies that the patient has sufficient information to understand:

1. The nature of and reason for surgery
2. Who will perform the surgery and whether others will be present during the procedure
3. All available options and the risks associated with each option
4. The risks associated with the surgical procedure and its potential outcomes
5. The risks associated with the use of anesthesia

! NURSING SAFETY PRIORITY: Action Alert

If you believe that the patient has not been adequately informed, contact the surgeon and request that he or she see the patient for further clarification. Document this request in the medical record.

- A competent adult has the right to refuse treatment for any reason, even when refusal might lead to death.
- Routine preoperative care includes:
  1. Determining the existence and nature of the patient's advance directives
  2. Implementing dietary restrictions
     a. Recommendations include NPO status (no eating or drinking), typically for 6 or more hours for easily digested solid food and 2 hours for clear liquids.
     b. Failure to adhere to NPO status can result in cancellation of surgery or increase the risk for aspiration during or after surgery.
  3. Administering regularly scheduled drugs
     a. Many oral drugs are held the morning before surgery or given IV.
     b. Others, especially for cardiac disease, respiratory disease, seizures, and hypertension, are usually allowed before surgery with a sip of water.
  4. Ensuring intestinal preparation
     a. Before abdominal, bowel or intestinal surgery, a simple enema, "enemas until clear," mild or potent laxatives (polyethylene glycol electrolyte solution [GoLYTELY] is an example of a potent laxative) may be prescribed to empty the large intestine to reduce the potential for contamination of the surgical field.
     b. Antibiotics may be administered immediately before abdominal surgery to reduce bacterial load in the gastrointestinal tract.

5. Performing skin preparation
   a. Confirm or assist the patient in the use of an antiseptic solution while showering and removal of oil and skin debris. This intervention reduces the number of organisms on the skin and the potential for a site infection.
   b. Remove hair at the surgical site with clippers.
6. Preparing the patient for tubes, drains, and vascular access
   a. Describe the purpose and placement of each device.
   b. Show the devices to the patient and family.
   c. Reassure the patient that these are temporary and that efforts will be made to reduce discomfort.
   d. Common devices include:
      (1) Foley catheter
      (2) Nasogastric (NG) tube
      (3) Drains (e.g., Penrose, Jackson-Pratt, Hemovac)
      (4) Vascular access
7. Teaching about procedures and exercises to prevent respiratory complications
   a. Deep diaphragmatic breathing
   b. Expansion breathing
   c. Incentive spirometry
   d. Coughing and splinting
   e. Turning
8. Teaching about procedures and exercises to prevent cardiovascular complications
   a. Assessing for venothromboembolism (VTE)
   b. Swelling in one leg
   c. Presence of calf pain that worsens with ambulation
   d. Antiembolism stockings (TEDs or Jobst stockings) and elastic (Ace) wraps
   e. Pneumatic compression devices
   f. Leg exercises to promote venous return
   g. Early ambulation
   h. Range-of-motion (ROM) exercises
9. Minimizing anxiety
   a. Assess the patient's knowledge about the surgical experience.
   b. Provide factual information.
   c. Allow ample time for questions.
   d. Respond to questions accurately or facilitate communication with the knowledgeable care provider.
   e. Incorporate family or supportive persons in communications.
   f. Provide prescribed antianxiety drugs.
   g. Promote rest and relaxation.
   h. Provide opportunity for distraction.

Final Preoperative Preparation
- Review the preoperative chart for:
  1. Completion of surgical informed consent form and any other special consent forms
     a. Patient's signature
     b. Date
     c. Witnesses' signatures
  2. Confirmation that the scheduled procedure is what is listed on the consent form

◥ NATIONAL PATIENT SAFETY GOAL

For surgical procedures that are site-specific, such as left, right, or bilateral, ask the competent patient to mark the site with a marker to ensure the correct site is used and the wrong site is avoided. At a minimum, the patient's identity, correct side and site, correct patient position, agreement on the proposed procedure, and availability of correct implants and equipment must be verified by all members of the surgical team.

  3. Documentation of allergies
  4. Accurate height and weight
  5. Documentation of the results of all laboratory, radiographic, and diagnostic tests in the chart
  6. Presence of autologous blood donor or directed blood donations slips (if appropriate)
  7. Documentation of current vital signs (within 1 to 2 hours of the scheduled surgery time)
  8. Documentation of any significant physical or psychosocial observations
  9. Communication of special needs, concerns, and instructions to the surgical team such as:
     a. Advance directives
     b. No use of blood products
     c. Presence of autologous blood products
     d. Communication difficulties (e.g., visually impaired, hearing impaired, does not speak the main language of the institution)
- Review patient preparation
  1. Appropriate clothing removal
  2. Application of prescribed antiembolism stockings or pneumatic compression devices
  3. Storage of valuables

4. Visible patient identification (e.g., identification band)
5. Removal and safekeeping of dentures, prosthetic devices, contact lenses, glasses, wigs, toupees, and hairpins and clips
6. Removal of dentures, dental prostheses (e.g., bridges, retainers), jewelry (including body piercing), eyeglasses, contact lenses, hearing aids, wigs, and other prostheses. Securely tape rings that cannot be removed.
7. Removal of nail polish and artificial nails if agency policy
8. Assurance that the patient has emptied his or her bladder
9. Siderails raised immediately before transport or after giving drugs that affect cognition or judgment
10. The call system within easy reach of the patient
11. The bed in a low position except during transport
- Correctly administer prescribed preoperative drugs:
    1. Positively identify the patient (using the armband and asking the patient to state his or her name).
    2. Ensure the correct drugs in the correct dosages via the correct route at the correct time are given and documented.
- Transfer the patient to the surgical suite.

INTRAOPERATIVE ISSUES

OVERVIEW
- The intraoperative period begins when the patient enters the surgical suite (operating room [OR]) and ends at the time of transfer to the postanesthesia recovery area, SDS unit, or intensive care unit (ICU).
- In the OR, a safe environment means:
    1. All members of the surgical team and other support personnel in the surgical suite are free of communicable diseases.
    2. Good personal hygiene is practiced, and no jewelry is worn.
    3. There is appropriate use of protective surgical attire (e.g., shirt and pants, cap or hood, shoe coverings, mask and eye protectors or face shields)
    4. Scrubbed team members also wear a sterile fluid-resistant gown and sterile gloves.
    5. Team members are trained and capable; nursing staff typically orients for 6 to 12 months.
- Surgical team members include:
    1. The *surgeon*, a physician who assumes responsibility for the surgical procedure and any surgical judgments about the patient

2. The *anesthesia provider*, who gives anesthetic drugs to induce and maintain anesthesia and delivers other drugs as needed to support the patient during surgery
   a. *Anesthesiologist*, a physician who specializes in giving anesthetic agents
   b. *Certified registered nurse anesthetist (CRNA)*, who is a registered nurse with additional education and credentials and who delivers anesthetic agents under the supervision of an anesthesiologist, surgeon, dentist, or podiatrist
3. *Perioperative nursing staff*, whose main concerns are the safety and advocacy for the patient during surgery
   a. *Holding area nurse*, who coordinates and manages the care of the patient in the presurgical holding area next to the main OR. This nurse assesses the patient's physical and emotional status, gives emotional support, answers questions, and provides additional education as needed.
   b. *Circulating nurse*, who is responsible for coordinating all activities within that particular OR. He or she sets up the OR and ensures that supplies, including blood products and diagnostic support, are available as needed. This nurse positions the patient, assists the anesthesia provider, inserts a Foley catheter if needed, and scrubs the surgical site before the patient is draped with sterile drapes. In the absence of a holding area nurse, the circulating nurse also provides holding area tasks. Other responsibilities include:
      (1) Monitoring traffic in the room
      (2) Assessing the amount of urine and blood loss
      (3) Reporting findings to the surgeon and anesthesia provider
      (4) Ensuring that sterile technique and a sterile field are maintained
      (5) Communicating information about the patient's status to family members
      (6) Documenting care, events, interventions, and findings
      (7) Completing documentation in the OR and nursing records about the presence of drains or catheters, the length of the surgery, and a count of all sponges, "sharps" (needles, blades), and instruments
   c. *Scrub nurse* sets up the sterile field, drapes the patient, and hands sterile supplies, sterile equipment, and instruments to the surgeon and the assistant. This person also maintains an accurate count of sponges, sharps,

instruments, and amounts of irrigation fluid and drugs used. An OR technician may also perform these tasks.

d. *Specialty nurse* may be in charge of a particular type of surgical specialty (e.g., orthopedic, cardiac, ophthalmologic) and is responsible for nursing care specific to patients needing that type of surgery.

- Types of anesthesia and complications
  1. *General anesthesia* is a reversible loss of consciousness induced by inhibiting neuronal impulses in several areas of the central nervous system (CNS). The patient is unconscious and unaware, and has loss of muscle tone and reflexes. Agents are administered by inhalation and IV injection.
     a. Complications include malignant hyperthermia (MH), an acute, life-threatening complication of certain drugs in which skeletal muscle exposed to specific agents increases calcium levels and metabolism leading to acidosis, cardiac dysrhythmias, and a high body temperature.
        (1) MH is a genetic disorder with an autosomal dominant pattern of inheritance and is most common in young, well-muscled men.
        (2) Drugs most associated with it are halothane, enflurane, isoflurane, desflurane, sevoflurane, and succinylcholine.
     b. Overdose of anesthesia can occur when the patient's metabolism and drug elimination are slower than expected, such as in an older patient or one who has liver or kidney problems.
     c. Unrecognized hypoventilation with failure to exchange gases adequately can lead to cardiac arrest, permanent brain damage, and death.
     d. Intubation complications from improper neck extension or anatomic differences in a patient can lead to broken or injured teeth and caps, swollen lip, or vocal cord trauma.
     e. Hemodynamic instability from medications, fluid loss, or dysrhythmias can contribute to brain or other organ damage.
  2. *Local or regional anesthesia* disrupts sensory nerve impulse transmission from a specific body area or region. The patient remains conscious and able to follow instructions.
     a. Local anesthesia is delivered topically (applied to the skin or mucous membranes of the area to be anesthetized) and by local infiltration.
     b. Regional anesthesia is a type of local anesthesia that blocks multiple peripheral nerves in a specific body region.

Regional anesthesia includes field block or nerve block and spinal or epidural routes of delivery.

c. Complications are associated with overdoses, inadvertent systemic drug delivery, or patient allergic reactions to the agent.

3. *Conscious sedation* is the IV delivery of sedative and opioid drugs to reduce the level of consciousness but allow the patient to maintain a patent airway and to respond to verbal commands. It is used most often in the emergency department or in procedures rooms before short but uncomfortable procedures.

PATIENT-CENTERED COLLABORATIVE CARE
Assessment

- Correct identification of the patient is the responsibility of every member of the health care team.
  1. Verify the patient's identity with two types of identifiers (e.g., name, birth date, medical record number, social security number) using the patient's identification bracelet.
     a. Ask the patient, "What is your name?" and "What is your birth date?"
  2. Validate that the surgical consent form has been signed and witnessed.
     a. Ask the patient, "What kind of operation are you having today?"
     b. Compare patient responses to the information on the operative permit and the operative schedule.
     c. When the procedure involves a specific site, validate the side on which a procedure is to be performed.
     d. Investigate any discrepancy and notify the surgeon.
- Validate that all aspects of the checklist are complete.
  1. Ask the patient about any allergies.
  2. Determine whether autologous blood was donated.
  3. Check the patient's attire to ensure adherence with facility policy.
  4. Ensure that all prostheses have been removed, including dentures, dental bridges or retainers, jewelry, contacts, and wigs.
- Review the medical record for:
  1. Advance directives (be prepared to implement do-not-resuscitate orders)
  2. Previous reactions to anesthesia or blood transfusions
     a. Allergies to iodine products or shellfish
     b. Latex allergies
  3. Laboratory and diagnostic test results
  4. Medical history and physical examination findings

✅ NATIONAL PATIENT SAFETY GOAL

Perform a time out before the procedure during which team members agree, at a minimum, on the correct patient identity, the correct site, and the procedure to be done.

Planning and Implementation
- Ensure proper positioning and prevent injury or pressure ulcer formation by:
    1. Padding the operating bed with foam or silicone gel pads, or both
    2. Properly placing the grounding pads
    3. Assisting the patient to a comfortable position
    4. Assessing the skin for pre-existing conditions and applying protective measures such as Duoderm, Tegaderm, or other skin protective product
    5. Modifying the patient's position according to the patient's safety and special needs
    6. Avoiding excessive joint abduction
    7. Securing the arms firmly on an armboard, positioned at shoulder level
    8. Supporting the wrist with padding and not overtightening wrist straps
    9. Placing safety straps above or below the nerve locations
    10. Maintaining minimal external rotation of the hips
    11. Supporting the lower extremities
    12. Not placing equipment on lower extremities
    13. Urging OR personnel to avoid leaning on the patient's lower extremities
    14. Maintaining the patient's extremities in good anatomic alignment by slightly flexing joints and supporting the patient with pillows, trochanter rolls, or pads
- Observe for complications of special positioning, such as wrist-drop or footdrop, loss of sensation, changes in extremity temperature or circulation, and inflammation.

✅ NATIONAL PATIENT SAFETY GOAL

Implement evidence-based practices for preventing surgical site infections, and monitor compliance with best practices. This includes practices related to the use of prophylactic antimicrobial agents, skin preparation, and hair removal.

- Reduce risk for infection by:
    1. Identifying patients with pre-existing health problems such as diabetes mellitus, immunodeficiency, obesity, and renal failure

   2. Performing prescribed skin preparation
   3. Protecting the patient's exposure to cross-contamination
   4. Ensuring the use of sterile surgical technique, protective
      drapes, skin closures, and dressings
   5. Administering preoperative antibiotics within 30 to 60 mi-
      nutes of the first incision
- Prevent complications from hypoventilation, hemodynamic
  instability and hypothermia by:
   1. Continuously monitoring the patient according to estab-
      lished standards, including:
      a. Breathing
      b. Circulation
      c. Cardiac rhythm
      d. Blood pressure
      e. Heart rate
      f. Oxygen saturation
   2. Evaluating core body temperature by:
      a. Maintaining core temperature at 95° to 98.6° F (35° to
         37° C)
      b. Determining the safe use of warming devices to effec-
         tively support normothermia

POSTOPERATIVE ISSUES

OVERVIEW
- Completion of surgery and transfer of the patient to either the
  postanesthesia care unit (PACU), the SDS unit (ambulatory care
  unit), or the ICU marks the beginning of the postoperative period.
- On arrival to the postoperative care unit, the anesthesia provider
  and the circulating nurse give the receiving nurse a verbal hand-
  off report to communicate the patient's condition and care
  needs.
- Discharge from the postoperative unit is based on the presence
  of a recovery score rating of at least 9 to 10 on an established
  recovery scale.

▼ NATIONAL PATIENT SAFETY GOAL
Effective communication among caregivers is the second prioritized National Patient Safety Goal established by The Joint
Commission. The language used by the report giver is clear
and cannot be interpreted in more than one way. Report
critical results from diagnostic procedures. Accurately and
completely reconcile medications, including short-term medications that will not be continued at discharge from the perioperative area.

- The handoff report should contain the following information:
  1. Type and extent of the surgical procedure
  2. Type of anesthesia and length of time the patient was under anesthesia
  3. Tolerance of anesthesia and the surgical procedure
  4. Allergies (especially to latex or drugs)
  5. Pathologic condition requiring surgery
  6. Oxygen saturation
  7. Status of vital signs
  8. Core body temperature
  9. Type and amount of IV fluids and drugs administered
  10. Estimated blood loss (EBL)
  11. Any intraoperative complications, such as a traumatic intubation
  12. Preoperative drugs and patient responses
  13. Primary language, any sensory impairments, any communication difficulties
  14. Anxiety level before receiving anesthesia
  15. Special requests that were verbalized by the patient preoperatively
  16. Preoperative and intraoperative respiratory function and dysfunction
  17. Pertinent medical history, including substance abuse
  18. Location and type of incisions, dressings, catheters, tubes, drains, or packing
  19. Intake and output, including current IV fluid administration and estimated blood loss
  20. Prosthetic devices
  21. Joint or limb immobility while in the OR, especially in the older patient
  22. Other intraoperative positioning that may be relevant in the postoperative phase
  23. Intraoperative complications, how managed, patient responses
  24. Any other important intraoperative occurrences

PATIENT-CENTERED COLLABORATIVE CARE
Assessment
- The initial assessment of the patient immediately after surgery includes level of consciousness, temperature, pulse, respiration, oxygen saturation, and blood pressure.
- Examine the surgical area for bleeding.
- Assess vital signs on admission and then at least every 15 minutes at least four times; then re-assess every 30 minutes four times, and then every 2 hours for 4 hours, then every 4 hours for 24 to 48 hours. If the patient has unstable or abnormal

findings, then the frequency of assessment does not advance. Frequency of assessment after 24 to 48 hours is then based on agency policy and patient responses.

- Routine postoperative monitoring and assessment includes:
    1. Respiratory status by assessing:
        a. Patent airway and gas exchange by oxygen saturation and end-tidal carbon dioxide levels
        b. Presence of an artificial airway (endotracheal tube, nasal trumpet, oral airway)
        c. Type of delivery device and the concentration or liter flow of the oxygen

! NURSING SAFETY PRIORITY: Critical Rescue

If the SpO_2 drops below the level of 95% or the patient's baseline, notify the surgeon or anesthesia provider. If it drops by 10 percentage points and there is certainty of an accurate measure, call the Rapid Response Team.

        d. Rate, pattern, and depth of breathing
        e. Lung fields for breath sounds by auscultation
        f. Degree of symmetry of breath sounds and chest movement
        g. Presence of snoring and stridor
        h. Assessment of skeletal muscle weakness by checking:
            (1) Inability to maintain a head lift
            (2) Weak hand grasps
            (3) Abdominal breathing pattern
    2. Cardiovascular status by assessing:
        a. Heart rate, quality, and rhythm
        b. Blood pressure
        c. Comparison of findings for trends

! NURSING SAFETY PRIORITY: Critical Rescue

Report blood pressure changes that are 25% higher or lower than values obtained before surgery (a 15- to 20-point difference, systolic or diastolic) to the anesthesia provider or the surgeon.

        d. Electrocardiography for dysrhythmias
        e. Comparison of distal pulses, color, temperature, and capillary refill on extremities
        f. Assessment of feet and legs for manifestations of deep vein thrombosis (DVT) (e.g., redness, pain, warmth, swelling)
        g. Maintain prescribed compression devices or antiembolic stockings applied in the preoperative or operative suite.

3. Neurologic status by assessing:
   a. Level of consciousness or awareness
   b. Presence of lethargy, restlessness, or irritability
   c. Patient responses to stimuli (calling the patient's name, touching the patient, and giving simple commands such as "Open your eyes" and "Take a deep breath")
   d. Degree of orientation to person, place, and time by asking the conscious patient to answer questions such as "What is your name?" (person), "Where are you?" (place), and "What day is it?" (time)
   e. Comparing the patient's baseline neurologic status (obtained before surgery) with the findings after surgery
4. Motor and sensory function status by:
   a. Asking the patient to move each extremity
   b. Assessing the strength of each limb and comparing the results on both sides
   c. Gradually elevating the patient's head and monitoring for hypotension
5. Assessing fluid, electrolyte, and acid-base balance by:
   a. Measuring intake and output (including IV fluid intake, emesis, urine, wound drainage, nasogastric tube drainage)
   b. Checking hydration status (e.g., inspecting the color and moisture of mucous membranes, the turgor, texture, and tenting of the skin, the amount of drainage on dressings, and the presence of axillary sweat)
   c. Comparing total output with total intake to identify a possible fluid imbalance
6. Renal or urinary status by:
   a. Measuring intake and output
   b. Assessing for urine retention by inspection, palpation, percussion of the lower abdomen for bladder distension, or use of a bladder scanner
   c. Performing prescribed intermittent catheterization
   d. Assessing urine for color, clarity, and amount
   e. Assessing voiding for frequency, amount per void, and any symptoms

■ NURSING SAFETY PRIORITY: Critical Rescue

Report a urine output of less than 0.5 mL/kg/hr for 2 or more hours or an average over 6 hours to the surgeon.

7. GI status by:
   a. Listening for bowel sounds in all four abdominal quadrants and at the umbilicus
   b. Assessing for nausea and vomiting
   c. Administering prescribed antiemetic drugs

    d. Assessing for manifestations of paralytic ileus (few or absent bowel sounds, distended abdomen, abdominal discomfort, vomiting, and no passage of flatus or stool)

    e. Assessing and recording the color, consistency, and amount of the NG tube drainage

    f. Checking NG tube placement

▉ NURSING SAFETY PRIORITY: Action Alert

After gastric surgery, do not move or irrigate the tube without an order from the surgeon.

8. Skin status by:
   a. Assessing the incision (if visible) for redness, increased warmth, swelling, tenderness or pain, and the type and amount of drainage
   b. Condition of the sutures or staples
   c. Presence of open areas
9. Dressings and drains for:
   a. Color, amount, consistency, and odor of drainage
   b. Leakage around or under the patient
   c. Patency of drains
   d. Any restriction of circulation or sensation
10. Pain
11. Psychosocial issues of anxiety, restlessness, fear

Planning and Implementation
- Airway management in the PACU or ICU may include:
   1. Monitoring for snoring or stridor that indicate obstruction
   2. Inserting an oral airway or a nasal airway (nasal trumpet) to keep the airway open
   3. Keeping the manual resuscitation bag and emergency equipment for intubation or tracheostomy nearby
   4. Positioning the patient in a side-lying position to prevent aspiration
   5. Suctioning the mouth, nose, and throat to keep the airway clear of mucus or vomitus as needed
   6. Keeping the patient's head flat to prevent hypotension and possible shock, unless this position is contraindicated by the condition or surgical procedure
   7. Applying prescribed oxygen by face tent, nasal cannula, or mask
   8. Raising the head of the bed (after the patient is fully reactive and stable)
   9. Assisting the patient to cough (with the incision splinted), breathe deeply, and use the incentive spirometer
   10. Performing mouth care after removing secretions

- Interventions for inpatients after PACU care may include:
  1. Encouraging the patient to continue coughing, deep breathing, and incentive spirometry exercises
  2. Assisting the patient out of bed and to ambulate as soon as possible
  3. Assisting the patient to turn at least every 2 hours (side to side)
  4. Offering prescribed pain medication 30 to 45 minutes before the patient gets out of bed

Nonsurgical Skin Management

- Wound care includes reinforcing the dressing, changing the dressing, assessing the wound for healing and infection, and caring for drains, including emptying, measuring, and documenting drainage features.
  1. The initial dressing is often changed by the surgeon.
     a. Reinforce the dressing (add more dressing material to the existing dressing) if it becomes wet from drainage.
     b. Document the added material and the color, type, amount, and odor of drainage fluid and time of observation.
  2. Routine wound care and dressing changes include:
     a. Changing gauze dressings at least once during a nursing shift or daily
     b. Cleaning the area with sterile saline or some other solution as prescribed
     c. Assessing the skin in areas where tape has been used for redness, rash, or blisters
     d. Assessing the incision for integrity, condition, and healing stage
     e. Assessing the incision for wound infection:
        (1) Redness, heat, and swelling
        (2) Drainage of purulent or foul-smelling material
     f. Removing sutures or staples according to agency policy and surgeon request
     g. Removing or advancing drains according to agency policy and surgeon request
     h. Administering prescribed antibiotic therapy

Surgical Management

- Poorly healing wounds, infected wounds, or complicated wounds may require surgical intervention.
- Management of *dehiscence*, which is opening of all or part of a wound down to the visceral peritoneum:
  1. Apply a sterile nonadherent (e.g., Telfa) or saline dressing to the wound and notify the surgeon.
  2. Instruct the patient to bend the knees and to avoid coughing.

3. The surgeon may reclose the wound or leave it open to heal by second intention.

- Management of *evisceration,* which is a wound opening with protrusion of internal organs. *This condition is a surgical emergency.*
    1. *Call for help.* Instruct the person who responds to notify the surgeon or Rapid Response Team immediately and to bring any needed supplies into the patient's room.
    2. Stay with the patient.
    3. Cover the wound with a nonadherent dressing premoistened with warmed, sterile normal saline.
    4. If premoistened dressings are not available, moisten sterile gauze or sterile towels in a sterile irrigation tray with sterile saline, and then cover the wound.
    5. If saline is not immediately available, cover the wound with gauze and then moisten with sterile saline using a sterile irrigation tray as soon as someone brings saline.
    6. Do not attempt to reinsert the protruding organ or viscera.
    7. While covering the wound, observe the patient's response and assess for manifestations of shock.
    8. Place the patient in a supine position with the hips and knees bent.
    9. Raise the head of the bed 15 to 20 degrees.
    10. Take vital signs and document them.
    11. Provide support and reassurance to the patient.
    12. Continue assessing the patient, including assessment of vital signs, every 5 to 10 minutes until the surgeon arrives.
    13. Keep dressings continuously moist by adding warmed sterile saline to the dressing as often as necessary. *Do not let the dressing become dry.*
    14. When the surgeon arrives, report your finding and your interventions. Then follow the surgeon's directions.
    15. Document the incident, the activity the patient was engaged in at the time of the incident, your actions, and your assessments.
    16. The surgeon performs surgery in the OR with the patient under general, regional, or local anesthesia to close the wound. Stay or retention sutures of wire or nylon are usually used in addition to or instead of standard sutures or staples.

Management of Surgical Pain
- Opioids and non-opioids are routinely given in the early postoperative period.
- Drugs are given IV initially and then are administered orally.

- Around-the-clock scheduling is more effective than on-demand scheduling because more constant blood levels are achieved.
- Patient-controlled analgesia (PCA) by IV infusion or internal pump (the catheter is sutured into or near the surgical area) may be used.
- Epidural analgesia can be given intermittently by the anesthesia provider or by continuous drip through an epidural catheter left in place after epidural anesthesia.
- See the "Pain" section on pp. 46–55 for an in-depth presentation of pain assessment and pain control interventions.

Prevent Hypoxemia

- The highest incidence of hypoxemia after surgery occurs on the second postoperative day. Those at highest risk are older adults and patients with lung disease.
- Monitor the patient's oxygen saturation (SpO_2) with pulse oximetry.
- Apply prescribed oxygen as needed.
- Prevent hypothermia.
- Implement a respiratory therapy assessor protocol to determine the need for respiratory treatments. Position the patient with the head of the bed elevated at 30 to 45 degrees unless contraindicated.
- Implement early progressive mobility within 6 to 48 hours of surgery.

Community-Based Care

- Discharge planning, teaching, and referral begin before surgery and continue after surgery.
- Provide written discharge instructions for the patient to follow at home.
- Assess the need for assistance with wound care and activities of daily living (ADLs).
- The teaching plan for the patient and family after surgery includes:
  1. Prevention of infection
  2. Care and assessment of the surgical wound
  3. Management of drains or catheters
  4. Nutrition therapy
  5. Pain management
  6. Drug therapy
  7. Progressive increase in activity
  8. Follow-up with the surgeon
- Ensure that appropriate referrals are made to a social worker, home care agency, skilled nursing care, Meals on Wheels, support groups, and homemaker services.

SUBSTANCE ABUSE

OVERVIEW

- Substance abuse is the excessive use of a chemical substance, such as drugs and alcohol, and the resulting physical and psychological dependence that interferes with life's activities.
- It is a documented nursing diagnosis when the patient:
  1. Loses control of use of the drug
  2. Ingests the drug even though the drug has caused adverse conditions in the body
  3. Demonstrates cognitive, behavioral, and physiologic disturbances with the abuse of drugs or inhalants
- *Dependence* is a condition that causes a habitual, compulsive, and uncontrollable urge to use a substance. Without the substance, the body experiences severe physiologic, psychological, and emotional disturbances.
- *Substance use* is taking chemicals for pleasure without dependence.
- *Substance misuse* occurs when people use chemicals for reasons other than their intended action.
- *Addiction* causes negative outcomes after abusers stop using the substances. It is a disease caused by changes in the brain that affect human behavior and is manifested by substance craving, seeking, and subsequent use.
- *Withdrawal syndrome* symptoms, such as hallucinations, severe irritability, and hyperactivity, may result if the drug is eliminated suddenly.
- Many people abuse substances for stress relief.
- Family history of substance abuse increases a person's risk for this behavior.

⊕ Cultural Awareness

- An understanding of the patient's culture helps avoid making assumptions about substance abuse.
- Some behaviors that are interpreted in Western society as negative responses are considered normal, even reverent in some cultures, as in the case of avoiding eye contact.

Genetic/Genomic Considerations

- Genetic factors appear to contribute to misuse, abuse, or dependence from illicit drug use, as evidenced by studies of twins showing genetic-associated susceptibility to drug abuse and dependence.
- Genes associated with illegal drug abuse are not the same as those associated with abuse of legal substances, such as alcohol and nicotine.

<u>Considerations for Older Adults</u>
- Substance abuse should not be overlooked in the older adult population; the potential is high because of the number of different drugs taken by this age group.
- Common substances abused by older adults include alcohol, drugs, over-the-counter (OTC) drugs, and herbal preparations.

TYPES OF DEPENDENCIES

ALCOHOL
- *Alcoholism (alcohol dependence)* is a disease in which the patient:
  1. Has a strong need (craving) or compulsion to consume alcohol
  2. Is unable to limit alcohol consumption once drinking has begun (loss of control)
  3. Experiences physical dependence
  4. Has a need to increase the amount of alcohol to get the desired effect (tolerance)
- *Alcohol dependence* is present when the person experiences alcohol withdrawal symptoms after habitual use is suddenly stopped, resulting in nausea, sweating, shakiness, and disorientation.
- *Alcohol abuse* exists when a person *does not* have a strong craving for alcohol, loss of control, or physical dependence but has problems resulting from alcohol use (e.g., failing to fulfill responsibilities at home, work, or school, drinking in unsafe situations, continuing to drink when problems have been caused or worsened by use of alcohol).
- *At-risk drinking* is five or more of these beverages for men or four or more for women:
  1. 12 ounces of beer
  2. 5 ounces of wine
  3. 1.5 ounces of 80-proof spirits

PATIENT-CENTERED COLLABORATIVE CARE
Assessment
- Tools to identify risk for alcohol problems
  1. CAGE
     Have you ever felt you should <u>C</u>ut down on your drinking?
     Have you ever been <u>A</u>nnoyed when people have commented on your drinking?
     Have you ever felt <u>G</u>uilty or badly about your drinking?
     Have you ever had an <u>E</u>ye opener first thing in the morning to steady your nerves or get rid of a hangover?
     Score one point for each "yes" answer. A score of 1 is associated with an 80% chance of addiction to alcohol; 2 is

associated with an 89% chance of addiction; 3 is associated with a 99% chance of addiction; and 4 is 100% associated with a diagnosis of addiction to alcohol.

2. Other tools: T-ACE or AUDIT. See www.niaaa.nih.gov/pub lications/arh28-2/78-79.htm for a detailed description.

- Blood alcohol levels (BALs)
  1. As found by a Breathalyzer test, a BAL of 0.08% is the legal limit in most states.
  2. Standard BALs
     a. 80 to 200 mg/dL (0.08 to 0.2%, mild to moderate intoxication), with mood and behavior changes, impaired judgment, poor motor coordination, and hypotension (levels greater than 100 mg/dL)
     b. 250 to 400 mg/dL (0.25 to 0.4%, marked intoxication), with staggering ataxia and emotional liability; may progress to confusion and stupor or coma
     c. Greater than 500 mg/dL (0.5%, severe intoxication), possible death from respiratory depression

- Symptoms of alcohol withdrawal can occur as late as 5 to 7 days after the last drink, particularly with a pattern of recurrent binge drinking.
  1. Mild (onset usually 6 to 24 hours after the last drink, persisting for 1 to 3 days)
     a. Restlessness, anxiety
     b. Low-grade fever, diaphoresis
     c. Tremors
     d. Headache
     e. Palpitations
     f. Mild hypertension
     g. Nausea, anorexia, and GI discomfort
     h. Insomnia
  2. More severe (onset usually 24 to 96 hours after the last drink, persisting for 1 to 5 days and may occur in addition to mild symptoms)
     a. Delirium tremens (DTs)
     b. Hallucinations (visual or auditory)
     c. Delirium
     d. Tachycardia and hypertension
     e. Low-grade fever and pronounced diaphoresis
     f. Agitation
     g. Vomiting
     h. Withdrawal seizures (tonic-clonic)

Interventions

- Priority during alcohol withdrawal is to protect the patient from self-harm and from harming others.
- Drug therapy

1. Benzodiazepines to prevent seizures
    a. Chlordiazepoxide (Librium)
    b. Lorazepam (Ativan)
2. Beta blockers to reduce cravings and decrease blood pressure
3. Alpha-adrenergic blockers to decrease withdrawal symptoms
4. IV fluids
5. Vitamins (e.g., thiamine, folic acid)

- Nursing interventions include:
    1. Using a protocol to monitor symptoms of withdrawal at regular intervals
    2. Creating a low-stimulation environment
    3. Monitoring vital signs during withdrawal
    4. Monitoring for DTs
    5. Administering prescribed anticonvulsants or sedatives, as appropriate
    6. Medicating to relieve physical discomfort, as needed
    7. Addressing hallucinations in a therapeutic manner
    8. Maintaining adequate nutrition and fluid intake
    9. Administering prescribed vitamin therapy
    10. Providing emotional support to the patient and family
    11. Providing reality orientation

NICOTINE

- Nicotine is one of the most addictive substances in the United States and is the addictive component of tobacco.
- Tobacco use remains the leading cause of preventable death in the United States and nicotine continues to be a major contributing factor to the occurrence of cardiovascular disease.
- Several nicotine products are available: cigarettes, pipe tobacco, snuff, chewing tobacco, and spit tobacco.
- Second-hand smoke contributes to the development of cardiovascular disease, pulmonary disease, and cancer in nonsmokers.
- The addictive power of nicotine is similar to that of cocaine, and withdrawal symptoms occur when nicotine is discontinued.

PATIENT-CENTERED COLLABORATIVE CARE

- Motivate the patient to quit using nicotine through education.
- Exhibit sensitivity to the actual addiction present with tobacco use.
- Refer patients to community-based support groups and smoking cessation programs, many of which use behavioral models, hypnosis, acupressure, or other modalities tailored to the individual.
- Drug therapy
    1. Bupropion (Zyban, Wellbutrin) can help diminish nicotine craving
    2. Varenicline (Chantix)
    3. Nortriptyline (Pamelor)

4. Clonidine (Catapres)
5. Nicotine patches, gums, lozenges, sprays, inhalants, or tablets
6. Low-dose naltrexone (ReVia, Depade) along with a nicotine patch

STIMULANTS
- *Stimulants* are drugs that excite the cerebral cortex of the brain, producing a variety of behavioral responses.
  1. Commonly used stimulants
     a. Amphetamines (street names include *black beauties, cross, hearts*)
     b. Methamphetamines (street names include *biker dope, chalk, speed, crank, crystal, glass, hillbilly crack, meth*)
     c. Cocaine
     d. Minor stimulants (caffeine, nicotine)
  2. Therapeutic effects of stimulants
     a. Improved sense of well-being
     b. Increased mental alertness
     c. Increased capacity to work
     d. Improved performance of motor skills
  3. Manifestations of overdose
     a. Respiratory distress
     b. Hypertension
     c. Ataxia
     d. Fever
     e. Myocardial infarction
     f. Convulsions
     g. Coma
     h. Stroke
     i. Death
  4. Emergency care for overdose
     a. Monitoring vital signs (especially heart rate, blood pressure, and temperature)
     b. Maintaining a safe environment
     c. Providing respiratory support
     d. Applying cooling blanket
     e. Administering anticonvulsants
     f. Administering anti-psychotics
     g. Administering ammonium chloride (to acidify urine for excretion of amphetamines [bases])
  5. Manifestations of stimulant withdrawal
     a. Fatigue
     b. Depression
     c. Agitation
     d. Apathy
     e. Anxiety

    f. Insomnia
    g. Disorientation
    h. Craving
6. Management of withdrawal focuses on drug therapy with:
    a. Antianxiety drugs
    b. Antidepressants
    c. Dopamine agonists (to reduce tremors)

❗ NURSING SAFETY PRIORITY: Critical Rescue

For the patient with an overdose of or withdrawal from cocaine, essential care includes observing for acute cardiac symptoms and assessing for depression and potential suicide gestures.

HALLUCINOGENS AND RELATED COMPOUNDS
- *Hallucinogens* are chemical substances that possess mind-altering or mental perception-altering properties.
- Lysergic acid (street names include *LSD, acid*)
  1. Manifestations
     a. Dilated pupils
     b. Tachycardia
     c. Palpitations
     d. Diaphoresis
     e. Tremors
     f. Poor coordination
     g. Elevated body temperature
     h. Increased pulse and respiration
     i. Psychological symptoms (paranoid ideas, anxiety, depression, sensory experiences, bizarre thoughts)
     j. Brain damage, psychosis, death
  2. Management involves one-to-one observation to keep the patient safe and to help the person sort reality as the effects subside and includes:
     a. Reducing environmental stimuli
     b. Administering prescribed antianxiety drugs (e.g., benzodiazepines or haloperidol)
- Phencyclidine (street names include *PCP, angel dust*)
  1. Manifestations
     a. Feelings of detachment
     b. Heart rate and blood pressure instability
     c. Eye flickering
     d. Flushing
     e. Increased perspiration
     f. Aggression

    g. Incoherence
    h. Seizures
    i. Progression to hallucinations, catatonia, coma, and death
  2. Management
    a. Calm environment
    b. Cardiac and respiratory support
  3. With long-term use, symptoms may persist for a year or cause permanent disabilities.
- Ketamine (street names include *businessman's LSD, Special K, K, Kat*)
  1. Manifestations of moderate doses
     a. Euphoria
     b. Loss of inhibition
     c. Confusion
     d. Ringing in the ears
     e. Quick burst of energy
     f. Drunken feeling
  2. Manifestations of overdose
     a. Tunnel vision
     b. Shortness of breath
     c. Loss of balance
     d. Numbness of the body
     e. Clinical depression
     f. No sense of time
     g. Seizures
     h. Coma
  3. Management
     a. Providing a calm and stimulus-free environment
     b. Respiratory support
- Methylenedioxymethamphetamine or MDMA (street names include *Adam, ecstasy, XTC, hug, beans, date rape drug*) is an altered amphetamine that produces hallucinogenic responses.
  1. Manifestations
     a. Development of trust in others
     b. Reduced inhibitions
     c. Increased confidence
     d. Euphoria
     e. Relaxation of voluntary muscles
     f. Heightened sexual experiences
     g. Amnesia
     h. Hyperthermia
     i. Psychological symptoms of depression, sleep disturbances, drug craving, severe anxiety, and paranoia
     j. Long-term use leads to parkinsonism, brain damage, multiorgan failure, and death

2. Management
   a. Symptom-based support
   b. Safe environment
   c. Reduction or elimination of adverse drug effects
- Marijuana (street names include *weed, smoke, pot, grass, Mary Jane, herb*)
  1. Manifestations
     a. Euphoria
     b. Sexual arousal
     c. Relaxation
     d. Increased heart rate and hypertension
     e. Impaired short-term memory
     f. Paranoia, panic attacks
     g. Increased appetite
     h. Impaired coordination
  2. Withdrawal symptoms
     a. Insomnia
     b. Decreased appetite
     c. Nausea
     d. Irritability
     e. Anxiety
  3. Management
     a. Frequent vital sign assessment
     b. Symptom management
     c. Pain control

DEPRESSANTS

- *Depressants* are drugs that reduce the activity of the central nervous system (CNS). They include the commonly prescribed drug categories of benzodiazepines and barbiturates, as well as many illicit drugs.
- All benzodiazepines can produce the same effects; however, some are much more potent than others and produce the effects at low doses.
- Flunitrazepam (Rohypnol) is a commonly abused benzodiazepine (street names include *rophies, roofies, ruffies, R2s, Mexican Valium, Rib, roach, Roches, Forget Me Pill, Forget Pill*).
  1. Manifestations
     a. Reduced anxiety
     b. Lowered inhibitions
     c. Lowered heart rate and blood pressure
     d. Lowered respirations
     e. Fatigue
     f. Poor concentration, confusion, impaired coordination, amnesia
     g. Impaired judgment

2. Manifestations of overdose
   a. Respiratory depression
   b. Excessive sedation
   c. Cardiac arrest
   d. Death
3. Management
   a. Respiratory support
   b. Close monitoring
   c. Symptomatic relief and comfort measures
   d. Drug therapy for acute overdose is flumazenil (Romazicon)
   e. Long-term therapy for abuse is detoxification with titrating doses

- Gamma hydroxybutyrate (street names include *GHB, liquid ecstasy*)
  1. Manifestations of low doses
     a. Reduced social inhibitions
     b. Increased libido
     c. Euphoria and anxiety
     d. Impaired judgment and loss of coordination
     e. Nausea
  2. Manifestations of higher doses and overdose
     a. Dizziness
     b. Respiratory depression
     c. Memory loss
     d. Muscle fatigue
     e. Coma and death
  3. Death is most common when the drug is combined with alcohol.

- Barbiturates are common drugs and include amobarbital (Amytal) and pentobarbital (Nembutal). Street names include *barbs, reds, red birds, phennies, tooies, yellows, yellow jackets.*
  1. Manifestations
     a. Sedation
     b. Drowsiness
     c. Decreased motor activity
  2. Manifestations of overdose
     a. Respiratory depression
     b. Pinpoint pupils
     c. Coma
  3. Manifestations of withdrawal
     a. Nausea, vomiting, abdominal cramping
     b. Seizures
     c. Variable behavioral responses

4. Management for overdose or withdrawal
   a. Drug tapering (for overdose to prevent withdrawal)
   b. Frequent vital signs checks
   c. Frequent neurologic checks
   d. Emotional support
   e. Food, fluids
   f. Calm environment

OPIOIDS

- *Opioids* is a broad term encompassing all drugs that are made from the Asian poppy or produced as a synthetic drug that causes the same effects as the opium plant.
- Other terms for opioids are *narcotics* and *narcs*. There are a variety of street names for opioids.
- Drugs included in this category are codeine, morphine, heroin, methadone, hydromorphone (Dilaudid), meperidine (Demerol), and oxycodone (OxyContin).
- Except for heroin, opioids are used for pain relief and have potential for abuse or addition.
- In patients who are opioid substance abusers, tolerance to pain relief effects may require high doses of opioids. Unrelieved pain in substance abusers can contribute to relapse or increase substance abuse. Withdrawal symptoms can occur when the substance abuser is given a partial opioid agonist or opioid antagonist.
  1. Manifestations of opiate intoxication
     a. Constricted pupils
     b. Decreased blood pressure
     c. Decreased respirations
     d. Drowsiness
     e. Slurred speech
     f. Initial euphoria followed by dysphoria (depression)
     g. Cognitive impairments resulting in judgment and memory losses
  2. Manifestations of opiate overdose
     a. Dilated pupils
     b. Respiratory depression
     c. Coma
     d. Shock
     e. Convulsions
     f. Respiratory arrest
     g. Death
  3. Manifestations of opiate withdrawal
     a. Yawning
     b. Insomnia
     c. Irritability

       d. Rhinorrhea
       e. Diaphoresis
       f. Abdominal cramps
       g. Nausea and vomiting
       h. Muscle aches
       i. Chills, cold flashes with goose bumps (referred to as *cold turkey*)
    4. Management of opiate overdose
       a. Drug therapy with anticonvulsants, opioid antagonists, and antianxiety agents
       b. Frequent vital sign and neurologic checks
       c. Supportive measures

INHALANT ABUSE

- *Inhalants* are breathable chemical vapors that produce psychoactive effects.
- Common or street names for these abused drugs include *glue, kick, bang, sniff, huffing, poppers, whippets,* and *Texas shoe-shine.*
  1. Commonly abused inhalants:
     a. Solvents such as paint thinners, gasoline, glues, paper correction fluid, felt-tip markers, and electronic contact cleaners
     b. Gases such as butane lighters, propane tanks, whipping cream aerosols, spray paints, hair or deodorant sprays, chloroform, ether, and nitrous oxide (laughing gas)
     c. Nitrites such as cyclohexyl nitrite, amyl nitrite, and butyl nitrite
  2. Manifestations of inhalant use
     a. Slurred speech
     b. Drunken, dizzy, or dazed appearance
     c. Chemical smell on the person
     d. Paint stains on the face or body
     e. Red eyes
     f. Rhinorrhea
  3. Management is supportive, based on manifestations.

STEROIDS

- *Anabolic-androgenic steroids* are synthetic substances that mimic the actions of testosterone and are sometimes abused by athletes to increase strength and performance.
- Their legal use is for people with hormonal difficulties such as delayed puberty or impotence.
- Street names include *roids, juice, hype,* and *pump.*
- Effects of steroid use
  1. In men
     a. Shrunken testicles
     b. Reduced sperm count

     c. Infertility
     d. Baldness
     e. Development of breasts
     f. Increased risk for cancer

2. In women
     a. Growth of facial hair
     b. Male pattern baldness
     c. Changes or cessation of menses
     d. Enlargement of the clitoris
     e. Deepened voice

3. General complications
     a. Negative emotional effects such as *roid rage*, with severe aggressive behavior with the potential for violence
     b. Mood swings
     c. Hallucinations, paranoia, anxiety or panic attacks, depression, or thoughts of suicide
     d. High blood pressure and heart disease
     e. Liver damage
     f. Stroke and blood clots
     g. Urinary and bowel problems such as diarrhea
     h. Headaches, muscle cramps, aching joints
     i. Sleep problems
     j. Increased risk of ligament and tendon injuries
     k. Severe acne

PART TWO

Diseases and Disorders

ABSCESS, ANORECTAL

- Anorectal abscesses result from obstruction of the ducts of glands in the anorectal region by feces, foreign bodies, or trauma.
- Stasis of the obstructing contents results in infection that spreads into adjacent tissue.
- Rectal pain is the first clinical manifestation.
- Local swelling, erythema, and tenderness on palpation appear a few days after the onset of pain.
- The diagnosis is made by physical examination and history.
- Simple perianal and ischiorectal abscesses can be excised and drained with local anesthesia; more extensive abscesses require incision using regional or general anesthesia.
- Intervention includes:
  1. Giving systemic antibiotics, particularly to immunocompromised patients such as those with diabetes
  2. Assisting the patient to maintain comfort and optimal perineal hygiene by providing warm sitz baths and analgesics, and by encouraging the patient to avoid constipation with bulk-forming agents, osmotic laxatives, or stool softeners
  3. Emphasizing the importance of ongoing perineal hygiene and the maintenance of a regular bowel pattern with a high-fiber diet

ABSCESS, BRAIN

OVERVIEW

- A *brain abscess* is an infection of the brain in which encapsulated pus forms in the extradural, subdural, or intracerebral area.
- A brain abscess is more likely to occur in patients with immunosuppression, organ transplantation, and acquired immune deficiency syndrome (AIDS).

- The causative organisms are most often bacteria, such as *Streptococcus* and *Staphylococcus*.
- Most brain abscesses occur in the frontal and temporal lobes.

PATIENT-CENTERED COLLABORATIVE CARE

- A brain abscess typically manifests with symptoms of a mass and of mildly increased intracranial pressure, including:
  1. Headache
  2. Fever
  3. Focal neurologic deficits
  4. Lethargy and confusion
  5. Visual field deficits
  6. Nystagmus and disconjugate gaze
  7. Generalized weakness, hemiparesis
  8. Ataxic gait
  9. Seizures
  10. Various degrees of aphasia with a frontal or temporal lobe abscess
  11. Elevated white blood cell (WBC) count
- Drug therapy includes:
  1. Antibiotics, typically administered IV or intrathecally
  2. Metronidazole (Flagyl, Novonidazol), if an anaerobic organism is the causative agent
  3. Antiepileptic drugs, as ordered, to prevent or treat seizures
  4. Analgesics, as ordered, to treat the patient's headache
- Surgical drainage of an encapsulated abscess, or an exploratory craniotomy may be performed

ABSCESS, HEPATIC

- Hepatic (liver) abscesses occur when the liver is invaded by bacteria or protozoa.
- Liver tissue is destroyed, producing a necrotic cavity filled with infected agents, liquefied liver cells and tissue, and leukocytes.
- Liver abscess occurs rarely and is associated with a high mortality rate.
- Pyrogenic abscesses are caused by bacteria such as *Escherichia coli*, *Klebsiella*, *Enterobacter*, *Salmonella*, *Staphylococcus*, and *Enterococcus*.
- Abscesses can result from acute cholangitis, liver trauma, peritonitis, or sepsis, or an abscess can extend to the liver after pneumonia or bacterial endocarditis.
- Amebic hepatic abscesses occur after amebic dysentery as a single abscess in the right upper quadrant of the liver.

- Assessment findings include:
  1. Right upper quadrant abdominal pain with a tender, palpable liver
  2. Anorexia
  3. Weight loss
  4. Nausea and vomiting
  5. Fever and chills
  6. Shoulder pain
  7. Dyspnea
  8. Pleural pain if the diaphragm is involved
  9. Jaundice
- Hepatic abscesses are usually diagnosed by contrast-enhanced computed tomography (CT) or ultrasound.
- Abscesses may be drained under CT or ultrasound guidance. Drainage is sent for laboratory analysis so optimal antibiotic treatment can be selected.

ABSCESS, LUNG

- A lung abscess is a localized area of lung destruction caused by liquefaction necrosis, which is usually related to pyogenic bacteria.
- Common causes are pneumonia, aspiration of mouth or stomach contents, and obstruction as a result of a tumor or foreign body.
- A lung abscess also can be caused by any condition that alters the ability to swallow, such as alcoholic blackouts, seizure disorders, other neurologic deficits, and swallowing disorders.
- Assessment findings include:
  1. Recent history of any pulmonary infection (influenza or pneumonia)
  2. Fever
  3. Cough and foul-smelling sputum
  4. Decreased breath sounds on affected side, crackles
  5. Fatigue and unplanned weight loss
  6. Abnormal chest x-ray
- Nursing diagnoses and interventions are similar to those for pneumonia.
- Medical management includes percutaneous drainage of the abscess and antibiotic therapy.

ABSCESS, PANCREATIC

- A pancreatic abscess consists of infected, necrotic pancreatic tissue.
- Pancreatic abscess usually occurs after severe acute pancreatitis, exacerbations of chronic pancreatitis, and biliary tract surgery.

- The problem may occur as a single abscess or multiloculated abscesses resulting from extensive inflammatory necrosis of the pancreas readily invaded by infectious organisms such as *Escherichia coli*, *Klebsiella*, *Bacteroides*, *Staphylococcus*, and *Proteus*.
- Temperature spikes may be as high as 104° F (40° C).
- The abscess is surgically drained; multiple drainage procedures are often required.
- Insulin-secreting beta cells may be destroyed with infection, leading to hyperglycemia.
- Antibiotic therapy alone does not resolve the abscess.
- Pleural effusions often accompany the abscess.

ABSCESS, PERITONSILLAR

- Peritonsillar abscess (PTA), or *quinsy*, is a complication of acute tonsillitis.
- The infection spreads from the tonsil to the surrounding tissue, forming an abscess.
- The most common cause is infection with group A beta-hemolytic streptococci.
- Signs of infection are pronounced on examination. Pus forms behind the tonsil and causes one-sided swelling with deviation of the uvula toward the unaffected side. The swelling causes drooling, severe throat pain radiating to the ear, a voice change, and difficulty swallowing.

■ NURSING SAFETY PRIORITY: Critical Rescue

Check the patient for respiratory obstruction, which may occur from swelling. If obstruction is present, notify the Rapid Response Team.

- Management includes:
  1. Percutaneous needle aspiration
  2. Antibiotics
  3. Analgesics
  4. Warm saline gargles or irrigations
  5. Ice collar
  6. Tonsillectomy after the abscess has healed

ABSCESS, RENAL

- A renal abscess is a collection of fluid and cells resulting from an inflammatory response to bacteria in the renal parenchyma, renal fascia, or flank.

- An abscess is suspected when fever and symptoms of kidney infection are unresponsive to antibiotic therapy.
- Symptoms include:
  1. Fever
  2. Flank pain
  3. General malaise
  4. Local edema
- Treatment includes:
  1. Broad-spectrum antibiotics
  2. Drainage by surgical incision or needle aspiration

ACIDOSIS, METABOLIC

OVERVIEW

- Acidosis is not a disease; it is a condition caused by a metabolic problem, a respiratory problem, or both.
- Four processes can result in metabolic acidosis: overproduction of hydrogen ions, underelimination of hydrogen ions, underproduction of bicarbonate ions, and overelimination of bicarbonate ions.
- It is reflected by the following arterial blood gas (ABG) values: pH below 7.35; bicarbonate (HCO_3) values below the normal range (below 22 mEq/L [mmol/L]).
- Metabolic acidosis often is accompanied by potassium excess (hyperkalemia).
- Common causes of metabolic acidosis include:
  1. Conditions that overproduce hydrogen ions
     a. Diabetic ketoacidosis
     b. Fever
     c. Heavy exercise
     d. Hypoxia, anoxia, or ischemia
     e. Starvation, carbohydrate-free diets
     f. Aspirin or other salicylate intoxication
     g. Ethanol, methanol, or ethylene glycol intoxication
  2. Conditions that cause underelimination of hydrogen ions (renal failure)
  3. Conditions that underproduce bicarbonate ions (liver failure, pancreatitis, or dehydration)
  4. Conditions that overeliminate bicarbonate (diarrhea)

PATIENT-CENTERED COLLABORATIVE CARE
Assessment

- Assessment findings include:
  1. Central nervous system (CNS) changes
     a. Decreased mentation (confusion, lethargy stupor, and coma)

2. Neuromuscular changes
   a. Hyporeflexia
   b. Skeletal muscle weakness leading to flaccid paralysis
3. Cardiovascular changes
   a. Delayed electrical conduction (bradycardia and heart block), manifested by prolonged PR interval and widened QRS complex
   b. Tall T waves
   c. Hypotension
   d. Thready peripheral pulses
4. Respiratory changes
   a. Increased respiratory rate
   b. Kussmaul pattern of respirations (greatly increased rate and depth of ventilation)
5. Skin changes
   a. Warm, flushed

Interventions

- Management focuses on:
  1. Correcting the underlying cause of the acid imbalance
  2. Administering IV fluids and maintaining IV access
  3. Monitoring ABG and serum potassium results and reporting critical values within 30 minutes to physician or prescribing health care provider
  4. Evaluating rate, rhythm, intervals and other components of cardiac monitoring
  5. Evaluating the balance of fluid intake and output and reporting significant imbalances (a difference greater than 500 to 1000 mL) over an 8-hour shift

ACIDOSIS, RESPIRATORY

OVERVIEW

- Acidosis is not a disease; it is a condition caused by a metabolic problem, a respiratory problem, or both.
- Respiratory acidosis results when respiratory function is impaired, leading to CO_2 retention.
- Respiratory acidosis results from only one mechanism: retention of CO_2, causing increased production of free hydrogen ions. It is always an *acid excess* acidosis.
- It can be an acute condition or a chronic condition.
- Acute respiratory acidosis is reflected by arterial blood gas (ABG) values indicating a pH below 7.35, normal HCO_3^-, low Po_2, and high Pco_2.
- Chronic respiratory acidosis is reflected by ABG values indicating a pH below 7.35, high HCO_3^-, low Po_2, and high Pco_2.

- Common causes of respiratory acidosis include:
  1. Respiratory depression
     a. Anesthetics
     b. Drugs (especially opioids and benzodiazepines)
     c. Brain injury
     d. Electrolyte imbalance
  2. Reduced alveolar-capillary diffusion
     a. Disease (emphysema, pneumonia, tuberculosis, fibrosis, or cancer)
     b. Pulmonary edema
     c. Atelectasis
     d. Pulmonary emboli
     e. Chest trauma
  3. Airway obstruction
     a. Foreign object in airway
     b. Disease (asthma, epiglottitis)
     c. Strangulation
     d. Regional lymph node enlargement
  4. Inadequate chest expansion
     a. Skeletal deformities (kyphosis, scoliosis), trauma (flail chest, broken ribs), spinal cord injury
     b. Hemothorax or pneumothorax
     c. Respiratory muscle weakness
     d. Obesity
     e. Abdominal or thoracic masses
     f. Ascites

Considerations for Older Adults

- The older adult is at higher risk for respiratory acidosis in the presence of comorbidities of cardiac, respiratory, and renal disease.
- The older adult is more likely to be taking drugs that interfere with acid-base balance, such as aspirin, diuretics, laxatives, antihypertensives, and cardiac glycosides.

PATIENT-CENTERED COLLABORATIVE CARE
Assessment

- Assessment findings include:
  1. Central nervous system (CNS) changes
     a. Decreased mentation (confusion, lethargy, stupor, and coma)
  2. Neuromuscular changes
     a. Hyporeflexia
     b. Skeletal muscle weakness leading to flaccid paralysis

3. Cardiovascular changes
   a. Delayed electrical conduction (bradycardia to heart block manifested by prolonged PR interval or widened QRS complex)
   b. Tall T waves
   c. Hypotension
   d. Thready peripheral pulses
4. Respiratory changes
   a. Rapid, shallow respirations.
   b. Diminished respiratory effort
5. Skin changes
   a. Cool, pale to cyanotic

Interventions

- Management focuses on:
  1. Ensuring adequate oxygenation:
     a. Assessing the airway and breathing effectiveness
     b. Administering oxygen as prescribed
     c. Positioning to provide maximal lung excursion, usually with a back rest elevation greater than 60 degrees.
  2. Administering inhaled bronchodilator drugs to improve ventilation and gas exchange, such as albuterol (Proventil, Ventolin), ipratropium (Atrovent, Apo-Ipravent ♣), theophylline (e.g., Elixophyllin, Theo-Dur, Uniphyl, Theolair)
  3. Monitoring respiratory status at least every 2 hours for response to therapy or worsening of breathing effectiveness
     a. Respiratory rate and depth
     b. Oxygen saturation (Spo_2) and arterial blood gas (ABG) values to maintain a normal range of oxygenation (Spo_2 greater than 90% to 92% and Pao_2 greater than 90 mm Hg)
     c. Effort of breathing, including use of accessory muscles
     d. Breath sounds
     e. Color of nail beds and mucous membranes
     f. Level of consciousness and mentation
     g. Fraction of inspired oxygen (Fio_2) with oxygen delivery system or ventilator settings

⚠ NURSING SAFETY PRIORITY: Critical Rescue

Notify the Rapid Response Team about any patient whose respiratory rate remains at less than 8 to 10 breaths/min with stimulation or whose oxygen saturation suddenly drops by 8 to 10 percentage points and does not improve within a few minutes after an intervention.

> **⚠ NURSING SAFETY PRIORITY: Critical Rescue**
>
> Avoid excessive oxygen flow rates for patients with chronic respiratory acidosis who are not being mechanically ventilated. High rates of delivered oxygen can interfere with the respiratory drive of a patient with a chronic lung condition.

ACUTE CORONARY SYNDROMES

- The term *acute coronary syndrome* (ACS) is used to describe patients who have either unstable angina or an acute myocardial infarction (MI).
- *Unstable angina* is chest pain or discomfort that occurs at rest or with exertion and causes severe activity limitation.
- MI occurs when myocardial tissue is abruptly and severely deprived of oxygen. When blood flow is quickly reduced by 80% to 90%, ischemia can lead to injury and necrosis of myocardial tissue if blood flow is not restored.
- In ACS, it is believed that the atherosclerotic plaque in the coronary artery ruptures, resulting in platelet aggregation ("clumping"), thrombus (clot) formation, and vasoconstriction
- For more information about assessment and management, go to "Coronary Artery Disease"

ACUTE RESPIRATORY DISTRESS SYNDROME

OVERVIEW
- Acute respiratory distress syndrome (ARDS) is acute respiratory failure with the following features:
  1. Hypoxemia that persists even when 100% oxygen is given
  2. Decreased pulmonary compliance
  3. Dyspnea
  4. Noncardiac-associated bilateral pulmonary edema
  5. Dense pulmonary infiltrates on x-ray (ground-glass appearance)
- ARDS is theorized to be the most pathologic on a continuum of acute lung injury (ALI). Injury can occur from both pulmonary and nonpulmonary causes such as sepsis, pneumonia, pulmonary embolism, shock, aspiration, acute pancreatitis, ascites, ovarian hyperstimulation, or inhalation injury.
- A local or systemic inflammatory response injures the alveolar-capillary membrane, causing protein-containing fluid to leak into alveoli. Fluid-filled alveoli cannot exchange oxygen and carbon dioxide.
- Fluid also leaks into the spaces between alveoli (interstitial edema), further compressing alveoli and reducing the capacity to exchange gases.

- ARDS also results in changes in the alveoli and respiratory bronchioles. Surfactant production is reduced, making the alveoli unstable and at risk for collapse, even when they are not filled with fluid.
- Lung volume and compliance are dramatically reduced, initially as a result of acute lung injury, and as nonfunctional alveoli are destroyed, with long-term consequences for prolonged illness and recovery.
- Poorly inflated alveoli receive blood but cannot oxygenate it, causing an increased pulmonary shunt known as $\dot{V}/\dot{Q}$ *mismatch*.
- Patients have a rapidly deteriorating respiratory status that does not respond to increased oxygen therapy. The mortality rate is high even when intensive interventions are used.

☑ NATIONAL PATIENT SAFETY GOAL

Reduce the risk of health care–associated respiratory infections that can contribute to the onset of ARDS by good handwashing and informing visitors to adhere to similar handwashing precautions.

⊞ NURSING SAFETY PRIORITY: Action Alert

A nursing priority in the prevention of ARDS is early recognition of patients at high risk for the syndrome. Two important areas for prevention are aspiration of gastric contents and prevention of sepsis. Use aspiration precautions such as elevating the head of bed greater than 30 to 45 degrees for patients receiving enteral feeding. Avoid oral intake in patients with problems that impair swallowing and gag reflexes. To reduce risk for sepsis, follow meticulous infection control guidelines, including handwashing, invasive catheter and wound care, and body substance precautions.

PATIENT-CENTERED COLLABORATIVE CARE
Assessment

- Assessment findings include:
    1. Decreasing oxygen saturation (SpO_2) or partial pressure of arterial oxygen (PaO_2)
    2. Increased respiratory rate
    3. Increased effort with breathing (grunting respiration, cyanosis, pallor, and intercostal retractions or substernal retractions)
    4. Diaphoresis
    5. Decreased breath sounds or crackles.
    6. If accompanied by sepsis or other systemic disease, hypotension, tachycardia and/or dysrhythmias, and symptoms of

infection (fever, increased sputum, elevated white blood cell [WBC] count)
7. Mental status changes
8. Fluid-filled pulmonary fields, manifested as "whited-out" areas on chest x-ray

Interventions
- Medical management includes drug therapy:
  1. Intubation and mechanical ventilation
  2. Anti-inflammatories such as corticosteroids, which may be used to reduce the inflammatory response and prevent fibrosis
  3. Antibiotics to manage identified infections
  4. Conservative IV fluid volume replacement to prevent hypotension and inadequate perfusion

---

◼ NURSING SAFETY PRIORITY: Action Alert

Avoid excessive IV fluid administration in these patients, because it leads to fluid overload and more edema in the pulmonary and systemic circulation.

---

  5. Enteral nutrition or parenteral nutrition as soon as possible to prevent malnutrition, loss of respiratory muscle function, and reduced immune response
- The course of ARDS and its management are divided into four phases:
  1. Phase 1 includes early changes of hypoxemia, dyspnea, and tachypnea. Early interventions involve supporting the patient and providing oxygen.
  2. In phase 2, patchy infiltrates form from increasing pulmonary edema. Interventions include intubation and mechanical ventilation and prevention of complications. Usually, positive end-expiratory pressure (PEEP) or continuous positive airway pressure (CPAP) is used. Patient positioning may include the prone position, continuously lateral rotation (CLRT) through automated bed technology, and chest vibration using a vest or other device. Sedation and paralysis may be needed for adequate ventilation and to reduce tissue oxygen needs.
  3. Phase 3 occurs over days 2 to 10. Interventions focus on maintaining adequate oxygen transport, preventing complications, and supporting the failing lung until it has had time to heal.

4. In phase 4, pulmonary fibrosis with progression occurs after 10 days. This phase is irreversible and is often called *late* or *chronic ARDS.* Patients who survive to this stage will have some permanent lung damage. Interventions focus on weaning the patient from the ventilator while preventing the complications from chronic critical illness such as multiorgan dysfunction, recurrent sepsis, weakness acquired during a stay in an intensive care unit, and cognitive deterioration from delirium.

ADRENAL INSUFFICIENCY (ADRENAL HYPOFUNCTION)

OVERVIEW

- Decreased production of adrenocortical steroids may occur as a result of inadequate secretion of adrenocorticotropic hormone (ACTH), dysfunction of the hypothalamic-pituitary control mechanism, or direct dysfunction of adrenal gland tissue.
- Primary hypofunction, or *Addison's disease,* develops gradually as adrenal function is reduced and can no longer supply normal levels of glucocorticoids or mineralocorticoids. Causes include tuberculosis, autoimmune factors, HIV/AIDS, adrenal tumors, hemorrhage, sepsis, irradiation of the adrenal glands, and adrenalectomy.
- The most common cause of secondary adrenal insufficiency is the sudden cessation of long-term, high-dose glucocorticoid therapy.
- Manifestations of adrenal hypofunction include:
  1. Hyperkalemia
  2. Hyponatremia
  3. Hypotension
  4. Hypoglycemia
  5. Shock
- Acute adrenal insufficiency, or *Addisonian crisis,* is a life-threatening event in which the need for cortisol and aldosterone is greater than the available supply. Manifestations may appear suddenly, without warning. Death from hypoglycemia, shock, and hyperkalemia-associated cardiac problems can occur unless interventions are implemented rapidly.

PATIENT-CENTERED COLLABORATIVE CARE

Assessment

- Obtain patient information about:
  1. Change in activity level
  2. Increased salt craving or intake
  3. GI problems, such as anorexia, nausea, vomiting, diarrhea, and abdominal pain

4. Unplanned weight loss
5. History of irradiation to the abdomen or head
6. Past or current medical problems (e.g., tuberculosis, previous intracranial surgery)
7. Past and current drugs, especially steroids, anticoagulants, opioids, or cytotoxic drugs
- Assess for and document:
  1. Manifestations of hypoglycemia (low blood glucose level, sweating, headaches, tachycardia, and tremors)
  2. Manifestations of hypovolemia (e.g., postural hypotension, dehydration)
  3. Cardiac problems from hyperkalemia (e.g., dysrhythmias, bradycardia, irregular heart rate, cardiac arrest)
  4. Skeletal muscle weakness
  5. Electrolyte abnormalities (elevated serum potassium and low serum sodium levels)
  6. Areas of increased pigmentation, decreased pigmentation, or patchy pigmentation
  7. Decreased alertness, forgetfulness, confusion
- Diagnosis is based on clinical manifestations and:
  1. Laboratory findings of low serum cortisol, low fasting blood glucose, low sodium, and elevated potassium levels
  2. Low urinary 17-hydroxycorticosteroid and 17-ketosteroid levels
  3. Skull x-rays, CT and MRI scans, and arteriograms
  4. CT scans of the adrenal gland
  5. ACTH stimulation testing

Interventions

- Cortisol and aldosterone deficiencies are corrected by replacement therapy with hydrocortisone (corrects glucocorticoid deficiency) and fludrocortisone (corrects aldosterone deficiency).
  1. For hydrocortisone therapy, divided doses are usually given, with two thirds given in the morning and one third in the late afternoon (or as prescribed).
  2. Dosage adjustment of fludrocortisone may be needed, especially in hot weather, when more sodium is lost because of excessive perspiration.
- Nursing interventions to promote fluid balance, monitor for fluid deficit, and prevent hypoglycemia include:
  1. Weighing the patient daily and recording intake and output
  2. Assessing vital signs every 1 to 4 hours
  3. Checking for dysrhythmias or postural hypotension
  4. Monitoring laboratory values to identify hemoconcentration (e.g., increased hematocrit, blood urea nitrogen [BUN])

⚠ NURSING SAFETY PRIORITY: Action Alert

Do not implement salt restriction or diuretic therapy for anyone with severe adrenal hypofunction because it may lead to an adrenal crisis.

ALKALOSIS, METABOLIC

OVERVIEW

- Alkalosis is not a disease; it is a condition caused by a metabolic problem, a respiratory problem, or both.
- Metabolic alkalosis is caused by any condition that creates the acid-base imbalance through either an increase of bases (base excess) or a decrease of acids (acid deficit).
- It is reflected by arterial blood gas (ABG) values indicating a pH above 7.45 and high HCO_3^-.
- Often, metabolic alkalosis is accompanied by a low serum potassium level (hypokalemia).
- An *actual metabolic alkalosis* occurs when a base (usually bicarbonate) is overproduced or undereliminated. This type of alkalosis is known as a *base excess alkalosis*.
- A *relative alkalosis* occurs when the amount or strength, or both, of the acids decreases, making the blood more basic than acidic as a result of overelimination or underproduction of acids. This type of alkalosis is known as an *acid deficit alkalosis*.
- Common causes of metabolic alkalosis include:
  1. Increase of base (especially bicarbonate)
     a. Excessive use of antacids or bicarbonate
     b. Milk-alkali syndrome
     c. Multiple transfusions of blood products
     d. IV administration of bicarbonate
     e. Total parenteral nutrition
  2. Acid loss
     a. Prolonged vomiting
     b. Continuous nasogastric suctioning
     c. Dehydration from excess diuretic use
     d. Hypercortisolism
     e. Hyperaldosteronism

PATIENT-CENTERED COLLABORATIVE CARE

Assessment

- Assessment findings include:
  1. Central nervous system (CNS) changes
     a. Light-headedness
     b. Decreased ability to concentrate
     c. Anxiety, irritability

   d. Paresthesia
   e. Positive Chvostek's sign
   f. Positive Trousseau's sign
   g. Tetany, seizures
  2. Neuromuscular changes
   a. Skeletal muscle weakness
   b. Muscle cramping and twitching
   c. Hyperreflexia
  3. Cardiac changes
   a. Weak, rapid pulse
   b. Hypotension (if hypovolemia is also present)
  4. Respiratory changes
   a. Decreased respiratory effort (a late manifestation of metabolic alkalosis, occurring as a result of weakness of respiratory skeletal muscles) leading to reduced oxygenation (low SpO_2 or PaO_2)

Interventions

- Management focuses on:
 1. Drug therapy to resolve the causes of alkalosis (e.g., antiemetics for severe vomiting)
 2. Oral or IV replacement to restore normal fluid, electrolyte, and acid-base balance
 3. Monitoring patient responses to therapy
  a. Respiratory effectiveness (rate, depth, oxygen saturation)
  b. Cardiac effectiveness (pulse, blood pressure)
  c. Intake and output
  d. Serum electrolytes and ABG values
  e. Hand grasps and deep tendon reflexes

ALKALOSIS, RESPIRATORY

OVERVIEW

- Respiratory alkalosis is not a disease; it is a condition caused by a respiratory problem that usually involves an excessive rate or depth of ventilation, or both.
- It is reflected by arterial blood gas (ABG) values indicating a pH above 7.45 and low PCO_2.
- Often, it is accompanied by a low serum potassium level (hypokalemia).
- Respiratory alkalosis occurs because of an excess loss of acids in the form of carbon dioxide.
- The main cause of respiratory alkalosis is hyperventilation, which leads to excessive exhalation of carbon dioxide. Common

conditions leading to hyperventilation include:
1. Anxiety or fear
2. Improper settings on mechanical ventilators (too high a ventilation rate, too great a tidal volume, or both)
3. Direct stimulation of central respiratory centers
   a. Fever
   b. Hyperthyroidism
   c. Drugs (e.g., salicylates, catecholamines, progesterone)
   d. High altitudes or low atmospheric oxygen levels

PATIENT-CENTERED COLLABORATIVE CARE
Assessment
- Assessment findings include:
  1. Central nervous system (CNS) changes
     a. Light-headedness
     b. Decreased ability to concentrate
     c. Anxiety, irritability
     d. Paresthesia
     e. Positive Chvostek's sign
     f. Positive Trousseau's sign
     g. Tetany, seizures
  2. Neuromuscular changes
     a. Skeletal muscle weakness
     b. Muscle cramping and twitching
     c. Hyperreflexia
  3. Cardiac changes
     a. Weak, rapid pulse

Interventions
- Management focuses on:
  1. Ensuring ventilator settings are appropriate for patient size
  2. Rebreathing exhaled air to increase carbon dioxide levels
  3. Calming the patient and working with him or her to control ventilation
  4. Administering drug therapy to resolve the causes of alkalosis (e.g., antipyretics for fever, anxiolytics for acute anxiety)
  5. Supporting oral or IV replacement to restore normal fluid and electrolyte levels
  6. Monitoring patient responses to therapy
     a. Respiratory effort (rate, depth, and oxygen saturation)
     b. Cardiovascular stability (heart rate and rhythm, pulse quality, and blood pressure)
     c. Intake and output

    d. Serum electrolytes, SpO_2 and, if obtained, ABG values

    e. Hand grasps and deep tendon reflexes

ALLERGY, LATEX

- Latex allergy is a type I hypersensitivity reaction; the specific allergen is a protein found in processed natural latex rubber products. Patients may report an allergy or skin irritation to adhesive bandages and balloons.
- Allergic reactions to latex vary from contact dermatitis (mild) to anaphylaxis (severe).
- People at greatest risk for latex allergy are those with a high-level exposure to natural latex products, such as patients with spinal bifida or congenital urinary tract abnormalities and health care workers who use latex health care products (e.g., gloves, syringes, BP cuffs).
- Individuals with a latex allergy often have a history of other allergies, especially to specific foods (e.g., banana, kiwi, avocado, passion fruit, chestnuts).

⚠ NURSING SAFETY PRIORITY: Critical Rescue

It is essential to use latex-free products in the care of a patient with a known latex allergy.

- Teach patients who are sensitive to latex to avoid products containing latex.
- When caring for a patient with a known latex allergy, the health care provider should:
  1. Remove any latex-containing product from his or her person (e.g., erasers, tourniquets, blood tubes).
  2. Use paper tape or other low-irritation adhesive products.
  3. Check syringes, medication vials, and IV tubing for latex and use alternatives if latex is present.
  4. Wash hands with soap and water (not alcohol-based rub) before entering the room or touching the patient to remove latex residue on the skin from health care products.

AMPUTATION

OVERVIEW

- Amputation is the removal of a part of the body.
- The psychosocial aspects of the procedure are often more devastating than the physical impairments that result. The loss is

- complete and permanent and causes a change in body image and often in self-esteem.
- *Traumatic amputation* occurs when a body part is severed unexpectedly, most often resulting from accidents. Depending on the extent of damage, body parts that are severed may be reattached or reimplanted.

❗ NURSING SAFETY PRIORITY: Critical Rescue

For prehospital care with any traumatic amputation:
- Call 911.
- Assess the patient for airway or breathing problems.
- Apply direct pressure to amputation site with layers of dry gauze or other cloth.
- Elevate the extremity above the patient's heart to decrease the bleeding.

❗ NURSING SAFETY PRIORITY: Critical Rescue

For prehospital care for amputation:
- Wrap the completely severed digit or limb in a dry, sterile gauze or clean cloth.
- Put the digit or limb in a watertight, sealed plastic bag.
- Place the bag in ice water—never directly on ice. Use one part ice and three parts water.
- Prevent contact between the digit or limb and the water.
- Keep semidetached parts of the digit or limb in contact with the digit or limb.
- Be sure that the amputated part goes with the patient to the hospital.

- *Surgical amputations* are planned, elective procedures performed for a variety of disorders and complications.
- Regardless of the reason for the surgical amputation, every effort is made to preserve maximum possible patient function.
- Loss of any or all of the small toes presents a minor disability.
- Loss of the great toe is significant, because it affects balance, gait, and push-off ability during walking.
- Midfoot amputations (e.g., Lisfranc, Chopart, or Syme amputation) remove most of the foot but retain the intact ankle so that weight bearing can be accomplished without the use of prosthesis and with reduced pain.
- Other lower extremity amputations are below-knee amputation (BKA), above-knee amputation (AKA), hip disarticulation, or removal of the hip joint, and hemipelvectomy (removal of half of the pelvis with the leg).

- The higher the level of amputation, the more energy is required for ambulation.
- Upper extremity (UE) amputations are rare and usually are more incapacitating than those of lower extremities. Early replacement with a prosthetic device is vital for the patient with UE amputation.
- Complications of elective or traumatic amputation include:
  1. Hemorrhage
  2. Infection
  3. Phantom limb pain
  4. Neuroma
  5. Flexion contractures
  6. Psychological maladjustment

⊕ Cultural Awareness

The incidence of lower extremity amputations is greater in the African American, Hispanic, and American Indian populations, because the incidence of major diseases leading to amputation, such as diabetes and arteriosclerosis, is greater in this population. Limited access to health care for these minority groups may also play a major role in limb loss.

PATIENT-CENTERED COLLABORATIVE CARE
Assessment
- Assess:
  1. Neurovascular status of extremity to be amputated
     a. Examine skin color, temperature, sensation, capillary refill, and pulses.
     b. Compare findings with those of the unaffected extremity.
     c. Check and document the presence of discoloration, edema, ulcerations, hair distribution, and any necrosis.
  2. Psychosocial responses
     a. Preparation for a planned amputation
     b. Presence of bitterness, hostility, depression
     c. Expectations of how the loss of a body part may affect employment, social relationships, and recreational activities
     d. Current self-concept and self-image
     e. Willingness and motivation to withstand prolonged rehabilitation after the amputation
     f. How he or she has dealt with previous life crises
  3. Family reaction to the surgery or trauma
  4. Patient's and family's coping abilities
  5. Patient's religious, spiritual, and cultural beliefs

6. Diagnostic assessment may include:
   a. Segmental limb blood pressures
   b. Ankle-brachial index (ABI)
   c. Blood flow by Doppler ultrasonography or laser Doppler flowmetry or use of transcutaneous oxygen pressure ($tcPo_2$)

⚐ NATIONAL PATIENT SAFETY GOAL

With the patient, identify the limb or digit to be amputated pre-operatively, and mark it with indelible ink. Follow time-out rules before amputation, so that the correct patient and digit or limb is identified by at least two people.

Interventions

- Monitor for signs indicating that there is sufficient tissue perfusion but no hemorrhage:
  1. Skin flap at the end of the residual limb should be pink in a light-skinned person and not discolored.
  2. Area is warm, not hot.
  3. Assess the closest proximal pulse for strength and compare it with that in the other extremity.
- Pain management for residual limb pain (RLP) is like that for any patient in pain.
- Phantom limb pain (PLP) management
  1. Recognize that the pain is real, and manage it promptly and completely.

❗ NURSING SAFETY PRIORITY: Action Alert

It is not helpful to respond to the patient with PLP by telling him or her that the limb is no longer present and therefore cannot be causing pain.

2. Handle the residual limb carefully to prevent stimulating PLP.
3. Opioid analgesics are usually not the first choice for PLP but can be used.
4. Common drugs for PLP are:
   a. IV infusions of calcitonin (Miacalcin, Calcimar)
   b. Beta-blocking agents such as propranolol (Inderal, Apo-Propranolol, Detensol) for constant, dull, burning pain
   c. Antiepileptic drugs, such as carbamazepine (Tegretol) and gabapentin (Neurontin), for knifelike or sharp, burning pain
   d. Antispasmodics such as baclofen (Lioresal) for muscle spasms or cramping
5. Complementary and alternative therapies
   a. Transcutaneous electrical nerve stimulation (TENS)

     b. Ultrasound therapy

A

     c. Massage
     d. Heat
     e. Biofeedback
     f. Relaxation therapy
     g. Hypnosis
     h. Psychotherapy

- Prevent infection
  1. Drug therapy with broad-spectrum prophylactic antibiotics may be used before, during, and after surgery.
  2. The initial pressure dressing and drains are usually removed by the surgeon 48 to 72 hours after surgery.
  3. Inspect the wound site for signs of inflammation (e.g., redness, swelling) and monitor the healing process.
  4. Record the characteristics of drainage, if present.
  5. Change the soft dressing every day until the sutures or staples are removed.
  6. Dressings usually include an elastic bandage wrapped firmly around the residual limb after application of a sterile gauze dressing over the incision.

- Promote mobility
  1. Coordinate with the physical therapist to begin exercises as soon as possible after surgery.
  2. For patients with AKAs or BKAs, teach range-of-motion (ROM) exercises for prevention of flexion contractures, particularly of the hip and knee.
  3. Ensure that a trapeze and an overhead frame are used to aid in strengthening the upper extremities and allow the patient to move independently in bed.
  4. Provide a firm mattress for the patient with a lower extremity amputation.
  5. Assist the patient into a prone position every 3 to 4 hours for 20 to 30 minutes if tolerated and not contraindicated.
  6. Instruct the patient to pull the residual limb close to the other leg and contract the gluteal muscles of the buttocks.
  7. For patients with BKAs, teach how to push the residual limb down toward the bed while supporting it on a pillow.
  8. Follow health care provider and agency policy for elevation of a lower leg residual limb on a pillow while the patient is in a supine position.

- Prepare for prosthesis
  1. Coordinate with a certified prosthetist-orthotist (CPO) for appropriate postoperative planning.
  2. Instruct the patient being fitted for a leg prosthesis to bring a sturdy pair of shoes to the fitting.

3. After surgery, apply the prescribed device, such as the Jobst air splint, or elastic bandages to shape and shrink the residual limb in preparation for the prosthesis. If elastic bandages are used, reapply the bandages in a figure-eight wrap every 4 to 6 hours or more often if they become loose.
   a. Decrease the tightness of the bandages while wrapping in a distal-to-proximal direction.
   b. After wrapping, anchor the bandages to the most proximal joint, such as above the knee for BKAs.

- Promote positive body image and lifestyle adaptation
  1. If possible, arrange for the patient to meet with a rehabilitated amputee who is about the same age as him or her.
  2. Assess the patient to determine what term for the remaining limb (e.g., *stump*) seems less offensive.
  3. Assess the patient's verbal and nonverbal references to the affected area.
  4. Ask the patient to describe his or her feelings about changes in body image and self-esteem.
  5. Check whether the patient looks at the area during a dressing change.
  6. Document behavior that indicates acceptance or nonacceptance of the amputation.
  7. Teach the patient and family about available resources and support from organizations such as the Amputee Coalition of America (ACA) (www.amputee-coalition.org) and the National Amputation Foundation (NAF) (www.nationalamputation.org).
  8. Stress the patient's personal strengths.
  9. Collaborate with a social worker or vocational rehabilitation specialist to evaluate the skills of a patient who may need to change employment.
  10. Discuss sexuality issues with the patient and the patient's partner together as needed.
  11. If appropriate, refer the patient and family for professional assistance from a sex therapist, intimacy coach, or psychologist.
  12. Help the patient and family set realistic desired outcomes and take one day at a time.
  13. Teach the patient and family how to care for the limb and the prosthesis if it is available.
  14. Teach the patient or family to care for the limb after it has healed by cleaning it each day with the rest of the body during bathing with soap and water.
  15. Teach the patient and family to inspect the limb every day for signs of inflammation or skin breakdown.

AMYOTROPHIC LATERAL SCLEROSIS (ALS)

- Amyotrophic lateral sclerosis (ALS), also known as *Lou Gehrig's disease,* is a progressive degenerative disease involving the motor tract of the central nervous system.
- The disease is characterized by atrophy of muscles used with talking, dysphagia, weakness of the hands and arms, nasal quality to speech, fasciculations of the face, and dysarthria.
- As the disease progresses, flaccid quadriplegia develops. Increased risk for pneumonia and respiratory failure result from paralysis of breathing muscles, including the diaphragm.
- There is no known cure.
- Treatment is symptomatic and directed toward the following: preventing complications of immobility, promoting comfort, providing ongoing support and counseling to the patient and family, and informing the patient about the need for advance directives such as a living will and durable power of attorney.
- The drug riluzole (Rilutek) is associated with increased survival time.

ANAL FISSURE

- An anal fissure is a tear in the anal lining.
- Acute anal fissures are superficial and heal spontaneously with conservative treatment.
- Chronic fissures recur, and surgical treatment may be needed.
- Pain during and after defecation is the most common symptom, but bleeding may also occur.
- Other symptoms associated with chronic fissures are pruritus, urinary frequency or retention, dysuria, and dyspareunia.
- Nonsurgical interventions include local symptomatic relief measures such as warm sitz baths, analgesics, and bulk-forming agents or osmotic laxatives.
- Topical anti-inflammatories are helpful if spasms are severe.
- Surgical repair under local anesthesia may be necessary if the fissures do not respond to nonsurgical management.

ANAL FISTULA

- An anal fistula, or *fistula in ano,* is an abnormal tract leading from the anal canal to the perianal skin.
- Most anal fistulas result from anorectal abscesses, but they can be associated with tuberculosis, Crohn's disease, cancer, or AIDs.

- Symptoms include pruritus, purulent discharge, and tenderness or pain aggravated by bowel movements.
- Because fistulas do not heal spontaneously, surgery (fistulotomy) is necessary.
- Pain relief measures such as sitz baths, flushable wipes, analgesics, and stool softeners are used to reduce tissue trauma and discomfort.
- Hygiene is important; patients should be instructed to clean the anal area after each bowel movement.
- Patients should avoid constipation and straining with stool.

ANAPHYLAXIS

OVERVIEW
- Anaphylaxis is the most dramatic and life-threatening example of a type I hypersensitivity reaction.
- It occurs rapidly and systemically, affecting many organs within minutes of allergen exposure.
- Anaphylaxis episodes vary in severity and can be fatal, particularly when treatment with epinephrine is delayed.

PATIENT-CENTERED COLLABORATIVE CARE
Assessment
- Assessment findings include:
  1. Demonstration of three clinical findings establish a clear anaphylactic reaction:
     a. Skin or mucus problems along with respiratory distress or ineffectiveness OR hypotension/reduced organ perfusion leading to dysfunction
     b. Onset within minutes to hours after exposure to allergen of more than two of the following symptoms:
        (1) Skin or mucus membrane problems
        (2) Respiratory distress or ineffectiveness;
        (3) Hypotension
        (4) GI distress
     c. Onset within minutes to hours of systolic blood pressure less than 9 mm Hg or 30% lower than patient's baseline
  2. History of anaphylactic response and documentation of allergen
  3. Subjective feelings of uneasiness, apprehension, weakness, and impending doom
  4. Generalized itching and urticaria (hives)
  5. Erythema
  6. Angioedema (diffuse swelling) of the eyes, lips, or tongue

7. Bronchoconstriction, mucosal edema, and excess mucus production
8. Nasal congestion and rhinorrhea
9. Dyspnea, increasing respiratory distress, audible wheezing
10. Crackles, wheezing, and reduced breath sounds on auscultation
11. Laryngeal edema (hoarseness, and stridor)
12. Respiratory failure with hypoxemia
13. Rapid, weak, irregular pulse
14. Dysrhythmias
15. Diaphoresis
16. Increasing anxiety and confusion

❗NURSING SAFETY PRIORITY: Critical Rescue

If a patient is suspected of having an anaphylactic reaction, immediately call the Rapid Response Team, because most anaphylactic deaths are related to treatment delay. If symptoms are not recognized immediately, the patient may lose consciousness and be unable to call for help. Dysrhythmias, shock, and cardiac arrest may occur within minutes. Anticipate the need for immediate administration of epinephrine (1:1000), 0.3 to 0.5 mL IM, IV, interosseous, or via an endotracheal tube.

Interventions

- Emergency respiratory management
  1. Immediately assess the respiratory status, airway, and oxygen saturation of patients who show any symptoms of an anaphylactic reaction.
  2. If the airway is compromised in any way, call the Rapid Response Team or (anesthesia and respiratory therapy if Rapid Response Team is not available) before proceeding in any other intervention.
  3. Apply oxygen using a high-flow, non-rebreather mask at 40% to 60%.
  4. Ensure that intubation and tracheotomy equipment is ready.
- Drug therapy
  1. Immediately discontinue the IV drugs of a patient having an anaphylactic reaction to that drug.

❗NURSING SAFETY PRIORITY: Action Alert

Do not remove the IV catheter, but change the IV tubing, and hang normal saline.

2. If the patient does not have an IV access, start one immediately, and run normal saline.

3. Anticipate the following:
    a. Epinephrine, 1:1000 concentration: 0.3 to 0.5 mL IV push (immediately); repeat as needed every 10 to 15 minutes until the patient responds
    b. Diphenhydramine: 25 to 50 mg IV push (immediately)
    c. Theophylline: 6 mg/kg IV over 20 to 30 minutes for severe, persistent bronchospasm
    d. Once stabilized, inhaled beta-adrenergic agonist such as metaproterenol (Alupent) or albuterol (Proventil) by means of a high-flow nebulizer every 2 to 4 hours
    e. Corticosteroids (IV) are not effective immediately but given as the patient stabilizes to maintain airway, breathing, and circulation
4. Document all drugs administered and observe patient responses to drugs.

- Supportive care
    1. Position the patient to maintain airway, breathing, and circulation. Elevate the back rest to 45 degrees unless hypotension is present.
    2. Raise the feet and legs to improve blood return to the heart.
    3. Monitor pulse oximetry and/or ABGs to determine oxygenation adequacy.
    4. Use suction to remove excess oral or nasal mucous secretions.
    5. Continually assess the patient's respiratory rate and depth.
    6. Stay with the patient.
    7. Reassure the patient that the appropriate interventions are being instituted.
    8. Observe the patient for fluid overload from the rapid drug and IV fluid infusions.
    9. Before discharge, instruct the patient to obtain and wear a medical alert bracelet or ID about the specific allergy.
    10. Teach the patient who carries an automatic epinephrine injector (EpiPen) how to care for, assemble, and use the device. Obtain a return demonstration.

ANEMIA

OVERVIEW

- Anemia is a reduction in either the number of red blood cells (RBCs), the amount of hemoglobin, or the hematocrit (percentage of packed RBCs per deciliter of blood). *Note: A patient who is fluid overloaded may have reduced hematocrit and NOT be anemic. With correction of vascular fluid excess, the hematocrit returns to a normal value.*

- It is a clinical sign, not a specific disease, because it occurs with many health problems.
- Anemia can be caused by increased destruction of RBCs as occurs with sickle cell disease, glucose-6-phosphate-dehydrogenase (G6PD) deficiency, and autoimmune hemolytic disease such as Fanconi's anemia.
- *Sickle cell disease* is an inherited disorder that results in defective hemoglobin synthesis.
- *G6PD deficiency* is an X-linked recessive deficiency of an enzyme needed for RBC glucose metabolism.
- *Autoimmune hemolytic anemia* occurs when an individual's white blood cells (WBCs) fail to recognize his or her own RBCs as self cells.
- Anemia can also be caused by decreased production of RBCs as occurs with iron, vitamin B_{12}, and folic acid deficiencies, or by aplastic anemia from bone marrow injury.
- *Iron deficiency anemia* is related to iron-deficient diets, chronic alcoholism, malabsorption syndromes, and partial gastrectomy. It can also occur during periods of rapid metabolism such as during adolescence or pregnancy or with severe infections and injury.
- *B_{12} deficiency anemia* can occur with dietary insufficiency and with failure to absorb vitamin B_{12} as a result of reduced intrinsic factor produced by the stomach. Anemia caused by failure to absorb vitamin B_{12} is called *pernicious anemia.*
- *Folic acid deficiency anemia* can occur as a result of dietary deficiency and in the presence of certain drugs, including oral contraceptives, antiepileptic drugs, and the immunomodulator drug, methotrexate, used to modulate the immune system and treat cancers..
- *Aplastic anemia* can occur with exposure to agents that damage the bone marrow such as radiation, insecticides, antineoplastic drugs, and some antibiotics.
- Anemia can also be caused by blood loss as with gastrointestinal bleeding or after surgery or trauma.

Assessment
- Assessment findings include:
  1. Weakness
  2. Pallor
  3. Shortness of breath from reduced oxygen-carrying capacity
  4. Petechiae or ecchymosis
  5. Chest pain related to reduced oxygen-carrying capacity in the presence of cardiac disease
  6. The complete blood count (CBC) shows reduced RBCs, hemoglobin, and hematocrit.
  7. Bone marrow biopsy may show abnormalities within this hematologic cell-forming organ.

Interventions
- Management includes:
  1. Blood transfusions when the anemia causes disability, including chest pain at rest or mild activity
  2. Immunosuppressive therapy with drugs such as prednisone and antineoplastic or immunomodulation drugs if the case is increased destruction of RBCs
  3. Splenectomy (removal of the spleen) when an enlarged spleen is destroying normal RBCs or suppressing their development.
  4. Hematopoietic stem cell transplantation (bone marrow transplantation) to replace defective bone marrow with aplastic anemia (although cost, availability, and complications limit this treatment of aplastic anemia)
  5. Implementation of dietary therapy
     a. For vitamin B_{12} deficiency, teach the patient to eat foods high in vitamin B_{12}, such as animal proteins, eggs, and dairy products. Provide vitamin B_{12} supplements.
        (1) For pernicious anemia, administer vitamin B_{12} parenterally on a regular basis (usually monthly for life). After pernicious anemia has been found to respond to parenteral vitamin B_{12}, the patient may start cyanocobalamin (CaloMist), which delivers vitamin B_{12} by nasal spray to maintain vitamin levels.
     b. For folic acid deficiency, provide scheduled folic acid replacement therapy.
     c. For iron deficiency, provide a scheduled iron supplement and instruct the patient to increase his or her oral intake of iron from common food sources, such as liver and other organ meats, red meat, kidney beans, whole wheat breads and cereals, green leafy vegetables, carrots, egg yolks, and raisins and other dried fruit.
  6. Teach the patient that iron preparations often change the color of stool to black and can promote constipation that can be treated with diet, stool softeners, osmotic laxatives, or bulk-forming agents.
  7. Provide transfusion therapy when ordered, using packed RBCs to maintain safe levels of oxygen-carrying hemoglobin.

◼ NURSING SAFETY PRIORITY: Critical Rescue

Be sure to follow institutional policy and national guidelines when implementing transfusion therapy. Use two patient identifiers and two providers to identify the patient and ensure a match between the prescribed therapy and the patient's blood type. Be familiar with common and severe transfusion reactions. Monitor the patient closely during the first 15 minutes of transfusion therapy to detect adverse reactions.

AORTIC ANEURYSM

OVERVIEW

- An aneurysm is a permanent, localized dilation of an artery accompanied by weakening of the vessel wall.
- An aneurysm forms when the media, or the middle layer of the artery, is weakened, producing a stretching effect in the intima (the inner layer) and adventitia (the outer layer of the artery).
- The effect of elevated blood pressure on the artery wall enlarges the aneurysm.
- The most common cause is atherosclerosis, or atheromatous plaque that weakens the intimal surface.
- Hypertension, hyperlipidemia, and cigarette smoking are contributing factors.
- Other causes are syphilis (a sexually transmitted disease), Marfan syndrome (a connective tissue disease), and Ehlers-Danlos syndrome (a rare genetic disorder). Chronic inflammation (aortitis) and blunt trauma, usually from motor vehicle crashes, can cause aneurysms in the descending thoracic aorta.
- Aneurysms can be classified as:
  1. Saccular, an outpouching from a distinct portion of the artery wall
  2. Fusiform, a diffuse dilation involving the total circumference of the artery
- Aneurysms can also be described as "true," meaning the arterial wall is weakened by congenital or acquired problems. False aneurysms occur as a result of vessel injury or trauma to all three layers of the arterial wall.
- Dissecting aneurysms, such as aortic dissections, differ from aneurysms in that they are formed when blood accumulates in the wall of an artery.
- Abdominal aneurysms are located between the renal arteries and the iliac bifurcation.
- Thoracic aneurysms develop between the origin of the left subclavian artery and the diaphragm.
- Aneurysms can thrombose, embolize, or rupture (rupture is the most common and life-threatening complication).

PATIENT-CENTERED COLLABORATIVE CARE

Assessment

- Most patients with abdominal or thoracic aneurysm are asymptomatic.
- Assess for clinical manifestations of abdominal aortic aneurysms:
  1. Abdominal, flank, or back pain that is usually steady, with a gnawing quality, is unaffected by movement, and may last for hours or days

   2. Prominent pulsation in the upper abdomen (do not palpate)
   3. Abdominal or femoral bruit
- Assess for clinical manifestations of thoracic aneurysms:
   1. Back pain
   2. Shortness of breath
   3. Hoarseness
   4. Difficulty swallowing
   5. Visible mass above the suprasternal notch (occasional)
- Assess for abdominal or thoracic aortic rupture:
   1. Pain that is described as tearing, ripping, and stabbing
   2. Pain that is located in the chest, back, and abdomen
   3. Symptoms of hypovolemic shock: hypotension, tachycardia, diaphoresis, and decreased mentation
   4. Nausea, vomiting
   5. Faintness, apprehension
   6. Decreased or absent peripheral pulses
- Also assess for:
   1. Presence of a distorted aortic profile on thoracic or abdominal x-ray or computed tomography (CT) scan
   2. Altered aortic profile by ultrasonography

Planning and Implementation

Nonsurgical Management

- Antihypertensive drugs are prescribed to maintain normal blood pressure and to decrease stress on an abdominal aneurysm that is smaller than 2 or 3 inches (6 cm) or when surgery is not feasible.
- Teach the patient the importance of keeping scheduled CT scan appointments to monitor size of the aneurysm for possible surgery.
- Review with the patient the clinical manifestations of aneurysms that need to be promptly reported and to avoid lifting or activity that increases abdominal pressure.
- The aneurysm may be manages with endovascular stent placement (see the following section).

Surgical Management

- Endovascular stent placement via an intra-aortic catheter avoids the need for an abdominal incision and can be done in the interventional radiology suite or operating room.
- Monitor the patient closely in the hospital and at home for the development of complications, such as bleeding, aneurysm rupture, peripheral embolization, and misdeployment of the stent graft. All of these complications require surgical intervention.
- Surgical removal of the aneurysm is reserved for symptomatic lesions or aneurysms larger than 3 inches (6 cm). The excised

portion of the aorta is replaced with a graft. Ruptures always require emergency surgery to replace the damaged aorta.

- Provide preoperative care:
  1. Maintain mean arterial pressure within prescribed ranges to promote tissue perfusion and avoid hypertension.
  2. Assess all peripheral pulses to serve as a baseline for comparison after surgery; mark where the pulse is heard.

☑NATIONAL PATIENT SAFETY GOAL

Before any procedure, use a time-out process to conduct a final verification of the procedure, patient, and site using active communication techniques and a checklist.

- Provide routine postoperative care:
  1. Care of the patient with an abdominal aneurysm repair is similar to that provided for patients undergoing other abdominal surgeries.
- In addition to routine postoperative care:
  1. Assess vital signs every hour to detect early signs of hypotension from graft leak.
  2. Assess circulation by checking pulses distal to the graft site when checking vital signs.
  3. Report signs of leak or occlusion immediately to the physician, such as pulse changes, severe pain, cool to cold extremities below the graft, white or blue extremities or flanks, abdominal distention, and decreased urinary output.
- Abdominal aortic aneurysm repair requires assessment of renal function and lower extremity movement and sensation, because the aorta is clamped during the repair, potentially compromising the blood flow to the kidneys and spinal cord.
- Additional postoperative care specific to abdominal aortic repair includes:
  1. Managing pain as for postoperative care by administering opioid analgesics for pain
  2. Avoiding nausea, vomiting, or other occasions of increased intra-abdominal pressure
  3. Monitoring electrocardiogram (ECG), ST segment, and patient symptoms for acute myocardial infarction; coagulopathy after vascular procedures increases the risk for acute coronary syndromes, including myocardial infarct
  4. Monitoring for less common complications such as respiratory distress and paralytic ileus
- Care of the patient undergoing thoracic aneurysm repair is similar to that for other thoracic surgeries. Additional postoperative care includes:

1. Reporting signs of hemorrhage obstruction immediately; assessing for bleeding and separation at the graft site by monitoring chest tube drainage for excess drainage such as more than 100 mL for 2 hours
2. Monitoring for cardiac dysrhythmias, paraplegia, acute kidney injury, and respiratory distress
3. Instructing the patient with thoracic aneurysm repair to report back pain, shortness of breath, difficulty swallowing, and/or hoarseness

■ NURSING SAFETY PRIORITY: Critical Rescue

Report signs of hemorrhage or graft occlusion to the physician immediately.

Community-Based Care

- Emphasize the importance of compliance with the schedule of CT scanning to monitor the size of the aneurysm in patients who have not had surgery.
- Emphasize the importance of controlling blood pressure.
- Educate the patient and family.
  1. Teach the patient to restrict activities (if surgery was performed), including:
     a. Avoiding lifting heavy objects for 6 to 12 weeks postoperatively
     b. Using discretion in activities that involve pulling, pushing, or straining, such as vacuuming, changing bed linens, moving furniture, mopping or sweeping, raking leaves, mowing grass, and chopping wood
     c. Avoiding hobbies such as tennis, swimming, golf, and horseback riding
     d. Deferring driving a car for several weeks
  2. Provide written and oral wound care instructions, if needed.
  3. Provide pain management instruction.
- Refer to home health nursing and other community agencies as needed.

APPENDICITIS

OVERVIEW

- Appendicitis is an acute inflammation of the vermiform appendix, the small finger-like pouch attached to the cecum of the colon.
- Inflammation of the appendix can occur when the lumen of the appendix is obstructed.

- Inflammation leads to infection as bacteria invade the wall of the appendix.
- Appendicitis is the most common cause of acute inflammation in the right lower abdominal quadrant.
- Appendicitis may occur at any age, but the peak incidence is between 20 and 30 years of age.

Considerations for Older Adults

- Appendicitis is not common in older adults, but when it occurs, perforation is a common complication.
- The diagnosis of appendicitis is difficult to establish for the older adult, because symptoms of pain and tenderness are not as pronounced as they are in younger persons.

PATIENT-CENTERED COLLABORATIVE CARE
Assessment
- Assessment findings include:
  1. Abdominal pain originating in the epigastric or periumbilical area and shifting to the right lower quadrant (McBurney's point); pain may not be localized
  2. Nausea and vomiting
  3. Anorexia after the initial diagnosis of pain
  4. Urge to defecate or pass flatus
  5. Muscle rigidity and rebound tenderness
  6. Normal or slightly elevated temperature
  7. Increased white blood cell (WBC) count with possible increased segmented neutrophils
- Abdominal pain that increases with cough or movement and is relieved by flexion of the right hip or knees suggests a perforated appendix with peritonitis.

Planning and Implementation
- Provide routine preoperative care; withhold oral fluids 2 to 4 hours preoperatively to surgical appendectomy (removal of the appendix).
- Keep the patient in a semi-Fowler's position so that abdominal drainage, if any, can be contained in the lower abdomen.
- Appendectomy may be performed as a traditional procedure through a small incision or, if not ruptured, by means of laparoscopy.
- Routine postoperative care for a traditional appendectomy includes:
  1. Assessing the abdominal drains for excess drainage; drains are placed only if an abscess is present
  2. Maintaining the patient's nasogastric tube or other drainage devices if inserted intraoperatively for peritonitis

3. Administering IV antibiotics
4. Assisting the patient out of bed on the evening of surgery
5. Typical postoperative pain management, including administering opioid analgesia
- Care after a laparoscopic procedure includes:
  1. Monitoring puncture sites for bleeding, foul or unusual drainage, or signs of infection
  2. Providing routine postoperative care, anticipating discharge within 24 hours of surgery

◼ NURSING SAFETY PRIORITY: Critical Rescue

A change in pain from localized to generalized abdominal pain may indicate that the appendix has ruptured. Immediately inform the surgeon of this finding, along with the patient's vital signs.

ARTERIOSCLEROSIS AND ATHEROSCLEROSIS

OVERVIEW

- Arteriosclerosis is a thickening or hardening of the arterial wall of the vascular system.
- Atherosclerosis, a type of arteriosclerosis, involves the formation of a plaque within the arterial wall and is the leading contributor to coronary artery disease (CAD) and cerebrovascular disease, which can lead to a stroke.
- The exact pathophysiologic mechanism of atherosclerosis is unknown but is thought to occur with inflammation of the vessel.
- Atherosclerosis begins as a fatty streak on the intimal surface of an artery and develops into a fibrous plaque that partially or completely occludes the blood flow of the artery.
- Plaques are either stable or unstable.
- When plaque ruptures, thrombosis and constriction obstruct the vessel lumen, causing inadequate perfusion and oxygenation to distal tissues. Unstable plaque rupture causes more severe injury.
- After the rupture occurs, the exposed underlying tissue causes platelet adhesion and rapid thrombus formation. The thrombus may suddenly block a blood vessel, resulting in ischemia and infarction (e.g., myocardial infarction).
- The rate of progression of plaque formation and rupture is thought to be influenced by genetic factors, certain diseases (e.g., diabetes mellitus), and certain lifestyle habits (e.g., smoking, eating habits, level of exercise).

PATIENT-CENTERED COLLABORATIVE CARE
Assessment

- Assess:
  1. Risk for cardiovascular disease, using history and standard tools
  2. Blood pressure in both arms and note any differences
  3. Pulses at all major sites and note any differences
  4. Presence of prolonged capillary refill
  5. Presence of temperature differences in lower extremities
  6. Presence of arterial bruits at carotid, abdominal, and femoral pulses
  7. Serum cholesterol (total, low-density lipoprotein [LDL], protective high-density lipoprotein [HDL]), and triglyceride levels.

Interventions

- Interventions include:
  1. Teaching the patient to adopt dietary habits (e.g., NCEP Therapeutic Lifestyle Changes diet for high-risk individuals) to reduce risk, including limiting dietary fat to fewer than 30% of total calories per day.
  2. Developing and reinforcing the plan for regular activity with at least 150 minutes weekly as a goal.
  3. Administering cholesterol-lowering drugs as prescribed for the patient
  4. Using evidence to assist patients to stop smoking (cigarette smoking lowers levels of HDL cholesterol) and informing nonsmokers to avoid secondhand smoke
     a. Offering patients who smoke behavior therapy, support group opportunities, a nicotine substitute, bupropion (Wellbutrin), or varenicline (Chantrix) to aid in smoking cessation.
     b. Offering complementary and alternative therapies to stop smoking, including acupuncture, hypnosis, and biofeedback
  5. Planning for follow-up and ongoing care with primary care provider at least annually

ARTHRITIS, RHEUMATOID

OVERVIEW

- Rheumatoid arthritis (RA) is a chronic, progressive, systemic inflammatory autoimmune disease process that damages and destroys synovial joints.
- Transformed autoantibodies (rheumatoid factors [RFs]) attack healthy tissue, especially synovium, causing inflammation.

- Onset may be acute and severe or slow and insidious, and the pattern of illness progression includes remissions and exacerbations.
- Permanent joint changes may be avoided or mitigated when RA is diagnosed early. Early aggressive treatment to suppress synovitis may lead to a remission.
- *Systemic* means that inflammatory factors related to this disease affect more than the joints. Affected body systems include cardiovascular (e.g., vasculitis, myocarditis, pericarditis), lung (e.g., pleurisy, pneumonitis), eyes, and skin. Inflammatory factors also contribute to anorexia, weight loss, and nutritional derangements.
- Genetic factors combine with environmental conditions and interact to trigger RA.
- Female reproductive hormones may influence the development of RA, because the disease affects more women than men.

PATIENT-CENTERED COLLABORATIVE CARE
Assessment
- Assess for early disease manifestations, including:
  1. Joint stiffness, swelling, pain (especially of the upper extremities); usually bilateral (affecting both sides) and symmetric (same joints) symptoms
  2. Fatigue, generalized weakness
  3. Anorexia, weight loss
  4. Persistent, low-grade fever
  5. Joint infection (one hot, swollen joint that has pain out of proportion to the other joints)

■ NURSING SAFETY PRIORITY: Critical Rescue
Refer the patient to the health care provider (usually the rheumatologist) immediately if manifestations of joint infection are present.

- Assess for late disease manifestations.
  1. Joints become progressively inflamed, puffy, and quite painful.
  2. Morning stiffness lasts longer than 45 minutes.
  3. Affected joints have a soft or a spongy feeling.
  4. Muscles atrophy above and below affected joints.
  5. Range of motion (ROM) decreases and can cause pain (e.g., carpal tunnel syndrome).
  6. Most or all of the synovial joints are eventually affected.
  7. Joint deformity may develop.

A

8. There may be Baker's cysts (enlarged popliteal bursae behind the knee).
9. There may be bone fractures.
10. Tendon rupture (especially the Achilles tendon) may occur.
11. Cervical vertebrae disease may result in subluxation that may be life threatening.

! NURSING SAFETY PRIORITY: Critical Rescue

Cervical pain with loss of ROM should be reported to the physician.

- Assess for systemic complications:
    1. Exacerbations, often called *flares*, manifested by increased joint swelling and tenderness
    2. Infection in affected joints and skin
    3. Moderate to severe weight loss
    4. Fever
    5. Extreme fatigue
    6. Subcutaneous nodules along muscles or tendons, which may become open and infected or interfere with activities of daily living (ADLs)
    7. Inflammation of blood vessels, resulting in vasculitis, particularly of small to medium-sized vessels
    8. Ischemic skin and nail lesions that appear in small groups as small, brownish spots
    9. Larger skin lesions, which appear on the lower extremities and may lead to ulceration, and which heal slowly as a result of vascular changes leading to poor peripheral circulation
    10. Peripheral neuropathy, causing footdrop and paresthesias
    11. Respiratory complications, including pleurisy, pneumonitis, diffuse interstitial fibrosis, and pulmonary hypertension
    12. Cardiac complications, including pericarditis and myocarditis
    13. Ocular involvement, such as iritis or scleritis
    14. Sjögren's syndrome (eye, mouth, and vaginal dryness)
    15. Felty's syndrome (enlarged liver and spleen, leukopenia)
    16. Caplan's syndrome (presence of rheumatoid nodules in the lungs and pneumoconiosis), which is found mainly in coal miners and asbestos workers
- Assess for psychosocial issues:
    1. Fear of becoming disabled and dependent, uncertainty about the disease process, altered body image, devaluation of self, frustration, and depression are common.

   2. Physical limitations may result in role changes in the family and society.
   3. Extreme fatigue often causes patients to desire an early bedtime and may result in a reluctance to socialize.
   4. Body changes may also cause poor self-esteem and body image.
   5. The patient may grieve, experience degrees of depression, or have feelings of helplessness caused by a loss of control over a disease that can "consume" the body.
   6. Evaluate the patient's support systems and resources.
- Assess laboratory data (none are specific for RA, but all are associated with it):
   1. Positive RF
   2. Positive antinuclear antibody test (ANA)
   3. Positive anti-Sjögren's syndrome antibodies, especially anti-SS-A (Ro)
   4. Decreased serum complement
   5. Elevated erythrocyte sedimentation rate
   6. Elevated high-sensitivity C-reactive protein (hsCRP) level
   7. Altered complete blood count (CBC) and platelet count (low hematocrit and hemoglobin levels, high white blood cell count)
- Other diagnostic assessments
   1. Joint x-rays
   2. Bone scan or joint scan
   3. Magnetic resonance imaging (MRI)
   4. Arthrocentesis, a procedure to aspirate a sample of the synovial fluid to relieve pressure and analyze the fluid for inflammatory cells and immune complexes, including RF

Interventions
- Drug therapy used to treat RA includes:
   1. Disease-modifying antirheumatic drugs (DMARDs) are used to slow the progression of mild rheumatoid disease before it progresses. They include:
      a. Methotrexate (Rheumatrex)
      b. Leflunomide (Arava)
      c. Hydroxychloroquine (Plaquenil)
      d. Sulfasalazine (Azulfidine)
   2. NSAIDs are often the drug of choice to relieve pain and inflammation on a short-term basis.
   3. Biological response modifiers (BRMs) interfere with the action of different inflammatory mediators.
      a. Etanercept (Enbrel)
      b. Infliximab (Remicade)

    c. Adalimumab (Humira)
    d. Anakinra (Kineret)
    e. Abatacept (Orencia)
    f. Rituximab (Rituxan)
    g. Tocilizumab (Actemra)
4. Steroidal anti-inflammatory drugs
    a. Prednisone (Deltasone, Medrol)
5. Other immunosuppressive drugs
    a. Azathioprine (Imuran)
    b. Cyclophosphamide (Cytoxan)
6. Analgesic drugs
    a. Acetaminophen (Tylenol, Exdol, Datril)

- Nonpharmacologic management:
  1. Other pain-relief measures: rest, positioning, ice, and heat
  2. Plasmapheresis (or plasma exchange) to remove the antibodies causing the disease
  3. Pain relief methods such as hypnosis, acupuncture, magnet therapy, imagery, or music therapy
  4. Stress management
  5. Nutrition to meet caloric and protein goals
  6. Nutritional supplementation including omega-3 fatty acid and antioxidant vitamins A, C, and E
- Promotion of self-care:
  1. Identify assistive devices to allow the patient as much independence as possible.
  2. Help the patients acquire household items with handles.
  3. Teach the patient to use larger muscle groups to perform tasks usually performed by fine muscle groups (e.g., use the flat of the hand to squeeze toothpaste tubes instead of the fingers).
  4. Refer the patient to an occupational or physical therapist or the Arthritis Foundation for special assistive and adaptive devices.
- Management of fatigue:
  1. Identify factors that contribute to fatigue (e.g., anemia, muscle atrophy, inadequate rest).
  2. Collaborate with the health care team to alleviate or manage contributing factors.
     a. Anemia
        (1) Administer iron, folic acid, vitamin supplements, or a combination of these.
        (2) Assess the patient for drug-related GI bleeding, such as that caused by NSAID therapy, by testing the stool for occult blood.

  b. Muscle atrophy
    (1) Collaborate with a physical therapist to develop and help the patient implement a personalized daily exercise program.
  c. Inadequate rest
    (1) Arrange for a quiet environment.
    (2) Encourage the patient to develop a bedtime routine for sleep hygiene, such as drinking a warm beverage before bedtime.
3. Teach principles of energy conservation.
  a. Pacing activities
  b. Setting priorities
  c. Planning rest periods
  d. Obtaining assistance when possible; delegating activities to the family
- Enhancement of body image:
  1. Identify factors to enhance body image.
  2. Determine the patient's perception of changes and the impact of the reactions of family and significant others.
  3. Communicate acceptance of the patient by establishing a trusting relationship.
  4. Encourage the patient to wear street clothes and his or her own nightclothes or bathrobe.
  5. Assist with grooming, such as shaving and makeup.

■ NURSING SAFETY PRIORITY: Action Alert

The patient may use strategies that range from denial or fear to anger and depression. Avoid labeling the patient as manipulative and demanding, because these behaviors may represent how he or she is trying to cope with the effects of the illness.

- Community-based care considerations for discharge include:
  1. Assisting the patient and family to identify structural changes needed in the home before discharge
  2. Reinforcing information about drug therapy
  3. Teaching the patient to consult with the health care provider before trying any over-the-counter or home remedies
  4. Teaching joint protection measures
  5. Teaching the patient to ask for help to prevent further joint damage and disease progression
  6. Reviewing energy conservation measures
  7. Reviewing the prescribed exercise program
  8. Referring the patient to local and national support groups such as the Arthritis Foundation

9. Referring the patient to the nutritionist, counselor, home health nurse, rehabilitation therapist, financial counselor, and local and state support groups as needed
10. Teaching the patient to check with the Arthritis Foundation for the latest information on arthritis myths and quackery

ASTHMA

OVERVIEW

- Bronchial asthma is an intermittent and reversible airflow obstruction affecting only the airways, not the alveoli.
- Airway obstruction occurs in two ways:
  1. Inflammation, obstructing the lumen (the inside) of airways, occurs in response to the presence of specific allergens; general irritants such as cold air, dry air, or fine airborne particles; microorganisms; and aspirin.
  2. Airway hyperresponsiveness, obstructing airways by constricting bronchial smooth muscle and causing a narrowing of the airway from the outside, can occur with exercise, an upper respiratory illness, and for unknown reasons.
- Many people with asthma have both problems at the same time.
- Severe airway obstruction can be fatal.
- Although asthma may be classified into different types based on the events known to trigger the attacks, the pathophysiology is similar for all types of asthma regardless of the triggering event.
- Asthma can occur at any age. About half of adults with asthma also had the disease in childhood. Asthma is more common in urban settings than in rural settings.

Considerations for Older Adults

Asthma occurs as a new disorder in about 3% of people older than 55 years. Another 3% of people older than 60 years have asthma as a continuing chronic disorder. Lung and airway changes as a part of aging make any breathing problem more serious in the older adult. One problem related to aging is a change in the sensitivity of beta-adrenergic receptors. When stimulated, these receptors relax smooth muscle and cause bronchodilation. As these receptors become less sensitive, they no longer respond as quickly or as strongly to agonists (e.g., epinephrine, dopamine) and beta-adrenergic drugs, which are often used as rescue therapy during an acute asthma attack. Teaching older patients how to avoid asthma attacks and to use preventive drug therapy correctly are nursing priorities.

Women's Health Considerations

The incidence of asthma is about 35% higher among women than men, and the asthma death rates are also higher among women. Obesity and hormonal fluctuations around the menstrual cycle are thought to contribute to the difference in incidence, and undertreatment of the disease is thought to be a factor in the higher death rate. Teaching women how to be a partner in asthma management and the correct use of preventive and rescue drugs remains a nursing priority in improving the outcomes of the disease.

PATIENT-CENTERED COLLABORATIVE CARE
Assessment

- Obtain the patient's personal history.
  1. Episodes of dyspnea, chest tightness, coughing, wheezing, and increased mucus production
  2. Specific patterns of dyspnea appearance (at night, with exercise, seasonally, or in association with other specific activities or environments)
  3. Other allergic symptoms such as rhinitis, skin rash, or pruritus, and whether other family members have asthma or respiratory problems
- Clinical manifestations during an attack include:
  1. Audible wheeze (at first, louder on exhalation)
  2. Increased respiratory rate
  3. Breathing cycle that is longer and requires more effort
  4. Coughing
  5. Inability to complete a sentence of more than five words
  6. Decreased oxygen saturation
  7. Pallor or cyanosis of oral mucous membranes and nail beds
  8. Tachycardia
  9. Changes in level of consciousness
  10. Use of accessory muscles (muscle retraction at the sternum, the suprasternal notch, and between the ribs)
- Physical changes from frequent asthma attacks include:
  1. Increased anteroposterior (AP) chest diameter
  2. Increased space between the ribs
- Laboratory assessment data changes during an asthma attack:
  1. Decreased Pao_2
  2. Decreased $Paco_2$ (early in attack)
  3. Elevated $Paco_2$ (later in attack)
- Laboratory assessment data changes from allergic asthma:
  1. Elevated serum eosinophil count
  2. Elevated immunoglobulin E (IgE) levels
  3. Sputum-containing eosinophils, mucus plugs, and shed epithelial cells (Curschmann's spirals)

- Diagnostic assessment:
  1. Pulmonary function tests (PFTs) measured using spirometry, especially:
     a. Forced vital capacity (FVC) (volume of air exhaled from full inhalation to full exhalation)
     b. Forced expiratory volume in the first second (FEV_1) (volume of air blown out as hard and fast as possible during the first second of the most forceful exhalation after the greatest full inhalation)
     c. Peak expiratory flow (PEF) (fastest airflow rate reached at any time during exhalation)
  2. Chest x-rays
  3. Blood levels of therapeutic drugs (theophylline)

Interventions

- The goals of asthma therapy are to improve airflow, relieve symptoms, and prevent episodes by making the patient an active partner in the management plan.
- Priority patient education focuses on:
  1. Teaching the patient to assess symptom severity at least twice daily with a peak flowmeter and adjust drugs to manage inflammation and bronchospasms to prevent or relieve symptoms
  2. Assisting the patient to establish a "personal best" peak expiratory flow (PEF) by measuring his or her PEF twice daily for 2 to 3 weeks when asthma is well controlled and using this value to compare against all other readings
  3. Instructing the patient to evaluate when to use a rescue inhaler (when PEF is between 50% and 80% of personal best) and when to seek emergency assistance (when PEF is below 50% of personal best)

⚠ NURSING SAFETY PRIORITY: Critical Rescue

Teach the patient who has a reading in the "red zone" in their flowmeter to use the rescue drugs immediately and seek emergency help.

  4. Teaching the patient to keep a symptom and intervention diary to learn his or her triggers of asthma symptoms, early cues for impending attacks, and personal response to drugs
  5. Stressing the importance of proper use of the asthma action plan for any severity of asthma
- Drug therapy focuses on prevention of asthma attacks (preventive therapy) and stopping attacks that have already started (rescue therapy).

- Many preventive and rescue drugs are delivered as dry powder inhalers (DPIs) or as aerosol metered dose inhalers (MDIs). Teach patients the proper ways to use and store these inhalers.
- Preventive therapy drugs are those used to change airway responsiveness to prevent asthma attacks from occurring. They are used every day, regardless of symptoms.

■ NURSING SAFETY PRIORITY: Critical Rescue

Teach patients using preventive therapy to take the prescribed drugs daily, even when asthma symptoms are not present.

1. Bronchodilators increase bronchiolar smooth muscle relaxation and include beta$_2$ agonists, cholinergic antagonists, and methylxanthines.
   a. Long-acting beta$_2$ agonists (LABAs) are delivered by inhaler directly to the site of action, the bronchioles. They need time to build up an effect, but the effects are longer lasting. The use of LABAs is recommended to be co-administered with inhaled steroids.

■ NURSING SAFETY PRIORITY: Drug Alert

These drugs are useful in preventing an asthma attack but have no value during an acute attack. Teach patients *not* to use LABAs to rescue them during an attack or when wheezing is getting worse.

   b. Cholinergic antagonists (anticholinergic drugs) are similar to atropine and block the parasympathetic nervous system, causing bronchodilation and decreased pulmonary secretions. Most are used by inhaler:
      (1) Ipratropium (Atrovent)
      (2) Tiotropium (Spiriva)
   c. Methylxanthines are used when other types of management are ineffective:
      (1) Theophylline (Theo-Dur)
      (2) Aminophylline (Truphylline)
      (3) Oxtriphylline (Choledyl)
      (4) Dyphylline (Dilor, Lufyllin)

■ NURSING SAFETY PRIORITY: Critical Rescue

Teach the patient who takes these drugs daily to keep all appointments for monitoring blood levels of the drug and not to self-increase the dose. These drugs have narrow safety ranges and have many dangerous side effects, especially cardiac and central nervous system stimulation.

2. Anti-inflammatory drugs decrease the inflammatory responses in the airways. Some are given systemically and have more side effects. Others are used as inhalants and have few systemic side effects.
   a. Inhaled corticosteroids (ICSs):
      (1) Fluticasone (Flovent)
      (2) Budesonide (Pulmicort)
      (3) Mometasone (Asmanex)
   b. Nonsteroidal anti-inflammatory drugs (NSAIDs):
      (1) Nedocromil (Tilade)
      (2) Cromolyn sodium (Intal)
   c. Leukotriene antagonists:
      (1) Montelukast (Singulair)
      (2) Zafirlukast (Accolate)
      (3) Zileuton (Zyflo)
   d. Immunomodulators:
      (1) Omalizumab (Xolair)

- Rescue therapy drugs are those used to actually stop an attack once it has started. Short-acting beta$_2$ agonists (SABAs) provide rapid but short-term relief. These inhaled drugs are most useful when an attack begins (rescue drug) or as premedication when the patient is about to begin an activity that is likely to induce an asthma attack.
  1. Albuterol (Proventil, Ventolin)
  2. Bitolterol (Tornalate)
  3. Levalbuterol (Xopenex)
  4. Pirbuterol (Maxair)
  5. Terbutaline (Brethaire)

█ NURSING SAFETY PRIORITY: Critical Rescue

Teach the patient to always carry the rescue drug inhaler with him or her and to ensure that there is enough drug remaining in the inhaler to provide a quick dose when needed.

- Regular exercise, including aerobic exercise, is a recommended part of asthma therapy.
  1. Teach patients to examine the conditions that trigger an attack and adjust the exercise routine as needed.
  2. Some patients may need to premedicate with inhaled SABAs before beginning activity.

- Supplemental oxygen with a high flow rate or high concentration is often used during an acute asthma attack. Oxygen is delivered by mask, nasal cannula, or endotracheal tube.
- Heliox, a mixture of helium and oxygen (often 50% helium and 50% oxygen) can help improve oxygen delivery to the alveoli.
- *Status asthmaticus* is a severe, life-threatening acute episode of airway obstruction that intensifies once it begins and often does not respond to usual therapy.
  1. Assess for manifestations, including:
     a. Extremely labored breathing and wheezing
     b. Use of accessory muscles
     c. Distention of neck veins are observed
     d. PEF below 50% of expected for patient's age, size, and gender
     e. Oxygen saturation less than 80%
  2. Apply oxygen.
  3. Immediate drug therapy includes:
     a. IV fluids
     b. Potent systemic bronchodilators
     c. IV steroids
     d. Parenteral epinephrine
  4. Prepare for emergency intubation.
  5. If the condition is not reversed, the patient may develop pneumothorax and cardiac or respiratory arrest.

BEDBUGS

- A common emerging parasite is the bedbug, *Cimex lectularius.* Increased infestation is attributed to travel and resistance to pesticides.
- Bedbugs do not carry disease but feed on human blood. The bite usually causes an itchy discomfort, and when a person is bitten extensively, anemia may result.
- The adult bedbug is the approximate size, shape, and color of an apple seed.
- Eradicating the infestation and preventing re-infestations require considerable effort, including the use of multiple powerful pesticides and extreme temperature.

BLINDNESS

See *Visual Impairment (Reduced Vision).*

BONE MARROW TRANSPLANTATION (HEMATOPOIETIC STEM CELL TRANSPLANTATION)

B

OVERVIEW

- Hematopoietic stem cell transplantation (HSCT) is the process of collecting stem cells from one person (the donor) and transplanting them into another person (the recipient) or into the same person at a later time.
- *Stem cells* are immature and undifferentiated cells that can mature into any blood cell type.
- Sources of stem cells include the bone marrow, circulating peripheral blood, and cord blood from newborns.
- When stem cells are obtained from the bone marrow, the process is called *bone marrow transplantation (BMT)*.
- When stem cells are transplanted into a recipient, the new cells go to the marrow and then begin the process of hematopoiesis, which results in normal, properly functioning white blood cells (WBCs), red blood cells (RBCs), and platelets.
- Disorders that can be cured by HSCT include acute leukemia, lymphoma, multiple myeloma, aplastic anemia, sickle cell disease, and many solid tumors.
- After successful HSCT, the recipient has the blood type and the immune function of the donor.
- The three types of transplantation are:
  1. *Allogeneic transplantation*, in which the stem cells are taken from a sibling or human leukocyte antigen (HLA)-matched, unrelated donor
  2. *Autologous transplantation*, in which the donor receives his or her own stem cells (collected before any cytotoxic treatment)
  3. *Syngeneic transplantation*, in which the stem cells are taken from the patient's own identical sibling

🌐 Cultural Awareness

About 70% of people on the bone marrow donor lists are white. The chance of finding an HLA-matched, unrelated donor is estimated at 30% to 40% for whites, but for African Americans the chance is less than 20%, because there are fewer African Americans among registered donors. Although blood types are common in all racial groups, tissue types can be very different among racial and ethnic groups. Nationally, efforts are made to publicize the need for donors from all cultural and ethnic backgrounds. Research in this area has identified several potential barriers to stem cell donation among African

Americans. These include fear of or not trusting the system, concern about costs to the donor, and concern that the recipient may be a drug abuser or a person who would not appreciate the sacrifice of a donation. Targeted education efforts may reduce these barriers.

- The five phases of HSCT are:
  1. *Stem cell obtainment,* which involves taking stem cells either from the patient directly (autologous stem cells) or from an HLA-matched person (allogeneic stem cells)
  2. *Conditioning regimen,* which involves either "wiping out" the patient's own bone marrow, thus preparing the patient for optimal graft take, or giving higher than normal doses of chemotherapy or radiotherapy to rid the person of cancer cells (myeloablation). Usually 5 to 10 days is required.
  3. *Transplantation,* which is the actual infusion of the stem cells through the patient's central catheter, like an ordinary blood transfusion
  4. *Engraftment,* which is the process of the transplanted cells moving into the recipient's bone marrow and beginning to make new, functioning blood cells
  5. *Post-transplantation recovery,* which is the time between when engraftment begins and full recovery of immune function, RBC function, and platelet function occur

PATIENT-CENTERED COLLABORATIVE CARE
- In addition to the recipient of an HSCT, allogeneic stem cell transplantation using bone marrow cells and plasma pheresis harvesting involves the donor as a patient.
- Patient care for the donor:
  1. Bone marrow harvest is a surgical procedure performed under general anesthesia.
  2. About 500 to 1000 mL of bone marrow is aspirated through multiple sites from the donor's iliac crests.
     a. After the procedure, monitor the donor for:
        (1) Pain
        (2) Fluid loss
        (3) Bleeding from harvest sites
     b. Teach the donor about:
        (1) Inspecting the harvest sites for bleeding
        (2) Taking prescribed analgesics for pain
  3. Peripheral blood stem cells (PBSCs) are stem cells that have been released from the bone marrow and circulate within the blood.

4. PBSC harvesting requires three phases: mobilization, collection by pheresis, and infusion or reinfusion.
   a. The *mobilization* phase involves giving the donor hematopoietic growth factors for several days before pheresis to increase the numbers of stem cells in the peripheral blood.
   b. *Pheresis* is the collection of stem cells by withdrawing whole blood, filtering out the cells, and returning the plasma to the patient. Between one and five pheresis procedures, each lasting 2 to 4 hours, are needed to obtain enough stem cells for transplantation.
   c. *Infusion* is the placement of collected stem cells into the recipient by infusion through a central venous catheter.
5. During pheresis, monitor the patient for:
   a. Hypotension
   b. Catheter clotting
   c. Hypocalcemia
      (1) Numbness or tingling in the fingers and toes or around the mouth
      (2) Abdominal or muscle cramping
      (3) Chest pain
- Patient care for the recipient:
  1. Conditioning:
     a. The day the patient receives the stem cells is day T-0. Before transplantation, the conditioning days are counted in reverse order from T-0, just like a rocket countdown. After transplantation, days are counted in order from the day of transplantation.
     b. The conditioning regimen is individually tailored to each patient and usually includes high-dose chemotherapy and sometimes includes total-body irradiation (TBI).
     c. A typical conditioning regimen is:
        (1) Days T-5 through T-4: high-dose chemotherapy to obliterate the patient's own bone marrow cells or to kill off any remaining cancer cells (if part of cancer treatment)
        (2) Days T-3 through T-1: delivery of TBI. The total radiation dose for TBI is 1200 rad given as 200 rad twice daily over 3 days.
     d. Immediate side effects from conditioning are intense or severe and include:
        (1) Nausea and vomiting
        (2) Mucositis
        (3) Capillary leak syndrome
        (4) Diarrhea

(5) Bone marrow suppression
    (i) Neutropenia
    (ii) Anemia
    (iii) Thrombocytopenia

∎NURSING SAFETY PRIORITY: Critical Rescue

During conditioning and before engraftment, the patient has no immune function and is at great risk for life-threatening infection. Infection protection is the priority for management at this time.

e. Late effects from the conditioning regimen are also common 3 to 10 years after transplantation. These problems include veno-occlusive disease (VOD), skin toxicities, cataracts, lung fibrosis, second cancers, cardiomyopathy, endocrine complications, and neurologic complications.
2. Transplantation:
    a. Frozen marrow, PBSCs, or umbilical cord blood cells are thawed and then infused.

∎NURSING SAFETY PRIORITY: Action Alert

Do not use blood administration tubing, because the cells can get caught in the filter and not enter the patient's body.

b. Side effects of all types of stem cell transfusions are similar and may include:
    (1) Fever
    (2) Hypertension
    (3) Fluid overload
    (4) Red urine (resulting from RBC breakage in the infused stem cells)
3. Engraftment:
    a. The successful acceptance of the transplanted cells in the patient's bone marrow is key to the whole transplantation process.
    b. Engraftment takes 8 to 12 days for PBSC transplantation and 12 to 28 days for bone marrow stem cell transplantation.
    c. To aid engraftment, growth factors, such as granulocyte colony-stimulating factor (G-CSF) or granulocyte-macrophage colony-stimulating factor (GM-CSF), may be given. When engraftment occurs, the patient's WBC, RBC, and platelet counts begin to rise.

 d. Nursing care focuses on prevention of complications, which include:
   (1) Infection
   (2) Bleeding
   (3) Failure to engraft (*If the transplanted cells fail to engraft, the patient will die unless another transplantation is successful.*)
   (4) Development of graft-versus-host disease (GVHD), in which the immunocompetent cells of the donated marrow recognize the patient's (recipient) cells, tissues, and organs as foreign and start an immunologic attack against them. GVHD occurs most often in the skin, intestinal tract, and liver, and more than 15% of the patients who develop GVHD die of its complications. Manifestations are:
     (i) Excessive peeling of the skin
     (ii) Profuse, watery diarrhea
     (iii) Liver tenderness, with jaundice
   (5) Development of veno-occlusive disease (VOD), which is the blockage of liver blood vessels by clotting and inflammation (phlebitis). Manifestations include:
     (i) Jaundice
     (ii) Pain in the right upper quadrant
     (iii) Ascites
     (iv) Weight gain
     (v) Liver enlargement
   (6) Depression (contributing factors include prolonged hospitalization, limited activity, intense therapy side effects, and uncertain treatment outcome)

BREAST CONDITION, FIBROCYSTIC

OVERVIEW

- The two main features of fibrocystic breast condition (FBC) are fibrosis and cysts. Areas of fibrosis are made up of fibrous connective tissue and are firm or hard. Cysts are spaces filled with fluid lined by breast glandular cells.
- This condition most often occurs in premenopausal women between 20 and 50 years of age.
- FBC is thought to be caused by an imbalance in the normal estrogen-to-progesterone ratio.
- Typical symptoms include breast pain and tender lumps or areas of thickening in the breasts. The lumps are rubbery, ill defined, and commonly found in the upper outer quadrant of the breast.

PATIENT-CENTERED COLLABORATIVE CARE
Interventions
- Management of FBC focuses on the symptoms of the condition:
  1. Supportive measures such as the use of mild analgesics or limiting salt intake before menses can help decrease swelling.
  2. Wearing a supportive bra can reduce pain by decreasing tension on the ligaments, although some women find that not wearing a bra is more comfortable.
  3. Local application of ice or heat may provide temporary relief of pain.
  4. If drug therapy is indicated, oral contraceptives may be prescribed to suppress oversecretion of estrogen, and progestins may be used to correct luteal insufficiency.

■ NURSING SAFETY PRIORITY: Drug Alert
Explain to women the benefits and risks associated with drug therapy for FBC, such as stroke, liver disease, and increased intracranial pressure. Teach them to seek medical attention immediately if any signs of symptoms of these complications occur.

  5. Vitamins C, E, and B complex may reduce cyst formation.
  6. Diuretics may be prescribed to decrease premenstrual breast engorgement.
  7. Reduction of dietary fat and caffeine has been suggested, although role of caffeine and fat in FBC is unclear.
  8. Teach patients to follow guidelines for self-breast examination, obtain breast examinations by a health care provider regularly, and undergo mammographic or magnetic resonance imaging (MRI) diagnostic testing.

BURNS

OVERVIEW
- A burn is an injury to the skin and other epithelial tissues as a result of exposure to temperature extremes, mechanical abrasion, chemical abrasion, radiation, and electrical currents.
- Local and systemic problems resulting from burns include fluid and protein losses, sepsis, and changes in metabolic, endocrine, respiratory, cardiac, hematologic, and immune functioning.
- Prevention of infection and closure of the burn wound are vitally important, because a lack of or delay in wound healing is a key factor for all systemic problems and a major cause of disability and death among patients who are burned.

- Burns are classified by their wound depth and severity:
    1. *Superficial-thickness wounds* have the least damage, because the epidermis is the only part of the skin that is injured. The epithelial cells and basement membrane, needed for total regrowth, remain. Common causes of superficial-thickness wounds are prolonged exposure to low-intensity heat (e.g., sunburn) or short (flash) exposure to high-intensity heat. Redness with mild edema, pain, and increased sensitivity to heat occur as a result. The area heals rapidly in 3 to 5 days without a scar or other complication.
    2. *Partial-thickness wounds* involve the entire epidermis and various depths of the dermis. Depending on the amount of dermal tissue damaged, partial-thickness wounds are further subdivided into superficial partial-thickness and deep partial-thickness injuries.
        a. *Superficial partial-thickness wounds* are caused by heat injury to the upper third of the dermis, leaving a good blood supply. Wounds are red, moist, and blanch (whiten) when pressure is applied. Blisters often form. Nerve endings are exposed, and any stimulation (touch or temperature change) causes intense pain. With care these burns heal in 10 to 21 days with no permanent scar, but some minor pigment changes may occur.
        b. *Deep partial-thickness wounds* extend deeper into the skin dermis, and fewer healthy cells remain. Blister formation does not usually occur. The wound surface is red and dry, with white areas in deeper parts. Edema is moderate, and the degree of pain is less than experienced with superficial burns, because more nerve endings have been destroyed.
    3. *Full-thickness wounds* occur with destruction of the entire epidermis and dermis, leaving no true skin cells to repopulate. The wounded tissue does not regrow, and whatever area of the wound not closed by wound contraction will require grafting. The wound has a hard, dry, leathery eschar that must slough off or be removed from the burn wound before healing can occur. The wound may be waxy white, deep red, yellow, brown, or black. Sensation is reduced or absent in these areas because of nerve ending destruction. Edema is severe under the eschar in a full-thickness wound.
        a. When the injury is circumferential (completely surrounds an extremity or the chest), blood flow and chest movement for breathing may be reduced by tight eschar.

  b. *Escharotomies* (incisions through the eschar) or *fascio-tomies* (incisions through eschar and fascia) may be needed to relieve pressure and allow normal blood flow and breathing.

 4. *Deep full-thickness wounds* extend beyond the skin into underlying fascia and tissues. Muscle, bone, and tendons are damaged and exposed. The wound is blackened and depressed, and sensation is completely absent.

- Common causes of burn injury and emergency interventions to limit injury
  1. *Dry heat injuries* result from open flames. The patient should stop, drop, and roll to smother the flames.
  2. *Moist heat (scald) injuries* are caused by contact with hot liquids or steam. Clothes that are saturated with hot liquids should be removed immediately.
  3. *Contact burns* occur when hot metal, tar, or grease contact the skin, often leading to a full-thickness injury. Removal of the hot substance limits the injury.
  4. *Chemical burns* occur as a result of accidents in the home or workplace. The severity of the injury depends on the duration of contact, the concentration of the chemical, the amount of tissue exposed, and the action of the chemical. Dry chemicals should be brushed off the skin and clothing. Wet clothing is removed. Depending on the specific agent, the skin may be flushed with water or covered with mineral oil.
  5. *Electrical injury burns* occur when an electrical current enters the body. These injuries have been called the "grand masquerader" of burn injuries, because the surface injuries may look small but the associated internal injuries can be huge. The longer the electricity is in contact with the body, the greater the damage. The patient should be removed from the source of the electricity in such a way that the care provider does not place himself or herself in danger (use a wooden pole, rather than a metal one, to separate the person from the electrical source). *The person must not be touched directly while he or she is in contact with the electrical source!*
  6. *Radiation injuries* occur when people are exposed to large doses of radioactive material. The most common type of tissue injury from radiation exposure occurs with therapeutic radiation. More serious injury occurs in industrial settings where radioactive energy is produced or radioactive isotopes are used. Removal of the patient from the source of radiation limits the injury.

- Compensatory responses to the stress of the injury and the direct tissue damage occur through the sympathetic nervous system and inflammatory responses. These result in specific and predictable changes in tissue and organ function:
  1. Inflammation
  2. Vital sign changes (decreased BP, tachycardia, increased respiratory rate and depth)
  3. Capillary leak with a *fluid shift* into the interstitial space. This fluid shift, also known as *third spacing* or *capillary leak syndrome*, is a continuous leak of plasma from the vascular space into the interstitial space. The loss of plasma fluids and proteins decreases blood volume and blood pressure. Leakage of fluid and electrolytes from the vascular space continues, causing extensive edema, even in areas that were not burned. Fluid shift with excessive weight gain usually occurs in the first 12 hours after the burn and can continue for 24 to 36 hours. Fluid returns to the vascular space within 48 to 72 hours.
  4. Decreased urine output
  5. Hemoconcentration (elevated hematocrit and hemoglobin values)
  6. Fluid and electrolyte imbalances (most commonly metabolic acidosis), hyperkalemia (high blood potassium levels), and hyponatremia (low blood sodium levels)
  7. Decreased to absent peristalsis, formation of Curling's ulcer
  8. Elevated blood glucose levels
  9. Hypermetabolism and body temperature variation
- Burn recovery occurs over the course of three phases. Each phase has unique manifestations and care requirements.

RESUSCITATION PHASE

- The resuscitation, or *emergent,* phase is the first phase of a burn injury. It begins at the onset of injury and continues to about 48 hours.
- The goals of management during the resuscitation/emergent phase are to:
  1. Secure the airway.
  2. Support circulation by fluid replacement.
  3. Keep the patient comfortable with analgesics.
  4. Prevent infection through careful wound care.
  5. Maintain body temperature.
  6. Provide emotional support.

PATIENT-CENTERED COLLABORATIVE CARE
Assessment

- During assessment, obtain the following injury-related information:
    1. Time of the injury
    2. Source of heat or injurious agent
    3. Detailed description of how and where the burn occurred
    4. Any interventions or other actions taken
    5. Whether drugs or alcohol may have been a factor
    6. Events occurring from the time of the burn to admission
    7. Any other events that could increase the burn injury or cause another injury or health problem
- Obtain the following personal patient information:
    1. Age
    2. Height and weight
    3. Medical history (especially cardiac or kidney disease, chronic alcoholism, substance abuse, diabetes mellitus)
    4. Use of prescribed, over-the-counter (OTC), or street drugs within the past 24 hours
    5. Smoking history
    6. Level of pain
    7. Allergies
    8. Immunization status (especially tetanus)
- Assess for:
    1. Direct airway injury:
        a. Changes in the appearance or function of the mouth, nose, or throat
        b. Facial burns; singed hair on the head, eyebrows, eyelids, or nose
        c. Blisters or soot on the lips, on oral mucosa, or in sputum
        d. "Smoky" smell of the breath
        e. Progressive hoarseness, wheezing, crowing, stridor
        f. Decreased oxygen saturation
        g. Drooling (inability to swallow oral secretions)

⚠ NURSING SAFETY PRIORITY: Critical Rescue

For a burn patient in the resuscitation phase who is hoarse, has a brassy cough, drools, has difficulty swallowing, or produces an audible breath sound on exhalation, immediately apply oxygen and notify the Rapid Response Team.

    2. Carbon monoxide poisoning:
        a. Headache
        b. Decreased cognitive functioning, confusion, coma

    c. Tinnitus

    d. Nausea

    e. Absence of cyanosis or pallor (lips and mucous membranes may appear bright red)

    f. Elevated carboxyhemoglobin levels

  3. Smoke poisoning/inhalation:

    a. Atelectasis, pulmonary edema

    b. Hemorrhagic bronchitis (6 to 72 hours after injury)

  4. Pulmonary fluid overload

    a. Dyspnea

    b. Hypoxia

    c. Moist breath sounds and crackles

  5. Cardiovascular changes:

    a. Hypovolemic and cardiogenic shock

    b. Circulatory overload with left-sided congestive heart failure

    c. Rapid, thready pulse

    d. Reduced peripheral pulses

    e. Slow or absent capillary refill

    f. Generalized edema

    g. Weight gain

    h. Baseline and continuous electrocardiographic tracings

  6. Renal or urinary changes:

    a. Decreased urine output (less than 0.5 to 1 mL/kg/hr)

    b. High urine specific gravity

    c. Proteinuria

    d. Absence of urine output

  7. Skin changes:

    a. Depth of injury

    b. Size of injury by the total body surface area (TBSA)

    c. Color and appearance

  8. Gastrointestinal changes:

    a. Decreased or absent bowel sounds

    b. Nausea, vomiting

    c. Abdominal distention

    d. Ulcer formation

    e. Gross or occult blood in vomitus or stool

- Laboratory assessment:
  1. Increased WBCs, especially the neutrophil percentage, followed by a rapid drop with a left shift
  2. Electrolytes
  3. Liver enzyme studies
  4. Clotting studies

⊕ Cultural Awarenesss

For African-American patients, a sickle cell preparation may be appropriate if sickle status is unknown. The trauma of a burn injury can trigger a sickle cell crisis in patients who have the disease and in those who carry the trait.

Planning and Implementation

- The priority problems for the patient with burn injuries in the resuscitation phase who have sustained a burn injury greater than 25% of the TBSA are:
  1. Potential for inadequate oxygenation related to upper airway edema, pulmonary edema, airway obstruction, or pneumonia
  2. Hypovolemic shock related to increase in capillary permeability, active fluid volume loss, electrolyte imbalance, and inadequate fluid
  3. Potential for organ ischemia (e.g., brain, heart, kidney, gastrointestinal) related to hypovolemia and hypotension
  4. Pain (acute and chronic) related to tissue injury, damaged or exposed nerve endings, débridement, dressing changes, invasive procedures, and donor sites
  5. Potential for acute respiratory distress syndrome (ARDS) related to inhalation injury.

INADEQUATE OXYGENATION
  Nonsurgical Management
- Interventions include airway maintenance, promotion of ventilation, monitoring gas exchange, oxygen therapy, drug therapy, positioning, and deep breathing.
  Surgical Management
- A tracheotomy may be needed when long-term intubation is expected. This procedure increases the risk for infection in burn patients even more than in nonburned patients. Emergency tracheotomies are performed when an airway becomes occluded and oral or nasal intubation cannot be achieved.

HYPOVOLEMIC SHOCK
Interventions are aimed at increasing blood fluid volume, supporting compensatory mechanisms, and preventing complications. Nonsurgical management is often sufficient for achieving these aims. Surgical management is required most often for full-thickness burns.

  Nonsurgical Management
- Fluid volume and tissue blood flow are restored through IV fluid therapy (rapid IV therapy is called *fluid resuscitation* and is guided by a well-established formula based on the size and depth of burn injury) and drug therapy. Priority nursing interventions

are carrying out fluid resuscitation and monitoring for indications of effectiveness or complications.

■ NURSING SAFETY PRIORITY: Action Alert

Avoid diuretic therapy (except in electrical injuries), because these drugs do not increase cardiac output; they instead decrease circulating volume and cardiac output by pulling fluid from the circulating blood volume to enhance diuresis. This effect reduces blood flow to other vital organs (especially the heart, lungs, and brain) and greatly increases the risk for severe shock.

Considerations for Older Adults

In older patients, especially those with cardiac disease, a complicating factor in fluid resuscitation may be heart failure or myocardial infarction. Drugs that increase cardiac output, such as dopamine (Intropin), or that strengthen the force of myocardial contraction, such as digoxin (Lanoxin), may be used along with fluid therapy.

Surgical Management

- An escharotomy may be needed when tight eschar impairs tissue perfusion.
- A fasciotomy (a deeper incision extending through the fascia) may be needed to relieve constriction from fluid buildup when a burn completely surrounds an extremity.

PAIN MANAGEMENT

Pain management is tailored to the patient's tolerance for pain, coping mechanisms, and physical status. The priority nursing actions include continually assessing the patient's pain level, using appropriate pain-reducing strategies, and preventing complications.

Nonsurgical Management

- Interventions for the patient having pain include drug therapy, complementary therapy measures, and environmental manipulation.
- Assess the patient's pain level hourly until pain is well controlled, then every 2 to 4 hours.
- Administer drug therapy with opioid and non-opioid analgesics (e.g., morphine, hydromorphone [Dilaudid], fentanyl). For the alert patients, consider using patient-controlled analgesia.

■ NURSING SAFETY PRIORITY: Critical Rescue

During the emergent postburn phase, the IV route is used for giving opioid drugs because of problems with absorption from the muscle and stomach. When these agents are given by the intramuscular or subcutaneous route, they remain in the tissue spaces and do not relieve pain. When edema is present, all the doses are rapidly absorbed at once when the fluid shift is resolving. This delayed absorption can result in lethal blood levels of analgesics.

- Provide a quiet environment to promote rest and sleep.
- Coordinate with all members of the health care team to ensure that most procedures are performed during the patient's waking hours.
- Use alternative and complementary pain management techniques, including relaxation techniques, meditative breathing, guided imagery, music therapy, massage, and healing or therapeutic touch.
  Surgical Management
- Surgical management for pain involves early surgical excision of the burn wound.
- There is potential for ARDS.
- Assess hourly for fluid overload (e.g., presence of lung crackles, distended neck veins, decreased cognition, decreased oxygen saturation, low urine output).
- Coordinate respiratory therapy and ventilation support to maintain airway.
- When the patient is receiving ventilatory support (noninvasive or invasive ventilation), interventions are aimed at increasing lung compliance and improving Pao_2 levels.
  1. Give prescribed positive end-expiratory pressure (PEEP) therapy to provide a continuous positive pressure in the airways and alveoli and enhance the diffusion of oxygen across the alveolar-capillary membrane. PEEP can be combined with intermittent mandatory volume.
  2. Assess and document the patient's response:
     a. Monitor oxygen saturation continuously; communicate decrements greater than 5% or values less than 92% immediately to prescribing health care provider and anticipate oxygen supplementation interventions.
     b. Evaluate arterial blood gas levels for low oxygenation (Pao_2 less than 90 mm Hg) or hypercarbia ($Paco_2$ greater than 46 mm Hg).

■ NURSING SAFETY PRIORITY: Critical Rescue

Immediately report any signs of respiratory distress or change in respiratory patterns to the health care team and the respiratory therapist.

  3. Administer prescribed neuromuscular blocking drugs to patients receiving mechanical ventilation to reduce oxygen consumption.

ACUTE PHASE

- The acute phase of burn injury begins about 36 to 48 hours after injury and lasts until wound closure is complete.
- A multidisciplinary approach to care will continue to be needed.
- Care focuses on continued assessment and maintenance of the cardiovascular and respiratory systems, as well as toward GI and nutritional status, burn wound care, pain control, and psychosocial interventions.
- Complications of this phase include pneumonia, malnutrition, loss of musculoskeletal function, infection, and sepsis.

PATIENT-CENTERED COLLABORATIVE CARE
Assessment
- Assess for:
  1. Cardiopulmonary dysfunction:
     a. Pneumonia
     b. Respiratory failure
  2. Metabolic dysfunction:
     a. Hypothermia
     b. Weight loss, negative nitrogen balance, malnutrition
  3. Immune system dysfunction:
     a. Local infection
     b. Systemic infection and sepsis
  4. Musculoskeletal dysfunction:
     a. Muscle atrophy
     b. Contracture formation
     c. Decreased range of motion (ROM)
  5. Wound healing impairment
  6. Body image changes
  7. Grieving
  8. Anxiety and fear

Planning and Implementation
- Priority nursing problems for patients with burn injuries greater than 25% TBSA in the acute phase of recovery are:
  1. Wound care management related to burn injury, skin grafting procedures, and immobilization
  2. Potential for infection related to open burn wounds, the presence of multiple invasive catheters, reduced immune function, and malnutrition
  3. Excessive weight loss related to increased metabolic rate, reduced calorie intake, and increased urinary nitrogen losses
  4. Reduced mobility related to open burn wounds, pain, and scars and contractures

5. Altered self-image related to trauma, changes in physical appearance and lifestyle, and alterations in sensory and motor function

WOUND CARE MANAGEMENT
Nonsurgical Management

- Assess all burn wounds at least daily for:
  1. Adequacy of circulation
  2. Size and depth of injury
  3. Presence of infection
  4. Effectiveness of therapy
- Participate in wound débridement procedures to remove debris and nonliving tissue from the burn wound.
  1. *Mechanical débridement* can be performed one or two times daily with hydrotherapy. The patient can be immersed in a tub, showered on a specially designed shower table, or have only small areas of the wound washed at the bedside. Nurses and skilled technicians use forceps and scissors to remove loose, nonviable tissue during hydrotherapy. Burn areas are washed thoroughly and gently with mild soap or detergent and water.
  2. *Enzymatic débridement* can occur naturally by autolysis or, more commonly, artificially by the application of exogenous agents. Topical agent are applied directly to the burn wound in once-daily dressing changes. The enzymes digest collagen in necrotic tissues.
  3. Dress the burn wound using standard wound dressings, biologic dressings, synthetic dressings, or artificial skin.
     a. *Standard wound dressings* involve cleansing the wound, applying a topical antimicrobial agent, and then applying multiple layers of gauze over the topical agents. The number of gauze layers depends on the depth of the injury, amount of drainage expected, area injured, patient's mobility, and frequency of dressing changes. The gauze layers are held in place with roller-type gauze bandages applied in a distal to proximal direction or with circular net fabrics. Dressings are reapplied every 8 to 24 hours.
     b. *Biologic dressings* are skin or membranes obtained from human tissue donors or animals. When applied over open wounds, a biologic dressing rapidly adheres and promotes healing or prepares the wound for permanent skin graft coverage. Types of biologic dressings include:
        (1) *Homografts (allografts)* are human skin obtained from a cadaver and provided through a skin bank.

(2) *Heterografts (xenografts)* are skin obtained from another species. Pig skin is the most common heterograft and is compatible with human skin.

(3) *Amniotic membrane* is another form of biologic dressing used on burn wounds. Its large size, low cost, and availability have helped with its success.

(4) *Cultured skin* can be grown from a small specimen of epidermal cells from an unburned area of the patient's body. Cells are grown in a laboratory to produce cell sheets that can be grafted on the patient to generate a permanent skin surface.

(5) *Artificial skin* is an alternative approach to closure of the burn wound. This substance has two layers: a Silastic epidermis and a porous dermis made from beef collagen and shark cartilage.

c. *Biosynthetic wound dressings* are a combination of biosynthetic and synthetic materials. Biobrane is the most common type and is made up of a nylon fabric that is partially embedded into a silicone film. Collagen is incorporated into both the silicone and nylon components. The nylon fabric comes into contact with the wound surface and forms an adherent bond until epithelialization has occurred. The porous silicone film allows exudates to pass through.

d. *Synthetic dressings* are made of solid silicone and plastic membranes (e.g., polyvinyl chloride, polyurethane). They are applied directly to the surface of a clean or surgically prepared wound and remain in place until they fall off or are removed. Many are transparent or translucent, allowing the wound to be inspected without removing the dressing.

Surgical Management

- Surgical management of burn wounds focuses on excision and wound covering. Surgical excision is performed early in the postburn period. Grafting may be performed throughout the acute phase as burn wounds are made ready and donor sites are available. Early grafting reduces the time patients are at risk for infection and sepsis. Wound covering by autografting involves taking healthy skin from an area of the patient's intact skin and transplanting it to an excised burn wound.

INFECTION

- Burn wound infection occurs through *autocontamination,* in which the patient's own normal flora overgrows and invades other body areas, and *cross-contamination,* in which organisms from other people or environments are transferred to the patient.

Nonsurgical Management
- Drug therapy for infection prevention:
  1. Tetanus toxoid, an IM vaccine, is routinely given when the patient is admitted to the hospital. Additional administration of tetanus immune globulin (human) (Hyper-Tet) is recommended when the patient's history of tetanus immunization is not known.
  2. Topical antimicrobial drugs are used at every dressing change or wound cleansing to prevent infection in burn wounds. The goal of this therapy is to reduce bacterial growth into the wound and prevent systemic sepsis. The most commonly used agents are silver sulfadiazine (Silvadene, Flamazine ✦) and mafenide (Sulfamylon).
- Drug therapy for treatment of infection:
  1. Systemic broad-spectrum antibiotics are used when burn patients have symptoms of an infection, including septicemia. After results of blood cultures and sensitivity status are available, specific drugs may be changed to those that are effective against the specific organisms causing the infection.
- Providing a safe environment:
  1. Use aseptic technique with all wound interventions.
  2. Ensure appropriate use of asepsis by all health care team members.
     a. Wear gloves during all contact with open wounds.
     b. Do not share equipment among patients.
     c. Use disposable items as much as possible.
     d. Ensure daily cleaning of patient's room and bathroom.
  3. Do not keep plants or flowers in patient's room; they are a source of microbes.
  4. Restrict visitors to healthy adults.
  5. Consider isolation therapy (less common).
- Monitoring for early recognition of infection by assessing the burn wounds at each dressing change for:
  1. Pervasive odor
  2. Color changes: focal, dark red, brown discoloration in the eschar
  3. Change in texture
  4. Purulent drainage
  5. Exudate
  6. Sloughing grafts
  7. Redness at the wound edges extending to nonburned skin

Surgical Management
- Infected burn wounds with colony counts of or approaching 10^5 colonies per gram of tissue are life threatening and may require surgical excision to control these infections.

EXCESSIVE WEIGHT LOSS

- Coordinate with a nutritionist to calculate the patient's current daily caloric needs and meet his or her desired nutrition status outcomes.
- Nutritional requirements for a patient with a large burn area can exceed 5000 kcal/day and include a diet high in protein for wound healing.
- Nasoduodenal tube feedings are often started within 4 hours of beginning fluid resuscitation to prevent nutritional deficits.
- Encourage patients who can eat solid foods to ingest as many calories as possible.
- Take the patient's preferences into consideration for diet planning and food selection.
- Encourage patients to request food whenever they feel they can eat, not just according to the hospital's standard meal schedule.
- Offer frequent high-calorie, high-protein supplemental feedings.
- Keep an accurate calorie count for foods and beverages that are ingested by the patient.

REDUCED MOBILITY

Nonsurgical Management

- Positioning:
  1. Maintain the patient in a neutral body position with minimal flexion.
  2. Use splints and other devices on the joints of the hands, elbows, knees, neck, and axillae to prevent contractures.
- ROM exercises:
  1. Work with the patient to perform these actively at least three times daily.
  2. Perform passive ROM exercises for patients who are unable to actively perform them.
  3. For burned hands, urge the patient to perform active ROM exercises for the hand, thumb, and fingers every hour while awake.
- Ambulation:
  1. Start ambulation as soon as possible after the fluid shifts have resolved.
  2. Assist patients to ambulate at least twice daily.
  3. Increase ambulation length each time.
- Pressure dressings:
  1. Apply pressure dressings after grafts heal to help prevent contractures and tight hypertrophic scars.
  2. Urge the patient to wear pressure dressings at least 23 hours every day until the scar tissue is mature (12 to 24 months).

Surgical Management
- Surgical management restores mobility rather than prevents immobility. Surgical release of contractures is most commonly performed in the neck, axilla, elbow flexion areas, and hand. Specific surgical procedures to improve movement vary for each patient.

ALTERED SELF-IMAGE
Nonsurgical Management
- Assess which stage of grief the patient is experiencing and help interpret his or her behavior.
- Reassure the patient that feelings of grief, loss, anxiety, anger, fear, and guilt are normal.
- Coordinate with other health care team members (e.g., psychologist, psychiatrist, social worker, clergy or religious leader) in addressing these problems.
- Accept the physical and psychological features of the patient.
- Present patients and families with realistic expected outcomes regarding the patient's functional capacity and physical appearance.
- Plan and encourage the patient's active participation in self-care activities.
- Urge families to include the patient in family decision making to the same degree that he or she participated in this process before the injury.
- Provide information sessions and counseling for the family to help identify effective patterns of support.
- Facilitate the patient's use of these systems and the development of new support systems.
- Make referrals to support groups.

Surgical Management
- Reconstructive and cosmetic surgery can restore function and improve the patient's appearance, often increasing his or her feelings of self-worth and promoting a positive body image. Teach the patient and family about expected cosmetic outcomes.

TECHNICAL REHABILITATIVE PHASE

- The technical rehabilitative phase begins with wound closure and ends when the patient returns to the highest possible level of functioning.
- The emphasis during this phase is the psychosocial adjustment of the patient, the prevention of scars and contractures, and the resumption of preburn activity, including resuming work, family, and social roles.

- This phase may take years or even last a lifetime as patients adjust to permanent limitations that may not be apparent until long after the initial injury.

PATIENT-CENTERED COLLABORATIVE CARE
Assessment
- Explore the patient's feelings about the burn injury.
- Ask the patient or a family member whether there is a history of psychological problems.
- Assess and document the type of coping mechanisms the patient has used successfully during times of stress to assist with a future plan of care.
- Assess the patient's family unit and the family members' history of interaction.
- Identify cultural and ethnic factors, and take these into consideration when planning psychosocial interventions.

Community-Based Care
- Discharge planning for the patient with a burn injury begins at the time of admission to the hospital or burn center.
- Help the patient adjust to the reaction of others to the sight of healing wounds and disfiguring scars.
- Teach the patient and family:
  1. How to perform dressing changes
  2. Signs and symptoms of infection
  3. Drug regimens
  4. Proper use of prosthetic and positioning devices
  5. Correct application and care of pressure garments
  6. Comfort measures to reduce pruritus
  7. Dates for follow-up appointments
- Additional common discharge needs of the patient with burns include:
  1. Financial assessment
  2. Evaluation of family resources
  3. Psychological referral
  4. Patient and family teaching (home care)
  5. Rehabilitation referral
  6. Home assessment (on-site visit)
  7. Medical equipment
  8. Home care nursing referral
  9. Evaluation of community resources
  10. Visit to referral agency
  11. Re-entry programs for school or work environment
  12. Nursing home placement
  13. Prosthetic rehabilitation

CANCER, BREAST

OVERVIEW

- Breast cancer is the most commonly diagnosed cancer in women and is second only to lung cancer as a cause of cancer death in women. Men account for less than 1% of breast cancers.
- Early detection through regular screening methods of breast self-examination (BSE), clinical breast examination, and mammography is the key to effective treatment and survival.
- It is a heterogeneous disease, having many forms with different clinical presentations and responses to therapy.
- Breast cancer is divided into two broad categories, noninvasive and invasive:
  1. *Noninvasive cancers* remain within the breast ducts and make up 20% of breast cancers. Ductal carcinoma in situ (DCIS) is a common, early, noninvasive breast cancer. Another type is lobular carcinoma in situ (LCIS).
  2. *Invasive cancers* penetrate the tissue surrounding the ducts and make up 80% of all breast cancers. The most common type of invasive breast cancer is infiltrating ductal carcinoma. Another type is inflammatory carcinoma.
     a. When the invasive breast tumor invades lymphatic channels, skin drainage is blocked, causing skin edema, redness, warmth, and an orange peel appearance of the skin ("peau d'orange").
     b. Invasion of the lymphatic channels carries cancer cells to the axillary lymph nodes. Pathologic examination of these nodes helps determine the stage of the disease.
     c. Invasive breast cancer can spread through the blood and lymph systems to distant sites, most commonly the bone, lungs, brain, and liver.
- There is no single cause of breast cancer, but many risk factors are associated with its development:
  1. Female gender
  2. Advancing age
  3. Family history, especially first-degree relatives, of breast cancer
  4. Previous exposure to high-dose ionizing radiation to the chest
  5. Early menarche (before 12 years of age) and late menopause (after 50 years of age)
  6. History of previous breast cancer
  7. Nulliparity (no pregnancies) or first birth after 30 years of age

Genetic/Genomic Considerations

- Inherited mutations in several genes are related to hereditary breast cancer. The most common known mutations that increase breast cancer risk are in the *BRCA1* and *BRCA2* genes. Mutations in these genes greatly increase breast cancer risk; however, only about 5% of all breast cancers are hereditary.
- Patients with these mutations have an increased risk for other cancers, including ovarian cancer and possibly colon cancer.
- Children of a patient with a *BRCA1* or *BCRA2* germline mutation have a 50% chance of inheriting that mutation.

⊕ Cultural Awareness

- Euro-American women older than 40 years are at a greater risk than other racial or ethnic groups, but African-American women younger than 40 have breast cancer more often than others in that age group.
- African-American women have a higher death rate at any age compared with other women with the disease. Research has found differences in tumor characteristics in some African-American women. For example, triple-negative breast cancer occurs more often in African-American women and younger women. In this type of breast cancer, cells lack receptors for estrogen, progesterone, and the protein Her2. Triple-negative breast cancer tends to be more aggressive than other types of breast cancer, and fewer effective treatments exist for it. Much research is ongoing to better understand this type of breast cancer.
- For American-Indian and Alaskan Native women, 5-year survivor rates for breast cancer are very poor. American Indian women are less likely than non-Hispanic white women to have mammography screening. Health promotion interventions to improve mammography rates should consider cultural customs, transportation, and social support.

PATIENT-CENTERED COLLABORATIVE CARE
Assessment

- Obtain patient information about:
  1. Age and race
  2. Personal and family history of breast cancer
  3. Age at menarche and menopause
  4. Number of children and age at first child's birth
  5. Health behaviors, including practice of BSE, clinical breast examination, and mammography

   6. How the mass was discovered and how long ago
   7. Whether other body changes have been noticed recently, especially bone or joint pain
   8. Brief nutritional history, including intake of fat and alcohol
- Assess for:
   1. Specific information about the mass:
      a. Location of the mass, described using the face-of-the-clock method
      b. Shape, size, consistency
      c. Whether it is mobile or fixed to the surrounding tissues
      d. Skin changes, such as dimpling, orange peel appearance, redness and warmth, nipple retraction, or ulceration
   2. Presence of enlarged axillary or supraclavicular lymph nodes
   3. Pain or soreness in the affected breast
   4. Psychosocial adjustment:
      a. Patient's current knowledge and need for information
      b. Patient's self-image
      c. Sexuality and current intimate relationships
      d. How the patient has successfully handled stress in the past
      e. Patient's feelings about the disease and expectations of treatment
      f. Myths or misconceptions the patient may have (and how to dispel them)
      g. Need for additional resources
   5. Imaging assessment for diagnosis and staging:
      a. Mammography or digital mammography
      b. Ultrasonography
      c. Breast-specific gamma imaging (BSGI)
      d. Chest x-ray
      e. Bone, liver, and brain scans
      f. Computed tomography (CT) scan of the chest and abdomen
      g. Magnetic resonance imaging (MRI)
   6. Pathologic examination of tissue for diagnosis and prognosis:
      a. Biopsy, which is the definitive test that proves cancer presence or absence
      b. Presence of estrogen and progesterone receptors (cancers that express receptors have a better treatment response)
      c. Protein expression profiling of tumor cells
      d. Size and location of tumors
      e. Lymph node involvement
      f. Presence of distant metastasis

Planning and Implementation

- Teach women ways to minimize surgical area deformity and enhance body image, such as the use of a breast prosthesis or the option of breast reconstruction.
- Address the reactions of family and significant others to the diagnosis of breast cancer; provide support and education.
- Assess benign lumps as mobile and round or oval; assess possible malignant lumps as fixed and irregularly shaped, often in the upper outer breast quadrant.
- After breast cancer surgery, assess vital signs, dressings, drainage tubes, and amount of drainage.
- Notify the health care team that the arm of the surgical mastectomy side should not be used for blood pressures, blood drawing, or injections.
- Assess the return of arm and shoulder mobility after breast surgery and axillary dissection.
- Assess for the presence of lymphedema, and assist the patient to perform therapeutic measures to reduce lymphedema in the affected arm.
- Teach the patient measures to prevent lymphedema after axillary node dissection.
- Observe for and report other complications of breast cancer surgery or breast reconstruction, especially infection and inadequate vascular perfusion.

Surgical Management
- To improve survival and to reduce the risk for local recurrence, the mass itself should be removed by one of several types of surgery.
- Removal of the axillary lymph nodes for staging purposes is usually performed for patients with palpable axillary lymph nodes.
- When nodes are not palpable, a sentinel lymph node biopsy (SLNB) may be performed during or before breast surgery. If no cancer cells are found in the sentinel node, it is not necessary to remove other lymph nodes in the chain.
- A large tumor may be treated with chemotherapy (neoadjuvant therapy) to shrink the tumor before it is surgically removed.
- Surgical approaches include:
  1. *Breast-conserving surgery*, in which the bulk of the tumor is removed (not the entire breast), is used mostly for stages I and II breast cancers and is usually followed with radiation therapy. Types of breast-conserving surgery include lumpectomy, wide excision, partial or segmental mastectomy, and quadrantectomy.
  2. *Modified radical mastectomy*, in which the affected breast, skin, and axillary nodes are completely removed, but the

underlying muscles remain intact, is indicated when tumor is present in different quadrants of the breast, when the patient may be unable to have radiation therapy, when the tumor is large and the breast is small, and when the patient prefers this approach.

- Provide preoperative care, including psychological preparation and preoperative teaching:
  1. Review the type of procedure planned.
  2. Assess the patient's current level of knowledge.
  3. Teach about postoperative information, including:
     a. The need for a drainage tube
     b. The location of the incision
     c. Mobility restrictions
     d. Length of hospital stay (if any)
     e. The possibility of adjuvant therapy
     f. Written materials for the patient and family to take home as references
     g. Body image issues
- Provide postoperative care, including:
  1. Performing routine postoperative care, including pain management, as described in Part One
  2. Placing a sign over the patient's bed to inform the staff to avoid using the affected arm for taking blood pressure measurements, giving injections, or drawing blood
  3. Assessing vital signs on a schedule of decreasing frequency, such as every 30 minutes for two times, every hour for two times, and then every 4 hours
  4. Assessing the dressing for bleeding and monitoring the amount and color of drainage
  5. Performing wound care:
     a. Observe the wound for signs of swelling and infection.
     b. Assess drainage tubes for patency.
  6. Positioning the patient for best drainage and comfort:
     a. Head of the bed up at least 30 degrees
     b. Arm on the same side as the axillary dissection elevated on a pillow while he or she is awake
  7. Working with the physical therapist to plan progressive exercises:
     a. Squeezing the affected hand around a soft, round object (a ball or rolled washcloth)
     b. Flexion and extension of the elbow
- Breast reconstruction is common for women without complications from the cancer surgery and may be performed during the cancer surgery or at a later time. It may involve one or more stages using skin flaps or prostheses.

- For patients with breast cancer at a stage for which surgery is the main treatment, follow-up with adjuvant radiation therapy, chemotherapy, hormone therapy, or targeted therapy may also be prescribed.
- The decision to follow the original surgical procedure with adjuvant therapy for breast cancer is based on:
  1. Stage of the disease
  2. Patient's age and menopausal status
  3. Patient's preferences
  4. Pathologic examination results
  5. Hormone receptor status
  6. Presence of a known genetic predisposition
- Radiation therapy is administered after breast-conserving surgery and may be delivered by any one of several methods. General management issues for care of patients undergoing radiation therapy are presented in Part One under *Cancer Therapy*.
  1. Traditional whole-breast irradiation is delivered by external beam radiation over 5 to 6 weeks.
  2. *Interstitial brachytherapy,* in which several catheters loaded with a radioactive source are inserted at the lumpectomy cavity and surrounding margin, is given over 4 to 5 days.
  3. *Balloon brachytherapy,* also known as *MammoSite,* involves the use of a single balloon-tipped catheter that is surgically placed near the tumor bed. The catheter is loaded with a radiation source and inflated to conform to the total cavity. A total of 10 treatments are given, with at least 6 hours between each treatment.
  4. *Intraoperative radiation therapy* uses a high single dose of radiation delivered during the lumpectomy surgery.
- Chemotherapy for breast cancer is delivered systemically with a combination of agents, usually for patients who have stage II or more advanced breast cancer. General management issues for care of patients undergoing radiation therapy are presented in Part One under *Cancer Therapy*.
- Targeted therapy for breast cancer involves the use of drugs that target specific features of cancer cells, such as a protein, an enzyme, or the formation of new blood vessels. These agents are useful only for cancers that overexpress a certain protein or enzyme. For breast cancer, a targeted biotherapy drug is trastuzumab (Herceptin) for cancers that overexpress the *HER2/NEU* gene product
- Hormonal therapy is used to reduce the estrogen available to breast tumors to stop or prevent their growth. Agents include:
  1. Luteinizing hormone-releasing hormone (LH-RH) gene agonists that inhibit estrogen synthesis

C

    a. Leuprolide (Lupron)
    b. Goserelin (Zoladex)
2. Selective estrogen receptor modulators (SERMs) that block the effect of estrogen in women who have estrogen receptor (ER)-positive breast cancer. One example is tamoxifen.
3. Aromatase inhibitors (AIs) to prevent the conversion of androgen to estrogen in the adrenal gland.
    a. Anastrozole (Arimidex)
    b. Exemestane (Aromasin)

Community-Based Care

- Make the appropriate referrals for care after discharge:
  1. Home care
  2. Reach to Recovery
  3. Social services
- Teach the patient and family about:
  1. Wound care: drains, dressings, avoidance of lotions or ointments in the area, keeping the affected arm elevated if a lymph node dissection was performed
  2. Initial activity restrictions, especially stretching or reaching for heavy objects, while continuing with activity to regain full range of motion (ROM)
  3. Measures to improve body image
  4. Information about interpersonal relationships and roles
  5. Essential follow-up, including annual health care provider visits and mammography or other imaging procedures
  6. Measures to avoid injury, infection, and swelling of the affected arm
- Prepare the patient and partner about psychosocial issues:
  1. Describe the expected postoperative appearance.
  2. Reassure her that scars will fade and edema will lessen with time.
  3. Encourage the woman to look at her incision before she goes home and offer to be present when she does so.
  4. Involve the partner or family in teaching.
  5. Discuss sexual concerns before discharge. Sexual dysfunction affects up to 90% of women treated for breast cancer, although it is an issue seldom discussed between patients and health care providers.
  6. Advise sexually active patients receiving chemotherapy or radiotherapy to use birth control during therapy.
  7. Suggest participation in local support groups or national organizations such as the American Cancer Society, the Susan G. Komen "Race for the Cure," the National Breast Cancer Coalition, Y-Me, Sisters Network, Young Survival Coalition, and Pink Ribbon Girls.

CANCER, CERVICAL

OVERVIEW

- Cervical cancer, a common female reproductive cancer that usually arises from the squamous cells on the outside of the uterine cervix, can be preinvasive or invasive.
- It generally takes years for the cervical cells to transform from normal to premalignant to invasive cancer.
- *Preinvasive* cancer is limited to the cervix.
- *Invasive* cancer has spread to other pelvic structures by direct extension to the vaginal mucosa, lower uterine segment, parametrium, pelvic wall, bladder, and bowel.
- Risk factors include:
  1. Infection with human papillomavirus (HPV)
  2. History of sexually transmitted disease
  3. Multiple sex partners
  4. Younger than 18 years of age at first intercourse
  5. Multiparity (multiple pregnancies)
  6. Smoking
  7. Oral contraceptive use
  8. Obesity, poor diet
- Vaccination with HPV vaccine, ideally before onset of intercourse, appears to protect against the high-risk HPV strains that are responsible for most cervical cancer.
- Cervical cancer can be detected at early stages, when cure is most likely, through periodic pelvic examinations and Papanicolaou (Pap) smears to screen. Teach women to avoid having this test during the menstrual period and to avoid these activities at least 48 hours before the test:
  1. Douching
  2. Sexual intercourse
  3. Tampon use
  4. Instillation of vaginal creams, jellies, or other drugs

PATIENT-CENTERED COLLABORATIVE CARE
Assessment

- Ask the patient if she has had or now has bleeding. It may start as spotting between menstrual periods or after sexual intercourse or douching. The classic symptom of invasive cancer is painless vaginal bleeding. As the cancer grows, bleeding increases in frequency, duration, and amount, and it may become continuous.
- Assess for later manifestations:
  1. Watery, blood-tinged vaginal discharge that becomes dark and foul-smelling (occurs as the disease progresses)
  2. Leg pain (along the sciatic nerve)

3. Swelling of one leg
4. Flank pain indicating hydronephrosis from tumor blocking a ureter, backing up the fluid into the kidney
- Assess for manifestations of recurrence or metastasis:
  1. Unexplained weight loss
  2. Dysuria (painful urination)
  3. Pelvic pain
  4. Hematuria (bloody urine)
  5. Rectal bleeding
  6. Chest pain
  7. Coughing
- Diagnosis is made by cytologic examination of the Pap smear. When Pap results are abnormal, an HPV-typing DNA test of the cervical sample can determine the presence of one or more high-risk types of the virus. Colposcopic examination may be performed to view the transformation zone and biopsy many areas of the cervix.

Interventions

Surgical Management: Early Stage

- Surgical management for small, early-stage cervical cancer:
  1. Loop electrosurgical excision procedure (LEEP) is a diagnostic procedure and a treatment. A thin loop-wire electrode that transmits a painless electrical current is used to cut away affected tissue.
  2. Laser therapy, in which a laser beam is focused on abnormal tissues, vaporizes cancerous cells without obtaining a tissue specimen for analysis.
  3. Cryotherapy, in which the entire cervix is frozen, produces necrosis of all superficial cells, including cancer cells.
- Teach patients who have these procedures to follow restrictions for about 3 weeks:
  1. Refrain from sexual intercourse.
  2. Do not use tampons.
  3. Do not douche.
  4. Take showers rather than tub baths.
  5. Avoid lifting heavy objects.
  6. Report or fever any heavy vaginal bleeding, foul-smelling drainage.

Surgical Management: Microinvasive Stage

- Surgical management at the microinvasive stage depends on the patient's health, desire for future childbearing, tumor size, stage, cancer cell type, and preferences.
- A *conization*, in which a cone-shaped area of cervix is removed surgically, can remove the affected tissue while preserving fertility.

1. Potential complications from this procedure include hemorrhage and uterine perforation.
2. Long-term follow-up care is needed, because new cancers can develop.

- A *total hysterectomy*, in which the cervix and body of the uterus are removed but the fallopian tubes and ovaries are spared, may be performed if fertility is not an issue. Care for patients undergoing hysterectomy is found in the *Uterine Leiomyoma* section.

C

- Provide preoperative care:
  1. Assess anxiety, concerns about sexual functioning, and the ability to adjust to an altered body image.
- Refer to *Cancer, Colorectal* for preoperative and postoperative care for the patient undergoing colostomy and to *Cancer, Urothelial (Bladder)* for preoperative and postoperative care for the patient undergoing ileal conduit.
- Provide routine preoperative care as outlined for surgical patients and for patients undergoing hysterectomy.

Nonsurgical Management

- Radiation therapy is reserved for invasive cervical cancer.
  1. *Intracavitary* and *external radiation therapies* are used in combination, depending on the extent and location of the lesion.
  2. General management issues for care of patients undergoing intracavitary (brachytherapy) or external (beam) radiation therapy are presented in Part One under *Cancer Therapy.*
- Chemotherapy with radiation therapy may be also be used for invasive cervical cancer.
  1. The most common agent used is cisplatin (Platinol). Paclitaxel (Taxol), carboplatin, and fluorouracil (5-FU) have also been used.
  2. General management issues for care of patients receiving combination chemotherapy are presented in Part One under *Cancer Therapy.*

CANCER, COLORECTAL

OVERVIEW

- Colorectal cancer (CRC), or cancer of the colon or rectum, is a common malignancy worldwide.
- Most CRCs are adenocarcinomas arising from the glandular epithelial tissue of the colon and develop as a multistep process, resulting in loss of key tumor suppressor genes and activation of certain oncogenes that alter colonic mucosa cell division.
- The increased proliferation of the colonic mucosa first forms polyps that can transform into malignant tumors.

- Tumors occur in all areas of the colon and can spread by direct invasion and through the lymphatic and circulatory systems.
- The most common sites of metastasis are the liver, lungs, brain, bones, and adrenal glands.
- Complications include bowel perforation with peritonitis, abscess or fistula formation, frank hemorrhage, and complete intestinal obstruction.
- Risk factors include:
  1. Age older than 50 years
  2. Genetic predisposition
  3. Personal or family history of cancer
  4. Personal history of diseases that predispose to cancer (e.g., familial adenomatous polyposis [FAP], hereditary nonpolyposis colorectal cancer [HNPCC])
  5. Personal history of inflammatory bowel diseases (IBDs)

Genetic/Genomic Considerations

- People with a first-degree relative (sister, sibling, or child) diagnosed with CRC have three to four times the risk of developing the disease.
- An autosomal dominant inherited genetic disorder known as FAP accounts for 1% of CRCs. People with mutation develop thousands of adenomatous polyps over 10 to 15 years that have an almost 100% chance of becoming malignant.
- Surgical prophylaxis with a colectomy can be performed for cancer prevention.
- HNPCC is another autosomal dominant disorder caused by mutations in the *MLH1* and *MLH2* genes. People with these mutations have an 80% chance of developing CRC at an average of 45 years of age.
- Genetic testing is available for both familial CRC syndromes, although they are the cause of fewer than 5% of CRCs.

PATIENT-CENTERED COLLABORATIVE CARE
Assessment

- Obtain patient information about:
  1. Age
  2. History of inflammatory or familial colon disease
  3. Personal history of breast, ovarian, or endometrial cancer
  4. Change in bowel habits with or without blood in stool
  5. Weight loss, pain, and abdominal fullness (late signs)
- Assess for:
  1. Rectal bleeding (the most common manifestation)
  2. Change in stool pattern or appearance

3. Anemia (low hemoglobin level and hematocrit; stool positive for occult blood)
4. Cachexia (late sign)
5. Guarding or abdominal distention (late sign)
6. Abdominal mass (late sign)

- Diagnostic assessment includes:
  1. Fecal occult blood test (FOBT)
  2. Carcinoembryonic antigen (CEA) blood test
  3. Colonoscopy
  4. Computed tomography (CT) or magnetic resonance imaging (MRI) of the chest, abdomen, pelvis, lungs, or liver

Planning and Implementation
POTENTIAL FOR COLORECTAL METASTASIS
Nonsurgical Management
- Radiation therapy:
  1. Preoperative radiation therapy is effective in providing local or regional control of the disease.
  2. Radiation is also used postoperatively as a palliative measure to reduce pain, hemorrhage, bowel obstruction, or metastasis.
  3. General management issues for care of patients undergoing radiation therapy are presented in Part One under *Cancer Therapy.*
- *Chemotherapy* is used after surgery to interrupt cancer cell division and improve survival. General management issues for care of patients undergoing chemotherapy are presented in Part One under *Cancer Therapy.*
  1. Common drugs include:
     a. 5-Fluorouracil (5-FU)
     b. Leucovorin (LV) (folinic acid)
     c. Capecitabine (Xeloda)
     d. Oxaliplatin (Eloxatin)
  2. Common side effects of this therapy are:
     a. Diarrhea
     b. Mucositis
     c. Leukopenia
     d. Mouth ulcers
     e. Peripheral neuropathy
- *Targeted biotherapy* approved for colorectal cancer may include:
  1. Bevacizumab (Avastin)
  2. Cetuximab (Erbitux)
Surgical Management
- In a colon resection, the bowel segment containing the tumor is resected (removed) along with several inches of bowel beyond

the tumor margin and regional lymph nodes, and an end-to-end anastomosis is performed. This procedure may be performed by the traditional open method or as minimally invasive surgery by laparoscopy.

- A colectomy (colon removal) with temporary or permanent colostomy may be needed.
- In an abdominal peritoneal (A-P) resection, the sigmoid colon and rectum are removed, the anus is closed, and a permanent colostomy is formed.
- Provide preoperative care:
  1. Implement routine preoperative care as presented in Part One.
  2. Reinforce the surgeon's explanation of the procedure.
  3. If a colostomy is planned, consult the enterostomal therapist (ET) to assist in identifying optimal placement of the ostomy and to instruct the patient about the rationale and general principles of ostomies.
  4. Instruct the patient to consume only clear liquids for a day or more before bowel surgery to minimize colonic contents.
  5. Administer laxatives, enemas, or an oral, liquid, large-volume laxative if ordered, the morning of surgery or the day before surgery to mechanically clean the bowel ("bowel prep").
  6. Give antibiotics preoperatively, as prescribed.
- Provide postoperative care, including:
  1. Implementing routine postoperative care as described in Part One.
  2. Providing nasogastric tube care, if needed
  3. Providing pain management
  4. Managing the colostomy, if present:
     a. If an ostomy pouch is not in place, cover the stoma with petroleum gauze to keep it moist, followed by a dry, sterile dressing.
     b. Place a pouch system on the stoma as soon as possible and in collaboration with the enterostomal therapist.
     c. Observe the stoma for color, discharge, and intactness of surrounding skin
     d. Check pouch system for proper fit and signs of leakage.
     e. Assess for colostomy functioning 2 to 4 days after surgery; stool is liquid immediately after surgery but becomes more solid.
     f. Empty the pouch when excess gas has collected or when it is one third to one half full of stool.

■ NURSING SAFETY PRIORITY: Action Alert

Report any of these problems related to the colostomy to the surgeon:

- Signs of ischemia and necrosis (dark red, purplish, or black color; dry, firm, or flaccid)
- Unusual bleeding
- Mucocutaneous separation (breakdown of the suture line securing the stoma to the abdominal wall)

5. Also assess the condition of the peristomal skin (skin around the stoma), and frequently check the pouch system for proper fit and signs of leakage. The skin should be intact, smooth, and without redness or excoriation.
6. Assessing the perineal wound, irrigating the site, and providing dressing changes to maintain hygiene. Copious serosanguineous drainage is expected.
7. Providing comfort measures for perineal itching and pain, such as antipruritic drugs (benzocaine) and sitz baths
8. Assessing for signs of infection, abscess, or other complications
9. Instructing the patient about activities such as assuming a side-lying position, avoiding sitting for long periods, and using a foam pad or pillow when in a sitting position
10. Consult with the skin care or ostomy specialist early and often during surgical recovery

ANTICIPATORY GRIEVING RELATED TO CANCER DIAGNOSIS
- Observe and identify:
  1. The patient's and family's current method of coping and effective sources of support
  2. The patient's and family's present perceptions of the patient's health problem
  3. Signs of anticipatory grief such as crying, anger, sadness, and withdrawal from usual relationships
- Encourage the patient to verbalize feelings about the diagnosis, treatment, and anticipated changes in body image if an ostomy is planned.
- Instruct the patient what to expect about the appearance and care of the colostomy.
- When the patient is physically able, encourage the patient to look at the ostomy (if performed), and to participate in colostomy care.
- Facilitate grief work by identifying the nature of and reaction to the loss.
- Invite the patient, family, social worker, or religious leader to participate in the discussion and decisions concerning potential lifestyle modifications, treatment, prognosis, and end-of-life decisions.
- Refer patients who are at risk for or have familial CRC for genetic counseling.

Community-Based Care

- Provide the patient with these verbal and written instructions:
  1. Avoid lifting heavy objects or straining on defecation to prevent tension on the anastomosis site.
  2. Avoid driving for 4 to 6 weeks.
  3. Note the frequency, amount, and character of the stool.
  4. For colon resection, watch for and report manifestations of bowel obstruction and perforation (e.g., cramping, abdominal pain, nausea, vomiting).
  5. Resume a normal diet, but avoid gas-producing foods and carbonated beverages.
- Teach the patient and family colostomy care, including:
  1. Normal appearance of a stoma
  2. Signs and symptoms of complications
  3. How to measure the stoma
  4. How to protect the skin adjacent to the stoma
  5. Dietary measures to control gas and odor
- Other discharge preparation includes:
  1. Inspection of the abdominal incision (and perineal wound if an A-P resection was performed) for redness, tenderness, swelling, and drainage
  2. Pain management, including drug therapy
  3. Tips on how to resume normal activities, including work, travel, and sexual intercourse
  4. Psychosocial preparation
- Provide these contacts for community and health resources, as needed:
  1. Social services
  2. Enterostomal therapist or certified wound ostomy continence specialist
  3. United Ostomy Association
  4. American Cancer Society
  5. Home health services
  6. Pharmacy or other medical supply source

CANCER, ENDOMETRIAL (UTERINE)

OVERVIEW

- Endometrial cancer (cancer of the uterus) is the most common gynecologic cancer.
- Adenocarcinoma is the most common type, accounting for 80% of all cases.
- It is slow-growing with initial growth in the uterine cavity, followed by extension into the myometrium and cervix.

- Risk factors associated with endometrial cancer include:
  1. Prolonged exposure to estrogen without the protective effects of progesterone
  2. Women in reproductive years
  3. Family history of endometrial cancer or hereditary non-polyposis colorectal cancer (HNPCC)
  4. Diabetes mellitus
  5. Hypertension
  6. Obesity
  7. Uterine polyps
  8. Late menopause
  9. Nulliparity (no childbirths)
  10. Smoking
  11. Tamoxifen (Nolvadex) given for breast cancer

PATIENT-CENTERED COLLABORATIVE CARE
Assessment
- Obtain patient information about:
  1. Age and ethnicity
  2. Risk factors of family history of cancer
  3. History of diabetes, obesity, or hypertension
  4. Childbearing status, pregnancies, births, infertility
  5. Prolonged estrogen use
- Assess for:
  1. Postmenopausal bleeding (the primary symptom)
  2. Watery, serosanguineous vaginal discharge
  3. Low back, abdominal, or pelvic pain
  4. Enlarged uterus
  5. Anemia from uterine bleeding
  6. CA (cancer antigen)-125 and alpha-fetoprotein (AFP), both of which may be elevated when ovarian (metastatic) cancer is present
  7. *Transvaginal ultrasound* and *endometrial biopsy* are the gold standard tests to determine the presence of endometrial thickening and cancer

Interventions
Surgical Management
- Surgical removal and cancer staging of the tumor is first-line therapy. Typically a total abdominal hysterectomy is done (see *Leiomyoma, Surgical Management, Hysterectomy*). Either a laparoscopic or open approach can be used.
Nonsurgical Management
- Radiation therapy and chemotherapy are used postoperatively and depend on the surgical staging.

- When intracavitary radiation therapy (IRT) (brachytherapy) is performed, an applicator is positioned within the uterus through the vagina. Implement these interventions for radiation safety and to prevent dislodgment of either the applicator or the radiation source:
  1. Maintain radiation precautions.
  2. Provide bedrest, laying the patient on her back, with her head flat or elevated less than 20 degrees. Restrict active movement to prevent dislodgment
  3. Assess for complications including cystitis, diarrhea, and mucosal or skin irritation.
- Instruct the patient undergoing external beam radiation to:
  1. Observe for signs of skin breakdown.
  2. Avoid sunbathing.
  3. Do not remove the markings that outline the treatment site.
  4. Recognize the complications of treatment, including cystitis, diarrhea, and nutritional alterations.
  5. Recognize that reactions to radiation therapy vary among patients and that some may feel unclean or radioactive after treatments.
- General management issues for the care of patients undergoing intracavitary (brachytherapy) or external (teletherapy) radiation therapy are presented in Part One under *Cancer Therapy.*
- Chemotherapy is used for stage 3 or 4 uterine cancer.
  1. Chemotherapeutic agents frequently used include doxorubicin (Adriamycin), cisplatin (Platinol), and paclitaxel (Taxol).
  2. General management issues for care of patients receiving combination chemotherapy are presented in Part One under *Cancer Therapy.*

Community-Based Care

- Provide verbal and written instructions on:
  1. Side effects that should be reported to the physician, including vaginal bleeding, rectal bleeding, foul-smelling discharge, abdominal pain or distention, and hematuria
  2. Dosages, scheduling, and side effects of prescribed drugs
- Inform the patient:
  1. High-dose radiation causes sterility.
  2. Vaginal shrinkage or dryness can occur with radiation and chemotherapy.
  3. Sexual partners cannot "catch" cancer.
  4. The patient is not radioactive (after the intracavitary radiation source is removed).

- After an abdominal hysterectomy, give the instructions and information to the patient as discussed under *Leiomyomas (Uterine Fibroids)*.
- Refer the patient to the local chapter of the American Cancer Society.

CANCER, HEAD AND NECK

OVERVIEW
- Head and neck cancers occur in structures within the larynx, the trachea, the throat, the oral cavity, or on the tongue, and they usually arise from the skin or mucosa as squamous cell carcinomas.
- Other origins of head and neck cancers include the salivary glands, the thyroid, and other structures.
- These cancers are slow-growing, with the tissue changes occurring in several stages.
  1. Premalignant lesions appear when the mucosa is chronically irritated, changing into tougher mucosa (squamous metaplasia), followed by mucosal thickening (acanthosis, or hyperplasia) and the development of a keratin layer (keratosis). The chronic irritation damages genes controlling cell growth, allowing enhanced growth of these abnormal cells, leading to:
     a. *Leukoplakia,* a thickened, white, firmly attached plaque
     b. *Erythroplakia,* a red, velvety patch
  2. With time, the premalignant lesions become cancerous and may spread (metastasize first into nearby structures, such as lymph nodes, muscle, and bone, and then to more distant sites, usually the lungs or liver).
  3. The degree of malignancy is determined by cellular analysis:
     a. Early-stage cancers are carcinoma in situ and well differentiated.
     b. Cancers that have progressed are moderately differentiated.
     c. Advanced cancers are poorly differentiated.

- The cause of head and neck cancers is unknown, but the two greatest risk factors are tobacco and alcohol use, especially in combination.
- Other risk factors include voice abuse, chronic laryngitis, exposure to industrial chemicals or hardwood dust, poor oral hygiene, and long-term or severe gastroesophageal reflux disease (GERD).

PATIENT-CENTERED COLLABORATIVE CARE
Assessment
- Obtain patient information about:
  1. Tobacco and alcohol use (quantify these)
  2. History of recurrent acute or chronic laryngitis or pharyngitis, oral sores, and lumps in the neck
  3. Exposure to environmental or occupational pollutants
- Assess for physical manifestations:
  1. Problems related to risk factors
  2. Dietary habits
  3. Weight loss
  4. Hoarseness
  5. Lumps on the head or in the neck
  6. Mouth sores
  7. Laryngeal abnormalities by laryngeal examination using a laryngeal mirror (physician or advanced practice nurse)
- Assess for psychosocial issues:
  1. Patient or family feelings of denial, guilt, blame, or shame
  2. Adequacy of support systems and coping mechanisms
  3. Social and family support systems
  4. Level of education or literacy of the patient and family to plan teaching before and after surgery
  5. Patient's use of speech for employment
- Diagnostic assessment may include:
  1. Laboratory tests, complete blood count (CBC), bleeding times, urinalysis, blood chemistries, protein levels, albumin levels, renal and liver function tests
  2. X-rays of the skull, sinuses, neck, and chest
  3. Computed tomography (CT) scan of the head and neck, with or without contrast media
  4. Magnetic resonance imaging (MRI)
  5. Brain, bone, and liver scans
  6. Positron emission tomography (PET) scans
  7. Direct and indirect laryngoscopy
  8. Panendoscopy (laryngoscopy, nasopharyngoscopy, esophagoscopy, and bronchoscopy)
  9. Biopsy

Planning and Implementation
The goal of treatment is to remove or eradicate the cancer while preserving as much normal function as possible. The specific treatment depends on the extent and location of the lesion.

Nonsurgical Management
- Radiation therapy for the treatment of small cancers involves external beam delivery of 5000 to 7500 rad (radiation absorbed dose), usually over 6 weeks and in daily or twice-daily doses.

1. Radiation therapy may be used alone or in combination with surgery. Because radiation therapy slows tissue healing, it may not be performed before surgery.
2. Complications of radiation therapy for head and neck cancer include increased hoarseness, dysphagia, skin problems, and dry mouth (leading to halitosis, taste changes, increased risk for dental caries and dental infection).
3. Dry mouth (xerostomia) is a long-term complication and may be permanent. Interventions include:
   a. Heavy fluid intake, particularly water
   b. Room humidification
   c. Use of artificial saliva (Salivart)
   d. Use of saliva stimulants (pilocarpine [Salagen] and cevimeline)
   e. Chewing gum and sucking hard candy
4. General management issues for care of patients undergoing radiation therapy are presented in Part One under *Cancer Therapy.*

- Chemotherapy can be used alone or in addition to surgery or radiation for head and neck cancer.
  1. Specific treatment regimens and drug combinations vary, but the most commonly used agents for head and neck cancer include cisplatin (Platinol), fluorouracil (5-FU), and gemcitabine (Gemzar).
  2. General management issues for care of patients undergoing chemotherapy are presented in Part One under *Cancer Therapy.*
- Targeted therapy for advanced head and neck cancers may include cetuximab (Erbitux).

Surgical Management

- Tumor size and location (according to tumor-nodes-metastasis [TNM] classification) determines the type of surgery needed for the specific head and neck cancer.
- Very small, early-stage tumors may be removed by laser therapy or photodynamic therapy, but few head and neck tumors are found at this stage, and most require extensive traditional surgery.
- Traditional surgical procedures for head and neck cancers include:
  1. Laryngectomy (total and partial): removal of the larynx
  2. *Tracheotomy:* creation of a new artificial airway by opening the wall of the trachea
  3. Oropharyngeal cancer resections
  4. *Cordectomy:* vocal cord removal
  5. Radical neck dissection, which is removal of the primary tumor along with lymph node dissection. It may involve removing skin, muscle, bone, and other structures.

      6. Composite resections are a combination of surgical procedures, including partial or total glossectomies, partial mandibulectomies, and, if needed, nodal neck dissections.
- Provide preoperative care:
    1. Give routine preoperative care, as described in Part One.
    2. Teach the patient about the probable location of the surgical incision, self-care of the airway, alternate methods of communication, suctioning, pain control methods, the critical care environment (including ventilators and critical care routines), nutritional support, feeding tubes, and goals for discharge.
    3. Help the patient to practice the use of an alternate form of communication (e.g., pen and pencil, "magic slate," picture or alphabet board, computerized word generator).
    4. Determine the communication method most preferred by the patient.
    5. Encourage the patient to express fears and concerns.
    6. Reinforce the surgeon's explanation of the surgical procedure.
- Provide postoperative care:
    1. Routine postoperative care, as described in Part One
    2. Airway maintenance and ventilation
        a. Ventilator management
        b. Suctioning
        c. Frequent swallowing as a sign of oropharyngeal bleeding, triggering the swallow reflex
        d. Oxygen therapy
        e. Humidification
        f. Coughing and deep breathing
        g. Laryngectomy or tracheostomy care (if surgery included tracheotomy or laryngectomy)

■ NURSING SAFETY PRIORITY: Critical Rescue

Secretions may remain blood-tinged for 1 to 2 days. Report any increase in bleeding to the surgeon.

      3. Wound management:
         a. Evaluate all grafts and flaps hourly for the first 72 hours.
         b. Monitor capillary refill, color, drainage, and Doppler activity of the major feeding vessel.
         c. Position the patient so that the side of the head and neck with the flaps is not dependent.
         d. Monitor drainage and record its amount and character.
         e. Report changes to the surgeon immediately, because surgical intervention may be needed.

4. Hemorrhage prevention:
   a. Observe for carotid artery leakage or rupture.
      (1) Rupture results in large amounts of bright red blood spurting quickly.
      (2) Leakage shows as oozing of bright red blood.

!NURSING SAFETY PRIORITY: Critical Rescue

If a carotid artery leak is suspected, call the Rapid Response Team, and do not touch the area, because additional pressure could cause an immediate rupture. If the carotid artery ruptures because of drying or infection, immediately place constant pressure over the site and secure the airway. Maintain direct manual continuous pressure on the carotid artery and immediately transport the patient to the operating room for carotid resection. Do not leave the patient. Carotid artery rupture has a high risk of stroke and death. Nursing response can save the patient's life.

5. Nutritional support:
   a. Collaborate with the dietitian to provide the patient with at least 35 to 40 kcal/kg of body weight daily.
   b. IV fluids or parenteral nutrition is used until the intestinal tract is functioning.
   c. Tube feeding by nasogastric, gastrostomy, or jejunostomy tube (usually remains in place for 7 to 10 days after surgery).
   d. Assess the patient's ability to swallow before removing the feeding tube.
6. Speech and language rehabilitation:
   a. Collaborate with the speech and language pathologist.
   b. Work with the patient and family toward developing an acceptable communication method:
      (1) Writing
      (2) Picture board
      (3) Computer
      (4) Artificial larynx
      (5) Esophageal speech
   c. Take time to understand the patient's communication.
   d. Celebrate every success.
   e. Arrange for a visit from a laryngectomee (a person who has had a laryngectomy).

DYSPHAGIA AND RISK FOR ASPIRATION
- Aspiration is not a problem for the patient who has had a total laryngectomy and a permanent tracheostomy.
- Observe the patient who has had a subtotal, vertical, or supraglottic laryngectomy for aspiration.

- Use these precautions for the patient with a feeding tube in place:
  1. Elevate the head of the bed 30 to 40 degrees.
  2. Strictly adhere to tube-feeding procedure.
  3. Check residual volume before each bolus feeding (or every 4 hours with continuous feeding and abdominal assessment).
  4. Evaluate the patient's tolerance of the tube feeding.
  5. If residual volume is high for 2 consecutive hours (i.e., > 200-250 mL), withhold the feeding and notify the physician.

❗NURSING SAFETY PRIORITY: Action Alert

Do not provide continuous enteral feedings any time the patient must be in a flat, supine position; maintain back rest elevation at 30 to 45 degrees.

- Use these precautions to prevent aspiration when feeding the patient or assisting him or her with eating:
  1. Avoid having meals when the patient is fatigued.
  2. Provide smaller and more frequent meals.
  3. Provide adequate time; do not hurry the patient.
  4. Provide close supervision if the patient is self-feeding.
  5. Keep emergency suctioning equipment close at hand and turned on.
  6. Avoid water and other "thin" liquids.
  7. Thicken all liquids, including water.
  8. Avoid foods that generate thin liquids during the chewing process, such as fruit.
  9. Position the patient in the most upright position possible.
  10. When present, completely (or at least partially) deflate the tracheal tube cuff during meals.
  11. Suction before and after initial cuff deflation to clear the airway and allow maximum comfort during the meal.
  12. Feed each bite or encourage the patient to take each bite slowly.
  13. Encourage the patient to "dry swallow" after each bite to clear residue from the throat.
  14. Avoid consecutive swallows of liquids.
  15. Provide controlled small volumes of liquids using a spoon.
  16. Encourage the patient to "tuck" his or her chin down and forward while swallowing.
  17. Allow the patient to indicate when he or she is ready for the next bite.
  18. If the patient coughs, stop the feeding until the patient indicates the airway has been cleared.

19. Continuously monitor tolerance to oral food intake by assessing respiratory rate, ease, pulse oximetry, and heart rate.

- Teach the patient the supraglottic method of swallowing:
   1. Inhaling and holding his or her breath (to close the vocal folds)
   2. Placing food or liquid in swallow position
   3. Swallowing while holding breath
   4. Coughing after swallowing and before inhaling (to clear any residue that may have entered the larynx)

ANXIETY
- Explore the reason for anxiety (e.g., fear of the unknown, lack of teaching, fear of pain, fear of airway compromise, fear of hospitalization, loss of control).
- Encourage the patient and family to express their feelings about the cancer diagnosis and uncertainty of treatment outcome.
- Dispel myths and correct misconceptions.
- Accept that different patients choose to deal with a cancer diagnosis in individual ways.
- Adjust your approach to care as the patient's emotional state changes.
- Integrate outside resources into the plan of care.
- Give prescribed antianxiety drugs.

DISTURBED BODY IMAGE
- The patient with head and neck cancer may have a permanent change in body image because of deformity, the presence of a stoma or artificial airway, speech changes, and a change in the method of eating.
- Help the patient set realistic goals, starting with involvement in self-care.
- Teach the patient alternate communication methods.
- Teach the family to ease the patient into a normal social environment.
- Use positive reinforcement and encouragement while demonstrating acceptance and caring behaviors.
- Refer the patient and family for counseling, as needed.
- Teach the patient tips for an enhanced appearance, including:
   1. The use of loose-fitting, high-collar shirts or sweaters, scarves, and jewelry to cover the laryngectomy stoma, tracheostomy tube, and other changes related to surgery
   2. The use of cosmetics to cover scars and skin disfigurement

Community-Based Care
- Ensure that the patient and family are able to perform tracheostomy or stoma care and participate in nutrition, wound care, and communication methods.

- Coordinate the efforts of the health care team in assessing the specific discharge needs and making the appropriate referrals to home care agencies.
- Coordinate the scheduling for chemotherapy or radiation therapy with the patient and family.
- Ensure that the home environment is assessed for general cleanliness, ease of patient access to toileting and living areas, need for increased humidity, and transportation.
- Teach the patient and family about:
  1. Stoma or tracheostomy or laryngectomy care
  2. Incision and airway care
  3. Safety
  4. Wearing a medical alert (Medic Alert) bracelet and carrying a special identification card
  5. Smoking cessation
  6. Community support agencies

CANCER, LUNG

OVERVIEW

- Lung cancer is a leading cause of cancer-related deaths worldwide.
- The overall 5-year survival rate for all patients with lung cancer is only 14%, because most lung cancers are diagnosed at a late stage, when metastasis is present.
- Lung cancers are classified as small cell lung carcinoma (SCLC) and non–small cell lung carcinoma (NSCLC), which includes epidermoid (squamous cell) cancer, adenocarcinoma, and large cell cancer.
- Metastasis (spread) of lung cancer occurs by direct extension, through the blood, and by invading lymph glands and vessels. Common sites of metastasis for lung cancer are the bone, liver, brain, and adrenal glands.
- Lung cancers occur as a result of repeated exposure to inhaled substances that cause chronic tissue irritation or inflammation. Cigarette smoking is the major risk factor and is responsible for 85% of all lung cancer deaths.
- Nonsmokers exposed to passive, or secondhand, smoke have a greater risk for lung cancer than nonsmokers.
- Additional environmental causes of lung cancer are chronic exposure to asbestos, beryllium, chromium, coal distillates, cobalt, iron oxide, mustard gas, petroleum distillates, radiation, tar, nickel, uranium, benzopyrone, and hydrocarbons.

<u>Genetic/Genomic Considerations</u>

- Variation is seen in lung cancer development among people exposed to similar environmental carcinogens and smoking use, suggesting that genetic factors can influence susceptibility. This variation may be the results of differences in gene products that activate carcinogens (a cancer susceptibility gene) and gene products that clear carcinogens from the body (a cancer resistance gene).
- Differences in a gene that regulates cell division, the *TP53* gene, may be the most important genetic susceptibility link for lung cancer development. Mutations in the alleles of this gene are known to increase the susceptibility to a wide variety of cancers with and without exposure to environmental risks, including lung cancer development among smokers and nonsmokers.

- Lung cancer interferes with oxygenation and tissue perfusion, including bronchial obstruction, airway compression, compression of alveoli, and compression of blood vessels.
- Common manifestations of lung cancer are associated with respiratory problems and include dyspnea, pallor or cyanosis, tachycardia, bloody sputum, and cough.
- Pain is common when lymph nodes are enlarged and press on nerves.

PATIENT-CENTERED COLLABORATIVE CARE
Assessment
- Obtain patient information about:
    1. Pack-year history and current smoking pattern
    2. Risk factors, including second-hand smoke and environmental exposures
    3. Cough, presence and triggers:
    4. Sputum:
        a. Amount
        b. Color
        c. Character
    5. Chest pain, tightness, or pressure:
        a. Location
        b. Severity
        c. Duration
        d. Quality
        e. Radiation
    6. Dyspnea:
        a. Duration
        b. Change in endurance
- Assess for pulmonary manifestations:

1. Hoarseness
2. Wheezing
3. Decreased or absent breath sounds
4. Breathing pattern abnormalities:
   a. Prolonged exhalation alternating with periods of shallow breathing
   b. Rapid, shallow breathing
5. Areas of tenderness or masses palpated on the chest wall
6. Increased fremitus (vibration) in areas of tumor
7. Decreased or absent fremitus on side with bronchial obstruction
8. Tracheal deviation
9. Pleural friction rub
10. Asymmetry of diaphragm movement
11. Use of accessory muscles
12. Retraction between ribs or at sternal notch

- Assess for nonpulmonary manifestations:
  1. Weight loss
  2. Muffled heart sounds
  3. Dysrhythmias
  4. Cyanosis of the lips and fingertips
  5. Clubbing of the fingers
  6. Bone pain
  7. Fever/chills related to pneumonitis, bronchitis, pneumonia
  8. Paraneoplastic endocrine syndromes caused by hormones secreted by tumor cells, such as syndrome of inappropriate antidiuretic hormone (SIADH).
- Assess for late manifestations, including fatigue, weight loss, anorexia, dysphagia, nausea and vomiting, lethargy, confusion, and personality changes.
- Assess for psychosocial issues of fear, anxiety, guilt, or shame:
  1. Convey acceptance; interact with patient in nonjudgmental way.
  2. Encourage the patient and family to express their feelings about the possible diagnosis of lung cancer.
- Diagnosis of lung cancer is made on the basis of:
  1. Direct examination of cancer cells obtained by biopsy
  2. Chest x-rays
  3. Computed tomography (CT) scan
  4. Fiberoptic bronchoscopy
  5. Thoracoscopy or thoracentesis
  6. Magnetic resonance imaging (MRI)
- Other tests used to determine extent of metastasis include radionuclide scans of the liver, spleen, brain, and bone and positron emission tomography (PET) scanning.

Nonsurgical Management

- Chemotherapy is often the treatment of choice for lung cancers, and it may be used alone or as adjuvant therapy in combination with surgery.
- The exact combination of drugs used depends on the response of the tumor and the overall health of the patient; however, most include platinum-based agents.
- Common side effects that occur with chemotherapy for lung cancer include:
  1. Chemotherapy-induced nausea and vomiting (CIN)
  2. Alopecia
  3. Mucositis
  4. Bone marrow suppression resulting in immunosuppression, anemia, and thrombocytopenia
  5. Peripheral neuropathy (PN)
- *Targeted therapy* is common in the treatment of later stage lung cancer and involves the use of drugs that target specific features of cancer cells, such as a protein, an enzyme, or the formation of new blood vessels. These agents are useful only for cancers that overexpress a certain protein or enzyme. These drugs cause fewer and less severe side effects for most patients compared with traditional antineoplastic agents. For lung cancer, targeted therapy drugs include:
  1. Erlotinib (Tarceva), an oral drug
  2. Bevacizumab (Avastin), which is given IV
- *Radiation therapy* may be used for locally advanced lung cancers confined to the chest. It is used in addition to surgery or chemotherapy and is most commonly given by external beam therapy daily over 5 to 6 weeks. General management issues for care of patients undergoing radiation therapy are presented in Part One under *Cancer Therapy.*
- Common side effects of radiation therapy for lung cancer are:
  1. Chest skin irritation and peeling
  2. Fatigue and taste changes
  3. Wheezing from inflamed airways
  4. Esophagitis
- *Photodynamic therapy (PDT)* may be used to remove small bronchial tumors when they are accessible by bronchoscopy. The patient is first injected with an agent that sensitizes cells to light. This drug enters all cells but leaves normal cells more rapidly than cancer cells, allowing it to concentrate in cancer cells. At about 48 hours, the patient goes to the operating room and is placed under anesthesia and intubated. A laser light is focused on the tumor. The light activates a chemical reaction

within the cells, retaining the sensitizing drug that induces irreversible cell damage. Some cells die and slough immediately; others continue to slough for several days.

- The photosensitizing drug has many effects that require special patient teaching and care both before and after the laser treatment. General management issues for care of patients undergoing PDT are presented in Part One under *Cancer Therapy.*
- When PDT is used in the airways, the patient usually requires a stay in the intensive care unit (ICU) for airway management.

Surgical Management

- Surgery is the main treatment for stage I and stage II NSCLC. Total removal of a non–small cell primary lung cancer is undertaken in hope of achieving a cure. If complete resection is not possible, the surgeon removes the bulk of the tumor.
- The specific surgery depends on the stage of the cancer and the patient's overall health and functional status. Surgeries include:
  1. Removal of the tumor only
  2. Removal of a lung segment (segmentectomy)
  3. Removal of a lobe (lobectomy)
  4. Removal of an entire lung (pneumonectomy)
- Procedures can be performed by open thoracotomy or thoracoscopy with minimally invasive surgery in selected patients.
- Provide preoperative care:
  1. Administer routine preoperative care, as described in Part One.
  2. Teach the patient about the probable location of the surgical incision or thoracoscopy openings, shoulder exercises, and about the chest tube and drainage system (except after pneumonectomy).
  3. Encourage the patient to express fears and concerns.
  4. Reinforce the surgeon's explanation of the surgical procedure.
- Provide postoperative care, as described in Part One:
  1. Respiratory management:
     a. Maintain a patent airway.
     b. Assess respiratory status at least every 2 hours for the first 12 to 24 hours:
        (1) Check the alignment of the trachea.
        (2) Assess oxygen saturation.
        (3) Assess the rate and depth of respiration.
        (4) Listen to breath sounds in all remaining lobes.
        (5) Assess the oral mucous membranes for cyanosis and the nail beds for rate of capillary refill.
     c. Perform oral suctioning as necessary.

  d. Provide oxygen therapy or mechanical ventilation as prescribed
  e. Assist the patient to a semi-Fowler's position or to sit up in a chair as soon as possible.
  f. For a patient with spontaneous respirations, encourage the patient to use the incentive spirometer every hour while awake.
  g. If coughing is permitted, help the patient cough by splinting any incision and ensuring that the chest tube does not pull with movement.
2. Pain management
3. Apply closed chest drainage (see *Closed Chest Drainage* and *The Patient Requiring Chest Tubes* in Appendix 8, The Patient Requiring Intubation and Ventilation).

Palliative Interventions

- Treatment may focus on symptom management, rather than cure.
- Dyspnea management is needed, because the patient with lung cancer tires easily and is often most comfortable resting in a semi-Fowler's position. Dyspnea is reduced with oxygen, drug therapy, radiation, management of pleural effusion, pain relief, and positioning for comfort. For example, the patient with severe dyspnea may be most comfortable sitting in a lounge chair or reclining chair.
- Oxygen therapy with humidification is prescribed to treat hypoxemia or to relieve dyspnea and anxiety.
- Drug therapy to improve oxygenation and relieve dyspnea includes:
  1. Bronchodilators and corticosteroids for the patient with bronchospasm
  2. Mucolytics to ease removal of thick mucus and sputum
  3. Antibiotics when bacterial infection is present
- Radiation therapy helps relieve hemoptysis, obstruction of the bronchi and great veins, dysphagia, and pain resulting from bone metastasis. Usually, radiation for palliation schedules higher doses for shorter periods than curative regimens. Complications are the same as those occurring with radiation therapy for cure.
- Thoracentesis and pleurodesis relieve pulmonary symptoms caused by pleural effusion.
  1. *Thoracentesis* is fluid removal by suction from the placement of a large needle or catheter into the intrapleural space.
  2. *Pleurodesis* is the deliberate development of an inflammation in the pleural space to cause the pleura to stick to the chest wall and prevent formation of effusion fluid. Agents

such as liquid sclerosing chemicals or talc are instilled in the chest by thoracentesis after the effusion fluid has been removed.

- Pain management may be needed for chest pain and pain radiating to the arm. The goal is to keep the patient as comfortable as possible.
  1. Morphine and related opioids relieve symptoms of dyspnea while also treating pain. Oral, parenteral, or transdermal preparations are all potentially effective.
  2. Analgesics are given around-the-clock and PRN (for breakthrough pain).
  3. Additional nonpharmacologic measures may include positioning, hot or cold compresses, distractions, and guided imagery.
  4. Perform ongoing pain assessment, as described in Part One.
  5. Evaluate the patient's response to the management strategies and collaborate with the health care team to make adjustments as necessary for improved patient comfort.
- Refer the terminal patient to hospice or other palliative care programs.
- Refer the family to the American Cancer Society and other community agencies as needed for support groups or the use of home care equipment.

CANCER, OVARIAN

OVERVIEW
- Ovarian cancer is the leading cause of death from female reproductive cancers.
- Most ovarian cancers are epithelial tumors that form on the surface of the ovaries.
- These tumors grow rapidly, spread quickly, and are often bilateral.
- Ovarian cancers metastasize by direct extension into nearby organs and through blood and lymph circulation to distant sites. Free-floating cancer cells also spread through the abdomen to seed new sites, usually accompanied by ascites.
- Women who have a mutation in the BRCA1 or BRCA2 genes are at high risk for developing ovarian cancer over their lifetime, although the actual number of women with these genes is relatively small.
- Survival rates are low, because ovarian cancer is so often not detected until its late stages.

PATIENT-CENTERED COLLABORATIVE CARE
Assessment
- Obtain patient information about risk factors for ovarian cancer:
  1. Family history of ovarian or breast cancer or hereditary non-polyposis colorectal cancer (HNPCC)
  2. Diabetes mellitus
  3. Nulliparity or infertility
  4. Older than 30 years at first pregnancy
  5. Personal history of breast or colorectal cancer
  6. *BRCA1* or *BRCA2* gene mutations
  7. Early menarche or late menopause
  8. Endometriosis
  9. Obesity or high-fat diet
- Ask the patient about manifestations of ovarian cancer:
  1. Abdominal pain, swelling, or bloating
  2. Vague GI disturbances such as dyspepsia (indigestion) and gas
  3. Urinary frequency or incontinence
  4. Unexpected weight loss
  5. Vaginal bleeding
- Assess for complications of metastatic cancer:
  1. Pleural effusion
  2. Ascites
  3. Lymphedema
  4. Intestinal obstruction
  5. Malnutrition
- Diagnosis and staging are performed by surgical exploration and biopsy analysis.
- Other assessment techniques helpful in staging the cancer and monitoring therapy progress include the CA-125 cancer antigen test, transvaginal ultrasonography, chest x-ray, and computed tomography (CT).

Interventions
- Nursing care of the patient with ovarian cancer is similar to that for endometrial or cervical cancer.
- Treatment options depend on the extent of the cancer and usually include surgery first, followed by chemotherapy. Radiation therapy is used for more widespread cancers.
  #### Surgical Management
- Total abdominal hysterectomy and bilateral salpingo-oophorectomy (BSO) are the surgical procedures for all stages of ovarian cancer.
- When cancer has spread to other abdominal organs or lymph nodes, the tumors can be removed during the surgery.

- After surgery, nursing care is similar to that of the patient undergoing a hysterectomy for uterine leiomyomas or care for the postoperative abdominal surgery patient and includes general postoperative care.

Nonsurgical Management

- For all stages of ovarian cancer, chemotherapy using cytotoxic drugs may be used. Drugs may include cisplatin (Platinol), carboplatin, and paclitaxel (Taxol). They may be given IV or intraperitoneally.

CANCER, PANCREATIC

OVERVIEW

- Pancreatic tumors are highly malignant and originate in the epithelial cells of the pancreatic ductal system.
- Primary tumors usually are adenocarcinomas and grow in well-defined, glandular patterns.
- These cancers grow rapidly and spread to surrounding organs (stomach, duodenum, gallbladder, and intestine) by direct extension and invasion of the lymphatic and vascular system.
- Pancreatic cancer may also result from metastasis from cancer of the lung, breast, thyroid, or kidney or from skin melanoma.
- Most pancreatic cancers are not diagnosed until the disease is advanced, and the overall survival rate is low.

PATIENT-CENTERED COLLABORATIVE CARE

Assessment

- Obtain patient information about:
  1. Jaundice (yellow discoloration) and pruritus (itching)
  2. Clay-colored stool and dark, frothy urine
  3. Abdominal pain described as a vague, constant dullness in the upper abdomen and nonspecific in nature; pain related to eating or activity; or back pain
  4. Weight loss (unplanned)
  5. Anorexia accompanied by early satiety, nausea, flatulence, and vomiting
- Assess for:
  1. High blood glucose levels
  2. Splenomegaly
  3. GI bleeding
  4. Leg or calf pain (from thrombophlebitis)
  5. Fatigue and weakness
  6. Dull sound on abdominal percussion indicating ascites

- Diagnostic assessment may include:
  1. Elevated levels of serum amylase, serum lipase, alkaline phosphatase, and bilirubin
  2. Elevated level of carcinoembryonic antigen (CEA)
  3. Elevated levels of serum markers: CA-19-9 and CA-242
  4. Abdominal ultrasound or computed tomography (CT)
  5. Endoscopic retrograde cholangiopancreatography (ERCP)
  6. Aspiration of pancreatic ascitic fluid

Interventions

- Management of the patient with pancreatic cancer is geared toward preventing tumor spread and decreasing pain. These measures are palliative, not curative. The cancers are often metastatic and recur despite treatment.

  Nonsurgical Management
- Drug therapy includes:
  1. High doses of opioid analgesia; dependency is not a consideration because of the poor prognosis
  2. Chemotherapy, which has limited success:
     a. Specific treatment regimens and drug combinations vary, but the most commonly used agents for pancreatic cancer include 5-fluorouracil (5-FU), gemcitabine (Gemzar), capecitabine (Xeloda), and docetaxel (Taxotere).
     b. General management issues for care of patients undergoing chemotherapy are presented in Part One under *Cancer Therapy.*
  3. Targeted therapy for pancreatic cancer may include erlotinib (Tarceva).
- *External beam radiation therapy* to shrink pancreatic tumor cells, alleviating obstruction and improving food absorption, may provide pain relief but has not increased survival rates.
- Implantation of radon seeds in combination with systemic or intra-arterial administration of floxuridine (FUDR) has also been used.
- Biliary stents may be inserted to relieve biliary obstruction.

  Surgical Management
- Surgery is the most effective form of management for pancreatic cancer.
- The classic surgery, the Whipple procedure, entails extensive surgical manipulation, including resection of the proximal head of the pancreas, the duodenum, a portion of the jejunum, the stomach (partial or total gastrectomy), and the gallbladder, with anastomosis of the pancreatic duct (pancreatojejunostomy), the common bile duct (choledochojejunostomy), and the stomach (gastrojejunostomy) to the jejunum. The spleen may also be removed (splenectomy). This surgery may be performed by the

traditional open abdominal method or by laparoscopic minimally invasive surgery (in select cancers).

- Palliative measures to relieve obstruction, such as cholecystojejunostomy, may be performed as a bypass procedure.
- Preoperative care and monitoring includes:
  1. Inserting the nasogastric (NG) tube for decompression
  2. Starting IV fluids or total parenteral nutrition to improve the patient's nutritional status before surgery
- Postoperative care and monitoring includes:
  1. Providing routine postoperative care as described in Part One
  2. Monitoring the drainage tubes placed during surgery to remove drainage and secretions from the area and to prevent stress on the anastomosis site
  3. Assessing the tubes and drainage devices for undue stress or kinking and maintaining tubes in a dependent position
  4. Monitoring drainage for color, consistency, and amount
  5. Observing for fistula formation (drainage of pancreatic fluids is corrosive and irritating to the skin, internal leakage causes peritonitis)
  6. Placing the patient in a semi-Fowler's position to reduce stress on the incision and anastomosis and to optimize lung expansion
  7. Maintaining fluid and electrolyte balance
  8. Closely monitoring vital signs for decreased blood pressure and increased heart rate, decreased vascular pressures, decreased hemoglobin and hematocrit levels, and electrolyte imbalances
  9. Assessing blood glucose levels for transient hyperglycemia or hypoglycemia resulting from surgical manipulation of the pancreas
  10. Monitoring the patient for pitting edema of the extremities and dependent edema in the sacrum and back
- Enteral feeding with a commercially prepared tube feeding is used while intestinal function is intact. A jejunostomy tube is inserted for late stages of pancreatic carcinoma; this method is preferred for lessening reflux and facilitating absorption.
- Hyperalimentation by TPN to optimize nutrition may be used as a single measure or in combination with tube feedings; a Hickman or other type of tunneled catheter may be required for long-term use.

Community-Based Care

- Many of the care measures are palliative and aimed at providing symptom relief.

CANCER, PROSTATE

OVERVIEW

- Prostate cancer is one of the most common types of cancer and men over 65 years old have the greatest risk for prostate cancer.
- Most prostate tumors are adenocarcinomas arising from epithelial cells located in the posterior lobe or outer portion of the gland, and most are androgen-sensitive (need testosterone to grow).
- These cancers are usually slow-growing and metastasize first into nearby lymph nodes and then to bones of the pelvis, sacrum, and lumbar spine.
- In advanced stages of the disease, additional metastatic sites may include the lungs, liver, adrenals, and kidneys.
- In some men, prostate tissue grows very rapidly, leading to noncancerous, high-grade prostatic intraepithelial neoplasia (HGPIN), creating a high risk for developing more aggressive prostate cancer.
- Many men with prostate cancer can be cured of the disease, and others may live 10 years or more with the disease.

Genetic/Genomic Considerations

Many gene mutations play a role in various types of prostate cancer. Some men with the most aggressive prostate cancers have *BCRA2* mutations similar to those in women who have *BCRA2*-associated breast and ovarian cancers. The most common genetic factor that increases the risk of prostate cancer is a mutation in the glutathione S-transferase (*GSTP1*) gene. This gene is normally part of the pathway that helps to prevent cancer.

PATIENT-CENTERED COLLABORATIVE CARE

Assessment

- Obtain patient information about:
  1. Age
  2. Race and ethnicity
  3. Family history of cancer
  4. Nutritional habits
  5. Problems with urination
     a. Difficulty in starting urination
     b. Frequent bladder infections
     c. Urinary retention
  6. Pain during intercourse, especially when ejaculating
  7. Any other pain (particularly bone pain)

- Assess for:
  1. Gross blood in the urine (hematuria)
  2. Pain in the pelvis, spine, hips, or rib
  3. Swollen lymph nodes, especially in the groin areas
- Assess for psychosocial issues:
  1. Anxiety, fear, and/or depression
  2. Assess the reaction of the patient to the diagnosis and ob-
     serve how his family or significant others react to the illness.
  3. Determine what support systems the patient has, such as
     family, spiritual leaders, or community group support, to
     help him through diagnosis, treatment, and recovery.
  4. Refer the patient with concerns related to sexuality and erec-
     tile dysfunction to his surgeon (urologist), sex therapist, or
     intimacy therapist, if available.
- Diagnostic assessment for cancer and metastasis may include:
  1. Digital rectal examination (DRE). A prostate that is found to
     be stony hard and have palpable irregularities or indurations
     is suspected to be malignant.
  2. Elevated levels of complexed prostate-specific antigen
     (cPSA) (greater than 3.4 ng/mL)
  3. Elevated levels of serum acid phosphatase
  4. Transrectal ultrasound (TRUS) of the prostate
  5. Prostate tissue biopsy
  6. Lymph node biopsy
  7. Computed tomography (CT) scan of the pelvis and
     abdomen
  8. Magnetic resonance imaging (MRI)

■ NURSING SAFETY PRIORITY: Action alert

Prostate-specific antigen (PSA) analysis should never be used as
a screening test without a DRE. Because other prostate problems
also increase the PSA level, it is not specifically diagnostic for
cancer, and some patients with prostate cancer have PSA levels
less than 4 ng/mL. The PSA should be drawn before the DRE is
performed, because the examination can increase the PSA level
as a result of prostate irritation.

Planning and Implementation

- Patients are faced with several treatment options, depending
  on the stage of the disease and their overall health. A urologist
  and an oncologist are needed to help them make the best
  decision.
- Because prostate cancer is slow-growing with late metastasis, older
  men who are asymptomatic and have an other illness may

choose observation without immediate active treatment, an option known as *watchful waiting*, or *expectant therapy.*
- Active treatment options are classified as local and systemic therapies. Local therapies include surgery and radiation. A variety of drugs is used for systemic therapy. Specific management is based on the extent of the disease and the patient's physical condition.

Surgical Management
- Surgery is the most common intervention for a cure. Minimally invasive surgery (MIS) or an open surgical technique for radical prostatectomy (prostate removal) is most often performed. Other surgeries for palliation may include:
  1. Transurethral resection of the prostate (TURP) to promote urination
  2. Bilateral orchiectomy (removal of both testicles) to slow the spread of cancer by removing the main source of testosterone
- *Laparoscopic radical prostatectomy (LRP)* is an MIS for cure of patients who have a PSA less than 10 ng/mL and who have had no previous hormone therapy or abdominal surgeries.
- *Traditional open radical prostatectomy* can be performed through a retropubic or perineal approach, but the retropubic method is done most often to preserve perineal nerves needed for penile erection.
- Provide preoperative care, including:
  1. Routine preoperative care, as described in Part One
  2. Teaching the patient about the probable location of the surgical incision, the use of an indwelling urinary catheter, placement of drains, and the possibility of temporary erectile dysfunction (ED)
- Provide postoperative care, including:
  1. Routine postoperative care, as described in Part One
  2. Encouraging the patient to use patient-controlled analgesia (PCA), as needed
  3. Helping the patient to get out of bed and into a chair on the night of surgery and to ambulate the next day
  4. Keeping an accurate record of intake and output, including drainage device drainage
  5. Keeping the urinary meatus clean using soap and water
  6. Avoiding rectal procedures or treatments
  7. Emphasizing the importance of not straining during bowel movement and advising the patient to avoid suppositories or enemas
  8. Reminding the patient about the importance of follow-up appointments with the physician to monitor progress

Nonsurgical Management

- Nonsurgical management is usually an adjunct to surgery but may be done as an alternative intervention if the cancer is widespread or the patient's condition or age prevents surgery.
- External or internal radiation therapy may be used in the treatment of prostate cancer or for palliation of late-stage symptoms.
  1. *External beam radiation therapy (EBRT)* comes from a source outside the body. Patients are usually treated 5 days each week for 6 to 9 weeks.
  2. Complications of EBRT may include:
     a. Erectile dysfunction
     b. Acute radiation cystitis
     c. Radiation proctitis
  3. *Internal radiation therapy (brachytherapy)* can be delivered by implanting low-dose radiation seeds directly into and around the prostate gland.
  4. General management issues for care of patients undergoing radiation therapy are presented in Part One under *Cancer Therapy.*
- Hormone therapy is often used for prostate tumors, because many are hormone-dependent, and these tumors can be reduced or have their growth slowed through androgen deprivation. Manipulating the patient's hormones may be accomplished in two ways:
  1. The testosterone influence can be removed by a bilateral orchiectomy (surgery).
  2. Luteinizing hormone-releasing hormone (LH-RH) agonists or antiandrogens (drugs) can be given.
  3. Side effects of hormone therapy may include:
     a. Hot flashes
     b. Gynecomastia (breast development)
- *Systemic cytotoxic chemotherapy* is an option for patients whose cancer has spread and for whom other therapies have not worked.
  1. Specific treatment regimens and drug combinations vary, but the most commonly used agents for prostate cancer include docetaxel (Taxotere), cisplatin (Platinol), and etoposide (VP-16, VePesid).
  2. General management issues for care of patients undergoing chemotherapy are presented in Part One under *Cancer Therapy.*
- *Cryotherapy (cryoablation)* is a minimally invasive procedure for patients whose disease is known to be confined to the prostate

gland. Transrectal cryoprobes are positioned around the prostate gland. Liquid nitrogen freezes the gland and results in prostate cell death.

Community-Based Care

- Include the patient's sexual partner in any teaching and discharge planning.
- Assess and address the patient's physical and psychosocial needs before hospital discharge and ensure their continued management in the community setting.
- Home care management of the patient after a radical prostatectomy includes:
  1. Collaborating with the case manager to coordinate the efforts of various health care providers, surgical unit nursing staff, and possibly a home care nurse
  2. Ensuring continuity of care during the weeks or months of therapies
  3. Health teaching about:
     a. Indwelling urinary catheter care if recovering from an open procedure, including:
        (1) Caring for the catheter
        (2) Using a leg bag
        (3) Identifying manifestations of urinary infection and other complications
     b. Determine restriction for activity or weight lifting. Restrictions may be as brief as 2 to 3 days for minimally invasive procedures and as long as 6 weeks for open surgical procedures.
     c. Kegel perineal exercises may reduce the severity of urinary incontinence after radical prostatectomy. Teach the patient to contract and relax the perineal and gluteal muscles
     d. Teach the patient to avoid straining at defecation.
     e. Teach the patient how to inspect the incision site daily for signs of infection.
     f. Stress the importance of keeping follow-up appointments.
- Refer the patient and partner to agencies or support groups, many of which can be found on the Internet through respected cancer organizations or government sites. Other personal and community support services, such as spiritual leaders or churches and synagogues, are also important to many patients.
- Refer men with ED to a specialist who can help with this problem.
- Refer patients with urinary incontinence to a urologist who specializes in this area.

CANCER, UROTHELIAL (BLADDER)

OVERVIEW

- Urothelial cancers are malignant tumors of the urothelium, which is the lining of transitional cells in the kidney, renal pelvis, ureters, urinary bladder, and urethra.
- Most urothelial cancers occur in the bladder; the term *bladder cancer* is the general term used to describe this condition.
- Most bladder cancers are transitional cell carcinomas of the bladder and are treated with surgical excision and chemotherapy. Chemotherapy is commonly instilled into the bladder and may require additional patient teaching about safe use of toilets for family members.
- New surgical techniques are being used to divert urine flow, including construction of a neobladder, to improve function of patients who have their bladder removed as part of cancer treatment.
- If the cancer is untreated, the tumor cells invade surrounding tissues, the cancer spreads to distant sites (liver, lung, and bone), and the condition ultimately leads to death.
- Causes of urothelial cancers include tobacco use; exposure to chemicals used in the hairdressing, rubber, paint, electric cable, and textile industries; *Schistosoma haematobium* (a parasite) infection; excessive use of drugs containing phenacetin; and long-term use of cyclophosphamide (Cytoxan, Procytox ✦).

PATIENT-CENTERED COLLABORATIVE CARE

Assessment

- Obtain patient information about:
  1. Age and gender
  2. Patient's perception of general health
  3. Active and passive exposure to cigarette smoke
  4. Occupation
  5. Description of change in color, frequency, amount of urine
  6. Presence of any abdominal discomfort
  7. Presence of dysuria, frequency, or urgency
- Assess:
  1. Overall appearance of the patient, especially skin color and general nutritional status
  2. Abdomen for asymmetry, tenderness, and bladder distention
  3. Urine for color, clarity, presence of blood (first sign of bladder cancer)
  4. Anxiety or fear
  5. Patient's methods of coping and the degree of support from family members

- Diagnostic assessment includes:
  1. Urinalysis
  2. Cystoscopy with retrograde urography
  3. Biopsy of visible bladder tumor
  4. Excretory urography
  5. Computed tomography (CT) scans
  6. Ultrasonography
  7. MRI for deep, invasive tumors

Interventions

Nonsurgical Management

- Prophylactic immunotherapy with intravesical instillation of bacille Calmette-Guérin (BCG) is used to prevent recurrence of superficial bladder cancers.
- Multiagent chemotherapy is successful in prolonging life after distant metastasis has occurred but rarely results in a cure.
- Radiation therapy is also useful in prolonging life.

Surgical Management

- The type of surgery for bladder cancer depends on the type and stage of the cancer and the patient's general health.
- Transurethral resection of the bladder tumor (TURBT) or partial cystectomy is performed for small, early, superficial tumors, and only a portion of the bladder is removed.
- Complete bladder removal (cystectomy) with additional removal of surrounding muscle and tissue offers the best chance of a cure for large, invasive bladder cancers. The ureters are diverted into one of several types of collecting reservoirs or a ureterostomy. The common types of alternative bladders are ileal conduit, continent pouch, bladder reconstruction (also known as *neobladder*), and ureterosigmoidostomy.
  1. *Ureterostomy* (or a *ureteroureterostomy*) results in the ureters placed on the skin surface as one or two stomas that drain urine into an external pouching system. This system is now less common.
  2. *Ileal conduit* results in the ureters surgically placed in the ileum, which is brought to the skin surface as a stoma. Urine is collected in a pouch on the skin around the stoma.
  3. *Ureterosigmoidostomy* results in the ureters surgically placed into a specially constructed segment of the sigmoid colon. No external pouching is needed.
  4. *Continent pouches* (e.g., Kock's pouch) are internal pouches constructed from an ileal segment. Although these pouches open to the outside of the abdomen, a fold prevents urine leakage. Urine is drained with intermittent catheterization, and an external pouch is not needed.

  5. *Neobladder* is reconstruction of the bladder from bowel tissue and connecting it to the urethra. Many patients learn to control voiding from the neobladder and neither external pouching nor intermittent catheterization is needed.
- Provide preoperative care, including:
  1. Implementing routine preoperative care, as presented in Part One
  2. Reinforcing the surgeon's explanation of the procedure
  3. Ensuring educational counseling about the specific urinary diversion and postoperative care requirements for self-care practices, methods of pouching, control of urine drainage, and management of odor
  4. Coordinating with the surgeon and enterostomal therapist (ET) for selection of the stoma
  5. Explore psychosocial concerns, including those about altered body image, sexuality, fear, and uncertainty.
- Provide postoperative care, including:
  1. Implementing routine postoperative care, as described in Part One
  2. Monitoring urine output and urine characteristics
  3. Working with the ET to focus care on the wound, the skin, and urinary drainage
  4. Managing external pouching systems for patients with cutaneous ureterostomy or ureteroureterostomy
  5. Managing the Penrose drain and plastic Medena catheter for patients who have had construction of a continent reservoir
  6. Performing initial irrigation and intermittent catheterization of the neobladder
  7. Teaching the patient with a neobladder how to use new cues to know when to void, such as voiding at prescribed times or noticing a feeling of neobladder pressure

Community-Based Care
- Provide health teaching to the patient and family about:
  1. Drugs, diet and fluid therapy, the use of external pouching systems, and the technique for catheterizing a continent reservoir
  2. Electrolyte replacement
  3. Avoiding foods that are known to produce gas (if the urinary diversion uses the intestinal tract)
  4. External pouch application, local skin care, pouch care, methods of adhesion, and drainage mechanisms
  5. Intermittent catheterization (with a continent reservoir)
- Assist the patient to prepare for the impact of urinary diversion on self-image, body image, sexual functioning, and self-esteem.

- Discuss issues related to sexuality.
- Refer patients and families to community support and information organizations such as the United Ostomy Association; the American Cancer Society; and the Wound, Ostomy, and Continence Nurses Society.

CARDIAC VALVE DISEASE

See *Stenosis* and *Regurgitation*.

CARDITIS, RHEUMATIC (RHEUMATIC ENDOCARDITIS)

- *Rheumatic carditis (rheumatic endocarditis)* is a sensitivity response that develops after an infection with group A beta-hemolytic streptococci.
- Inflammation is evident in all layers of the heart and results in impaired contractile function of the myocardium, thickening of the pericardium, and inflamed endocardium, leading to valvular damage.
- Common manifestations include:
  1. Symptoms of streptococcal infection, leading to endocarditis
     a. Evidence of an existing streptococcal infection: fever, sore throat, tachycardia, and elevated serum findings of antideoxyribonuclease B titer, antistreptolysin O titer, complement assay, C-reactive protein
     b. New-onset murmur, pericardial friction rub, precordial pain, and/or extreme fatigue
     c. Acute electrocardiogram (ECG) changes indicating pericarditis
  2. Symptoms of cardiac scarring and cardiac valve disease after acute infection or recurrent infection.
  3. Cardiomegaly
  4. Development of a new murmur or change in existing murmur
  5. ECG changes such as prolonged PR interval or left ventricular hypertrophy
  6. Symptoms of heart failure
- Treatment includes:
  1. Giving antibiotics, usually penicillin or erythromycin (Eryc, Erythromid) with strep infection
  2. Managing fever by maintaining hydration, administering antipyretics
  3. Encouraging the patient to obtain adequate rest with cardiac dysfunction

4. Teaching the patient that antibiotic prophylaxis to prevent infective endocarditis is considered for dental and invasive procedures throughout life, although it is not always prescribed

CARDIOMYOPATHY

OVERVIEW

- Cardiomyopathy is a subacute or chronic heart muscle disease of unknown cause.
- Cardiomyopathy is divided into four categories on the basis of abnormalities in structure and function:
  1. *Dilated cardiomyopathy (DCM),* the most common type, involves extensive damage to the myofibrils and interference with myocardial metabolism; it is characterized by dilation of both ventricles and impairment of systolic function.
  2. Asymmetric ventricular hypertrophy and disarray of the myocardial fibers are cardinal features of *hypertrophic cardiomyopathy (HCM).* Left ventricular (LV) hypertrophy leads to a stiff left ventricle that results in diastolic filling abnormalities. In about 50% of patients, HCM is transmitted as a single-gene autosomal dominant trait.
  3. *Restrictive cardiomyopathy (RCM),* the least common of the four cardiomyopathies, results in restriction of filling of the ventricles. It is caused by endocardial or myocardial disease and produces a clinical picture similar to that of constrictive pericarditis.
  4. *Arrhythmogenic right ventricular (ARV) cardiomyopathy* is a condition that results from replacement of myocardial tissue with fibrous and fatty tissue, usually as a familial condition.
- Sudden death may be the first and only manifestation of cardiomyopathy.

PATIENT-CENTERED COLLABORATIVE CARE

Assessment

- Assess for clinical manifestations of DCM:
  1. Signs of left ventricular failure at onset of disease, progressing to biventricular failure (see Heart Failure on p. 349)
  2. Progressive dyspnea on exertion
  3. Orthopnea
  4. Palpitations
  5. Activity intolerance
  6. Atrial fibrillation

- Assess for clinical manifestations of HCM:
  1. Exertional dyspnea
  2. Angina
  3. Syncope
  4. Atypical chest pain that occurs at rest, is prolonged, has no relation to exertion, and is not relieved by nitrates
  5. Ventricular dysrhythmias
- Assess for clinical manifestations of RCM:
  1. Exertional dyspnea
  2. Weakness
  3. Exercise intolerance
  4. Palpitations
  5. Syncope
- Assess of clinical manifestations of ARV cardiomyopathy:
  1. Dizziness, syncope or palpitations, particularly with aerobic effort
  2. Irregular pulse, abnormal conduction with ECG

Interventions
Nonsurgical Management
- Care of the patient with cardiomyopathy is similar to that for patients with heart failure (see *Heart Failure*) and dysrhythmias.
- Treatment includes:
  1. Administering an angiotensin-converting enzyme inhibitor or angiotensin receptor blocker and a beta blocker to block the neurohormonal contributions to cardiomyopathy. Diuretics, vasodilators, and cardiac glycosides may be used as substitutes or as adjuncts as the disease progresses.
  2. Anticipating procedure to implant automatic cardiac defibrillator to promote synchronous ventricular emptying and control ventricular dysrhythmias
  3. Teaching the patient to abstain from alcohol because of its cardiac depressant effects
  4. Teaching the patient to report any palpitations, dizziness, or fainting that may indicate a dysrhythmia
- Management of HCM includes beta-adrenergic blocking agents (carvedilol); strenuous exercise is prohibited.
Surgical Management
- The type of surgery performed depends on the type of cardiomyopathy.
- The most commonly performed surgery for HCM is excision of a portion of the hypertrophied ventricular septum to create a widened outflow tract.
- Cardiomyoplasty is used when cardiac transplantation is not an option and the patient is asymptomatic at rest.

- Heart transplantation is the treatment of choice for patients with severe DCM; a donor heart from a person of comparable body weight and ABO compatibility is transplanted into a recipient within 6 hours of procurement.
- Criteria for candidates for heart transplantation include:
  1. Life expectancy less than 1 year
  2. Age younger than 65 years (variable)
  3. New York Heart Association Class III or IV (poor functional status)
  4. Normal or only slightly increased pulmonary vascular resistance
  5. Absence of active infection
  6. Stable psychosocial status
  7. No evidence of drug or alcohol abuse
- Nursing interventions include:
  1. Providing postoperative care similar to that provided for patients having open heart surgery (see surgical management of *Coronary Artery Disease*)
  2. Monitoring carefully for occult bleeding into the pericardial sac with the potential for cardiac tamponade
  3. Teaching the patient to change positions slowly because of the potential of orthostatic hypotension
  4. Monitoring the patient closely for infection and respiratory distress
  5. Maintaining invasive hemodynamic monitoring devices safely and effectively during evaluation and while awaiting transplant
- Provide discharge teaching:
  1. Teach the patient to report signs and symptoms of rejection, such as hypotension, dysrhythmias, weakness, fatigue, dizziness, respiratory distress, weight gain, or edema (initial episode of acute rejection usually occurs in the first 3 months after transplantation).
  2. Inform the patient that the surgeon will perform endomyocardial biopsy at regularly scheduled intervals to detect rejection.
  3. Teach the patient the importance of taking immunosuppressants for life to prevent transplant rejection.
  4. Encourage the patient to follow a lifestyle similar to that of patients with coronary artery disease.
  5. Encourage the patient to participate in an exercise program, allowing at least 10 minutes of warm-up and cool-down for the denervated heart to adjust to changes in activity level.
  6. Provide information about discharge drugs and diet.

⚠ NURSING SAFETY SRIORITY: Action Alert

Avoid fluid overload in patients with cardiomyopathy, and use daily weights to assess fluid balance. A gain of 1 kg is equivalent to an extra liter of fluid.

CARPAL TUNNEL SYNDROME

C

OVERVIEW

- Carpal tunnel syndrome (CTS) is a condition in which the median nerve in the wrist becomes compressed, causing pain and numbness.
- Risk factors include common repetitive strain injury (RSI), synovitis, excessive hand exercise, edema or hemorrhage into the carpal tunnel, or thrombosis of the median artery, Colles' fracture of the wrist, and hand burns. CTS is also a common complication of certain metabolic and connective tissue diseases.
- People at risk are those whose jobs require repetitive hand activities involving pinch or grasp during wrist flexion, such as factory workers, computer operators, and jackhammer operators.
- CTS most often occurs in women between the ages of 30 and 60 years.

PATIENT-CENTERED COLLABORATIVE CARE

Assessment

- Assess for:
  1. Nature, location, and intensity of patient-reported hand pain and numbness and whether symptoms are worse at night
  2. Presence of paresthesia (painful tingling) in the hand or hands
  3. Positive results for the Phalen maneuver, producing paresthesia in the palmar side of the thumb, index, and middle finger and radial half of the ring finger within 60 seconds (patient is asked to relax the wrist into flexion or place the back of the hands together and flex both wrists simultaneously)
  4. Positive results for the Tinel sign, which is the same response as for the Phalen maneuver, elicited by tapping lightly over the area of the median nerve in the wrist
  5. Weak pinch, clumsiness, and difficulty with fine movements that progresses to muscle weakness
  6. Muscle wasting in the affected hand
  7. Wrist swelling

   8. Autonomic changes such as skin discoloration, nail brittleness, and increased or decreased palmar sweating
- Diagnostic assessment may include any of these: standard x-rays, electromyography (EMG), magnetic resonance imaging (MRI), and ultrasonography.

Interventions

Nonsurgical Management

- Drug therapy
   1. NSAIDs
   2. Corticosteroid injections
- Wrist immobilization with a splint or brace to place the wrist in a neutral position or slight extension during the day, during the night, or both

Surgical Management

- Surgery is performed to relieve the pressure on the median nerve by providing nerve decompression through either open carpal tunnel release (OCTR) or endoscopic carpal tunnel release (ECTR).
- When CTS is a complication of rheumatoid arthritis, a synovectomy (removal of excess synovium) through a small inner wrist incision may be performed.
- Provide preoperative care, including:
   1. Reinforcing the teaching provided by the surgeon regarding the nature of the surgery
   2. Reviewing postoperative care so that the patient knows what to expect
- Provide postoperative care, including:
   1. Monitoring vital signs
   2. Checking the dressing for drainage and tightness
   3. Checking the neurovascular status of the digits every hour during the immediate postoperative period
   4. Encouraging the patient to move all fingers of the affected hand at least every hour
   5. Administering pain medication, as needed
   6. Teaching patients who have had the endoscopic procedure to keep the hand and arm elevated above heart level for several days
   7. Explaining that certain hand movements, including lifting heavy objects, may be restricted and a wrist-hand splint worn for 4 to 6 weeks after surgery
   8. Reminding the patient that weakness and discomfort may last for weeks or months
   9. Teaching the patient how to assess neurovascular status
   10. Ensuring that assistance is available in the home for routine daily tasks and ADLs

CATARACTS

OVERVIEW

- A cataract is an opacity of the lens that distorts the image projected onto the retina.
- Types of cataracts include:
  1. *Age-related cataracts,* which are most common and usually affect people older than 65 years
  2. *Traumatic cataracts* that are caused by blunt trauma to or around the eye, penetrating eye injury, and exposure to excessive heat, x-rays, ultraviolet light, or radioactive material
  3. *Toxic cataracts,* which occur after long-term exposure to drugs, such as corticosteroids, chlorpromazine, beta blockers, or miotic drugs
  4. *Associated cataracts,* which occur with other diseases, such as diabetes mellitus, hypoparathyroidism, and Down syndrome
  5. *Complicated cataracts* that develop as a complication of intraocular disease such as retinitis pigmentosa, glaucoma, and retinal detachment

PATIENT-CENTERED COLLABORATIVE CARE

Assessment

- Assess patient information about:
  1. Age
  2. Recent or past trauma to the eye
  3. Exposure to radioactive materials, x-rays, or ultraviolet light
  4. Systemic disease (e.g., diabetes mellitus, hypoparathyroidism, Down syndrome, atopic dermatitis)
  5. Prolonged use of corticosteroids, chlorpromazine, or miotic drugs
  6. Intraocular disease (e.g., recurrent uveitis)
- Ask the patient to describe his or her vision, specifically about:
  1. Blurred vision
  2. Decreased color perception
  3. Double vision
  4. Reduced visual acuity
- Assess the eye for:
  1. Loss of red reflex
  2. Presence of white pupil (late stage)

Planning and Implementation

- Surgery is the only cure for cataracts. However, patients often live with reduced vision for years before the cataract is removed. Driving privileges may be restricted or withheld during this period of reduced vision.

- Interventions for enhanced communication, safety, and independence before surgery are described later in *Visual Impairment (Reduced Vision)*. The patient with cataracts is at high risk for falls.

  Surgical Management

- The most common surgical procedure is removal of the lens by phacoemulsification and replacement with a clear plastic lens for specific vision correction.
- Provide preoperative care:
  1. Assess how the patient's vision affects ADLs, especially dressing, eating, and ambulating.
  2. Reinforce the information provided by the ophthalmologist, and teach about the nature of cataracts, their progression, and their treatment.
  3. Stress that care after surgery requires the instillation of different types of eyedrops several times each day for 2 to 4 weeks.
  4. Assess the patient's ability to evaluate eye appearance and instill eyedrops.
  5. If the patient is unable to perform these tasks, help him or her make arrangements for this care.
- Provide postoperative care:
  1. Teach him or her to wear dark glasses outdoors or in brightly lit environments until the pupil responds to light.
  2. Teach the patient and family members how to instill the prescribed eyedrops.
  3. Create a written schedule for the timing and the order of eyedrop administration.
  4. Stress the importance of keeping all follow-up appointments.
  5. Teach the patient and family about expected manifestations (mild eye itching; a "bloodshot" appearance; slightly swollen eyelid; creamy white, dry, crusty drainage on the eyelids and lashes).
  6. Suggest the use of cool compresses and a mild analgesic such as acetaminophen (Abenol ✿, Tylenol) for control of discomfort.
  7. Remind him or her to avoid aspirin because of its effects on blood clotting.
  8. Instruct the patient to notify the ophthalmologist if there is significant swelling or bruising around the eye; pain occurring with nausea or vomiting; increasing redness of the eye, a change in visual acuity, tears, and photophobia; and yellow or green drainage.

⚑ NURSING SAFETY PRIORITY: Critical Rescue

Teach the patient to report any reduction in vision immediately to the ophthalmologist.

9. Teach the patient to avoid activities that can increase intra-ocular pressure, including:
   a. Bending from the waist
   b. Lifting objects weighing more than 10 pounds (22 kg)
   c. Sneezing, coughing
   d. Blowing the nose
   e. Straining to have a bowel movement
   f. Vomiting
   g. Having sexual intercourse
   h. Keeping the head in a dependent position
   i. Wearing tight shirt collars

Community-Based Care

- If the patient has difficulty instilling eyedrops, a supportive neighbor, friend, or family member can be taught the procedure. Eyedrops are often prescribed for 2 to 4 weeks after cataract surgery.
- Remind the patient that he or she may wash his or her hair 1 or 2 days after surgery, but only with the head tilted back, such as in a beauty salon or barber shop, to avoid getting water in the eye. Teach the patient to stand in the shower with the face away from the showerhead for the first week after surgery.
- Teach the patient about activity restrictions. Cooking and light housekeeping are permitted, but vacuuming should be avoided for several weeks because of the forward flexion involved and the rapid, jerky movements required.
- Advise him or her to refrain from operating machinery and participating in certain sports, such as golf, until given specific permission from the ophthalmologist.

CELIAC DISEASE

- Celiac sprue is thought to be caused by a genetic immune hypersensitivity response to gluten or its breakdown products or to result from the accumulation of gluten in the diet with peptidase deficiency.
- Celiac disease causes a disruption to the gut mucosa and can result in inflammation and malabsorption, potentially leading to malnutrition.
- Symptoms of celiac disease are the result of malabsoption and/or malnutrition.

- Malabsorption occurs early in the condition and persists. Malabsorption symptoms include diarrhea, malodorous flatulence, abdominal bloating, and steatorrhea.
- Malnutrition symptoms occur over time when nutrients cannot be absorbed due to digestive enzyme deficiencies. Patients may have muscle weakness, anemia, osteoporosis, peripheral neuropathy, infertility, weight loss, fluid retention, easy bruising.
- The xylose absorption test can be diagnostic if malabsorption in the small intestine is present; a biopsy is performed for diagnostic confirmation.
- Gluten-free diets are available for those with celiac sprue.
- Steroids are sometimes given in celiac disease to decrease inflammation.

CEREBROVASCULAR ACCIDENT (CVA)

See *Stroke (Brain Attack)*.

CHLAMYDIAL INFECTION

OVERVIEW

- *Chlamydial trachomatis* is an intracellular bacterium that causes genital chlamydial infection, which is the most common sexually transmitted disease (STD) in the United States.
- The incubation period ranges from 1 to 3 weeks, but the pathogen may be present in the genital tract for months without producing symptoms.
- The main manifestation in men is urethritis with dysuria, frequent urination, and a watery, mucoid discharge. Complications include epididymitis, prostatitis, infertility, and reactive arthritis (also known as Reiter's syndrome).
- Many women may have no symptoms or a mucopurulent cervicitis that occurs with a change in vaginal discharge, easily induced cervical bleeding, urinary frequency, and abdominal discomfort or pain. Complications include salpingitis, pelvic inflammatory disease (PID), ectopic pregnancy, and infertility.
- Chlamydia infections are reportable to the local health department.

PATIENT-CENTERED COLLABORATIVE CARE
Assessment
- Obtain patient information about:
  1. Presence of symptoms, including vaginal or urethral discharge, dysuria (painful urination), pelvic pain, irregular bleeding

2. Any history of STDs
3. Whether sexual partners have had symptoms or a history of STDs
4. Whether patient or partner has had any unprotected intercourse

⚠ NURSING SAFETY PRIORITY: Action Alert

For men, ask about dysuria, frequent urination, and a mucoid discharge that is more watery and less copious than a gonorrheal discharge. These manifestations indicate urethritis, the main symptom of chlamydia in men.

- Diagnostic assessment requires sampling cells from the endocervix and/or urethra and laboratory testing:
  1. Gram staining (to rule out gonorrhea)
  2. Tissue culture for *Chlamydia*
  3. Gene amplification tests or DNA amplification tests (ligand chain reaction [LCR] and polymerase chain reaction [PCR])
  4. Enzyme-linked immunoassay (ELISA)
  5. Direct fluorescent antibody (DFA)

Interventions

- Antibiotic therapy provides a cure. The most common, effective antibiotic is azithromycin (Zithromax), but other agents can be used.
- Test and treat sexual partners.
- Educate patients about:
  1. The mode of disease transmission
  2. The incubation period
  3. Manifestation, including the possibility of asymptomatic infections
  4. Essential elements of treatment with antibiotic
  5. The need for abstinence from sexual intercourse until the patient and partner have completed treatment
  6. No test of cure is required, but all women should be rescreened 3 to 4 months after treatment because of the high risk for PID if reinfection occurs.
  7. The need for the patient and partner to return for evaluation if symptoms recur or new symptoms develop
  8. Possible complications of an untreated or inadequately treated infection, such as PID, ectopic pregnancy, or infertility

CHOLECYSTITIS

OVERVIEW
- Cholecystitis is an inflammation of the gallbladder that can occur as an acute or chronic process.
- Acute calculous cholecystitis usually develops in association with cholelithiasis (gallstones). About one half of the adult U.S. population has asymptomatic gallstones.
- Acalculous cholecystitis occurs in the absence of gallstones and is associated with biliary stasis caused by any condition that affects the regular filling or emptying of the gallbladder, such as decreased blood flow to the gallbladder, or anatomic problems, such as kinking of the gallbladder neck or cystic duct that can result in pancreatic enzyme reflux into the gallbladder and cause inflammation.
- Chronic cholecystitis results when repeated episodes of cystic duct obstruction result in chronic inflammation, and the gallbladder becomes fibrotic and contracted, resulting in decreased motility and deficient absorption.
- Complications of cholecystitis include pancreatitis and cholangitis (inflammation and inflection of the common bile ducts).
- Cholangitis is usually associated with choledocholithiasis (common bile duct stones).
- Jaundice (yellow discoloration of body tissues) and icterus (yellow discoloration of the sclera) can occur in acute disease but are most commonly seen in the chronic phase of cholecystitis. Jaundice results from increased bilirubin in the body that collects in the skin and sclera. Itching and a burning sensation result.

PATIENT-CENTERED COLLABORATIVE CARE
Assessment
- Record patient information:
  1. Height and weight, body mass index, and waist circumference
  2. Gender, age, race, and ethnic group
  3. Food preferences and intolerances and related GI symptoms, including flatulence, dyspepsia (indigestion), eructation (belching), anorexia, nausea, vomiting, and abdominal pain in relation to fatty food intake
  4. Exercise routine or daily activities
  5. Family history of gallbladder disease
  6. In women, history of estrogen replacement therapy
- Assess for:
  1. Abdominal pain of varying intensity in the right upper abdominal quadrant, including radiation to the right upper

shoulder; ask the patient to describe the intensity, duration, precipitating factors, and relief measures
2. Other GI symptoms, including nausea, vomiting, dyspepsia, flatulence, eructation, and feelings of abdominal heaviness
3. With right subcostal palpation, increasing pain with deep inspiration (Murphy's sign)
4. Guarding, rigidity, rebound tenderness (Blumberg's sign)
5. Sausage-shaped mass in the right upper quadrant
6. Late symptoms seen in chronic cholecystitis, such as jaundice, clay-colored stools, and dark urine
7. Steatorrhea (fatty stools)
8. Elevated temperature with tachycardia and dehydration from fever and vomiting
9. Results of serum liver enzyme and bilirubin tests (may be elevated); amylase (may be elevated if pancreas is involved
10. Increased white blood cell (WBC) count

Considerations for Older Adults

- Older adults and patients with diabetes mellitus have atypical manifestations, including the absence of pain and fever. Localized tenderness may be the only presenting sign.
- The older adult may become acutely confused.

Planning and Implementation

Nonsurgical Management

- Patients with chronic cholecystitis are encouraged to consume small-volume, low-fat meals.
- If gallstones are causing an obstruction of bile flow, fat-soluble vitamins and bile salts may be prescribed to facilitate digestion and vitamin absorption.
- Food and fluids are withheld during nausea and vomiting episodes; nasogastric (NG) decompression is initiated for severe vomiting.
- Drug therapy includes:
  1. Opioid analgesics to relieve pain and reduce spasm
  2. Antiemetics to provide relief from nausea and vomiting

Surgical Management

- A percutaneous transhepatic biliary catheter may be inserted to decompress obstructed extrahepatic ducts so bile can flow.
- An endoscopic retrograde cholangiopancreatography (ERCP) may be performed.
- Cholecystectomy (removal of the gallbladder) is the usual surgical treatment:

1. Laparoscopic laser procedure (performed more often than the traditional surgical approach)
2. Traditional open surgical approach for complicated or infected sites
   a. A T-tube drain is surgically inserted when the common bile duct is explored to ensure patency of the duct.
3. Newer techniques, such as natural orifice transluminal endoscopic surgery (NOTES), are becoming more commonly used in large tertiary care centers.

- Provide routine preoperative care.
- Provide postoperative care for laparoscopic patients:
  1. Teach the patient the importance of early ambulation to absorb the carbon dioxide that is retained in the abdomen.
  2. Inform the patient that shoulder pain is both expected and common; the pain decreases as the gases expanding the abdomen are dissipated.
  3. Inform the patient that he or she can return to usual activities 1 to 3 weeks after the procedure.
- Provide postoperative care for traditional surgery patients:
  1. Administer IV (by patient-controlled analgesia [PCA]) for pain relief, as ordered.
  2. Administer antiemetics for relief of postoperative nausea and vomiting, as ordered.
  3. Advance the diet from clear liquids to solid foods, as tolerated by the patient.
  4. Maintain the patient's T-tube:
     a. Keep the drainage system below the level of the gallbladder.
     b. Assess the amount, color, consistency, and odor of drainage (bile output is approximately 400 mL/day).
     c. Administer synthetic bile salts such as dehydrocholic acid (Decholin), as ordered.
     d. Report to the physician sudden increases or output of more than 1000 mL in 24 hours in bile output.
     e. Assess for foul odor and purulent drainage and report changes in drainage to the physician.
     f. Inspect the skin around the T-tube insertion site for signs of inflammation.
     g. Never irrigate, aspirate, or clamp the T-tube without a physician's order.
     h. Assess the drainage system for pulling, kinking, or tangling of the tubing.
     i. Place the patient in a semi-Fowler's position when in bed.

    j. Assist the patient with early ambulation.

    k. Teach patient to observe stools for brown color 7 to 10 days postoperatively.

◪NURSING SAFETY PRIORITY: Action Alert

Before the start of any invasive procedure, conduct a final verification process using active communication to confirm the correct patient, procedure, and site.

Community-Based Care

- If traditional surgery is performed, give the patient written postoperative instructions on:
  1. Inspection of the abdominal incision for redness, tenderness, swelling, and drainage
  2. Dressing change, wound care, and T-tube drain care instructions
  3. Pain management, including prescriptions
  4. Signs and symptoms of infection, including when to call the physician (elevated temperature and increased pain)
  5. Activity limitations, including avoiding lifting a weight greater than 25 pounds (11.4 kg) and restricting driving for 2 to 4 weeks
- Provide diet therapy instructions based on the patient's tolerance of fats. Instruct the patient to add one food at a time to trial tolerance and weight reduction after healing from surgery, if indicated.
- Provide information to the patient and family about the potential for postcholecystectomy syndrome, manifested by jaundice of the skin or sclera, darkened urine, light-colored stools, pain, fever, and chills.
- Refer to home health nursing if needed.

CHRONIC OBSTRUCTIVE PULMONARY DISEASE (COPD)

OVERVIEW

- Chronic obstructive pulmonary disease (COPD) is an irreversible chronic lung disease that includes both emphysema and chronic bronchitis.
- The major features of *emphysema* that lead to dyspnea are:
  1. Loss of lung elasticity
  2. Hyperinflation of the lung (air trapping)
- Emphysema is classified as panlobular, centrilobular, or paraseptal, depending on the pattern of destruction and dilation

of the gas-exchanging units (acini). Each type can occur alone or in combination in the same lung. Most are associated with smoking or chronic exposure to other inhalation irritants.

- *Bronchitis* is an inflammation of the bronchi and bronchioles caused by chronic exposure to irritants, especially tobacco smoke. It affects only the airways.
- The major features of chronic bronchitis are:
  1. Increased number and size of mucous glands, which produce large amounts of thick mucus
  2. Thickening of bronchial walls that impairs airflow
  3. Poor gas exchange with decreased Pao_2 (hypoxemia) and increased $Paco_2$ (respiratory acidosis)
- Risk factors for COPD include cigarette smoking, alpha$_1$-antitrypsin (AAT) deficiency, and air pollution.

🌐 Cultural Awareness

The prevalence of smoking remains higher among African Americans, blue collar workers, and less educated people than the overall population of the United States. Smoking prevalence is highest among northern plains American Indians and Alaskan Natives. The overall prevalence of smoking for men and women has decreased over the past 2 decades, but the decrease for women has been less than it has been for men. Development of culturally appropriate smoking cessation programs and research examining barriers to cessation in these populations may help reduce this disparity.

Genetic/Genomic Considerations

The gene for AAT has many known mutations, some of which increase the risk for emphysema. Variation of mutations (polymorphisms) results in different levels of AAT deficiency. This variation is one reason why the disease is more severe for some people than for others. The most serious mutation for an increased risk for emphysema is the Z mutation, although others also increase the risk but to a lesser degree.

- Complications of COPD include:
  1. Hypoxemia
  2. Acidosis
  3. Respiratory infection
  4. Pneumothorax
  5. Cardiac failure
  6. Dysrhythmias

PATIENT-CENTERED COLLABORATIVE CARE
Assessment

- Obtain and record patient information:
  1. Age, gender, occupational history, ethnic-cultural background, and family history
  2. Smoking history, including the length of time the patient has smoked and the number of packs smoked daily
  3. Current breathing problems:
     a. Does the patient have difficulty breathing while talking? Can he or she speak in complete sentences, or is it necessary to take a breath between every one or two words?
     b. Ask about the presence, duration, or worsening of wheezing, coughing, and shortness of breath, and what activities trigger these problems.
     c. If the cough is productive, what is the sputum color and amount, and has the amount increased or decreased?
     d. What is the relationship between activity tolerance and dyspnea? How is the patient's activity level and shortness of breath now compared with a month earlier and a year earlier? Is he or she having any difficulty with eating, sleeping, or performing ADLs?
  4. How are the patient's weight and general appearance? The patient with increasingly severe COPD is thin, with loss of muscle mass in the extremities, enlarged neck muscles, has a barrel-shaped chest, and is slow moving and slightly stooped.
- Assess for:
  1. Respiratory changes:
     a. Breathing rate and pattern, especially rapid, shallow respirations, paradoxical respirations, or use of accessory muscles
     b. Abnormal chest retractions and asymmetric chest expansion
     c. Limited diaphragmatic movement (excursion) and diaphragm position
     d. Hyperresonant chest sounds on percussion
     e. Wheezes and other abnormal sounds
     f. Degree of dyspnea using a Visual Analog Dyspnea Scale (VADS)
  2. Cardiovascular changes:
     a. Heart rate and rhythm
     b. Swelling of feet and ankles
     c. Cyanosis, or blue-tinged, dusky appearance
     d. Delayed capillary refill
     e. Clubbing of the fingers

3. Psychosocial issues:
   a. Social isolation
   b. Exposure to smoke or crowded living conditions
   c. Work, family, social, and sexual roles that may change and affect self-esteem
   d. Anxiety and fear related to dyspnea that may reduce the patient's ability to participate in a full life
   e. Patient's and family's expression of their feelings about the limitations on lifestyle and disease progression
   f. Patient's and family's awareness and use of support groups and services
4. Economic issues:
   a. The patient may not be able to work or might have had to change jobs, resulting in reduced income or changes in health insurance coverage.
   b. Drugs, especially the metered dose inhalers (MDIs) and dry powder inhalers (DPIs), are expensive, and many patients with limited incomes may use them only during exacerbations and not as prescribed.
5. Diagnostic and laboratory tests:
   a. Serial arterial blood gas (ABG) values for hypoxemia and hypercarbia
   b. Oxygen saturation by pulse oximetry
   c. Sputum cultures
   d. Hematocrit and hemoglobin for polycythemia
   e. Serum electrolyte levels for hypophosphatemia, hyperkalemia, hypocalcemia, and hypomagnesemia, which reduce muscle strength
   f. Serum AAT levels in patients with a family history of COPD
   g. Chest x-rays
   h. Pulmonary function test (PFT) changes
   i. Peak expiratory flow rates
   j. Carbon monoxide diffusion test

Planning and Implementation
HYPOXEMIA

- Hypoxemia with hypercapnia related to alveolar-capillary membrane changes, reduced airway size, ventilatory muscle fatigue, excessive mucus production, airway obstruction, diaphragm flattening, fatigue, and decreased energy

  Nonsurgical Management
- Assess breath sounds and oxygen saturation routinely as part of physical assessment and before and after interventions.
- Maintain a patent airway:
  1. Keep the patient's head, neck, and chest in alignment.
  2. Assist the patient to clear the airway of secretions.

- Position to provide lung expansion with elevated back rest, pillows, and chair-sitting.
- Monitor for changes in respiratory status in the hospitalized patient with COPD at least every 2 hours.
- Identify factors that may contribute to the increased work of breathing, such as respiratory infection.
- Interventions aim to improve the patient's breathing efforts and decrease the work of breathing. Teach breathing techniques:
  1. Diaphragmatic or abdominal breathing
  2. Pursed-lip breathing
- Enhance coughing effectiveness:
  1. Assist the patient to a sitting position with head slightly flexed, shoulders relaxed, and knees flexed.
  2. Teach the patient to take a deep breath, hold it for 2 seconds, and cough two or three times in succession.
  3. Teach the patient to follow coughing with several maximal inhalation breaths.
- Oxygen therapy:
  1. Provide oxygen as prescribed, usually a flow rate of 2 to 4 L/min by nasal cannula or up to 40% by Venturi mask.
  2. Ensure that there are no open flames or other combustion hazards in rooms where oxygen is in use.

!NURSING SAFETY PRIORITY: Critical Rescue

Assess the respiratory status of the patient with COPD who is receiving oxygen therapy at least hourly for respiratory depression. Oxygen therapy can alter the stimulus for breathing.

- Drug therapy includes:
  1. Inhaled bronchodilator drugs, such as albuterol (Proventil, Ventolin), ipratropium (Atrovent, Apo-Ipravent ✤), tiotropium (Spiriva), theophylline (Elixophyllin, Theo-Dur, Uniphyl, Theolair, many others)
  2. Inhaled or systemic anti-inflammatory drugs, such as fluticasone (Flovent), prednisone (Deltasone, Medrol)
  3. Mucolytic drugs, such as acetylcysteine (Mucosil, Mucomyst ✤) or dornase alfa (Pulmozyme)
  4. Stepped therapy for patients with chronic bronchitis or emphysema who are aware of their disease and are able to participate in symptom management
  5. Teaching patients and family members the correct techniques for using inhalers and how to care for them properly
- Pulmonary rehabilitation can improve function and endurance in patients with COPD:

1. Teach patients about the need for exercise training to prevent general and pulmonary muscle deconditioning.
2. Collaborate with the physical therapist and patient to plan an individualized exercise program.
3. Remind the patient to perform planned exercises at least two or three times each week.
4. Teach patients whose symptoms are severe to modify the exercise by using a walker with wheels or, if needed, to use oxygen therapy during the exercise period.

Surgical Management

- Lung transplantation may be performed for select patients with end-stage COPD.
- Lung reduction surgery can improve gas exchange through removal of the hyperinflated lung tissue areas that are useless for gas exchange.
- Preoperative care includes:
  1. Pulmonary rehabilitation to maximize lung and muscle function
  2. Testing with pulmonary plethysmography, gas dilution, or perfusion scans to determine the location of greatest lung hyperinflation and poorest lung blood flow
  3. Standard preoperative care and teaching, as described in Part One
- Postoperative care includes:
  1. Routine postoperative care, as described in Part One
  2. Pain management
  3. Close monitoring for continuing respiratory problems
  4. Chest tube management
  5. Maintenance of bronchodilator and mucolytic therapy
  6. Pulmonary hygiene with incentive spirometry 10 times per hour while awake, chest physiotherapy starting on the first day after surgery, and hourly pulmonary assessment

WEIGHT LOSS

- Weight loss is related to dyspnea, excessive secretions, anorexia, and fatigue.
- The patient with COPD often has food intolerance, nausea, early satiety, loss of appetite, and meal-related dyspnea.
- The increased work of breathing raises calorie and protein needs and leads to protein-calorie malnutrition.
- Malnourished patients have reduced effective breathing because of loss of total body mass, ventilatory muscle mass and strength, lung elasticity, and alveolar-capillary surface area.
- Identify patients at risk for or who have this complication and request nutritional consultation.

- Monitor patient weight and other indicators of nutrition, such as skin condition and serum prealbumin levels.
- Manage dyspnea to reduce the shortness of breath that interferes with eating.
  1. Urge the patient to rest before meals.
  2. Teach the patient to plan the biggest meal of the day for the time when he or she is most hungry and well rested. Four to six small meals each day may be preferred to three larger ones.
  3. Suggest the use of a bronchodilator 30 minutes before the meal.
- Collaborate with the patient and dietitian for food selection to prevent weight loss and improve appetite (foods that are easy to chew, high in calories and protein, and not gas-forming).
  1. Suggest dietary supplements, such as Pulmocare, that provide nutrition with reduced carbon dioxide production.
  2. If early satiety is a problem, advise the patient to minimize drinking fluids before and during meals.

ANXIETY
- Anxiety is related to dyspnea, a change in health status, and situational crisis.
- Patients with COPD often have increased anxiety during acute dyspneic episodes, especially if they feel as though they are choking on excessive secretions. Anxiety has been shown to cause dyspnea.
- Help the patient develop a written plan that states exactly what to do if symptoms flare.
- Stress the use of pursed-lip and diaphragmatic breathing techniques during periods of anxiety or panic.
- Recommend professional counseling, if needed, as a positive suggestion. Stress that talking with a counselor can help identify techniques to maintain control over the dyspnea and feelings of panic.
- Explore other approaches to control dyspneic episodes and panic attacks, such as progressive relaxation, hypnosis therapy, and biofeedback.

ACTIVITY INTOLERANCE
- Activity Intolerance is related to fatigue, dyspnea, and an imbalance between oxygen supply and demand (NANDA).
- Teach energy conservation techniques to plan and pace activities for maximal tolerance and minimal discomfort.
  1. Work with the patient to develop a personal daily schedule for activities and rest periods.
  2. Encourage the patient to avoid working with the arms raised or reaching above the head.

3. Teach the patient to adjust work heights to reduce back strain and fatigue.
4. Remind him or her to keep arm motions smooth and flowing to prevent jerky motions that waste energy.
5. Teach about the use of adaptive tools for housework, such as long-handled dustpans, sponges, and dusters, to reduce bending and reaching.
6. Suggest how to organize work spaces so that items used most often are within easy reach.
7. Teach the patient not to talk when engaged in other activities that require energy, such as walking.
8. Teach him or her to avoid breath-holding while performing any activity.

- Assist with ADLs of eating, bathing, and grooming based on assessment of the patient's needs and fatigue level.
- Assess the patient's response to activity by noting skin color changes, pulse rate and regularity, blood pressure, and work of breathing.
- Suggest the use of supplemental oxygen during periods of high energy use, such as bathing or walking.

PNEUMONIA
- The patient has a potential for pneumonia or other respiratory infections.
- Patients with COPD who have excessive secretions or who have artificial airways are at increased risk for respiratory tract infections.
- Teach patients to avoid large crowds and anyone who is ill.
- Stress the importance of receiving a pneumonia vaccination and a yearly influenza vaccination.

Community-Based Care
- Coordinate with all members of the health care team to individualize plans for the patient to be discharged to home.
- Determine what equipment and assistance will be needed in the home setting.
- Teach the patient and family about:
  1. The disease and its course
  2. Drug therapy
  3. Manifestations of infection
  4. Avoidance of respiratory irritants
  5. Nutrition therapy regimen
  6. Stress and anxiety management
  7. Breathing and coughing techniques
  8. Energy conservation measures while maintaining self-care activities

- Collaborate with the care manager and social worker to obtain needed home services:
  1. Oxygen and nebulizer
  2. Hospital-type bed
  3. Home health nurse or aide
  4. Financial assistance
- Provide appropriate referrals, as needed:
  1. Home care visits
  2. Housekeeping assistance and meal preparation
  3. Support groups
  4. Smoking cessation programs

CIRRHOSIS

OVERVIEW

- Cirrhosis is extensive, irreversible scarring of the liver, usually caused by a chronic reaction to hepatic inflammation and necrosis. Diffuse fibrotic bands of connective tissue distort the normal architectural anatomy of the liver, resulting in disturbed metabolic processes and circulatory pathology.
- Cirrhosis of the liver can be divided into several common types, depending on the cause of the disease:
  1. *Postnecrotic cirrhosis* is caused by viral hepatitis, especially hepatitis C, and certain drugs or other toxins. Worldwide, hepatitis B and hepatitis D are the leading causes of this condition.
  2. *Laennec's cirrhosis,* or *alcoholic cirrhosis,* is caused by chronic alcoholism. The long-term use of illicit drugs, such as cocaine, has similar effects on the liver.
  3. *Biliary cirrhosis* also called *cholestatic cirrhosis* is caused by chronic biliary obstruction or autoimmune disease.
- Complications of cirrhosis include:
  1. *Portal hypertension:* A persistent increase in pressure within the portal vein develops as a result of increased resistance or obstruction to flow. Blood flow backs into the spleen, causing splenomegaly. Veins in the esophagus, stomach, intestines, abdomen, and rectum become dilated. Dilated vessels have thinner walls and are more likely to leak, causing hemorrhage.
  2. *Ascites:* Free fluid containing almost pure plasma accumulates within the peritoneal cavity. Increased hydrostatic pressure from portal hypertension results in venous congestion of the hepatic capillaries, causing plasma to leak directly from the liver surface and portal vein. Other contributing

factors include reduced circulating plasma protein and increased hepatic lymphatic formation.

3. *Esophageal varices:* Fragile, thin-walled, distended esophageal veins become tortuous, and fragile. Varices occur most often in the lower esophagus and can rupture, resulting in upper gastrointestinal bleeding.

4. *Coagulation defects:* Decreased synthesis of bile fats in the liver prevents the absorption of fat-soluble vitamins. Without vitamin K and clotting factors II, VII, IX, and X, the patient is susceptible to bleeding and easy bruising. Splenomegaly (enlarged spleen) results from the backup of blood into the spleen. The enlarged spleen destroys platelets, causing thrombocytopenia (low serum platelet count) and increased risk for bleeding.

5. *Jaundice,* which is caused by one of two mechanisms:
   a. In *hepatocellular jaundice,* the liver is unable to effectively excrete bilirubin.
   b. In *intrahepatic obstruction,* edema, fibrosis, or scarring of the hepatic bile duct channels and bile ducts interferes with normal bile and bilirubin excretion. Patients with jaundice often report pruritus (itching).

6. *Hepatic encephalopathy* (also called *portal-systemic encephalopathy [PSE]*): This is a complex, cognitive syndrome manifested by neurologic symptoms. It is associated with elevated serum ammonia levels. Early symptoms include sleep disturbance, mood disturbance, mental status changes, and speech problems. Later, altered level of consciousness, impaired thinking processes, and neuromuscular disturbances (e.g., "liver flap") are common symptoms.

7. *Hepatorenal syndrome:* Progressive, oliguric kidney failure is associated with hepatic failure, resulting in functional impairment of kidneys with normal anatomic and morphologic features. It is manifested by a sudden decrease in urinary flow and elevated serum urea nitrogen and creatinine levels, with abnormally decreased urine sodium excretion and increased urine osmolarity.

8. Spontaneous bacterial peritonitis manifestations include fever, chills, and abdominal pain and tenderness.

PATIENT-CENTERED COLLABORATIVE CARE
Assessment
- Record patient information:
  1. Age, gender, and race
  2. Employment history, including working conditions exposing the patient to harmful chemical toxins

3. History of individual and family liver disease
4. Previous medical conditions, including jaundice, acute viral hepatitis, biliary tract disease, viral infections, blood transfusions, autoimmune disorders, and history of heart disease or respiratory disorders
5. Sexual history
6. History of or present substance use

- Assess for:
  1. Generalized weakness, fatigue
  2. Weight changes (loss or gain)
  3. GI symptoms, including loss of appetite, early morning nausea and vomiting, dyspepsia, flatulence, and changes in bowel habits
  4. Abdominal pain or tenderness
  5. Jaundice of the skin and sclera
  6. Dry skin, rashes, pruritus
  7. Petechiae or ecchymosis
  8. Palmar erythema
  9. Spider angiomas on the nose, cheeks, upper thorax, and shoulders
  10. Hepatomegaly palpated in the right upper quadrant, confirmed by palpation, ultrasound, or radiographic imaging
  11. Ascites revealed by bulging flanks and dullness on percussion of the abdomen
  12. Protruding umbilicus
  13. Dilated abdominal veins (caput medusae)
  14. Hematemesis or melena
  15. Fetor hepaticus (the fruity, musty breath odor of chronic liver disease)
  16. Amenorrhea in women
  17. Testicular atrophy, gynecomastia, and impotence in men
  18. Changes in mentation and personality
  19. Asterixis (liver flap), a coarse tremor characterized by rapid, nonrhythmic extension and flexions in the wrist and fingers
  20. Elevated serum liver enzyme and serum bilirubin levels
  21. Decreased hemoglobin, total serum protein, and albumin levels
  22. Elevated serum globulin level
  23. Altered coagulation factors; prolonged bleeding times
  24. Elevated serum ammonia level

Planning and Implementation
EXCESS FLUID VOLUME
  Nonsurgical Management
- Monitor respiratory status to avoid complications from pulmonary edema.

1. Monitor SpO_2 with vital signs.
2. Elevate the head of the bed to minimize shortness of breath and position for comfort.

- Provide diet therapy:
    1. Provide a low-sodium diet initially, restricting sodium to 500 mg to 2 g/day.
    2. Suggest alternatives to salt, such as lemon, vinegar, parsley, oregano, and pepper.
    3. Collaborate with the dietitian to explain the purpose of diet and meal planning; suggest elimination of table salt, salty foods, canned and frozen vegetables, and salted butter and margarine.
    4. Restrict fluid intake to 1000 to 1500 mL/day if the serum sodium level falls.
    5. Supplement vitamin intake with thiamine, folate, and multivitamin preparations.
- Provide drug therapy:
    1. Give diuretics to reduce intravascular fluid and to prevent cardiac and respiratory impairment.
    2. Monitor intake and output carefully.
    3. Weigh the patient daily.
    4. Measure abdominal girth daily.
    5. Monitor serum electrolytes.
- Paracentesis may be indicated if dietary restrictions and drug administration fail to control ascites:
    1. Explain the procedure and verify informed consent obtained.
    2. Obtain vital signs and weight, and check allergies.
    3. Assist the patient to an upright position at the side of the bed.
    4. Monitor vital signs every 15 minutes during the procedure; rapid, drastic removal of ascitic fluid leads to decreased abdominal pressure, which may contribute to vasodilation and shock.
    5. Measure and record drainage; send samples to laboratory if ordered.
    6. Position the patient in a semi-Fowler's position in bed, and maintain bedrest until vital signs are stable.

Surgical Management

- A peritoneovenous shunt may be placed for severe ascites. Ascites are drained through a one-way valve into a silicone rubber tube that terminates in the superior vena cava.
- Preoperative care is aimed at optimizing the patient's physical state.

- Provide preoperative care by treating underlying medical conditions:
  1. Treat abnormal coagulation with fresh-frozen plasma or vitamin K.
  2. Correct electrolyte imbalances.
  3. Ensure that packed red blood cells (RBCs) are available for surgery.
  4. Provide routine preoperative care.
- Provide postoperative care:
  1. Provide routine postoperative care.
  2. Auscultate breath sounds for the presence of crackles, indicating excessive lung fluid.
  3. Assess for excess fluid volume and hemodilution.
  4. Administer diuretics for volume excess.
  5. Monitor coagulation study results.
  6. Perform daily abdominal girth measurements.
  7. Record accurate fluid intake and output daily.
  8. Weigh the patient daily.

POTENTIAL FOR HEMORRHAGE
- Portal hypertension causes bulging and weakening of venules and veins along the esophagus and antrum of the stomach.
  1. Administer antihypertensive medications.
  2. Monitor hemoglobin and hematocrit for decreased levels, which indicates bleeding.
  3. Monitor stool for occult or visible blood.
  4. Evaluate postural blood pressure (orthostatic BP) and heart rate to determine the presence of hypovolemia.
- Determine the acceptable range of systolic and mean arterial blood pressure and communicate out-of-range findings to the prescribing health care provider.
- Esophageal bleeding is controlled by:
  1. Gastric intubation to lavage the stomach until the fluid returned is clear
  2. Esophagogastric balloon tamponade to compress bleeding vessels with a tube called a *tamponade tube*
     a. The tube is inserted through the nose and into the stomach. The large esophageal balloon compresses the esophagus; a smaller gastric balloon helps anchor the tube and exerts pressure against bleeding varices at the distal esophagus and the cardia of the stomach. A third lumen terminates in the stomach and is connected to suction, allowing the aspiration of gastric contents and blood.
     b. Check balloons for integrity and leaks; label each lumen to prevent errors in adding or removing pressure and volume.

    c. Keep tube taped and secure.

    d. Keep an extra tube and scissors at the bedside.

    e. Monitor the patient for respiratory distress caused by obstruction from the esophageal balloon or aspiration; if distress occurs, cut both balloon ports to allow for rapid balloon deflation and tube removal.

3. Administering blood products (RBCs and fresh-frozen plasma) and IV fluids.

4. Giving vasopressin intra-arterially or IV to lower pressures in the portal venous system to decrease bleeding

5. Injection sclerotherapy, which may be performed during endoscopy to sclerose bleeding esophageal varices:

    a. Monitor the patient's vital signs and assess for chest pain.

    b. Administer pain drug and report severe pain to the physician.

    c. Assess lung sounds to determine presence of pneumonia or pleural effusion.

6. Endoscopic band ligation procedure, which uses bands to ligate the bleeding varices

7. Transjugular intrahepatic portal-systemic shunting, a nonsurgical procedure whereby the physician implants a shunt, passed through a catheter, between the portal vein and the hepatic vein to reduce portal venous pressure and therefore control the bleeding

8. *Esophagogastroduodenoscopy (EGD)* to directly visualize the upper GI tract and to detect the presence of bleeding or oozing esophageal varices, stomach irritation and ulceration, or duodenal ulceration and bleeding. EGD is performed by introducing a flexible fiberoptic endoscope into the mouth, esophagus, and stomach while the patient is under moderate sedation. A camera attached to the scope permits direct visualization of the mucosal lining of the upper GI tract.

9. An *endoscopic retrograde cholangiopancreatography (ERCP)* uses the endoscope to inject contrast material via the sphincter of Oddi to view the biliary tract and allow for stone removals, sphincterotomies, biopsies, and stent placements if required

◾ NURSING SAFETY PRIORITY: Action Alert

Avoid placing or manipulating the nasogastric or orogastric tube in a patient who is at high risk for or diagnosed with esophageal varices, because tube movement can injure a dilated vessel, causing it to rupture and bleed.

Surgical Management

- Surgical management of portal hypertension and esophageal varices is a last resort intervention associated with high mortality from coagulation abnormalities, infection, poor tolerance to anesthesia, and ascites.

POTENTIAL FOR HEPATIC ENCEPHALOPATHY
Nonsurgical Management

- Provide a safe environment.
  1. Altered mentation places patient at risk for falls, aspiration, and pressure ulcer formation from prolonged immobility. Institute institutional interventions to avoid these adverse events.
  2. Coagulopathy and high blood pressure can place the patient at significant risk for hemorrhage. Institute frequent monitoring, and communicate observations related to increased risk for hemorrhage immediately.
- Provide diet therapy:
  1. Patient has increased nutritional requirements: high-carbohydrate, moderate-fat, and high-protein foods.
  2. Patients with PSE usually have protein intake limited in the diet to reduce excess protein breakdown by intestinal bacteria leading to ammonia formation.
- Provide drug therapy:
  1. Administer lactulose to promote excretion of fecal ammonia.
     a. Oral lactulose can be diluted to help the patient tolerate the sweet taste. Lactulose can also be given via retention enema if the patient is unable to safely swallow.
     b. Dosing is titrated to serum ammonia levels. The desired effect of lactulose is two to five soft stools per day; watery diarrheal stools may complicate the drug regimen and contribute to electrolyte abnormalities. Evaluate daily ammonia levels and communicate with other health care team members about patient responses to lactulose administration.
  2. Be aware of reduced metabolism of many drugs, especially opioids, sedatives, and other central nervous system (CNS) agents.

Community-Based Care

- Health teaching is individualized for the patient, depending on the cause of the disease.
- Identify if the patient needs a family member or friend to help with drugs, or needs a home health care nurse or aide.
- Teach the patient and family to:
  1. Follow the prescribed diet.
  2. Restrict sodium intake if ascites occur.

3. Restrict protein intake if the patient is susceptible to encephalopathy.
4. Take diuretics as prescribed, report symptoms of hypokalemia, and consume foods high in potassium.
5. Take H_2 receptor antagonist agent or proton pump inhibitor for GI bleeding.
6. Avoid all nonprescription drugs.
7. Avoid alcohol (refer to Alcoholics Anonymous if patient is addicted to alcohol).
8. Recognize signs and symptoms of PSE.
9. Notify the patient's health care provider immediately in case of GI bleeding or PSE.
10. Keep follow-up visits with the physicians.

COLITIS, ULCERATIVE

OVERVIEW

- Ulcerative colitis (UC) creates widespread inflammation of mainly the rectum and rectosigmoid colon but can extend to the entire colon
- UC is characterized by hyperemic intestinal mucosa (increased blood flow) with resultant edema. In more severe inflammation, the lining can bleed and small erosions, or ulcers, occur. Abscesses can form in these ulcerative areas and result in tissue necrosis. Continued edema and mucosal thickening can lead to a narrowed colon and possibly a partial bowel obstruction.
- Complications of the disease include intestinal perforation with peritonitis and fistula formation, toxic megacolon, hemorrhage, increased risk for colon cancer, malabsorption, and extraintestinal clinical manifestations.
- The patient's stool typically contains blood and mucus. Patients report tenesmus (an unpleasant and urgent sensation to defecate) and lower abdominal colicky pain relieved with defecation. Malaise, anorexia, anemia, dehydration, fever, and weight loss are common.

PATIENT-CENTERED COLLABORATIVE CARE
Assessment

- Record patient information:
  1. Family history of inflammatory bowel disease
  2. Previous and current therapy for illnesses, including surgeries
  3. Diet history, including usual patterns and intolerances of food

4. History of weight changes
5. Presence of abdominal pain, cramping, urgency, and diarrhea
6. Bowel elimination patterns; color, consistency, and character of stools and the presence or absence of blood
7. Relationship between the occurrence of diarrhea and the timing of meals, pain, emotional distress, and activity
8. Extraintestinal symptoms such as arthritis, mouth sores, vision problems, and skin disorders

- Assess for:
  1. Abdominal cramping, pain, and distention
  2. Bloody diarrhea, tenesmus
  3. Low-grade fever, tachycardia
  4. Patient's understanding of the disease process
  5. Psychosocial impact of the disease
     a. Factors that produce symptoms
     b. Family and social support systems
     c. Concerns regarding the possible genetic basis and associated cancer risks of the disease
  6. Abnormal laboratory values: hematocrit, hemoglobin, WBC count, erythrocyte sedimentation rate, C-reactive protein, and electrolytes
  7. Results from most recent colonoscopy

Planning and Implementation
DIARRHEA AND POTENTIAL FOR INCONTINENCE
  Nonsurgical Management
- Management of ulcerative colitis is aimed at relieving the symptoms and reducing intestinal motility, decreasing inflammation, and promoting intestinal healing.
- At the onset of treatment, activity is restricted to promote comfort and intestinal healing.
- Diarrhea management:
  1. Record patient responses to interventions, noting changes in the color, volume, frequency, and consistency of stools.
  2. Monitor the skin in the perianal area for irritation and ulceration resulting from loose, frequent stools.
  3. Monitor immune function and results of stool or other cultures.
- Drug therapy:
  1. Aminosalicylates are used to reduce inflammation.
  2. Glucocorticoids are used during exacerbations of the illness.
  3. Antidiarrheal drugs are given to provide symptomatic management of diarrhea; they are given cautiously, because they can precipitate colonic dilation and toxic megacolon.

   4. Immunomodulators are given to alter the immune response
      and are commonly given with glucocorticoids. Infliximab
      (Remicade) or adalimumab (Humira) may be given for re-
      fractory disease or for severe complications such as toxic
      megacolon.
- Diet therapy may include:
   1. NPO status for the patient with severe symptoms
   2. Total parenteral nutrition (TPN) while NPO
   3. Elemental formulas, which are absorbed in the upper bowel,
      thereby minimizing bowel stimulation
   4. Avoiding high-fiber foods such as nuts and fresh fruits or
      vegetables
   5. Avoiding carbonated beverages, pepper, nuts and corn, dried
      fruits, and smoking, because these are common GI stimu-
      lants that could cause discomfort.
- Ensure that the patient has easy access to the bedside commode
  or bathroom.
- Explore psychosocial concerns such as body image, fear, and
  anxiety.
- Complementary and alternative therapies used as a supplement
  to traditional therapies may include herbs such as flaxseed, se-
  lenium, vitamin C, biofeedback, yoga, acupuncture, and Ayur-
  veda (combination of diet, herbs, and breathing exercises).
  Surgical Management
- The need for surgery is based on the patient's response to medical interventions.
- Surgical procedures include
   1. *Total proctocolectomy with permanent ileostomy,* in which the
      colon, rectum, and anus are removed and the anus closed.
      The end of the terminal ileum forms the stoma, which is lo-
      cated in the right lower quadrant. Postoperatively, the nurse
      provides skin and ostomy care.
      a. Oral or parenteral antibiotics may be given preopera-
         tively as a bowel antiseptic.
      b. Usually, the patient wears an ostomy pouch at all times.
      c. Initial output from the ileostomy is a loose, dark green
         liquid; over time, the volume decreases, becomes thicker,
         and turns yellow-green or yellow-brown.
      d. Any foul or unpleasant odor may be a symptom of some
         underlying problem (blockage or infection).
   2. *Total colectomy* with a continent ileostomy (Kock's ileostomy)
      or ileal reservoir. An intra-abdominal pouch or reservoir is
      constructed from the terminal ileum where stool can be stored
      until the pouch is drained by the nurse or patient. The pouch
      is connected to the stoma with a nipple-like valve constructed

from an intussuscepted portion of the ileum; the stoma is flush with the skin.

  a. Immediately postoperatively, a Foley catheter is placed in the pouch and connected to low intermittent suction and irrigated, as ordered.

  b. Monitor the character and quality of drainage.

  c. Teach the patient to drain the stoma. When the pouch needs to be emptied, the patient experiences a sense of fullness.

3. Creation of an ileoanal reservoir, a procedure known as *Restorative Proctocolectomy with Ileal Pouch Anal Anastomosis (RPC-IPAA)*. It is usually a two-stage procedure that first includes the removal of the colon and most of the rectum. The anus and anal sphincter remain intact. The surgeon surgically creates an internal pouch (reservoir) using the last 1.5 feet of the small intestine. The pouch, sometimes called a J-pouch, S-pouch, or pelvic pouch, is then connected to the anus. In the second surgical stage, the loop ileostomy is closed. The time interval between the first and second stage varies, but many patients have the second surgical stage to close the ileostomy within 1 to 2 months of the first surgery.

4. Specific nursing care interventions as determined by the procedure performed, including ostomy or perineal wound care

5. Opportunity for patient to interact with the certified wound, ostomy, continence nurse (CWOCN) or enterostomal therapist (ET) preoperatively and postoperatively and at follow-up appointments or at home.

▉ NURSING SAFETY PRIORITY: Critical Rescue

The ileostomy stoma is usually placed in the right lower quadrant of the abdomen below the belt line. It should not be prolapsed or retract into the abdominal wall. Assess the stoma frequently. It should be pinkish to cherry red to ensure an adequate blood supply. *If the stoma looks pale, bluish, or dark, report these findings to the health care provider immediately.*

PAIN MANAGEMENT

- Assess the patient for changes in complaints and responses to pain that may indicate disease complications, such as increased inflammation, obstruction, hemorrhage, or peritonitis.
- Assess for pain, including its character, pattern of occurrence (e.g., before or after meals, during the night, before or after bowel movements), and duration.
- Assist the patient to reduce or eliminate factors that can precipitate or increase the pain.

- Take measures to relieve irritated skin caused by contact with diarrheal stool.
- Assist the patient to use other pain relief measures such as biofeedback and music therapy.

POTENTIAL FOR LOWER GI BLEEDING

- Monitor the patient for signs and symptoms of GI bleeding.
- Notify the health care provider immediately of GI bleeding, because surgical interventions may be necessary.

◼ NURSING SAFETY PRIORITY: Critical Rescue

Monitor stools for blood loss. The blood may be bright red (frank bleeding) or black and tarry (melena). Monitor hematocrit, hemoglobin, and electrolyte values, and assess vital signs. Prolonged slow bleeding can lead to anemia. Observe for fever, tachycardia, and signs of fluid volume depletion. Changes in mental status may occur, especially among older adults, and may be the first indication of dehydration or anemia.

Community-Based Care

- Health teaching includes the following:
  1. Provide information on the nature of the disease, including acute episodes, remissions, and symptom management.
  2. The patient with ulcerative colitis provides self-management at home. Home care management focuses on controlling clinical manifestations and monitoring for complications.
  3. Provide additional information for the patient with an ostomy regarding:
     a. Ostomy care
     b. Pouch care
     c. Skin care
     d. Special issues related to drugs (e.g., to avoid taking enteric-coated drugs and capsule drugs); the patient should inform health care providers and the pharmacist that he or she has an ostomy.
     e. Symptoms to watch for, such as increased or no drainage; stomal swelling; color of stoma
     f. Activity limitations, including avoidance of heavy lifting
     g. Importance of maintaining adequate fluid intake, especially during periods of high ostomy/liquid output
- Refer the patient to home health care ostomy or outpatient clinics.
- Refer the patient to support groups such as the United Ostomy Association and the Crohn's and Colitis Foundation of America.

COMPARTMENT SYNDROME

OVERVIEW

- Compartments are areas in the body where muscles, blood vessels, and nerves are contained within fascia, especially in extremities.
- Fascia is an inelastic tissue that surrounds groups of muscles, blood vessels, and nerves in the body.
- *Acute compartment syndrome (ACS)* is a serious condition in which increased pressure from tissue swelling as a result of blood or fluid collection within one or more compartments causes massive compromise of circulation to the area.
- It is usually a complication of musculoskeletal trauma in the lower leg and forearm, but it can be seen with severe burns, extensive insect bites, or massive infiltration of IV fluids and with abdominal swelling.
- Pressure to the compartment can also occur from an external source, such as tight, bulky dressings and casts.
- If the condition is not treated, cyanosis, tingling, numbness, pain, paresis, and permanent tissue damage can occur.
- Complications of ACS can include infection, persistent motor weakness in the affected extremity, contracture, and myoglobinuric renal failure.
- In extreme cases, amputation becomes necessary.

PATIENT-CENTERED COLLABORATIVE CARE

- Nursing care includes:
  1. Identifying patients who may be at risk
  2. Monitoring for early signs of ACS by assessing for the "six Ps," which include:
     a. Pain
     b. Pressure
     c. Paralysis
     d. Paresthesia
     e. Pallor
     f. Pulselessness
  3. Invasive monitoring of compartment pressure in patients at especially high risk for ACS using a handheld device with a digital display or a pressure monitor such as that used for abdominal compartment syndrome evaluation.
  4. When external conditions are causing the syndrome, implementing interventions to relieve the pressure:
     a. Loosening dressings or tape
     b. Following agency protocol about cutting a tight cast

🛑 NURSING SAFETY PRIORITY: Critical Rescue

When manifestations indicate compartment syndrome, notify the surgeon immediately, because irreversible damage can occur within a few hours.

- Surgical intervention is a fasciotomy (opening in the fascia) made by incising through the skin and subcutaneous tissues into the fascia of the affected compartment to relieve the pressure and restore circulation to the affected area.
- After fasciotomy, the open wound is packed and dressed on a regular basis until secondary closure occurs.
- Débridement and skin grafting may be required.

CORNEAL ABRASION, INFECTION, AND ULCERATION

OVERVIEW

- A *corneal abrasion* is a painful scrape or scratch of the cornea that disrupts the integrity of this structure, most commonly caused by the presence of a small foreign body, trauma, and contact lens use.
- The abrasion provides a portal of entry for organisms, leading to *corneal infection*, which can lead to corneal ulceration.
- *Corneal ulceration* is a deeper disruption of the corneal epithelium, often occurring with bacterial, fungal, or viral infection. *This problem is an emergency and can lead to permanently impaired vision.*

PATIENT-CENTERED COLLABORATIVE CARE

Assessment

- Assess for these problems in the affected eye:
  1. Severe pain
  2. Reduced vision
  3. Photophobia
  4. Eye secretions
  5. Cloudy or purulent fluid on eyelids or eyelashes
  6. Hazy, cloudy cornea with a patchy area of ulceration
  7. Damaged areas appear green with fluorescein stain

Interventions

- Drug therapy delivered as eyedrops:
  1. Antibiotics, antifungals, and antivirals are prescribed to reduce or eliminate the organisms. Usually, a broad-spectrum antibiotic is prescribed first, and it may be changed when culture results are known.

2. Usually the anti-infective therapy involves instilling eye-drops every hour for the first 24 hours.
3. Steroids may be used with antibiotics to reduce the inflammatory response in the eye.
4. Anesthetic drops can be used to decrease pain.
5. Teach the patient how to apply the eyedrops correctly.
6. Teach the patient to not use the drug in the unaffected eye.
7. Teach the patient to wash hands after touching the affected eye and before touching or doing anything to the healthy eye.
8. If both eyes are infected, separate bottles of drugs are needed for each eye and are clearly labeled *right eye* and *left eye.*
9. Teach the patient to completely care for one eye, then wash the hands and, using the drugs for the remaining eye, care for that eye.
10. Teach the patient to not wear contact lenses during the entire time that these drugs are being used.

⬛ NURSING SAFETY PRIORITY: Critical Rescue

Stress the importance of applying the drug as often as prescribed, even at night. Stopping the infection can save the patient's vision in the infected eye.

CORNEAL OPACITIES, KERATOCONUS, AND CORNEAL TRANSPLANTATION

OVERVIEW

- The cornea can permanently lose it shape, become scarred or cloudy, or become thinner, reducing refraction and interfering with useful vision.
- *Keratoconus* is the degeneration of the corneal tissue resulting in an abnormal corneal shape that can occur with trauma or may occur as part of an inherited disorder.

PATIENT-CENTERED COLLABORATIVE CARE

- Management for a permanent corneal disorder that obscures vision is a *keratoplasty* (corneal transplant), the surgical removal of diseased corneal tissue and replacement with tissue from a human donor cornea. For a misshaped cornea that is still clear, surgical management involves a corneal implant that adjusts the shape of the cornea.
- Provide preoperative care:
  1. Assess the patient's knowledge of the surgery and of expected care before and after surgery.

2. Examine the eyes for signs of infection and report any redness, drainage, or edema to the ophthalmologist.
3. Instill antibiotic drops into the eye.
4. Obtain IV access.
5. Inform the patient that local anesthesia usually is used.

- Provide postoperative care:
  1. The eye is covered with a pressure patch and a protective shield. This dressing is left in place until the next day, when the patient returns to the surgeon.
  2. Notify the ophthalmologist of changes in vital signs or of drainage on the dressing.
  3. Perform patient and family teaching about:
     a. Applying an eye patch
     b. Wearing an eye shield at night and whenever around small children or pets
     c. Instilling eyedrops
     d. Examining the eye daily for the presence of infection or graft rejection
     e. Reporting immediately to the surgeon the presence of purulent discharge, a continuous leak of clear fluid from around the graft site (not tears), or excessive bleeding
     f. Reporting manifestations of graft rejection to the surgeon that include redness starting in the donor cornea near the graft edge and moving toward the center, reduced vision, and corneal clouding
     g. Avoiding activities that promote rapid or jerky head motions or increase intraocular pressure for several weeks after surgery

CORONARY ARTERY DISEASE

OVERVIEW

- Coronary artery disease (CAD) is a broad term that includes *chronic angina* and *acute coronary syndromes (ACS)*. (See *ACS.*)
- CAD affects the arteries that provide blood, oxygen, and nutrients to the myocardium.
- CAD causes ischemia when insufficient oxygen is supplied to meet the requirements of the myocardium. *Infarction* (necrosis or cell death) occurs when severe ischemia is prolonged, resulting in irreversible damage to tissue.
- The most common cause of CAD is atherosclerosis, which is characterized by a lesion that narrows the vessel lumen or obstructs blood flow (see *Arteriosclerosis and Atherosclerosis*).

- The most common symptom of CAD is angina. *Angina* is a sign of myocardial ischemia, a temporary imbalance between the ability of the coronary arteries to supply oxygen and the demand of the myocardium for it.
  1. Stable angina is chest discomfort that occurs with exertion in a pattern that is familiar to the patient and that has not increased in frequency, duration, or intensity of symptoms during the past several months; it is usually associated with a stable atherosclerotic plaque.
  2. Unstable angina is chest pain or discomfort that is new or newly occurs at rest or with minimal exertion or an increase in the number of episodes ("attacks"), or an increase in the quality or intensity of pain.

Women's Health Considerations
- Many women experience atypical angina, described as a choking sensation that occurs with exertion, indigestion, pain between the shoulders, or an aching jaw.
- Angina is more likely to be the primary presenting symptom of CAD in women than in men.
- Women have higher morbidity and mortality rates after myocardial infarction (MI) than men do.
- Angina is twice as common as MI in women.

- MI occurs when coronary blood flow is stopped and the myocardial muscle is abruptly and severely deprived of oxygen. Ischemia and necrosis (infarction) of the myocardial tissue result if blood flow is not restored. Generally, an MI is caused by an unstable plaque that initiates the inflammatory cascade and leads to thrombus formation. The clot is the cause of coronary artery blood flow cessation. The patient's response to an MI depends on which coronary arteries were obstructed and which part of the left ventricular wall was damaged: anterior, lateral, septal, inferior, or posterior.
  1. Patients with obstruction of the left anterior descending artery have anterior or septal MIs, or both; patients with anterior MIs are most likely to experience left ventricular heart failure and ventricular dysrhythmias.
  2. Patients with obstruction of the circumflex artery may experience a posterior wall or a lateral wall MI and sinus dysrhythmias.
  3. Patients with obstruction of the right coronary artery often have inferior MIs; these patients are likely to experience bradydysrhythmias or atrioventricular

conduction defects, especially transient second-degree heart block.
- Nonmodifiable risk factors that contribute to the onset and progression of CAD include age, gender, family history, and ethnic background.
- Modifiable risk factors include elevated serum cholesterol levels, cigarette smoking, hypertension, impaired glucose tolerance, obesity, physical inactivity, and stress.

PATIENT-CENTERED COLLABORATIVE CARE
Assessment
- Collection of historical data is delayed until interventions for pain, vital sign instability, and dysrhythmias are initiated and the discomfort resolves.
- Record the patient's family history and risk factors.
- Assess for clinical manifestations of angina and MI:
  1. Quality, onset, duration, and alleviating and aggravating factors related to chest pain
     a. Presence and quality of atypical pain, including jaw pain, back pain, or extreme fatigue, particularly in women and in patients with diarrhea
  2. Nausea and vomiting
  3. Diaphoresis
  4. Dizziness
  5. Weakness
  6. Palpitations
  7. Shortness of breath
  8. Diminished or absent pulses
  9. Dysrhythmias such as tachycardia, premature beats, irregular rhythm
  10. Abnormal blood pressure
  11. S_3 gallop or S_4 heart sound
  12. Increased respiratory rate
  13. Crackles or wheezes (if concurrent heart failure occurs)
  14. Elevated temperature
  15. Denial (early reaction to chest discomfort)
  16. Fear and anxiety
  17. Elevated serum cardiac enzyme levels:
     a. Myoglobin
     b. Troponin
     c. Creatine kinase (CK-MB isoenzyme)
  18. Electrocardiography (ECG) changes:
     a. In angina, ST depression or elevation or T-wave inversion that manifests on the ECG

    b. In MI, ST elevation, T-wave inversion, and abnormal Q wave in two or more contiguous leads (this is also known as an ST elevation MI or STEMI)

    c. An MI can occur in the absence of ECG changes (this is known as a non-ST elevation MI or NSTEMI).

19. Results of exercise tolerance test (stress test), thallium scan, contrast-enhanced magnetic resonance (CMR), multigated acquisition (MUGA) scan, and cardiac catheterization, if performed

C

Considerations for Older Adults

- About 25% of older adults and patients with diabetes who experience MI complain primarily of shortness of breath; chest discomfort may be mild or absent.
- Many older patients do not typically experience chest discomfort but have disorientation or confusion as the primary manifestation.

Women's Health Considerations

- Chest discomfort is often not the initial symptom.
- Women may initially have atypical symptoms such as heart "flutters" without pain, shortness of breath, fatigue, and depression.
- As the MI progresses, women usually report atypical chest discomfort: arm and shoulder pain, back pain, or an aching jaw, neck, or tooth.

⊕ Cultural Awareness

Modifiable risk factors vary for people of different racial and ethnic backgrounds. Some of the differences may be explained by lack of access to health care or genetic factors. American Indians, for example, have limited access to care or language barriers in a predominantly English-speaking, Euro-American health care system. Nutritional preferences may explain some of the differences. For instance, high cholesterol is more common in African-American and Hispanic populations. Diets higher in fat and cholesterol are often less expensive and may be a factor in explaining differences, and obesity is more common in these groups. Genetic factors may also contribute to the differences among ethnic groups.

❗NURSING SAFETY PRIORITY: Action Alert

Do not delay in reporting the patient's chest pain. Prompt diagnostic testing and treatment can lead to reperfusion of the myocardium and optimal outcomes.

Planning and Implementation

- For the patient with CAD, planning and intervention focus on restoring perfusion through the coronary arteries.

ACUTE PAIN

- Related to an imbalance between myocardial oxygen supply and demand
- Management of acute pain includes both pain relief and interventions to reduce the thrombosis and oxygen demands:
  1. Supplemental oxygen to provide additional oxygen to the ischemic myocardium; a nasal cannula at 2 to 4 L is usually sufficient.
  2. Nitroglycerin (sublingually), used for angina, to increase collateral blood flow, redistributing blood flow toward the subendocardium; if three repeated doses given 5 minutes apart do not relieve discomfort, the patient may be experiencing an MI and needs immediate evaluation in a heart center.
  3. Nitroglycerin (IV), administered in a specialized unit to carefully monitor the patient's blood pressure; hypotension is a serious side effect of this drug.
  4. Morphine sulfate (IV) for patients unresponsive to nitroglycerin
  5. Aspirin (325 mg, chewed), to reduce platelet aggregation and prevent clot extension in coronary arteries
  6. Metoprolol, a beta blocker to reduce heart rate, decrease sympathetic stimulation of the compromised myocardium, and prevent life-threatening dysrhythmias
  7. Initiating *heparin* IV continuously to prevent clot extension in the coronary arteries until the patient can be transported to the cardiac catheterization laboratory for definitive treatment

⬛ NURSING SAFETY PRIORITY: Drug Alert

Heparin is one of 10 medications most commonly associated with adverse events in the hospital setting. If you are unsure about calculations or dosage, ask the pharmacist for verification.

- Other interventions include:
  1. Obtaining a 12-lead ECG to determine the location of compromised coronary artery blood flow
  2. Placing the patient in a semi-Fowler's position for comfort
  3. Maintaining a quiet, calm environment to the extent possible
  4. Maintaining continuous monitoring and preparing for a cardiac arrest situation by placing the crash cart close to the patient room.

INEFFECTIVE CARDIAC TISSUE PERFUSION

- Definitive treatment is percutaneous coronary intervention (PCI), which typically involves placement of a stent to open the clotted coronary artery. Care after PCI includes:
    1. Monitoring for potential problems after the procedure, including acute closure of the vessel, reaction to the dye used in angiography, hypotension, hyperkalemia, and dysrhythmias
    2. Instructing the patient to report the development of chest pain immediately
    3. Frequently monitoring the insertion site for bleeding or vessel occlusion by palpating pulses, observing skin color and warmth of the limb, and marking the circumference of any hematoma where the catheter was inserted
        a. Apply manual pressure if there is bleeding from the insertion site.
        b. Report bleeding or changes in perfusion immediately to the physician.
    4. Maintaining immobilization of the affected limb for at least 6 hours
    5. Maintaining pressure dressing
    6. Elevating the head of the bed slowly, per hospital protocol
    7. Instructing the patient to:
        a. Return to usual activities in 1 to 2 weeks or when instructed by the physician.
        b. Avoid heavy lifting for several weeks.
        c. Apply manual pressure if there is bleeding from the insertion site and notify the physician if the bleeding is extensive or if oozing persists for more than 15 minutes.
        d. Take nitrates, aspirin, beta blockers, angiotensin-converting enzyme (ACE) inhibitors, and statin, as prescribed.
- If an interventional radiologist is not available to place a stent, then thrombolytic agents are given IV or by an intracoronary route during cardiac catheterization to dissolve thrombi in the coronary arteries and to restore myocardial blood flow. Examples include tissue plasminogen activator (TPA; alteplase [Activase]), reteplase (Retavase), and tenecteplase (TNKase).
- Fibrinolytic agents are most effective when used within 6 hours of a coronary event.
- Interventions after administration of fibrinolytic agents include monitoring the patient for signs of obvious and occult bleeding and reporting indications of bleeding immediately to the physician (most common in women who receive thrombolytic therapy):
    1. Monitor the patient for indications of cerebrovascular bleeding.

C

2. Observe all IV sites for bleeding and patency.
3. Monitor clotting studies.
4. Observe for signs of internal bleeding (watching hematocrit and hemoglobin).
5. Test stool, urine, and emesis for occult blood.

- Glycoprotein (GP) IIb/IIIa inhibitors prevent fibrin from attaching to activated platelets at the site of a thrombus after PCI or fibrinolysis.
  1. GP IIb/IIIa is used particularly in unstable angina and non-Q-wave MI and before and during PCI to ensure patency of the newly opened artery.
  2. If GP IIb/IIIa inhibitors are used with fibrinolytic agents, then the dose of the thrombolytic should be reduced.
- Monitor for indications of coronary artery reperfusion, including abrupt cessation of chest pain or discomfort, sudden onset of ventricular dysrhythmias, and resolution of ST segment depression, and reduction of markers of myocardial damage over 12 hours.
- IV heparin and aspirin may be given after thrombolytic therapy to reduce additional clot formation; monitor activated partial thromboplastin time (aPTT).

ACTIVITY INTOLERANCE FROM MYOCARDIAL DAMAGE

- Promote rest and provide assistance in ADLs to minimize oxygen demands during episodes of chest pain.
- Progress patient mobility with supervision, starting with having the patient dangle the legs at the side of the bed and proceeding to ambulation.
- Assess the patient's vital signs and level of fatigue with each higher level of activity.
- Notify the health care provider if there are indications of activity intolerance such as orthostatic hypotension, hypertension with activity, or complaints of dyspnea, chest pain, or dizziness.
- Consider initiating cardiac rehabilitation if the patient has not participated previously. Cardiac rehabilitation is divided into three phases:
  1. Phase 1 begins with acute illness and ends with discharge from the hospital.
  2. Phase 2 begins after discharge and continues through convalescence at home.
  3. Phase 3 involves long-term conditioning.

POTENTIAL FOR INEFFECTIVE COPING

- Potential for Ineffective Coping is related to effects of acute illness and major changes in lifestyle

- Direct interventions toward assisting the patient to take personal actions to manage lifestyle stressors related to CAD:
    1. Assess the patient's understanding of the disease process.
    2. Assess the patient's coping mechanisms (commonly denial, anger, and depression) and level of anxiety.
    3. Provide simple, repeated explanations of therapies, expectations, and surroundings.
    4. Help the patient identify the information that is most important to obtain.
    5. Denial that results in a patient's "acting out" and refusing to follow treatment regimen can be harmful.
        a. Remain calm and avoid confronting the patient.
        b. Clearly indicate when a behavior is not acceptable and is potentially harmful.
    6. Anger may be the result of a patient's attempt to regain control of his or her life.
        a. Encourage patient to verbalize frustrations.
        b. Provide opportunities for decision making and control.
    7. Depression may be a patient's response to grief.
        a. Listen to the patient, and do not offer false or general reassurances.
        b. Acknowledge depression, but expect the patient to perform ADLs and other activities within restrictions.
- For the patient who experiences an MI, planning and interventions focus on identifying and treating complications from the damage to the heart. After an MI, the following drugs are often prescribed:
    1. Aspirin taken daily to prevent platelet aggregation at the site of obstruction
    2. Beta-adrenergic agents to prevent pathologic cardiac remodeling and prevent dysrhythmias:
        a. Monitor heart rate rhythm, and blood pressure.
    3. An ACE inhibitor or an angiotensin receptor blocker (ARB) to prevent ventricular remodeling and the development of heart failure:
        a. Monitor for decreased urinary output, hypotension, cough, and changes in serum potassium, creatinine, and blood urea nitrogen.
    4. A statin (antilipemic) to reduce serum cholesterol, which contributes to plaque formation, and to provide anti-inflammation:
        a. Monitor liver enzymes and serum cholesterol.
    5. Calcium channel blockers for patients with variant angina or for those who are hypertensive and continue to have angina despite therapy with beta blockers

POTENTIAL FOR DYSRHYTHMIAS
- If a dysrhythmia occurs, the following actions are taken:
  1. Identify the dysrhythmia.
  2. Assess the patient's hemodynamic status, including blood pressure and peripheral with level of consciousness.
  3. Evaluate the patient for chest discomfort.
- Dysrhythmias are treated when they are causing hemodynamic compromise, are increasing myocardial oxygen requirements, or are predisposing to lethal ventricular dysrhythmias (see *Dysrhythmias*).

POTENTIAL FOR HEART FAILURE
- Heart failure is a relatively common complication after MI; the most severe form of heart failure, cardiogenic shock, accounts for most in-hospital deaths after MI.
- See *Heart Failure* for detailed assessment and management.

Nonsurgical Management
- Decreased cardiac output related to heart failure is a common complication after MI.
- Assess the patient with left ventricular failure for low mean arterial pressure or reduced pulse pressure, pulmonary edema, reduced urine output, and other symptoms of poor systemic perfusion.
- Medical management of heart failure includes:
  1. Oxygen therapy (intubation and mechanical ventilation may be necessary)
  2. Diuretics, nitroglycerin, or nitroprusside to reduce preload
  3. IV morphine to decrease pulmonary congestion and relieve pain
  4. Information from hemodynamic monitoring, which is used to titrate drug therapy
- Patients who do not respond to drug therapy may require an intra-aortic balloon pump (IABP) or left ventricular assistive device, which is used to improve myocardial perfusion, reduce afterload, and facilitate ventricular emptying.
- Immediate reperfusion may be performed after a left-sided cardiac catheterization for diagnosis. If the patient has a treatable lesion, the surgeon performs a PCI or the patient undergoes a coronary artery bypass grafting (CABG).
- The goal of medical management of right-sided heart ventricular failure is to improve right ventricular stroke volume:
  1. Provide IV fluids (as much as 200 mL/hr) to increase right atrial pressure (central venous pressure [CVP]) to 20 mm Hg.
  2. Monitor pulmonary artery wedge pressure (goal is maintaining values of 15 to 20 mm Hg).
  3. Auscultate the lungs to detect early left-sided heart failure.
  4. Monitor cardiac output to ensure that fluid administration has the desired effect.

POTENTIAL FOR RECURRENT SYMPTOMS
AND EXTENSION OF INJURY

- Recurrent chest pain despite medical therapy is a major indicator for surgery.

  Surgical Management

- PCI, an invasive but technically nonsurgical technique, is performed to provide symptom reduction for patients with chest discomfort without a significant risk of complications. PCI is performed by introducing a balloon-tipped catheter into the area of the coronary artery occlusion. When the balloon is inflated, it presses the atherosclerotic plaque against the vessel wall to reduce or eliminate the occlusion.

- Techniques used to ensure patency of the vessel are laser angioplasty, stents, and atherectomy devices.

- Nursing interventions after PCI are described above.

- CABG surgery is indicated when other treatments have been unsuccessful in managing CAD and ACS. This procedure is performed while the patient is under general anesthesia and undergoing cardiopulmonary bypass surgery. The graft to the saphenous vein or the internal mammary artery bypasses the occluded vessel to restore blood supply to the myocardium.

- Preoperative care includes:
  1. If surgery is performed as an elective procedure, familiarizing the patient and family with the cardiac surgical critical care environment
  2. Teaching the patient how to splint the chest incision, cough and deep-breathe, perform arm and leg exercises, what to expect during the postoperative period, and how pain will be managed

- Provide immediate postoperative care in a specialized unit:
  1. Maintain mechanical ventilation for 3 to 6 hours.
  2. Monitor chest tube drainage system.
  3. Monitor pulmonary artery and arterial pressures.
  4. Frequently assess vital signs and cardiac rate and rhythm.
  5. Ensure that pain is appropriately managed.
  6. Treat symptomatic dysrhythmias according to unit protocols or physician's order.
  7. Monitor for complications of open heart surgery, including:
     a. Fluid and electrolyte imbalances
     b. Hypotension
     c. Hypothermia
     d. Hypertension
     e. Bleeding
     f. Cardiac tamponade
     g. Altered cerebral perfusion

C

- Provide continued postoperative care:
  1. Encourage deep breathing and coughing every 2 hours while splinting incision after extubation.
  2. Assist the patient in resuming activity and ambulation.
  3. Monitor for dysrhythmias, especially atrial fibrillation.
  4. Assess for wound or sternal infection (mediastinitis), such as prolonged fever (more than 4 days), reddened sternum, purulent incisional drainage, and an elevated white blood cell (WBC) count.
  5. Observe for indications of postpericardiotomy syndrome: pericardial and pleural pain, pericarditis, friction rub, elevated temperature and WBC count, and dysrhythmias; the problem may be self-limiting or may require treatment for pericarditis.
- Minimally invasive direct coronary arterial bypass (MIDCAB) is indicated for patients with a lesion of the left anterior descending artery. Cardiopulmonary bypass is not required.
  1. Assess the patient for postoperative chest pain and electrocardiographic changes, because occlusion of the internal mammary artery graft occurs acutely in 10% of patients.
  2. Encourage the patient to cough and deep-breathe (chest tube and thoracotomy incision).
- Transmyocardial laser revascularization, for patients with unstable angina and inoperable CAD with area of reversible myocardial ischemia, involves the creation of 20 to 24 long narrow channels through the left ventricular muscle to the left ventricle, which eventually allows oxygenated blood to flow.
- Robotic heart surgery allows surgeons to operate endoscopically through 8- to 10-mm long incisions in the chest wall, eliminating tremors that can exist with human hands, increasing the ability to reach inaccessible sites, and improving depth perception and visual acuity.

◼ NURSING SAFETY PRIORITY: Critical Rescue

Monitoring the ECG and using the bedside alarms to notify about changes in ST from baseline can provide an early warning of coronary artery occlusion after any of the radiologic or surgical interventions for CAD. Immediately notify the physician about new-onset dysrhythmias, ST elevation, and other changes in the ECG indicating ischemia, injury, or infarct.

Community-Based Care

- Assignment to case manager at the beginning of the hospitalization can promote discharge goals achievement (e.g., guideline adherence) and assist with the transition to home or subacute care center.
- Most patients are still recovering from their illness or surgery when discharged from the hospital; home health services may be required.
- Teach the patient and family about:
    1. The pathophysiology of angina and MI
    2. Risk factor modification
        a. Smoking cessation
        b. Dietary changes (e.g., decreasing fat intake)
        c. Blood pressure control
        d. Blood glucose control
    3. Gradual increase in physical and sexual activity, according to cardiac rehabilitation protocol
    4. Cardiac drugs
    5. Occupational considerations, if any
    6. Complementary and alternative therapies such as progressive relaxation, guided imagery, music therapy, pet therapy
- Teach the patient to seek medical assistance if they experience:
    1. Pulse rate that remains 50 or less while awake
    2. Wheezing or difficulty breathing
    3. Weight gain of 3 pounds in (6.6 kg) 1 week, or 1 to 2 pounds (2.2 to 4.4 kg) overnight
    4. Slow, persistent increase in nitroglycerin use
    5. Dizziness, faintness, or shortness of breath with activity
- Patients should call for emergency transportation to the hospital if they experience the following:
    1. Chest discomfort that does not improve after 20 minutes or after taking three nitroglycerin tablets
    2. Extremely severe chest or epigastric discomfort with weakness, nausea, or fainting
    3. Other angina symptoms that are particular to the patient, such as fatigue or nausea
- Other important discharge plans include:
    1. Referring the patient to the American Heart Association for information
    2. Referring the patient for continued cardiac rehabilitation
    3. Referring the patient who has had CABG surgery to Mended Hearts, a nationwide program that provides education and support to patients and their families

CROHN'S DISEASE

OVERVIEW

- Crohn's disease, or *regional enteritis,* is an idiopathic inflammatory disease that occurs anywhere in the GI tract but most often affects the terminal ileum with patchy lesions that extend through all bowel layers.
- Chronic nonspecific inflammation of the entire intestinal tract occurs, and eventually deep fissures and ulcerations develop and often extend through all bowel layers, predisposing the patient to development of bowel fistulas.
- Chronic pathologic changes include thickening of the bowel wall, resulting in narrowing of the bowel lumen and strictures.
- Complications of Crohn's disease include malabsorption, fistulas, hemorrhage, abscess formation, bowel obstruction, and increased risk for cancer. Because of small intestine involvement, patient's with Crohn's disease can develop severe malnutrition.

PATIENT-CENTERED COLLABORATIVE CARE

Assessment

- Assess for:
  1. Fever, abdominal pain, loose stools
  2. Frequency, consistency, and presence of blood in the stool
  3. Periumbilical pain before and after bowel movements
  4. Weight loss (indicates serious nutritional deficiencies)
  5. Family history of the disease
  6. Distention, masses, or visible peristalsis
  7. Ulcerations or fissures of the perianal area
  8. Bowel sounds diminished or absent in the presence of severe inflammation
  9. High-pitched or rushing sounds over the areas of narrowed bowel loops
  10. Diarrhea with steatorrhea (stool does not usually contain blood but is fatty, frothy, foul-smelling)
  11. Psychosocial issues related to coping skills and support systems
  12. Results of barium enema and upper GI series that show narrowing, ulcerations, strictures, and fistulas consistent with Crohn's disease
  13. Results of laboratory studies, especially WBC count and electrolytes

Interventions

- The care of the patient with Crohn's disease is similar to care for the patient with ulcerative colitis (see *Colitis, Ulcerative*).
- Drug therapy includes:

1. Aminosalicylates used for anti-inflammation
2. Glucocorticoids during diseases exacerbation
3. Immunomodulatory therapy, used for patients with refractory disease:
   a. Azathioprine (Imuran), mercaptopurine (Purinethol), or methotrexate may be given to suppress the immune system, but they can lead to serious infections.
   b. Infliximab (Remicade), adalimumab (Humira), natalizumab (Tysabri), and certolizumab pegol (Cimzia), anti-tumor necrosis agents to decrease the inflammatory response may be used. However, they can lead to opportunistic infections.
4. Metronidazole (Flagyl, Novonidazol) can be helpful for patients with fistulas.

! NURSING SAFETY PRIORITY: Action Alert

Adequate nutrition and fluid and electrolyte balance are priorities in the care of the patient with a fistula. GI secretions are high in volume and rich in electrolytes and enzymes. The patient is at high risk for malnutrition, dehydration, and hypokalemia (decreased serum potassium). Assess for these complications, and collaborate with the health care team to manage them. Monitor urinary output. A decrease indicates possible dehydration, which should be treated immediately by providing additional fluids.

- Malnutrition can result in poor fistula and wound healing, loss of lean muscle mass, decreased immune system response, and increased morbidity and mortality.
  1. Monitor tolerance to diet.
  2. Assist the patient to select high-calorie, high-protein, high-vitamin, low-fiber meals.
  3. Offer oral supplements such as Ensure and Vivonex.
  4. Record food intake and accurate calorie count.
  5. Total parenteral nutrition (TPN) may be needed for severe exacerbations while the patient is NPO.
- Electrolyte therapy includes:
  1. Fluid and electrolyte replacement by oral liquids and nutrients, as well as IV fluids
  2. Cautious use of antidiarrheal agents to decrease fluid loss
  3. Strict monitoring of intake and output
- Impaired skin integrity results from fistula formation. The degree of associated problems is related to the location of the fistula, the patient's general health status, and the character and amount of fistula drainage.

1. In collaboration with the enterostomal therapist, apply a pouch to the fistula to prevent skin irritation and to measure the drainage.
2. Cover the area around the fistula with skin barriers, such as Stomahesive or DuoDerm, and apply a wound drainage system over the fistula, securing it to the protective barriers.
3. Clean adjacent skin and keep it dry. The wound drainage should never be allowed to have direct skin contact without prompt cleaning, because intestinal fluid enzymes are caustic.
4. Observe for subtle signs of infection or sepsis such as fever, abdominal pain, or change in mental status.

- Some patients with Crohn's disease require surgery such as a bowel resection and anastomosis with or without a colon resection to improve the quality of life (see *Surgical Management* under *Cancer, Colorectal*).
- Stricturoplasty may be performed for bowel strictures.

Community-Based Care
See *Community-Based Care* under *Colitis, Ulcerative*.

CYSTIC FIBROSIS

OVERVIEW
- Cystic fibrosis (CF) is a genetic disease present from birth that affects many organs and lethally impairs pulmonary function.
- The underlying problem of CF is blocked chloride transport in cell membranes, causing the formation of thick and sticky mucus.
- This mucus plugs up glands in the lungs, pancreas, liver, salivary glands, and testes, causing atrophy and organ dysfunction.
- Nonpulmonary problems include pancreatic insufficiency with malnutrition and intestinal obstruction, poor growth, male sterility, and cirrhosis of the liver.
- Life expectancy is over 30 years for a patient with typical manifestations of CF. The primary cause of death in the patient with CF is respiratory failure.
- The disorder is most common among white individuals, and about 4% are carriers. It is very rare among African Americans or Asians. Males and females are affected equally.

Genetic/Genomic Considerations
- CF is an autosomal recessive disorder in which both gene alleles must be mutated for the disease to be expressed. The CF gene is located on chromosome 7 and produces a protein that controls chloride movement across cell membranes.

- There is great variation in the severity of CF. Life expectancy is considerably reduced when there is pulmonary involvement.
- People with one mutated allele are carriers and have few or no symptoms of CF but can pass the abnormal allele on to their children.
- More than 1700 different mutations have been identified. The inheritance of different mutations is responsible for the wide variation in disease severity.

PATIENT-CENTERED COLLABORATIVE CARE
Assessment
- The major diagnostic test is sweat chloride analysis, and additional genetic testing can be performed to determine which specific mutation a person may have.
- Assess for these nonpulmonary manifestations: abdominal distention, gastroesophageal reflux, rectal prolapse, foul-smelling stools, steatorrhea (excessive fat in stools), small stature, and underweight for height.
- Assess for these common pulmonary manifestations: frequent or chronic respiratory infections, chest congestion, limited exercise tolerance, cough, sputum production, use of accessory muscles, and decreased pulmonary function (especially forced vital capacity [FVC] and forced exhalation volume over 1 second [FEV_1]).

Interventions
Nonsurgical Management
- Nutritional management focuses on weight maintenance, vitamin supplementation, diabetes management, and pancreatic enzyme replacement (enzymes must be taken with food).
- Pulmonary management is focused on preventive maintenance and management of pulmonary exacerbation.
  1. Preventive or maintenance therapy involves the use of a regimen of chest physiotherapy, positive expiratory pressure, active cycle breathing technique, and an individualized regular exercise program. Drug therapy includes bronchodilators, anti-inflammatory agents, mucolytics, and antibiotics.
  2. Exacerbation therapy is needed when the patient with CF has a change in manifestations from baseline. Management focuses on mucus clearance, oxygenation, and antibiotic therapy:
     a. Supplemental oxygen
     b. Heliox delivery of 50% oxygen and 50% helium
     c. Airway clearance techniques (ACTs) four times each day

      d. Intensified bronchodilator and mucolytic therapies; glucocorticoids; and IV antibiotics

⚠ NURSING SAFETY PRIORITY: Critical Rescue

Strict procedures approved by the Cystic Fibrosis Foundation should be used when cleaning clinic rooms, pulmonary function laboratories, and respiratory therapy equipment to reduce the risk of contamination between CF patients who are often colonized with pathogens that can contribute to disease exacerbation and mortality.

3. Teach patients about protecting themselves by avoiding direct contact of bodily fluids such as saliva and sputum. Teach them not to routinely shake hands or kiss people in social settings. Handwashing is critical because the organism also can be acquired indirectly from contaminated surfaces such as sinks and tissues.

Surgical Management
- The surgical management of the patient with CF involves lung and/or pancreatic transplantation.
- Lung transplantation procedures include two lobes or a single lung transplantation, as well as double-lung transplantation. Most often the patient with CF has a bilateral lobe transplant from a cadaver donor or living related donor.
- Provide preoperative care:
  1. Teach the patient the expected regimen of pulmonary hygiene to be used in the period immediately after surgery.
  2. Assist the patient in a pulmonary muscle strengthening and conditioning regimen.
- Provide postoperative care:
  1. The patient is intubated for at least 48 hours and has chest tubes and arterial lines in place. Much of the care needed is the same as that for any thoracic surgery.
  2. Assess for bleeding, infection, and transplant rejection.
  3. Anti-rejection drug regimens must be started immediately after surgery, which increases the risk for infection. The drugs generally used for routine long-term rejection suppression after organ transplantation are combinations of:
     a. Very specific immunosuppressants (cyclosporine [Sandimmune])
     b. Less specific immunosuppressants (azathioprine [Imuran] or mycophenolate mofetil [CellCept])
     c. One of the corticosteroids (prednisone [Apo-Prednisone ✦, Deltasone ✦] or prednisolone [Delta-Cortef]).

CYSTITIS (URINARY TRACT INFECTION)

OVERVIEW

- *Cystitis* is an inflammation of the urinary bladder with both infectious and noninfectious causes. Infectious causes are bacteria, viruses, fungi, and parasites. Noninfectious causes are chemical exposure, radiation therapy, and immunologic responses in chronic inflammatory disease.
- *Interstitial cystitis* is a chronic inflammation of the entire lower urinary tract (bladder, urethra, and adjacent pelvic muscles) that is not the result of infection and can lead to pyelonephritis and sepsis.
- *Urosepsis* is the spread of infection from the urinary tract to the bloodstream.
- *Escherichia coli* normally found in the GI tract account for most cases of bacterial cystitis.
- Other factors that contribute to the development or recurrence of cystitis, or urinary tract infections (UTIs), include:
  1. Structural or functional abnormalities of the urinary tract
  2. Use of indwelling urinary catheters

❗NURSING SAFETY PRIORITY: Action Alert

Avoid use of indwelling urinary catheters for longer than 3 days to reduce catheter-related UTIs.

  3. Sexual intercourse, diaphragm use, and pregnancy in women
  4. Prostate disease

Considerations for Older Adults

- UTIs occur more often in older adults than in younger adults, with women more commonly affected than men.
- Older patients are at greater risk than others of having an overwhelming and generalized infection, known as *urosepsis*.

◪NATIONAL PATIENT SAFETY GOAL

Timely reporting of abnormal complete blood count (CBC) results (especially an elevated white blood cell [WBC] count), abnormal urinalysis results (especially positive nitrogen and leukocyte esterase), and positive urine culture reports are essential to initiating and evaluating effective antibiotic treatment.

❗NURSING SAFETY PRIORITY: Critical Rescue

A decrease in mental status or increase in heart rate combined with a decrease in blood pressure can indicate clinical instability or urosepsis, requiring immediate intervention.

PATIENT CENTERED COLLABORATIVE CARE
Assessment
- Record patient information:
  1. History of UTIs
  2. History of renal or urologic problems, such as kidney stones, structural disease, or functional problems with voiding
  3. History of impaired immune response, such as diabetes mellitus or inflammatory and autoimmune disease
- Assess for:
  1. Increased frequency in voiding
  2. Urgency to void
  3. Pain or discomfort on urination
  4. Change in urine color, clarity, or odor; presence of WBCs or red blood cells (RBCs)
  5. Presence of nitrogen or leukocyte esterase with urinalysis
  6. Positive urine culture
  7. Elevated plasma WBCs (occasional)
  8. Abdominal or back pain
  9. Bladder distention
  10. Feelings of incomplete bladder emptying
  11. Voiding in small amounts
  12. Difficulty in initiating urination
  13. Complete inability to urinate
  14. Urinary meatus inflammation
  15. Prostate gland changes or tenderness

Considerations for Older Adults
- The only symptoms of UTI may be as vague as increasing mental confusion or unexplained falls.
- Sudden onset of or worsening of incontinence may be an early symptom.
- Fever, tachycardia, tachypnea, and hypotension even without any urinary symptoms may be signs of urosepsis.
- Loss of appetite, nocturia, and dysuria are common symptoms.

Planning and Implementation
- Drug therapy includes:
  1. Antibiotics: In uncomplicated, acute bacterial cystitis in healthy, ambulatory patients, a 3-day course of oral antibiotic treatment may be adequate. A 7- to 14-day course of oral or parenteral antibiotics may be needed for complex, chronic, or recurring infections and for urosepsis.

2. Analgesics or antipyretics may be used to promote comfort.
3. Urinary antiseptics such as nitrofurantoin (Macrodantin, Nephronex ✺) and trimethoprim (Proloprim, Trimpex) may be prescribed.
4. Antispasmodics may be used to decrease bladder spasm and promote complete bladder emptying.
5. Antifungal agents such as amphotericin B in daily bladder instillations and ketoconazole (Nizoral) in oral form may also be used.

- Diet therapy includes:
  1. Ensure sufficient fluid intake to maintain clear or light yellow urine (1.5 to 2.5 L/day), unless contraindicated.
  2. Cranberry juice or tablets taken daily may reduce the frequency of recurrent UTI but should be avoided with interstitial cystitis.
- Other therapy includes providing warm sitz baths to relieve perineal discomfort.

  Surgical Management
- Surgical interventions for management of cystitis include urologic procedures for structural abnormalities or endourologic procedures to manipulate or pulverize kidney stones if these conditions are associated with cystitis.

🚩 NATIONAL PATIENT SAFETY GOAL

Anticipate fall prevention interventions for older patients to reduce the risk of patient harm when confusion accompanies cystitis.

Community-Based Care

- Teach the patient to:
  1. Self-administer drugs and complete all of the prescribed drug.
  2. Expect changes in color of urine with some treatments.
  3. Use appropriate techniques to prevent discomfort with sexual activities and how to prevent postcoital infections.
  4. Consume liberal fluid intake to maintain urine color as clear or light yellow.
  5. Clean the perineum after urination.
  6. Empty the bladder as soon as the urge is felt.
  7. Avoid known irritants such as caffeine, carbonated beverages, tomato products, chemicals in bath water (e.g. bubble baths), vaginal washes, and scented toilet tissue.
  8. Wear cotton underwear.
  9. Seek prompt medical care if symptoms recur.

10. Pregnant women with cystitis require prompt and aggressive antibiotic treatment, because this infection can lead to preterm labor and premature birth.
- Refer patients with interstitial cystitis to the Interstitial Cystitis Foundation.

CYSTOCELE

- A cystocele is a protrusion of the bladder through the vaginal wall resulting from weakened pelvic structures.
- Causes include obesity, advanced age, childbearing, or genetic predisposition.
- Assess for:
  1. Difficulty in emptying the bladder
  2. Urinary frequency and urgency or other symptoms of urinary tract infection
  3. Stress urinary incontinence
  4. Bulging of the anterior vaginal wall, especially when the woman is asked to bear down during a pelvic examination
- Diagnostic tests may include cystography, measurement of residual urine, IV urography (IVU), voiding cystourethrography (VCUG), cystometrography, and uroflowmetry.
- Management of patients with mild symptoms is conservative and may include:
  1. Use of a pessary for bladder support
  2. Application of intravaginal estrogen to prevent atrophy and weakening of vaginal walls
  3. Kegel exercises to strengthen perineal muscles
- Surgical intervention for severe symptoms is usually a vaginal sling or an anterior colporrhaphy (anterior repair) to tighten the pelvic muscles for better bladder support (see *Prolapse, Vaginal*).

DEHYDRATION

OVERVIEW

- Dehydration is a state in which fluid intake or fluid retention is less than what is needed to meet the body's fluid needs, resulting in a fluid volume deficit.
- It may be an actual decrease in total body water caused by either too little intake of fluid or too great a loss of fluid; or it can occur as a relative dehydration, without an actual loss of total body water, such as when water shifts from the plasma into the interstitial space.

Considerations for Older Adults

Older patients are at high risk for dehydration, because they have less total body water than younger adults. Many older adults have decreased thirst sensation and may have difficulty with walking or other motor skills needed for ingesting fluids. Other older adults may voluntarily cut back fluid intake because of concerns about incontinence. Older adults also may take drugs such as diuretics, antihypertensives, and laxatives that increase the amount of fluid excreted and, at times, experience overdiuresis.

D

- *Isotonic dehydration* is the most common type of fluid volume deficit, in which fluid is lost only from the extracellular fluid (ECF) space, including both the plasma and the interstitial spaces.
- Circulating blood volume is decreased (hypovolemia) and leads to inadequate tissue perfusion.
- Causes include:
    1. Hemorrhage
    2. Vomiting, diarrhea
    3. Profuse salivation
    4. Fistulas, draining abscesses
    5. Profuse diaphoresis
    6. Burns and other severe wounds
    7. Long-term NPO status
    8. Diuretic therapy
    9. Continuous GI or nasogastric (NG) suctioning
    10. Impaired motor skills, preventing self-care and fluid intake

PATIENT-CENTERED COLLABORATIVE CARE

Assessment

- Obtain and record patient information:
    1. Nutritional history
    2. Fluid history
        a. Intake and output volumes
        b. Weight (a weight change of 1 pound corresponds to fluid volume change of about 500 mL)
    3. Presence of excessive sweating, diarrhea
    4. Drug therapy (especially diuretics and laxatives)
    5. Medical history
        a. Diabetes
        b. Kidney disease
    6. Level of consciousness and functional status
    7. Amount of strenuous physical activity
    8. Exposure to high environmental temperatures
    9. Dizziness or light-headedness when standing

- Assess for:
  1. Vital signs, including orthostatic heart rate (HR) and blood pressure (BP) if patient is able to sit or stand
  2. Cardiovascular changes:
     a. Tachycardia at rest
     b. Weak peripheral pulses
     c. Low systolic or mean arterial BP
     d. Decreased pulse pressure
     e. Flat neck and hand veins in dependent position
  3. Respiratory changes:
     a. Increased respiratory rate
     b. Increased respiratory depth
  4. Skin changes:
     a. Dry mucous membranes
     b. Tongue has a pastelike coating or fissures
     c. Dry, flaky skin
     d. Poor skin turgor (skin "tents" when pinched)

Considerations for Older Adults

Assess skin turgor in an older adult by pinching the skin over the sternum or on the forehead, rather than the back of the hand, because these areas more reliably indicate hydration. As a person ages, the skin loses elasticity and tents on hands and arms even when the person is well hydrated.

  5. Neurologic changes:
     a. Alterations of mental status (especially confusion)
     b. Low-grade fever
  6. Renal changes:
     a. Decreased output
     b. Increased urine concentration (specific gravity greater than 1.030, dark amber, strong odor)

■ NURSING SAFETY PRIORITY: Critical Rescue

Urine output below 500 mL/day for any patient without kidney disease is cause for concern and should be reported to the health care provider.

- Diagnostic assessment: No single laboratory test result confirms or rules out dehydration. Instead, it is determined by laboratory findings along with clinical manifestations. Common laboratory findings for dehydration include:
  1. Elevated levels of hemoglobin and hematocrit
  2. Increased serum osmolarity, glucose, protein, blood urea nitrogen, and various electrolytes

Hemoconcentration is not present when dehydration is from hemorrhage. Therefore do not rely only on laboratory values to identify dehydration.

Interventions

- Management of dehydration aims to prevent injury, prevent further fluid losses, and increase fluid compartment volumes to normal ranges.
  1. Patient safety issues (to prevent falls):
     a. Monitor vital signs, especially heart rate and blood pressure.
     b. Assess muscle strength, gait stability, and level of alertness.
     c. Instruct the patient to get up slowly from a lying or sitting position and to immediately sit down if he or she feels light-headed.
     d. Implement the falls precautions.
  2. Fluid replacement:
     a. Oral fluid replacement is used for correction of mild to moderate dehydration if the patient is alert enough to swallow and can tolerate oral fluids. Commercial solutions for adults include Equalyte, Oralyte, and Rehydralyte.
     b. IV fluid replacement is used when dehydration is severe and when the patient is not alert enough to swallow or cannot tolerate oral fluids.
     c. Measure fluid intake and output.
     d. Monitor pulse rate and quality.
  3. Drug therapy may correct some causes of the dehydration:
     a. Antidiarrheal drugs
     b. Antiemetics
     c. Antipyretics

DEMENTIA

OVERVIEW

- Dementia is a chronic, progressive, degenerative disease that is characterized by memory loss and cognitive impairment.
- *Alzheimer's disease (AD)* and *dementia, Alzheimer's type (DAT)*, account for 60% of the dementias occurring in persons older than 65 years.
- Dementia is also seen in people in their 40s and 50s, which is referred to as *early dementia*, or *presenile DAT*.

- AD is characterized by neurofibrillary tangles and neuritic plaques of beta-amyloid proteins in the brain.
- The exact cause of AD is unknown; genetic predisposition, chemical changes, environmental agents, and immunologic alterations have been implicated in the pathology.
- Other causes of dementia are stroke or cerebrovascular impairment, head injury, Lewy body formation, and human immunodeficiency virus (HIV) infection.

PATIENT-CENTERED COLLABORATIVE CARE
Assessment
- Record patient information:
  1. Age
  2. Current employment status and work history
  3. Self-management skills for daily living
  4. Ability to complete independent activities such as grocery shopping, laundry, meal planning, and financial transactions
  5. Driving ability
  6. Oral and written communication skills
  7. Behavior
  8. Family history of AD
  9. Medical history, with particular attention to head trauma, viral illness, or exposure to metal or toxic waste
  10. Available support systems (spouse, adult children)
- Assess for:
  1. Indicators of the stages of the disease:
     a. *Early (stage I) AD* is characterized by forgetfulness, misplacing household items, mild memory loss, short attention span, decreased performance, loss of judgment, subtle changes in personality and behavior, and the inability to travel alone to new destinations. There are no associated social or employment problems.
     b. *Middle (stage II) AD* is characterized by severe impairments in all cognitive functions; gross intellectual impairments; complete disorientation to time, place, and event; physical impairment; loss of ability to care for self; visual-spatial deficits; speech-language problems; and incontinence.
     c. *Late (stage III) AD* is characterized by lost motor and verbal skills and by severe physical and cognitive deterioration and total dependence for the ADLs.
  2. Cognitive changes, such as changes in attention, concentration, judgment, perception, learning, and short-term memory
  3. Alterations in communication and language skills

4. Changes in behaviors and personality, such as aggressiveness, paranoia, inappropriate social interactions, rapid mood swings, and increased confusion at night or when fatigued

5. Changes in self-management requiring assistance in hygiene, dressing, following directions, or completing familiar activities

- Genetic testing specifically for apolipoprotein E (apo-E) may be helpful as an ancillary test (not a predictive test) for the differential diagnosis of AD.

- A variety of laboratory or radiographic tests are performed to rule out other treatable causes of dementia or delirium, including serum levels of beta-amyloid.

D

Planning and Implementation
CHRONIC CONFUSION

- Confusion is related to neuronal degeneration in the brain.

- Collaborate with the health care team to prevent overstimulation and provide a structured and orderly environment.

   1. Provide a safe environment with adequate lighting, and remove items that can obstruct walking.

   2. Implement falls precautions in the acute care setting.

   3. Place the patient within easy view of the staff, preferably in a private room.

   4. Arrange the patient's schedule to provide as much uninterrupted sleep at night as possible. Fatigue increases confusion and behavioral problems such as agitation and aggression.

   5. Establish a daily routine, explaining changes in routine before they occur and again immediately before they take place.

   6. Place familiar objects, clocks, and single-date calendars in easy view of the patient. Encourage the family to provide pictures of family members and close friends that are labeled with the person's name on the picture.

   7. Regularly reorient the patient to the environment (during early stages).

   8. Use validation therapy for later stages of the disease to prevent agitation.

   9. Collaborate with the physical and occupational therapist to assist the patient to maintain independence in ADLs as long as possible through the use of assistive devices (grab bars in the bathroom) and exercise programs.

   10. Develop an individualized bowel and bladder program for the patient.

   11. Attract the patient's attention before conversing, then use short, clear sentences.

12. Allow sufficient time for the patient to respond.
13. In the home environment, place complete outfits on a single hanger for the patient to choose from; encourage the family to include the patient in meal planning, grocery shopping, and other household routines as he or she is able.
14. Provide drug therapy:
    a. Cholinesterase inhibitors are approved for symptomatic treatment of AD.
    b. Selective serotonin reuptake inhibitors are used to treat depression; tricyclic antidepressants should not be used because of their anticholinergic effect.
    c. Psychotropic drugs, also called *antipsychotic* and *neuroleptic drugs*, should be reserved for a patient with emotional and behavioral health problems that may accompany dementia, such as hallucinations and delusions.
15. Use activities and recreation such as art, dance, and music in the long-term care setting to minimize agitation.

RISK FOR INJURY

- The risk for injury is related to wandering or elder abuse.
- The following nursing planning and implementation steps are used to decrease the risk for injury:
    1. Ensure that the patient always wears an identification bracelet or badge that cannot be removed by the patient. Devices that use global positioning system (GPS) can be embedded in the bracelet or badge to provide tracking abilities.
    2. Ensure that alarms or other barriers to outside doors are working properly at all times.
    3. Check on the patient often.
    4. Take the patient for walks several times each day, and encourage the patient to participate in activities to decrease his or her restlessness.
    5. Talk calmly and softly, redirecting the patient as needed and using diversion.
    6. Keep the patient busy with structured activities such as music, recreation, and art therapy.
    7. Remove and secure all sharp objects and medications.
    8. Implement seizure precautions if there is a history of seizures.
    9. Keep an updated photograph of the patient that can be used if the patient wanders away.
    10. Inform the patient's family about the Safe Return program, a national government-funded program of the Alzheimer's Association that assists in the identification and safe, timely return of individuals with AD and related dementias who wander off and become lost.

CAREGIVER ROLE STRAIN
- The following nursing planning and implementation steps are used to increase family coping and decrease caregiver role strain:
  1. Advise the family to seek legal counsel regarding the patient's competency and the need to obtain guardianship or durable power of attorney.
  2. Refer the family to a local support group affiliated with the Alzheimer's Association.
  3. Assess the family and other caregivers for signs of stress, such as anger, social withdrawal, anxiety, depression and lack of concentration, sleepiness, irritability, and health problems; refer them to their health care provider.
  4. Encourage the family to maintain its own social network and to obtain respite care periodically.
  5. Assist the family to identify and develop strategies to cope with the long-term consequences of the disease.

▼ NATIONAL PATIENT SAFETY GOAL
Evaluate and report critical laboratory values in a timely manner so that reversible causes of delirium receive effective interventions, such as hemoglobin or electrolyte replacement therapy.

Community-Based Care
- When possible, the patient should be assigned to a case manager who can assess the patient's need for health care resources and facilitate appropriate placement throughout the continuum of care.
- The patient is usually cared for in the home until late in the disease process. Therefore teach the patient and family:
  1. How to assist the patient with ADLs
  2. How to use adaptive equipment
  3. With dietary consultation, how to select and prepare food that the patient is able to chew and swallow
  4. How to prevent the patient from wandering
  5. What to do if the patient has a seizure
  6. How to protect the patient from injury
  7. Drug information (if drugs are prescribed) and how to secure drugs so the patient does not take them inappropriately
  8. How to implement the diversion, including activity or exercise
  9. How to obtain respite services
  10. Strategies that caregivers can use to reduce their stress, including:

    a. Maintaining realistic expectations for the person with AD
    b. Taking one day at a time
    c. Trying to find positive aspects of each incident or situation
    d. Using humor with the person who has AD
    e. Setting aside time each day for rest or recreation, away from caregiving duties if possible
    f. Seeking respite care periodically
    g. Exploring alternative care settings early in the disease process for possible use later
    h. Establishing advance directives with the person who has AD early in the disease process
    i. Taking care of themselves by watching their diet, exercising, and getting plenty of rest
    j. Being realistic about what they can do, and getting and accepting help from family, friends, and community resources
- Refer the patient's family and significant others to the local chapter of the Alzheimer's Association.

DIABETES INSIPIDUS

OVERVIEW
- Diabetes insipidus (DI) is a water metabolism problem caused by an antidiuretic hormone (ADH) deficiency (a decrease in ADH synthesis or an inability of the kidneys to respond to ADH). ADH deficiency results in the excretion of large volumes of dilute urine.
- DI is classified into four types, depending on whether the problem is caused by too little ADH or an inability of the kidneys to respond to ADH.
  1. *Nephrogenic DI*: an inherited disorder in which the renal tubules do not respond to the actions of ADH, which results in inadequate water absorption by the kidney
  2. *Primary DI*: results from a problem in the hypothalamus or pituitary gland resulting in lack of ADH production or release
  3. *Secondary DI*: results from tumors in or near the hypothalamus or pituitary gland, head trauma, infectious processes, surgical procedures, or metastatic tumors (usually from the lung or breast)
  4. *Drug-related DI*: most often caused by lithium (Eskalith, Lithobid, Carbolith ♣) and demeclocycline (Declomycin), which can interfere with the kidney response to ADH

PATIENT-CENTERED COLLABORATIVE CARE
Assessment
- Assess patient information:
  1. History of known causes, such as recent surgery, head trauma, or drugs
  2. Excretion of large amounts of dilute urine (more than 4 L in 24 hours) in excess of fluid intake
  3. Dehydration manifestations (e.g., poor skin turgor, dry mucous membranes, or weight loss in excess of 1 pound/day)
  4. Increased or excessive thirst
  5. Low urine specific gravity (below 1.005) and urine osmolality (50 to 20 0 mOsm/kg)
  6. Indications of circulatory collapse, shock (e.g., low blood pressure; rapid, thready pulse; increased respiratory rate; and decreased pulse pressure)
  7. Neurologic changes such as irritability, lethargy, or decreased cognition

Interventions
- Drug therapy may include:
  1. Desmopressin (DDAVP), a synthetic form of vasopressin given intranasally in a metered spray or as an oral tablet; frequency of dosing depends on the patient's response
  2. Aqueous vasopressin for short-term therapy or when the dosage must be changed often; given parenterally
  3. Chlorpropamide (Diabinese, Insulase), an antidiabetic drug that also decreases urine output by an unknown mechanism; given orally
- Nursing interventions include:
  1. Replacing fluids by encouraging the patient to drink fluids equal to the amount of urinary output (If the patient is unable to do so, provide IV, as prescribed.)

◾ NURSING SAFETY PRIORITY: Critical Rescue
Patients with this condition are at risk for severe dehydration and circulatory collapse. Provide ongoing access to oral or IV fluids and monitor patient response to intake and output every 4 hours around the clock.

  2. Monitoring accurately intake and output and communicating imbalances in a timely manner.
  3. Monitoring for vital sign changes indicating poor tissue perfusion (e.g., low blood pressure; rapid, thready pulse; decreased consciousness)

4. Monitoring for indications of dehydration, including dry skin, poor skin turgor, and dry or cracked mucous membranes
5. Measuring urine specific gravity at least once daily
6. Monitoring therapy effectiveness by weighing the patient every day; a loss of 1 kg is equivalent to losing 1 L of fluid.

- Patient education includes:
  1. Teaching the patient that polyuria and thirst are signals for the need for another drug dose
  2. Teaching the patient to use daily weights to estimate dehydration (and need for additional vasopressin) or overhydration (reduce medication)
  3. Teaching about the side effects of nasal sprays, including ulceration of the mucous membranes, allergy, sensation of chest tightness, and inhalation of the spray into the lungs, which precipitates pulmonary problems
  4. Teaching what to do if side effects occur or if an upper respiratory infection develops
  5. Teaching the patient going home on vasopressin how to self-inject the drug
  6. Encouraging the patient with chronic DI to wear a medical alert bracelet or necklace at all times

DIABETES MELLITUS

OVERVIEW

- Diabetes mellitus (DM) is a metabolic disease that results from problems with insulin secretion, insulin action, or both.
- The main metabolic effects of insulin are to stimulate glucose uptake in skeletal muscle and heart muscle, and to suppress liver production of glucose and very-low-density lipoprotein (VLDL). Overall, insulin keeps blood glucose levels from becoming too high and helps keep blood lipid levels in the normal range. Insulin is needed for metabolism of carbohydrates, proteins, and fats.
- Movement of glucose into some cells requires the presence of specific carrier proteins, glucose transport proteins (GLUTs), and insulin. As glucose from the blood enters the cells, the blood glucose level goes back to normal (euglycemia). The glucose in the cell can be used immediately to make adenosine triphosphate (ATP) if the cell needs more chemical energy. If the cell already has enough ATP, the glucose is stored for later use.
- The lack of insulin in DM from a lack of production or a problem with insulin use at its cell receptor prevents some cells from

using glucose for energy. Without insulin, the body enters a serious state of cellular starvation, breaking down body fat and protein.

- DM is diagnosed with either a blood glucose measurement or a test of glycosylated hemoglobin (A_{1c}) levels.
- Acute manifestations of DM are hyperglycemia (elevated blood glucose levels), polyuria (excessive urination), polydipsia (excessive thirst and drinking), and polyphagia (hunger).
- Chronic complications of DM result from changes in large blood vessels *(macrovascular)* and small blood vessels *(microvascular)* in tissues and organs, leading to poor tissue circulation and cell death. Macrovascular complications include coronary heart disease, cerebrovascular disease, peripheral vascular disease, and early death. Microvascular complications lead to *nephropathy* (kidney dysfunction), *neuropathy* (nerve dysfunction), and *retinopathy* (vision problems).
- DM is classified according to the cause of the disease and the severity of insulin lack. The three most common types of DM are type 1, type 2, and gestational diabetes.
  1. *Type 1 diabetes* is an autoimmune disorder in which beta cells of the pancreas are destroyed in a genetically susceptible person and no insulin is produced. Type I diabetes:
     a. Is abrupt in onset
     b. Requires insulin injections to prevent hyperglycemia and ketosis and to sustain health
     c. Represents fewer than 10% of all people who have diabetes
     d. Occurs primarily in childhood or adolescence but can occur at any age
     e. Causes patients to be thin and underweight
     f. May follow a viral infection; viral infection can trigger autoimmune antibody formation
     g. Can lead to ketoacidosis
  2. *Type 2 diabetes* is a problem resulting from a reduction in the ability of most cells to respond to insulin (insulin resistance), poor control of liver glucose output, and decreased beta cell function. Type 2 diabetes:
     a. Is generally slow in onset
     b. May require oral antidiabetic drug therapy or insulin to correct hyperglycemia
     c. Is usually found in middle-aged and older adults but may occur in younger people
     d. May be part of the metabolic syndrome
     e. Occurs more often among obese people
     f. Is usually not associated with ketoacidosis

D

      g. Represents about 90% of all people who have diabetes

      h. May be present for years before it is diagnosed

  3. Gestational diabetes mellitus (GDM):

      a. Carbohydrate intolerance noted during pregnancy and confirmed by an oral glucose tolerance test

      b. Is suspected when a first baby weighs more than 9 pounds

      c. Leaves women at high risk for type 2 diabetes after pregnancy

- Acute complications of DM include:

  1. Diabetic ketoacidosis (DKA):

      a. DKA occurs in people with type 1 DM and is most often precipitated by illness, especially infection.

      b. Patients have acidosis and severe dehydration.

      c. Laboratory diagnosis is based on serum glucose level equal to or greater than 300 mg/dL (16.7 mmol/L), arterial pH less than 7.35, arterial bicarbonate level less than 15 mEq/L, blood urea nitrogen level greater than 20 mg/dL, creatinine level greater than 1.5 mg/dL, and ketonuria.

      d. Clinical manifestations of dehydration and acidosis include decreased skin turgor, dry mucous membranes, hypotension, tachycardia, tachypnea, Kussmaul respirations, abdominal pain, nausea, and vomiting; central nervous system depression results in changes in consciousness varying from lethargy to coma.

      e. Death occurs in 1% to 10% of these cases even with appropriate treatment. Mortality is highest for older patients who also have infection, stroke, myocardial infarction (MI), vascular thrombosis, intestinal obstruction, or pneumonia.

  2. Hyperglycemic-hyperosmolar state (HHS):

      a. HHS is a hyperosmolar state caused by hyperglycemia of any origin; it differs from DKA by the relative absence of ketosis and by much higher blood glucose levels (may exceed 600 mg/dL) and blood osmolarity levels (may exceed 320 mOsm/L).

      b. Dehydration is the most common cause of HHS and becomes worse with the disorder.

      c. HHS occurs almost exclusively in patients with type 2 DM.

      d. It occurs most often in older adults and those who are unaware of their diabetic condition.

      e. Conditions such as silent myocardial infarction (MI), sepsis, pancreatitis, and stroke, and drugs such as glucocorticoids, diuretics, phenytoin sodium, propranolol, and calcium channel blockers may precipitate HHS.

Considerations for Older Adults

Older adults with DM are at the greatest risk for dehydration and subsequent HHS. The onset of HHS is slow and may not be recognized. The older patient often seeks medical attention later and is sicker than younger patients. The mortality rate for HHS is as high as 40% to 70% among older adults.

🔳 NURSING SAFETY PRIORITY: Action Alert

HHS does not occur in people who are adequately hydrated. Take steps to avoid dehydration in susceptible patients.

3. Hypoglycemia:
   a. Hypoglycemia is a blood glucose level lower than 70 mg/dL.
   b. It can be caused by excessive insulin, some oral antidiabetic drugs, insufficient food intake, and increased physical activity.
   c. *Neurogenic symptoms* of hypoglycemia, which result from autonomic nervous system stimulation triggered by hypoglycemia, include hunger, diaphoresis, weakness, and nervousness. These symptoms occur when there is an abrupt decrease in the blood glucose level.
   d. *Neuroglycopenic symptoms,* which result directly from brain glucose deprivation and include headache, confusion, slurred speech, behavioral changes, and coma, occur with a more gradual decline in blood glucose level.
   e. If not managed properly, hypoglycemia can lead to brain damage and death.

- The classic signs and symptoms of hypoglycemia may not appear in older patients with DM; changes in levels of consciousness may be slow and progress through confusion and bizarre behavior. Coma may come without warning.
- Chronic complications of DM result from blood vessel changes related to hyperglycemia. These changes lead to serious health problems and early death. Although nothing prevents the complications, they can be slowed significantly by maintaining serum glucose between 60 and 150 mg/dL ("tight control"). The chronic complications can be divided into macrovascular (large vessel) and microvascular (small vessel) problems.
  1. Macrovascular complications include:
     a. Coronary heart disease
     b. Peripheral vascular disease (often leading to amputation)
     c. Cerebrovascular disease

2. Microvascular complications include:
   a. Ocular complications (can lead to blindness) such as diabetic retinopathy, retinal detachment, macular degeneration, myopia, cataracts, and glaucoma
   b. Diabetic neuropathy (damage to peripheral and autonomic nerves), including cardiac autonomic neuropathy leading to reduced heart rate variability, orthostatic hypotension, and heart failure
   c. Diabetic nephropathy (renal failure)
   d. Male erectile dysfunction

⊕ Cultural Awareness

- DM is a significant problem for African Americans, American Indians, and Mexican Americans.
- In all populations, prevalence of type 2 DM rises with age and obesity.
- Minority group members have a higher risk for complications such as hypertension, retinopathy, neuropathy, and nephropathy, than whites, even after adjusting for differences in blood glucose control.

PATIENT-CENTERED COLLABORATIVE CARE

Assessment

- Ask about and record patient information:
  1. Age
  2. Birth weight of children
  3. Weight change
  4. Occurrence of a recent illness or extreme stress
  5. Omission of insulin or oral antidiabetic drugs if the patient is known to have DM
  6. Change in eating habits
  7. Change in exercise schedule or activity level
  8. Presence and duration of polyuria, polydipsia, polyphagia, and loss of energy
  9. History of small skin injuries becoming infected more easily or taking a longer time to heal
  10. In women, frequency and duration of vaginal infections
  11. Presence of cardiovascular disease such as dysrhythmias, heart failure, hypertension, or stroke
  12. Presence of diabetes in a parent or sibling
  13. History of higher than normal fasting blood glucose levels
- Assess for:
  1. Elevated fasting blood glucose level (higher than 126 mg/dL) or random blood glucose level (higher than 200 mg/dL)

2. Abnormal oral glucose tolerance test
3. Glycosylated hemoglobin assay (HbA_{1c}) results greater than 7.5%
4. Positive results for urinary ketones; presence of albumin and glucose in the urine
5. Abdominal pain, nausea, and vomiting (in DKA)
6. Dehydration (e.g., poor skin turgor, dry mucous membranes, hemoconcentration with elevated hematocrit and hemoglobin levels, decreased urine output, dark and strong-smelling urine)

Planning and Implementation
RISK FOR INJURY RELATED TO HYPERGLYCEMIA
  Nonsurgical Management
- Drug or insulin therapy is indicated when a patient with type 2 DM cannot achieve blood glucose control with dietary modification, regular exercise, and stress management.
  1. *Sulfonylureas*: The most common drugs in this class are glipizide (Glucotrol) and glyburide (DiaBeta). These oral drugs are used for patients who still have some pancreatic beta cell function; hypoglycemia is the most serious complication; other side effects include hematologic reactions, allergic skin reactions, and GI effects.
  2. *Meglitinide analogues*: Repaglinide (Prandin) and nateglinide (Starlix) are oral drugs that have actions and side effects similar to sulfonylurea agents. Adverse effects include hypoglycemia, GI disturbances, upper respiratory infections, arthralgia, back pain, and headache.
  3. *Biguanides*: Metformin (Glucophage) is the major drug in this class. This drug does not cause hypoglycemia.

❗ NURSING SAFETY PRIORITY: Drug Alert

Metformin can cause lactic acidosis in patients with renal insufficiency and should not be used by anyone with kidney disease. To prevent kidney damage, the drug should be withheld for 48 hours before and after using contrast material or any surgical procedure requiring anesthesia.

---

  4. *Alpha-glucosidase inhibitors*: These oral drugs include acarbose (Precose) and miglitol (Glyset). They reduce hyperglycemia after meals by slowing digestion and absorption of carbohydrate within the intestine. Drugs in this class do not cause hypoglycemia. Side effects include abdominal discomfort related to undigested carbohydrate in the intestinal tract.

5. *Thiazolidinediones (TZDs)*: These oral drugs include rosiglitazone (Avandia) and pioglitazone (Actos). They work by increasing the sensitivity of insulin receptors, promoting glucose utilization in peripheral tissues. Liver function studies should be done at the start of therapy and at regular intervals while the patient is receiving therapy.

⚠ NURSING SAFETY PRIORITY: Drug Alert

Rosiglitazone has been associated with an increased risk for heart-related deaths and should not be used in patients with serious cardiac problems.

6. *Combination agents*: These are combinations from two different classes of drugs, such as Glucovance, which combines glyburide with metformin. Remember that the side effects of combination agents include those of all drugs contained in the combination.

7. *Amylin analogues*: The drug in this class is pramlintide (Symlin), which is similar to amylin, a naturally occurring hormone produced by beta cells in the pancreas, that works with and is co-secreted with insulin in response to blood glucose elevation. It works in at least three different ways to reduce blood glucose levels and is injected subcutaneously. This drug can be used for patients with either type 1 or type 2 DM.

⚠ NURSING SAFETY PRIORITY: Drug Alert

Assess the patient for severe hypoglycemia, because pramlintide can lower blood glucose levels below normal.

8. *Incretin analogues*: The drug in this class is exenatide (Byetta) and is injected subcutaneously. It mimics a hormone produced in the small intestine in the presence of food that works with insulin to lower plasma glucose levels. This drug is approved for use only in combination with a sulfonylurea, metformin, or both in patients with type 2 DM.

⚠ NURSING SAFETY PRIORITY: Drug Alert

When exenatide is used with a sulfonylurea, assess the patient for hypoglycemia.

9. *DPP-4 inhibitors*: The drugs in this class are sitagliptin (Januvia) and liraglutide (Victoza). It is an oral drug that increases the body's natural incretin hormone levels and reduces high

blood glucose levels. Side effects include stuffy or runny nose, sore throat, upper respiratory infection, GI disturbances, and renal insufficiency.

- Insulin therapy is necessary for type 1 DM and for moderate to severe type 2 DM.
  1. Insulin is available in rapid-, short-, intermediate-, and long-acting forms, which may be injected separately, and some can be mixed in the same syringe.
  2. Insulin regimens try to duplicate the normal release pattern of insulin from the pancreas, including single daily injections, two-dose protocol, three-dose protocol, four-dose protocol, combination therapy, and intensified insulin regimens.
  3. Teach the patient that insulin type, injection techniques, site of injection, and individual response can all affect absorption, onset, degree, and duration of insulin activity and reinforce that changing insulin may affect blood glucose control.
  4. Complications of insulin therapy include:
     a. Hypoglycemia
     b. *Dawn phenomenon,* a fasting hyperglycemia thought to result from the nocturnal release of growth hormone secretion that may cause blood glucose elevations around 5 to 6 AM and is managed or prevented by providing more insulin for the overnight period
     c. *Somogyi's phenomenon,* a morning hyperglycemia resulting from an effective counterregulatory response to nighttime hypoglycemia, which is managed or prevented by ensuring adequate dietary intake at bedtime and evaluating the insulin dose and exercise program.
     d. *Hypertrophic lipodystrophy,* a spongy swelling at or around injection sites
     e. *Lipoatrophy,* a loss of subcutaneous fat in areas of repeated injection that is treated by injection of human insulin at the edges of the atrophied area
     f. *Lipohypertrophy,* an increased swelling of fat that occurs at the site of repeated injections and is prevented by rotating injection sites
  5. Insulin may be administered by:
     a. Intermittent subcutaneous injection, typically with a syringe; some patients may use a prefilled cartridge or syringe
     b. Continuous subcutaneous infusion of insulin using an externally worn pump containing a syringe and reservoir with rapid or short-acting insulin connected to the patient by an infusion set

D

      c. Insulin pumps implanted into the peritoneal cavity where insulin can be absorbed in a more physiologic manner

6. Teach the patient about storage, dose preparation, injection procedures, and complications associated with drug therapy.

7. Instruct the patient to always buy the same type of syringes and use the same gauge and needle length; short needles are not used for an obese patient.

- The patient needs to know how to perform all aspects of self-monitoring of blood glucose (SMBG) and understand several issues:

  1. Accuracy of the results depends on the accuracy of the specific blood glucose meter, operator proficiency, and test strip quality. Help the patient select a meter based on cost of the meter and strips, ease of use, availability of repair and servicing.

  2. Results are influenced by the amount of blood on the strip, the calibration of the meter to the strip currently in use; environmental conditions of altitude, temperature, and moisture; and patient-specific conditions of hematocrit, triglyceride level, and presence of hypotension.

  3. Teach the patient how to clean the equipment to prevent infection.

  4. Instruct the patient not to use alternative site testing (forearm, upper arm, abdomen, thigh, and calf) in the following situations:
     a. When patient is hypoglycemic or susceptible to hypoglycemia (at time of peak activity of basal insulin)
     b. After exercise
     c. During an illness
     d. When blood glucose levels are changing rapidly
     e. Before driving

  5. *Continuous blood glucose monitoring* (CGM) systems monitor glucose levels in interstitial cavities. The system consists of three parts: a disposable sensor that measures glucose levels, a transmitter that is attached to the sensor, and a receiver that displays and stores glucose information. A thin plastic sensor is inserted into subcutaneous tissue.

     NOTE: Continuous glucose monitoring is meant to supplement, not replace, fingerstick tests. Insulin should be given only after confirming the results of any of the continuous glucose monitoring systems.

- Diet therapy:

  1. Collaborate with the patient, physician, and nutritionist to formulate an individualized meal plan for the patient.

2. Day-to-day consistency in the timing and amount of food eaten helps control blood glucose. Patients taking insulin need to eat at consistent times that are coordinated with the timed action of insulin.
3. Base the meal plan on blood glucose monitoring results, total blood lipid levels, and glycosylated hemoglobin.
4. Dietary guidelines are based on individual needs of the patient.
   a. Carbohydrates should make up 45% to 65% of daily calories.
   b. A protein intake of 15% to 20% of total daily calories is appropriate for patients with normal kidney function. In patients with microalbuminuria, reduction of protein to 10% of calories may slow progression of kidney failure.
   c. Less than 7% of total daily calories should be from saturated fat, and cholesterol intake should be limited to 200 mg.
   d. Foods high in *trans*-fat acids are avoided or severely restricted.
   e. High-fiber diets improve carbohydrate metabolism and lower cholesterol levels. High-fiber foods are added to the patient's diet gradually to prevent cramping, loose stools, and flatulence.
   f. Suggest artificial sweeteners, such as sucralose, saccharin, aspartame, and acesulfame K, instead of sugar to enhance dietary compliance.
   g. Warn the patient that fat "substitutes" or replacements may increase carbohydrate content in foods.
5. Teach the patient that alcohol may be taken in moderation only if DM is well controlled.
6. Explain and reinforce how to read food labels.
7. Reinforce dietary teaching such as how to follow the exchange system for meal planning and how to perform carbohydrate counting.
8. Support and reinforce information provided by the nutritionist regarding how to make adjustments in nutritional intake during illness, planned exercises, and social occasions.

Considerations for Older Adults
- A realistic approach to diet therapy is essential for older patients with DM.
- Attempts to change long-time eating habits may be difficult.
- Patients who live alone, do their own food preparation, and have physical limitations may have difficulty following the diet recommended by the American Diabetes Association.

- Socioeconomic factors may also affect a patient's ability to prepare the proper foods.

- Regular physical exercise is a recommended component of a comprehensive DM treatment plan:
  1. Collaborate with the patient and rehabilitation specialist to develop an exercise program.
  2. Instruct the patient to have a complete physical examination before starting an exercise program at home.
  3. Instruct the patient to wear proper footwear with good traction and cushioning and to examine the feet after exercise.
  4. Discourage exercise in extreme heat or cold or during periods of poor glucose control.
  5. Advise the patient to stay hydrated.
  6. Patients with type 1 DM should perform vigorous exercise only if blood glucose levels are between 80 and 250 mg/dL and no ketones are present in the urine.
  7. Teach the patient about the risks and complications related to exercise, such as prolonged alterations in blood glucose levels, vitreous hemorrhage, retinal detachment in patients with proliferative retinopathy, and increased proteinuria and foot and joint injury in patients with peripheral neuropathy.

Surgical Management
- Whole-pancreas transplantation can be performed in one of three ways: pancreas transplantation alone (PTA) in the preuremic patient, pancreas transplantation after successful kidney transplantation (PAK), and simultaneous pancreas-kidney (SPK) transplantation.
  1. Immunosuppressive therapy is needed for life to prevent rejection of the transplanted pancreas.
  2. Complications include venous thrombosis, rejection, and infection.

ENHANCE SURGICAL RECOVERY
- Surgery is a physical and emotional stressor, making the diabetic patient more at risk for intraoperative and postoperative complications.
- Provide preoperative care:
  1. Discontinue antidiabetic drugs:
     a. Chlorpropamide (Diabinese) 36 hours before surgery
     b. Metformin (Glucophage) 48 hours before surgery
     c. All other oral antidiabetic drugs on the day of surgery
  2. Restart oral antidiabetic drugs only after renal function has been re-evaluated and found to be normal.

   3. Start IV fluids to maintain hydration when the patient is
      admitted.
   4. Monitor blood glucose results and administer insulin to
      maintain serum glucose at less than 18 mg/dL.
- Intraoperative IV administration of short-acting insulin in 5%
  to 10% glucose is recommended for all insulin-treated patients
  and for drug-treated or diet-treated patients who are undergoing general anesthesia and whose DM is poorly controlled.
- Provide postoperative care:
   1. Monitor vital signs, especially temperature; hypothermia
      may cause high blood glucose levels.
   2. Monitor fluid and electrolyte balance; patients with azote-
      mia may have problems with fluid management.
   3. Maintain tight glycemic control throughout the postopera-
      tive phase.
   4. Provide pain management, ideally with patient-controlled
      analgesia (PCA) pump.
   5. Monitor for postoperative complications, including:
      a. Myocardial infarction (MI)
      b. Hypoglycemia and hyperglycemia; monitor at least four
         times daily
      c. Hyperkalemia or hypokalemia
      d. Impaired wound healing or wound infection; an unan-
         ticipated episode of hyperglycemia may indicate a new
         infection.
      e. Acute kidney injury or progression of chronic kidney
         disease

RISK FOR INJURY RELATED TO NEUROPATHY
- Nonhealing foot wounds cause more inpatient hospital days
  than any other complication of diabetes.
- Loss of pain, pressure, and temperature sensation in the foot increases the risk for injury and ulceration.
- Foot deformities common in diabetic neuropathy may lead to
  callus formation, ulceration, and increased areas of pressure.
- Foot care education includes:
   1. Teaching preventive foot care to the patient; sensory neurop-
      athy, ischemia, and infection are the leading causes of foot
      disease.
   2. Recommending that the patient have shoes fitted by an ex-
      perienced shoe fitter such as a certified podiatrist, and
      instructing the patient to change shoes at midday and in
      the evening and to wear socks or stockings with shoes
   3. Instructing the patient on how to care for wounds
- Refer the patient to a specialist for orthotic devices to eliminate
  pressure on infected or open wounds of the foot.

- Topical application of growth factors may be used to accelerate tissue healing for long-standing foot ulcers.
- Wound care for diabetic ulcers includes a moist wound environment, débridement of necrotic tissue, and offloading or elimination of pressure.

MANAGING PAIN

- Drug therapy may include:
  1. Anticonvulsants for pain secondary to diabetic neuropathy
  2. Tricyclic antidepressants, particularly amitriptyline (Elavil, Levate ♣), nortriptyline (Pamelor), or selective serotonin and norepinephrine reuptake inhibitors, such as duloxetine (Cymbalta), as prescribed, to alleviate peripheral neuropathic pain
  3. Capsaicin cream, 0.075% (e.g., Axsain ♣, Zostrix-HP) topically to relieve neuropathic pain
- Use other nondrug pain management techniques as appropriate, such as bed cradles, warm baths, and backrubs.

PREVENTING INJURY FROM REDUCED VISION

- Encourage all patients to have a baseline ophthalmic examination and yearly follow-up examinations.
- Advise the patient to seek a retinal specialist if problems are present.
- Collaborate with the rehabilitation specialist to recommend strategies to improve the patient's visual abilities; strategies include improving lighting, placing dark equipment against a white background, coding objects such as insulin vials with bright colors or felt-tip markers, and using large-type books and newspapers.
- Various stages of diabetic retinopathy can be treated with laser therapy or surgery.
- Teach the patient with limited vision the following strategies for using adaptive devices to self-administer insulin:
  1. Ensuring proper placement of the device on the syringe
  2. Holding the insulin bottle upright when measuring insulin
  3. Avoiding air bubbles in the syringe by pulling a small amount of insulin into the syringe, moving the plunger in and out three times, and measuring insulin on the fourth draw

REDUCING THE RISK FOR KIDNEY DISEASE

- Stress the importance of maintaining a normal blood glucose level, maintaining a blood pressure level below 130/85 mm Hg, and being screened annually for microalbuminuria.
- Teach the patient to limit protein to 0.8 g/kg of body weight per day if he or she has overt nephropathy.

PROMOTE CONTROL OF SERUM LIPID LEVELS
- Teach the patient about the signs and symptoms of urinary tract infection.
- The health care provider should adjust the insulin dosage for patients undergoing dialysis.
- Advise the patient not to take any over-the counter (OTC) drugs, especially NSAIDs, without checking with the health care provider.

POTENTIAL FOR HYPOGLYCEMIA
- Monitor glucose levels before administering hypoglycemic agents, before meals, at bedtime, and when the patient is symptomatic.
- Treat the patient with mild hypoglycemia (hungry, irritable, shaky, weak, headache, fully conscious, blood glucose less than 60 mg/dL [3.4 mmol/L]) and who is able to swallow with 15 to 20 g of glucose such as *one* of these:
  1. 2 or 3 glucose tablets
  2. 4 oz of fruit drink
  3. 4 oz of regular soft drink
  4. 8 oz of skim milk
  5. Six saltines
  6. 3 graham crackers
  7. 6 to 10 hard candies
  8. Four cubes of sugar
  9. 2 teaspoons of sugar
- The blood glucose level should be tested after 15 minutes.
- Treat the patient with moderate hypoglycemia (cold and clammy skin, pale, rapid pulse, rapid shallow respirations, marked changes in mood, drowsiness, blood glucose less than 40 mg/dL [2.2 mmol/L]) with 15 to 30 g of rapidly absorbed carbohydrates and additional food such as low-fat milk or cheese after 10 to 15 minutes.

■ NURSING SAFETY PRIORITY: Critical Rescue

For the patient with severe hypoglycemia (unable to swallow, unconscious or convulsing, blood glucose usually less than 20 mg/dL [1.0 mmol/L]), treat by this approach:
- Administer 50% dextrose (25 to 50 mL) IV or glucagon, 1 mg subcutaneously or IM.
- Repeat the dose in 10 minutes if the patient remains unconscious.
- Notify the primary health care provider immediately, and follow instructions.

- Teach the patient to prevent the four common causes of hypoglycemia: excess exercise, excess insulin, alcohol use, and deficient food intake.
- Encourage the patient to wear an identification (medical alert) bracelet.

POTENTIAL FOR DIABETIC KETOACIDOSIS

- Monitor the patient for signs and symptoms of diabetic ketoacidosis (DKA).
- Give insulin bolus as indicated, followed by a continuous drip.
- Check the patient's blood pressure, pulse, and respirations every 15 minutes until stable.
- Monitor the patient for hypokalemia (symptoms are muscle weakness, abdominal distention or paralytic ileus, hypotension, and weak pulse); before administering potassium, ensure that the patient's urine output is at least 30 mL/hr.
- Replace both fluid volume and ongoing losses, monitoring for heart failure symptoms and pulmonary edema if large volume of IV fluid is administered.
- Record urine output, temperature, and mental status every hour.
- Assess the patient's level of consciousness, hydration status, fluid and electrolyte balance, and blood glucose levels every hour until stable; once stable, assess every 4 hours.
- Instruct the patient about how to prevent future episodes of DKA by contacting the primary health care provider when the blood glucose is greater than 250 mg/dL, when ketonuria is present for more than 24 hours, when he or she is unable to take food or fluids, and when illness persists for more than 1 to 2 days.

POTENTIAL FOR HYPERGLYCEMIC-HYPEROSMOLAR STATE (HHS)

- Administer IV fluids and insulin as indicated, and monitor and assess the patient's response to therapy.
- Assess for signs of cerebral edema and immediately report change in level of consciousness; change in pupil size, shape, or reaction to light; or seizure activity to the physician.

Community-Based Care

- Discharge planning includes:
  1. Ensuring that the patient understands the significance, symptoms, causes, and treatment of hypoglycemia and hyperglycemia
  2. Assisting the patient to identify the items needed for the administration of insulin and for glucose monitoring
  3. Teaching the patient how to monitor blood sugar level
  4. Teaching the patient how to administer drugs and prevent hypoglycemia

5. In collaboration with the nutritionist, teaching the patient basic survival skills associated with drugs, diet, exercise, and complications
6. Referring the patient to a diabetes educator for the necessary education
7. Helping the patient adapt to DM, including teaching stress management techniques and identifying coping mechanisms
8. Referring the patient to the American Diabetes Association and its resources
9. Providing information about community resources, such as diabetic education programs

DIVERTICULA, ESOPHAGEAL

OVERVIEW

- Diverticula are sacs resulting from the herniation of esophageal mucosa and submucosa into surrounding tissue.
- Patients with esophageal diverticula are at risk for esophageal perforation.
- The most common form of diverticulum is Zenker's diverticulum, which is usually located near the hypopharynx and occurs most often in older adults.

PATIENT-CENTERED COLLABORATIVE CARE

Assessment

- Assessment findings include:
  1. Dysphagia
  2. Regurgitation
  3. Feelings of fullness or pressure
  4. Halitosis
  5. Nocturnal cough

Interventions

- Diet therapy and positioning are the primary interventions for controlling symptoms related to diverticula.
- Nursing interventions include:
  1. Collaborating with the dietitian to determine the size and frequency of meals and the texture and consistency that can best be tolerated by the patient
  2. Elevating the head of the bed for sleep to avoid reflux of gastric contents onto diverticula
  3. Teaching patient to avoid the recumbent position and vigorous exercising for at least 2 hours after eating to prevent reflux
  4. Teaching patient to avoid restrictive clothing at the abdomen and thorax and to minimize stooping or bending to reduce reflux

- Surgical management is aimed at excision of the diverticula.
- Postoperative care
  1. Monitor for bleeding and perforation.
  2. Do not irrigate the nasogastric (NG) tube used for decompression unless specifically ordered by the physician.
  3. Maintain hydration and nutrition through IV fluids and enteral feedings until oral intake is permitted; NPO status may be several days' duration to allow esophageal healing.
  4. Manage the patient's postoperative pain.
  5. Teach the patient to observe for complications such as infection or poor wound healing.
  6. Teach the patient measures to take to reduce reflux (e.g., elevating head of bed and avoiding recumbent position).

DIVERTICULAR DISEASE

OVERVIEW
- Diverticular disease includes diverticulosis and diverticulitis.
  1. *Diverticulosis* is pouchlike herniations of the mucosa through the muscular wall of any portion of the gut, but it most commonly refers to diverticula of the colon. They can occur in any part of the intestine but are most common in the sigmoid colon. High intraluminal pressure forces the formation of a pouch in the weakened area of the mucosa, commonly near blood vessels. Without inflammation, diverticula are asymptomatic.
  2. *Diverticulitis,* or inflammation of one or more diverticula, results when the diverticulum retains undigested food, which compromises the blood supply to that area and facilitates bacterial invasion of the diverticular sac, which may then perforate. A perforated diverticulum can progress to intra-abdominal perforation with generalized peritonitis.

PATIENT-CENTERED COLLABORATIVE CARE
Assessment
- Patients with diverticulosis are usually asymptomatic; a minor history of left quadrant pain or constipation may be reported.
- Diverticula may be identified on colonoscopy, barium enema (rectal), or upper GI tract series (small intestine).
- Assess for clinical manifestations of diverticulitis:
  1. Abdominal pain that may begin as intermittent and may progress to continuous:

    a. Pain may be localized to the left lower quadrant and increase with coughing, straining, or lifting.

    b. Generalized abdominal pain is a sign of perforation and peritonitis.

2. Fever
3. Nausea and vomiting
4. Abdominal distention
5. Palpable, tender abdominal or rectal mass
6. Blood in the stool (microscopic to larger amounts)
7. Elevated WBC; reduced hematocrit and hemoglobin if bleeding occurs
8. Hypotension and dehydration occur if massive bleeding occurs (see *Hypovolemic Shock*).
9. Signs of septic shock occur if peritonitis has occurred
10. Flat plate x-ray to evaluate for free air and fluid outside the GI tract
11. Computed tomography (CT) scan to diagnose abscess or thickening of lumen caused by repeated inflammation and injury
12. Serum electrolytes
13. Intake, output, and patient fluid status
14. If a nasogastric tube (NGT) is used for gastric decompression or to manage vomiting, check output for amount and quality or color.

Interventions

- Drug therapy is used to treat inflammation from diverticulitis.
  1. Administer broad-spectrum antibiotics such as metronidazole (Flagyl) plus trimethoprim/sulfamethoxazole (Bactrim, Septra), or ciprofloxacin (Cipro).
  2. Implement management for mild or moderate pain; if pain is severe, use opioids.
  3. Laxatives and enemas are not given, because they increase intestinal motility.
- A NGT is inserted if nausea, vomiting, or abdominal distention is severe. Report the appearance of output.
- Recommend rest.
- Diet therapy:
  1. Provide IV fluids for hydration during the acute phase of the disease or when the patient is NPO.
  2. Consult with a dietitian to promote healthy food choices.

Surgical Management

- Patients with diverticulitis need emergent surgery if one of the following occurs:
  1. Rupture of the diverticulum with subsequent peritonitis
  2. Pelvic abscess

    3. Bowel obstruction
    4. Fistula
    5. Persistent fever or pain after 4 days of medical treatment
    6. Uncontrolled bleeding

- Surgical management includes a colon resection with an end-to-end anastomosis or temporary or permanent colostomy.
- Preoperative care includes:
  1. Reinforcing physician teaching about the possible need for a temporary or permanent colostomy
  2. Administering IV fluids, antibiotics, and pain medications, if prescribed
  3. Maintaining NPO status with a NGT in place for patients having emergency surgery
- Postoperative care includes:
  1. Maintaining drainage system at the abdominal incision site
  2. If a colostomy was created, monitoring colostomy stoma for color and integrity, anticipating that a gray or black color or separation between the mucous membranes and skin is indicative of poor healing and requires immediate communication with the surgeon
  3. Providing the patient with an opportunity to express feelings about the colostomy
  4. Consulting with the wound or ostomy specialist
  5. Providing written postoperative instructions on:
     a. Inspection of the incision for redness, tenderness, swelling, and drainage
     b. Dressing change procedures, if necessary
     c. Avoidance of activities that increase intra-abdominal pressure, including straining at stool, bending, lifting heavy objects, and wearing restrictive clothing
     d. Pain management, including prescriptions
- Teach the patient and family to:
  1. Follow dietary considerations for diverticulosis, which include consultation with the dietitian. Keep a food diary to note food associations with symptoms and to implement the following:
     a. Eat a diet high in cellulose and hemicellulose, which are found in wheat bran, whole-grain breads, and cereals. Foods containing seeds or indigestible material that may block a diverticulum, such as nuts, corn, popcorn, cucumbers, tomatoes, figs, and strawberries, may be eliminated.
     b. Use a bulk-forming laxative such as psyllium (Metamucil) to increase fecal size and consistency if the recommended fiber requirements cannot be tolerated.
     c. Encourage fluids to prevent bloating that may accompany a high-fiber diet.

   d. Avoid alcohol, which has an irritant effect on the bowel.

   e. Do not exceed a fat intake of 30% of the total daily caloric intake.

2. Avoid all fiber when symptoms of diverticulitis are present, because high-fiber foods are then irritating.

3. Monitor for signs and symptoms of diverticulitis (e.g., fever, abdominal pain, and bloody stools).

4. Avoid enemas and irritant or stimulant laxatives.

DUCTAL ECTASIA

- Ductal ectasia is a benign breast problem in women approaching menopause, caused by thickening and dilation of breast ducts.
- The ducts are blocked, becoming distended and filled with cellular debris, which activates an inflammatory response.
- Manifestations are a hard and tender mass with irregular borders; greenish brown nipple discharge; enlarged axillary nodes; and redness and edema over the mass.
- Ductal ectasia does not increase breast cancer risk, but the mass may be difficult to distinguish from breast cancer. Because the risk for breast cancer is increased among women in the menopausal age group, accurate diagnosis is vital.
- Nipple discharge is examined microscopically for any atypical or malignant cells.
- Warm compresses and antibiotics may be helpful in relieving symptoms and improving drainage. The affected area may be excised.
- Nursing interventions focus on reducing the anxiety and providing support through the diagnostic and treatment procedures.

DYSRHYTHMIAS, CARDIAC

OVERVIEW

- Cardiac dysrhythmias are abnormal rhythms of the heart's electrical system that are caused by disturbances of cardiac electrical impulse formation, conduction, or both.
- Many cardiac diseases cause dysrhythmia, including congenital heart disease, myocardial injury or infarction, cardiomyopathy, left or right ventricular dysfunction.
- Contributing factors can also cause and worsen dysrhythmias. Electrolyte imbalance, hypoxemia, serum acidosis and alkalosis, and drug toxicity are the most common contributing factors.

- *Tachydysrhythmias* are heart rates greater than 100 beats/min.
  1. Signs and symptoms include palpitations, chest discomfort; pressure or pain from myocardial ischemia or infarction; restlessness; anxiety; pale, cool skin; and syncope from hypotension.
  2. They may cause heart failure as indicated by dyspnea, orthopnea, pulmonary crackles, distended neck veins, fatigue, and weakness.
- *Bradydysrhythmias* are characterized by a heart rate less than 60 beats/min.
  1. The patient may tolerate a low heart rate if blood pressure is adequate.
  2. Symptomatic bradydysrhythmias lead to hypotension, myocardial ischemia or infarction, other dysrhythmias, and heart failure.
- *Premature complexes* are early complexes that occur when a cardiac cell or group of cells other than the sinoatrial (SA) node becomes irritable and fires an impulse before the next sinus impulse is generated.
  1. *Bigeminy* occurs when normal complexes and premature complexes occur alternately in a repetitive two-beat pattern, with a pause occurring after each premature complex so that complexes occur in pairs.
  2. *Trigeminy* is a repetitive three-beat pattern, usually occurring as two sequential normal complexes followed by a premature complex and a pause, with the same pattern repeating itself in triplets.
  3. *Quadrigeminy* is a repetitive four-beat pattern, usually occurring as three sequential normal complexes followed by a premature complex and a pause, with the same pattern repeating itself in a four-beat pattern.
- Dysrhythmias are further classified according to their site of origin.
- Sinus dysrhythmias include:
  1. *Sinus tachycardia,* which occurs when the SA node discharge exceeds 100 beats/min. Treatment is based on identifying the underlying cause (e.g., angina, fever, hypovolemia, pain); beta-adrenergic blocking agents may be prescribed.
  2. *Sinus bradycardia,* a decreased rate of SA node discharge of less than 60 beats/min. If the patient is symptomatic, treatment includes atropine, a pacemaker, and avoidance of parasympathetic stimulations such as prolonged suctioning.
- Atrial dysrhythmias
  1. *Premature atrial complex (PAC)* occurs when atrial tissue becomes irritable. This ectopic focus fires an impulse before the next sinus impulse is due.

   a. No intervention is generally needed except to treat the cause, such as heart failure or valvular disease.
2. *Supraventricular tachycardia (SVT)* involves the rapid stimulation of atrial tissue at a rate of 100 to 280 beats/min.
   a. No intervention is generally needed except to treat the cause.
   b. Sustained SVT may need to be treated with radiofrequency catheter ablation.
   c. Oxygen therapy, antidysrhythmic drugs, or synchronized cardioversion may also be needed.
3. *Atrial flutter* is a rapid arterial depolarization occurring at a rate of 250 to 350 times/min.
   a. Drug treatment includes ibutilide (Corvert), amiodarone (Cordarone), and diltiazem (Cardizem).
   b. Synchronized cardioversion is done if the patient is hemodynamically compromised.
   c. Rapid atrial overdrive pacing or radiofrequency catheter ablation may be needed if none of these treatments are successful.
4. *Atrial fibrillation (AF)* consists of rapid atrial impulses at a rate of 350 to 600 times/min.
   a. Treatment is the same as for atrial flutter.
   b. Anticoagulants are given, because this rhythm places the patient at high risk for emboli formation in the atrial appendage. The clot can break off and travel through major arteries causing stroke, myocardial infarction (MI), pulmonary emboli, deep vein thrombosis, and other thrombotic disease.
- Junctional dysrhythmias may occur when the cells in the atrioventricular (AV) junctional node generate an impulse. Junctional rhythms usually do not persist beyond the acute disease that caused slowing or absence of SA pacemaker function.
   1. If treatment is needed, generally atropine is used to speed up the junctional rhythm (Advanced Cardiac Life Support [ACLS] bradycardic algorithm).
   2. A pacemaker is used for definitive treatment.
- Ventricular dysrhythmias
   1. *Idioventricular rhythm* occurs when the ventricular cells become the pacemakers of the heart, usually in the absence of pacemaking above the bundle of His.
      a. This bradycardic rhythm is often symptomatic, with hypotension or decreased or absent peripheral pulses.
      b. With symptoms, initiate the ACLS bradycardic algorithm.
   2. *Premature ventricular complexes (PVCs)* result from increased irritability of the ventricular cells. PVCs are early

ventricular complexes followed by a pause and often occur in repetitive rhythms.

   a. The patient may be asymptomatic or may experience palpitations, chest discomfort, or diminished or absent peripheral pulses.

   b. If there is no underlying heart disease, PVCs are not treated other than by eliminating any contributing cause.

   c. In the presence of myocardial ischemia or infarction, symptomatic PVCs are treated with oxygen and amiodarone (Cordarone); other drugs are prescribed if an MI occurs.

3. *Ventricular tachycardia (VT),* or "V tach," occurs with repetitive firing of an irritable ventricular ectopic focus, usually at a rate of 140 to 180 beats/min.

   a. Symptoms depend on ventricular rate; the patient may be hemodynamically compromised and in cardiac arrest.

   b. Medications used to treat VT are oxygen, amiodarone, lidocaine, or magnesium sulfate.

   c. Unstable VT is treated with emergency defibrillation followed by oxygen and antidysrhythmic therapy.

   d. With pulseless VT, immediately begin cardiopulmonary resuscitation (CPR) and defibrillate as soon as possible. If the patient remains pulseless, continue CPR and other resuscitative measures.

   e. After the patient has been successfully defibrillated, attention is given to treating the reversible causes of VT.

4. *Ventricular fibrillation (VF),* sometimes called "V-fib," is the result of electrical chaos in the ventricles.

   a. The patient immediately loses consciousness, becoming pulseless and apneic. Within minutes, death occurs unless there is prompt restoration of an organized rhythm.

   b. Immediate defibrillation is performed and the ACLS algorithm is followed.

5. *Ventricular asystole* is the complete absence of any ventricular rhythm. The patient is in full cardiac arrest and is treated with CPR and by following the ACLS algorithm.

- *Atrioventricular (AV) conduction blocks* exist when supraventricular impulses are excessively delayed or totally blocked in the AV node or intraventricular conduction system.

1. *First-degree AV block:* All sinus impulses eventually reach the ventricles; conduction is slowed.

   a. The patient usually has no symptoms, and no treatment is needed.

    b. If caused by drug therapy, the offending drug is withheld and the health care provider notified.

    c. If associated with symptomatic bradycardia, oxygen is administered.

2. *Second-degree AV block type I (AV Wenckebach or Mobitz type I):* Each successive sinus impulse takes a little longer to conduct through the AV node, until one impulse is completely blocked and fails to depolarize the ventricles. The symptomatic patient is treated with oxygen and atropine; a pacemaker may be needed.

3. *Second-degree AV block type II (Mobitz type II):* The block is infranodal, occurring below the bundle of His, and involves a constant block in one of the bundle branches; the impulse fails to reach the ventricle.

    a. Symptoms depend on the frequency of the dropped rate.

    b. If the patient is symptomatic, he or she is treated with prophylactic pacing to avert the threat of sudden third-degree heart block.

    c. A permanent pacemaker may be required.

4. *Third-degree heart block (complete heart block):* None of the sinus impulses conducts to the ventricles.

    a. Clinical manifestations depend on the overall ventricular rate and cardiac output and may have hemodynamic consequences such as light-headedness, confusion, syncope, seizures, hypotension, or cardiac arrest.

    b. Oxygen and atropine are given to the patient who is symptomatic; prophylactic pacing may be initiated.

5. *Bundle branch block:* A conduction delay or block occurs within one of the two main bundle branches below the bifurcation of the bundle of His.

    a. There are no clinical manifestations and no specific interventions.

    b. A new bundle branch block may be an indicator of a recent MI; be alert to symptoms of acute coronary syndrome.

PATIENT-CENTERED COLLABORATIVE CARE
Interventions
DECREASED CARDIAC OUTPUT AND INEFFECTIVE TISSUE PERFUSION

- The major interventions are to assess for complications and monitor the patient for response to treatment.

1. Monitor the patient's electrocardiogram (ECG) and assess for signs and symptoms of dysrhythmias.

2. Assess apical and radial pulses for a full minute for any irregularity.

3. Management includes:
   a. Drug therapy
   b. Vagal maneuvers such as carotid sinus massage and Valsalva maneuvers
   c. Cardioversion
   d. Temporary or permanent pacing
   e. CPR or ACLS
   f. Defibrillation
   g. Radiofrequency catheter ablation
   h. Aneurysmectomy
   i. Coronary artery bypass grafting
   j. Insertion of an implantable cardioverter-defibrillator (ICD)

◼ NURSING SAFETY PRIORITY: Critical Rescue

Call the Rapid Response Team for an increase or onset in irregular pulses or rhythm when it is associated with a deterioration in consciousness or blood pressure. It may be an early sign of electrolyte disturbance, drug toxicity, or new myocardial injury.

Community-Based Care

- A case manager or care coordinator identifies the need for health care resources at home and coordinates access to the services.
- Discharge planning and health care resources:
  1. Provide information on lifestyle modifications including activity restrictions.
  2. Teach the patient and family the name, dosage, schedule, and side effects of drugs.
  3. Teach and observe the patient and family taking a pulse.
  4. Stress the importance of reporting chest discomfort, shortness of breath, and change in heart rhythm and rate to the health care provider.
  5. Post emergency numbers.
  6. Encourage the patient to adhere to diet instructions.
  7. Instruct the patient to keep all appointments with the health care provider.
  8. Encourage family members to learn CPR.
  9. Refer to the American Heart Association (AHA) or the provincial affiliate of the Heart and Stroke Foundation in Canada and other community agencies.
- Give the following special instructions to a patient with a pacemaker or ICD device:
  1. Give instructions on how to care for the pacemaker or ICD and how it functions (if appropriate) and the importance of reporting any fever or any redness, swelling, or drainage at the pacemaker or ICD insertion site.

2. Keep the ICD identification card in a wallet and consider wearing a medical alert bracelet.

3. Do not wear tight clothing or belts that could cause irritation over the site.

4. Keep handheld cellular phones at least 6 inches away from the generator, with the handset on the ear opposite the side of the generator.

5. Avoid sources of strong electromagnet fields such as large electrical generators and radio or television transmitters and radar.

6. If a patient feels symptoms when he or she is near any device, he or she should move 5 to 10 feet away from it and check your pulse.

7. Notify all health care providers, including dentist, that a pacemaker or ICD device is in use.

8. Notify airport security personnel before passing through a metal detector (screening device) that a pacemaker or ICD is in use, and show them the ICD identification card.

9. MRI is contraindicated.

- Give the following special instructions to a patient with a pacemaker:

  1. Take your pulse for 1 minute at the same time each day, and record the rate in your pacemaker diary.

  2. Take your pulse any time you feel symptoms of possible pacemaker failure, and report your heart rate and symptoms to your health care provider.

  3. Know the rate at which your pacemaker is set, and know the rate changes to report to your physician.

  4. Know the indications of battery failure, and report these findings to your health care provider.

  5. Check your pulse, and report any of the following symptoms to your health care provider: difficulty breathing, dizziness, fainting, chest pain, weight gain, and prolonged hiccupping.

  6. Do not operate electrical appliances directly over your pacemaker site, because they may cause it to malfunction. Be sure electrical appliances are properly grounded.

  7. Do not lean over electrical or gasoline engines or motors.

- Give the following special instructions to a patient with an ICD:

  1. Sit or lie down immediately if you feel dizzy, faint, or lightheaded.

  2. Avoid activities that involve rough contact with the ICD implantation site.

  3. Avoid sources of strong electromagnet fields such as large electrical generators and radio or television transmitters

because they may inhibit tachydysrhythmia detection and therapy or alter pacing or shock settings. If beeping tones are heard coming from the device, move away from the electromagnetic field immediately before the inactivation sequence is completed, and notify the health care provider.

4. Report symptoms such as fainting, nausea, weakness, blackout, and rapid pulse to your health care provider.
5. Know how to perform cough CPR as instructed.
6. Notify your health care provider if your ICD device discharges.
7. Avoid strenuous activities that may cause your heart rate to meet or exceed the rate cutoff of your ICD device, because this causes the device to discharge inappropriately.

■ NURSING SAFETY PRIORITY: Action Alert

Teach the patient to keep all appointments to assess the function of the ICD device. Many of these devices also maintain records that can be accessed at the cardiology visit; the device can be "interrogated" to provide a record of the type, frequency, and duration of dysrhythmias so that therapeutic adjustments to the device or medications can be made.

■ NURSING SAFETY PRIORITY: Drug Alert

Many antidysrhythmic drugs have a narrow safety range and dangerous side effects, and many interact with other medications. Avoid adding over-the-counter (OTC) or prescribed drugs to the patient's regimen without first ensuring that the prescriber is aware of the antidysrhythmic drug used.

ENCEPHALITIS

OVERVIEW

- Encephalitis, an inflammation of the brain parenchyma (brain tissue) and often the meninges, is most often caused by infective organisms:
  1. Arboviruses transmitted through the bite of an infected tick or mosquito
  2. Enteroviruses associated with mumps and chickenpox
  3. Herpes simplex virus type 1, which is the most common nonepidemic type
  4. Amoebae such as *Naegleria* and *Acanthamoeba*, found in warm freshwater, which may also be involved
- Encephalitis can be life-threatening or lead to persistent neurologic problems such as learning disabilities, epilepsy, memory, or fine motor deficits.

PATIENT-CENTERED COLLABORATIVE CARE
Assessment
- Assessment findings include:
  1. Fever
  2. Nausea and vomiting
  3. Stiff neck; nuchal rigidity
  4. Decreased level of consciousness and impaired cognition
  5. Motor dysfunction
  6. Focal neurologic deficits
  7. Symptoms of increased intracranial pressure
  8. Ocular palsies
  9. Facial weakness
  10. Abnormal cerebrospinal fluid analysis
  11. Elevated white blood cell (WBC) count

E

> **⚠ NURSING SAFETY PRIORITY: Critical Rescue**
> Level of consciousness is the most sensitive indicator of neurologic status. Inform the physician of worsening cognition or decreased arousal, because this may mean worsening of acute neurologic disease.

Interventions
- The treatment for encephalitis is similar to that for meningitis.
  1. Maintain a patent airway; avoid aspiration.
  2. Encourage and assist the patient to reposition and deep-breathe frequently; suction if respiratory status is compromised.
  3. Monitor vital signs and neurologic signs, such as level of consciousness, orientation, pupil responses, and motor movement.
  4. Elevate the head of the bed 30 to 45 degrees.
  5. Administer acyclovir (Zovirax) for herpes encephalitis; no specific drug therapy is available for infection by arboviruses or enteroviruses.
  6. If there are neurologic disabilities, the patient may be discharged to a rehabilitation setting or a long-term care facility.

ENDOCARDITIS, INFECTIVE

OVERVIEW
- Infective endocarditis (previously called *bacterial endocarditis*) refers to a microbial infection (virus, bacterium, fungus) involving the endocardium.
- Infective endocarditis occurs primarily in patients who are IV drug abusers, have had cardiac valve replacements, have experienced systemic infection, or have structural cardiac defects.

- Portals of entry for infecting organisms include:
  1. Oral cavity, especially if dental procedures have been performed
  2. Skin rashes, lesions, or abscesses
  3. Infections (cutaneous, genitourinary or gastrointestinal, systemic)
  4. Surgical or invasive procedures, including IV line placement

PATIENT-CENTERED COLLABORATIVE CARE
Assessment
- Assessment findings include:
  1. Signs of infection, including fever, chills, malaise, night sweats, and fatigue:
     a. Older adults may remain afebrile.
  2. Heart murmurs, usually regurgitant in nature
  3. Right-sided heart failure, evidenced by:
     a. Peripheral edema
     b. Weight gain
     c. Anorexia
  4. Left-sided heart failure, evidenced by:
     a. Fatigue
     b. Shortness of breath
     c. Crackles
  5. Evidence of arterial embolization from fragments of vegetation on valve leaflets, which may travel to other organs and compromise function. Manifestations of acute embolization include:
     a. Splenic emboli, evidenced by sudden abdominal pain and radiation to the left shoulder
     b. Kidney infarction, evidenced by flank pain that radiates to the groin and is accompanied by hematuria or pyuria
     c. Mesenteric emboli, evidenced by diffuse abdominal pain, often after eating and abdominal distention
     d. Brain emboli, in which the patient shows signs of stroke, confusion, reduced concentration, and difficulty speaking
     e. Pulmonary emboli, evidenced by pleuritic chest pain, dyspnea, and cough
  6. Petechiae of the neck, shoulders, wrists, ankles, mucous membranes, or conjunctivae
  7. Splinter hemorrhages, or black longitudinal lines or small red streaks in the nail bed
  8. Osler's nodes (reddish, tender lesions with a white center on the pads of the fingers, hands, and toes)
  9. Janeway's lesion (nontender hemorrhagic lesion found on the fingers, toes, nose, and earlobes)
  10. Positive blood culture

11. Low hemoglobin level and hematocrit
12. Abnormal transesophageal echocardiogram

Interventions
- Interventions include:
  1. Administering IV antimicrobial therapy
  2. Monitoring the patient's tolerance to activity; anticipating pacing activities more slowly or clustering activities to increase duration of rest if patient tires
  3. Protecting the patient from contact with potentially infective organisms
  4. Informing the Rapid Response Team if there are symptoms of embolization. Collaborate and communicate to prevent complications from embolization, particularly decreased oxygenation, brain injury, and acute coronary syndromes.
- Surgical intervention includes removal of the infected valve, repair or removal of congenital shunts, repair of injured valves and chordae tendineae, and draining abscesses in the heart or elsewhere.
- Preoperative and postoperative care for the patient having surgery involving the valves is similar to that described for patients undergoing a coronary artery bypass grafting or valve replacement.

Community-Based Care
- Teach the patient and family:
  1. Information on the cause of the disease and its course, drug regimens, signs and symptoms of infection, and practices to prevent future infections
  2. How to administer IV antibiotic and care for the IV site, ensuring that all supplies are available to the patient discharged to home
  3. The importance of good personal and oral hygiene, such as using a soft toothbrush, brushing the teeth twice each day, and rinsing the mouth with water after brushing
  4. To avoid the use of dental irrigation devices and dental floss
  5. To inform health care providers and dentists about the history of endocarditis so that prophylactic antibiotics are given before treatment

ENDOMETRIOSIS

OVERVIEW
- Endometriosis occurs when the endometrial (inner uterine) tissue implants outside the uterine cavity, most commonly on the ovaries and the cul-de-sac (posterior rectovaginal wall) and less commonly on other pelvic organs and structures.
- This tissue responds to cyclic hormonal stimulation just as if it were in the uterus.

- Monthly cyclic bleeding occurs at the site of implantation, where it is trapped, causing pain, irritation, scarring, and adhesion formation in the surrounding tissue.
- When endometriosis is on an ovary, a brown swelling known as a "chocolate cyst" can form.
- The cause of endometriosis is unknown.
- The disorder is most often found in women during their reproductive years and can lead to infertility.

PATIENT-CENTERED COLLABORATIVE CARE
Assessment
- Obtain patient information about:
  1. Menstrual history, sexual history, and bleeding characteristics
  2. Pain, which is the most common symptom of endometriosis
  3. Dyspareunia (painful sexual intercourse)
  4. Painful defecation
  5. Low backache
  6. Infertility
  7. GI disturbances
- Assess for and document:
  1. Pelvic tenderness
  2. Tender nodules in the posterior vagina and limited movement of the uterus
  3. Anxiety, because of uncertainty about the diagnosis and potential infertility
- Diagnostic studies may include tests to rule out other diagnoses such as:
  1. Pelvic inflammatory disease (PID) caused by chlamydia or gonorrhea
  2. Ovarian cancer detected by serum cancer antigen CA-125
  3. Pelvic masses detected by transvaginal ultrasound
  4. Laparoscopy and biopsy to determine endometrial tissue typing

Interventions
Nonsurgical Management
- Hormonal contraceptives for cycle control
- Heat packs, relaxation techniques, yoga, and biofeedback to improve blood flow to painful areas
- Calcium and magnesium, which may relieve muscle cramping for some patients

Surgical Management
- Surgical management of endometriosis with laser therapy through laparoscopy removes the implants and adhesions, allowing the woman to remain fertile.
- In women with intractable pain, severing a pelvic nerve may provide relief.

- If the patient does not wish to have children, the uterus and ovaries may be removed.
- Nursing care is similar to that for a woman undergoing a vaginal hysterectomy (see *Surgical Management* under *Leiomyomas, Uterine*).

EPIDIDYMITIS

OVERVIEW
- Epididymitis is an inflammation of the epididymis, which may result from an infectious (most common) or noninfectious source such as trauma.
- Main manifestations include pain along the inguinal canal and along the vas deferens, followed by pain and swelling in the scrotum and the groin.
- It can be a complication of a sexually transmitted disease (STD), such as gonorrhea or chlamydia.
- If untreated, the infection can spread and an abscess may form, requiring an orchiectomy (removal of one or both testes). If both testes are affected, sterility may result.
- Less often, it can be a complication of long-term use of an indwelling urinary catheter, prostatic surgery, or a cystoscopic examination.

E

PATIENT-CENTERED COLLABORATIVE CARE
Assessment
- Obtain patient information about:
  1. Pain along the inguinal canal
  2. Pain and swelling of the scrotum and groin
- Assess for and document:
  1. Pyuria, bacteria
  2. Regional lymph node swelling
  3. Signs of infection such as fever, chills and elevated white blood cell (WBC) count
- Diagnosis is made on the basis of manifestations and a smear or culture of the urine or prostate secretions to identify the causative organism.

Interventions
- Interventions include:
  1. Drug therapy
     a. Antibiotics
     b. NSAIDs to decrease inflammation and promote comfort
  2. Comfort measures, including:
     a. Elevating or supporting the swollen scrotum (use a jock strap)

b. Applying cold compresses or ice to the scrotum intermittently
c. Taking sitz baths
d. Avoiding lifting, straining, or sexual activity until the infection is under control (which may take as long as 4 weeks)

- The sexual partner should be treated if the infection is caused by an STD.
- An epididymectomy (excision of the epididymis from the testicle) may be needed if the problem is recurrent or chronic.
- An ultrasound study can rule out an abscess or tumor.

ERECTILE DYSFUNCTION

OVERVIEW

- Erectile dysfunction (ED) is the inability to achieve or maintain an erection for sexual intercourse. There are two major types of ED, organic and functional
- *Organic ED* is a gradual deterioration of function. The man first notices diminishing firmness and a decrease in frequency of erections. Causes include:
  1. Inflammation of the prostate, urethra, or seminal vesicles
  2. Surgical procedures such as prostatectomy
  3. Pelvic fractures
  4. Lumbosacral injuries
  5. Vascular disease, including hypertension
  6. Chronic neurologic conditions, such as Parkinson's disease or multiple sclerosis
  7. Endocrine disorders, such as diabetes mellitus or thyroid disorders
  8. Smoking and alcohol consumption
  9. Drugs
  10. Poor overall health that prevents sexual intercourse
- *Functional ED* usually has a psychological cause. Men with functional ED have normal nocturnal (nighttime) and morning erections. Onset is usually sudden and preceded by a period of high stress.

PATIENT-CENTERED COLLABORATIVE CARE

- Assess the medical, social, and sexual history to help determine the cause of ED.
- Hormone testing is used for patients who have a poor libido, small testicles, or sparse beard growth.
- Duplex Doppler ultrasonography may be performed to determine the adequacy of arterial and venous blood flow to the penis.

Nonsurgical Management
- Functional ED is managed by sexual counseling and drugs that increase penile blood flow.
- Nonsurgical management of organic ED may include:
  1. Drug therapy to improve penile blood flow, phosphodiesterase-5 (PDE-5) inhibitors such as:
     a. Sildenafil (Viagra)
     b. Vardenafil (Levitra)
     c. Tadalafil (Cialis)

◪ NURSING SAFETY PRIORITY: Drug Alert

Instruct patients taking PDE-5 inhibitors to abstain from alcohol before sexual intercourse, because it may impair the ability to have an erection. Common side effects of these drugs include dyspepsia (heartburn), headaches, facial flushing, and stuffy nose. If more than one pill a day is being taken, leg and back cramps, nausea, and vomiting also may occur. Teach men who take nitrates to avoid these drugs, because the vasodilation effects can cause a profound hypotension and reduce blood flow to vital organs. For patients who cannot take these drugs or do not respond to them, other methods are available to achieve an erection.

E

  2. Vacuum devices:
     a. A vacuum device is a cylinder that fits over the penis, and a vacuum is created with a pump. The vacuum draws blood into the penis to maintain an erection.
     b. The advantage of this procedure is that the device is easy and safe to use regardless of what drugs the patient may be taking.
  3. Intracorporal injections:
     a. Vasoconstrictive drugs can be injected directly into the penis to reduce blood outflow and make the penis erect.
     b. Common agents are papaverine, phentolamine (Regitine), and alprostadil.
     c. Adverse effects include priapism (prolonged erection), penile scarring, fibrosis, bleeding, bruising at the injection site, pain, infection, and vasovagal responses.

Surgical Management
- Penile implants can be surgically placed when other modalities fail. Devices include semirigid, malleable, or hydraulic inflatable and multicomponent or one-piece instruments.
- Advantages include the man's ability to control his erections.
- The major disadvantages include device failure and infection.

FATIGUE SYNDROME, CHRONIC

- Chronic fatigue syndrome (CFS), also known as chronic fatigue and immune dysfunction syndrome (CFIDS), is characterized by severe fatigue for 6 months or longer, usually following flulike symptoms.
- For a diagnosis of CSF, four or more of the following criteria must be met:
  1. Sore throat
  2. Substantial impairment in short-term memory or concentration
  3. Tender lymph nodes
  4. Muscle pain
  5. Multiple joint pain with redness or swelling
  6. Headaches of a new type, pattern, or severity (not familiar to the patient)
  7. Unrefreshing sleep
  8. Postexertional malaise lasting more than 24 hours
- There is no test to confirm the disorder, and the cause is unknown.
- Management is supportive and focuses on alleviation or reduction of symptoms:
  1. NSAIDs for body aches and pain
  2. Low-dose antidepressants for promoting sleep and preventing or treating depression
  3. Teaching the patient to follow healthy practices:
     a. Adequate sleep
     b. Proper nutrition
     c. Regular exercise (but not excessive enough to increase fatigue)
     d. Stress management
     e. Energy conservation
  4. Use of complementary and alternative therapies that include acupuncture, tai chi, massage, and herbal supplements
- Refer the patient to support groups and reputable Internet sites for information and Web-based support.

FIBROMYALGIA SYNDROME

OVERVIEW

- Fibromyalgia syndrome (FMS) is chronic, noninflammatory syndrome manifested by pain and tenderness at specific sites in the back of the neck, upper chest, trunk, low back, and extremities.

- The tender points (trigger points) can be palpated to elicit pain in a predictable, reproducible pattern. Other sensations of numbness and tingling also occur.
- Secondary FMS can accompany any connective tissue disease, particularly lupus and rheumatoid disease.
- Other symptoms include:
  1. Fatigue with or without sleep disturbances
  2. Gastrointestinal (GI) disturbances, including abdominal pain, diarrhea and constipation, and heartburn
  3. Genitourinary manifestations, including dysuria, urinary frequency, urgency, and pelvic pain
  4. Cardiovascular symptoms, including dyspnea, chest pain, and dysrhythmias
  5. Visual disturbances, including blurred vision and dry eyes
  6. Neurologic symptoms, including forgetfulness and concentration problems
- Interventions include:
  1. Antidepressant drugs approved for fibromyalgia nerve pain e.g., pregabalin [Lyrica] and duloxetine [Cymbalta])
  2. Tricyclic antidepressive agents to promote sleep and reduce pain or muscle spasms (amitriptyline [Elavil, Apo-Amitriptyline ✦], trazodone [Desyrel], or nortriptyline [Pamelor])
  3. NSAIDs
  4. Physical therapy
  5. Regular exercise, which includes stretching, strengthening, and low-impact aerobic exercise
- Refer the patient to the National Chronic Fatigue Syndrome and Fibromyalgia Association for additional information.

FLAIL CHEST

OVERVIEW

- Flail chest is the inward movement of the thorax during inspiration, with outward movement during expiration, usually involving only one side of the chest.
- It results from multiple rib fractures or ribs fractured in more than one place caused by blunt chest trauma, leaving a segment of the chest wall loose.
- Flail chest often occurs in high-speed vehicular crashes. Another cause is bilateral separations of the ribs from their cartilage connections without an actual rib fracture during cardiopulmonary resuscitation (CPR).
- Gas exchange, the ability to cough, and the ability to clear secretions are impaired.

PATIENT-CENTERED COLLABORATIVE CARE
Assessment
- Assess the patient for and document:
  1. Paradoxical chest movement ("sucking inward" of the loose chest area during inspiration and a "puffing out" of the same area during expiration)
  2. Pain
  3. Dyspnea
  4. Cyanosis
  5. Tachycardia
  6. Hypotension

Interventions
- Interventions include:
  1. Humidified oxygen
  2. Pain management
  3. Promotion of lung expansion through deep breathing and positioning
  4. Secretion clearance by coughing and tracheal aspiration
  5. Psychosocial support
  6. Intubation with mechanical ventilation and positive end-expiratory pressure (PEEP)
  7. Surgical stabilization (only in extreme cases of flail chest)
- Monitor the patient's:
  1. Vital signs
  2. Oxygen saturation and arterial blood gases
  3. Fluid and electrolyte balance
  4. Central venous pressure (CVP)

FLUID OVERLOAD

OVERVIEW
- Fluid overload, also called *overhydration,* is an excess of body fluid, not a disease. It is a clinical sign of a problem in which fluid intake or retention is greater than the body's fluid needs.
- The most common type of fluid overload is hypervolemia, because the problems result from excessive fluid in the extracellular fluid (ECF) space.
- Most problems caused by fluid overload are related to fluid volume excess in the vascular space or to dilution of specific electrolytes and blood components.
- Causes of fluid overload are related to excessive intake or inadequate excretion of fluid and include:
  1. Excessive fluid replacement
  2. Kidney failure (late phase)

3. Heart failure
4. Long-term corticosteroid therapy
5. Syndrome of inappropriate antidiuretic hormone (SIADH)
6. Psychiatric disorders with polydipsia
7. Water intoxication

PATIENT-CENTERED COLLABORATIVE CARE
Assessment
- Assess for and document:
  1. Cardiovascular changes:
     a. Bounding pulse quality
     b. Peripheral pulses full
     c. Elevated blood pressure
     d. Decreased pulse pressure
     e. Elevated central venous pressure
     f. Distended neck and hand veins
     g. Engorged varicose veins
     h. Weight gain
  2. Respiratory changes:
     a. Respiratory rate increased
     b. Shallow respirations
     c. Dyspnea increases with exertion or in the supine position
     d. Moist crackles present on auscultation
  3. Skin and mucous membrane changes:
     a. Pitting edema in dependent areas as well as joints and skin around bony prominences (elbows, metacarpals, metatarsals)
     b. Skin pale and cool to touch. Skin and puncture sites from needle sticks may "weep" as fluid tries to escape through the skin.
  4. Neuromuscular changes:
     a. Altered level of consciousness
     b. Headache
     c. Visual disturbances
     d. Skeletal muscle weakness
     e. Paresthesias
  5. Gastrointestinal changes:
     a. Increased motility
     b. Enlarged liver
- Diagnosis of fluid overload is based on assessment findings and the results of laboratory tests. Usually, serum electrolyte values are normal, but decreased hemoglobin, hematocrit, and serum protein levels may result from excessive water in the vascular space (hemodilution).

F

Interventions
- Management of patients with fluid overload aims to ensure patient safety, restore normal fluid balance, provide supportive care until the imbalance is resolved, and prevent future fluid overload.
  1. Monitor patients to prevent fluid overload or prevent worsening of fluid overload:
     a. Assess particularly for symptoms of pulmonary edema and heart failure.
     b. Evaluate for the presence of bounding pulses, engorged neck veins, unbalanced intake and output, and daily weight.
     c. Collaborate with health care team members to set a daily output goal and inform the physician when goals are at risk for not being met.

     ■ NURSING SAFETY PRIORITY: Critical Rescue

     Pulmonary edema can occur very quickly and can lead to death. Notify the health care provider of any change that indicates the fluid overload is not responding to therapy or is becoming worse.

     d. Reduce risk for pressure ulcers in patients with edema by using a pressure-reducing or pressure-relieving overlay on the mattress and over bony prominences (e.g., heel protectors, padding at elastic bands for holding oxygen delivery devices in place).
     e. Assess skin pressure areas, especially the coccyx, elbows, hips, and heels, daily for signs of redness or open areas and document findings.
     f. Assist the patient to change positions at least every 2 hours.
  2. Drug therapy focuses on removing the excess fluid (diuretics, conivaptan [Vaprisol]):
     a. Monitor the patient's response to drug therapy:
        (1) A weight gain or loss of 1 kg in less than 24 hours is a gain or loss of 1 L of fluid.
        (2) Compute intake/output balance every 8 hours and set goals such as "negative 500 mL," indicating a desired urine output 500 mL greater than intake. Notify the health care provider when reduced urine output occurs.
     b. Observe for manifestations of electrolyte imbalance:
        (1) Changes in electrocardiographic patterns
        (2) Changes in sodium and potassium values

3. Nutritional therapy:
   a. Sodium restriction
   b. Fluid restriction

FOOD POISONING

- Food poisoning is caused by ingestion of infectious organisms in food. Unlike gastroenteritis, food poisoning is not directly communicable from person to person and incubation periods are shorter.
- Prevention occurs with good handwashing and properly handling and processing food. Food poisoning is caused by over 250 pathogens.
- Examples of food poisoning are:
  1. Staphylococcal food poisoning:
     a. *Staphylococcus* grows in meats and dairy products and can be transmitted by human carriers.
     b. Symptoms of staphylococcal infection include abrupt onset of vomiting, diarrhea, and abdominal cramping, usually 2 to 4 hours after the ingestion of contaminated food.
     c. The diagnosis is made when stool culture yields 100,000 enterotoxin-producing staphylococci.
     d. Treatment includes oral or IV fluids if the fluid volume is grossly depleted.
  2. *Escherichia coli* infection:
     a. Some strains cause disease by making a substance called *Shiga toxin*. The bacteria that make these substances are called *Shiga toxin-producing E. coli*, or *STEC* for short Enterohemorrhagic strains of *E. coli* (EHEC) and STEC can cause serious complications, such as hemorrhagic colitis and hemolytic-uremic syndrome.
     b. Symptoms include vomiting, diarrhea, abdominal cramping, and fever.
     c. Treatment includes IV fluids.
  3. Botulism:
     a. Botulism is a severe, life-threatening food poisoning associated with a high mortality rate; it is most commonly acquired from improperly processed canned foods.
     b. The incubation period is 18 to 36 hours, and the illness may be mild or severe.
     c. *Clostridium botulinum* enters the bloodstream from the intestines and causes symptoms of diplopia, dysphagia, dysphonia, respiratory muscle paralysis, nausea, vomiting, and diarrhea or constipation.

F

d. The diagnosis is made by the history and stool culture revealing *C. botulinum*; the serum may be positive for toxins.

e. Treatment of botulism includes trivalent botulism antitoxin (types A, B, and E), stomach lavage, IV fluids, and tracheostomy with mechanical ventilation if respiratory paralysis occurs.

❗NURSING SAFETY PRIORITY: Action Alert

To prevent botulism, teach patients the importance of discarding cans of food that are punctured or swollen or that have defective seals. Remind them to check for expiration dates and to not use any canned food that has expired. Containers for home-canned foods must be sterilized by boiling for 20 minutes to destroy *C. botulinum* spores before canning.

4. *Salmonellosis* is a bacterial infection:
   a. Incubation is 8 to 48 hours after ingestion of contaminated food or drink.
   b. Fever, nausea, vomiting, cramping abdominal pain, and severe diarrhea, which may be bloody, last 3 to 5 days.
   c. Diagnosis is made by stool culture.
   d. Treatment is based on symptoms; antibiotics are used if the patient becomes bacteremic.
   e. Salmonellosis can be transmitted by the *five Fs*: Flies, Fingers, Food, Feces, and Fomites; strict handwashing is essential to avoid transmission.

FRACTURE, NASAL

OVERVIEW

- A nasal fracture often results from injuries received during falls, sports activities, motor vehicle accidents, or physical assaults.
- Bone or cartilage displacement can cause airway obstruction or cosmetic deformity and is a potential source of infection.

PATIENT-CENTERED COLLABORATIVE CARE
Assessment

- Assess for and document:
  1. Deviation or malalignment of the nasal bridge
  2. Change in nasal breathing

3. Crackling of the skin (crepitus) on palpation
4. Midface bruising and pain
5. Blood or clear cerebrospinal fluid (CSF) draining from one or both nares

■ NURSING SAFETY PRIORITY: Critical Rescue

CSF drainage may indicate a skull fracture. When CSF dries on a piece of filter paper, a yellow halo appears as a ring at the dried edge of the fluid. Immediately report positive findings to the health care provider.

Interventions

- Management for a simple fracture is usually a closed reduction performed by the health care provider, using local or general anesthesia, within the first 24 hours after injury.
- Teach the patient to use cold compresses for pain relief and to reduce swelling.
- Management of more severe fractures may require surgery:
  1. Rhinoplasty, a surgical reconstruction of the nose for cosmetic purposes and to improve airflow:
     a. Packing is in place with a "moustache" dressing (or drip pad) under the nose.
     b. A splint or cast may cover the nose for better alignment and protection.
  2. Teach the patient to:
     a. Stay in semi-Fowler's position and move slowly.
     b. Use cool compresses on the nose, eyes, or face.
     c. Limit Valsalva maneuvers (e.g., forceful coughing, straining during a bowel movement).
     d. Not to sniff upward or blow the nose.
  3. Nasoseptoplasty or submucous resection (SMR) straightens a deviated septum. Nursing care is similar to that for a rhinoplasty.

FRACTURES

OVERVIEW

- A fracture is a break or disruption in the continuity of a bone.
- Fractures are classified as complete or incomplete:
  1. *Complete fracture:* The break is across the entire width of the bone in such a way that the bone is divided into two distinct sections.

    2. *Incomplete fracture:* The fracture does not divide the bone into two portions, because the break is through only part of the bone.
- Fractures can also be described by the extent of associated soft-tissue damage:
  1. A *simple fracture* does not extend through the skin and therefore has no visible wound.
  2. An *open (compound) fracture* has a disrupted skin surface that causes an external wound.
- Fractures are also defined by their cause:
  1. *Pathologic (spontaneous) fractures* occur after minimal trauma to a bone that has been weakened by disease.
  2. *Fatigue (stress) fractures* result from excessive strain and stress on the bone.
  3. *Compression fractures* are produced by a loading force applied to the long axis of cancellous bone.
- Bone healing occurs in five stages:
  1. Stage 1 occurs within 24 to 72 hours after the injury, with hematoma formation at the site of the fracture.
  2. Stage 2 occurs in 3 days to 2 weeks, when granulation tissue begins to invade the hematoma, stimulating the formation of fibrocartilage.
  3. Stage 3 of bone healing usually occurs within 2 to 6 weeks as a result of vascular and cellular proliferation. The fracture site is surrounded by new vascular tissue known as a *callus* that begins the nonbony union.
  4. Stage 4 usually takes 3 to 6 months and results in gradual resorption of the callus, with transformation into bone.
  5. Stage 5 consists of bone consolidation and remodeling. This stage may start as early as 6 weeks after fracture and can continue for up to 1 year.

Considerations for Older Adults

- Bone formation and strength rely on adequate nutrition, especially calcium, phosphorus, vitamin D, and protein.
- For women, the loss of estrogen after menopause is detrimental to the body's ability to form new bone tissue.

- Other diseases, such as arteriosclerosis, reduce arterial circulation to bone. The bone receives less oxygen and reduced amounts of nutrients, both of which are needed for repair.
- Acute complications of fractures:
  1. *Acute compartment syndrome (ACS)* is a serious condition in which increased pressure within one or more tissue compartments causes massive compromise of circulation to

the area. The most common sites for the problem in patients experiencing musculoskeletal trauma are the compartments in the lower leg and forearm. Edema fluid forms and is trapped within the compartment pressing on nerves (causing pain) and blood vessels, preventing adequate tissue perfusion and oxygenation. Without treatment, ACS can lead to infection, loss of motor function, contracture formation, and release of myoglobin, leading to renal failure. Treatment is by surgical fasciotomy.

■ NURSING SAFETY PRIORITY: Critical Rescue

Myoglobinuric renal failure from muscle breakdown is a potentially fatal complication of compartment syndrome. It occurs when large or multiple compartments are involved. Injured muscle tissues release myoglobulin (muscle protein) into the circulation, where it can clog the renal tubules and cause acute renal failure. Monitor urine output and report oliguria, as well as discolored urine; both are signs of acute kidney injury.

2. *Crush syndrome (CS)* results from an external crush injury that compresses one or more compartments in the leg, arm, or pelvis. It is a potentially life-threatening, systemic complication that results from hemorrhage and edema after a severe fracture injury. Management involves early recognition and adequate IV fluids, diuretics, and low-dose dopamine to enhance renal perfusion. When not managed, results of this syndrome include:
   a. ACS
   b. Hypovolemia
   c. Hyperkalemia
   d. Rhabdomyolysis (myoglobulin released from skeletal muscle into the bloodstream)
   e. Acute tubular necrosis (ATN) and kidney failure
   f. Dark brown urine
   g. Muscle weakness and pain
3. *Hypovolemic shock* may occur with a fracture as a result of damage to bone blood vessels or the severing of nearby arteries.
4. *Fat embolism syndrome (FES)* is a serious complication in which fat globules are released from the yellow bone marrow into the bloodstream within 12 to 48 hours after an injury. These emboli clog small blood vessels that supply vital organs, most commonly the lungs, and impair organ perfusion. FES usually results from long bone fractures and pelvic bone or fracture repair, but it is occasionally seen in

patients who have a total joint replacement. Manifestations include decreased level of consciousness, anxiety, respiratory distress, tachycardia, tachypnea, fever, hemoptysis, and petechiae, a macular, measles-like rash that may appear over the neck, upper arms, or chest and abdomen.

5. *Venous thromboembolism (VTE)* includes deep vein thrombosis (DVT) and its major complication, pulmonary embolism (PE). It is the most common complication of lower extremity surgery or trauma and the most common fatal complication of musculoskeletal surgery.

6. Infection is possible with fractures, because the trauma disrupts the body's defense system. Wound infections may range from superficial skin infections to deep wound abscesses. Bone infection, or osteomyelitis, is most common with open fractures in which skin integrity is lost and after surgical repair of a fracture.

- Chronic complications of fractures:
  1. *Ischemic necrosis*, sometimes referred to as *aseptic* or *avascular necrosis (AVN)* or *osteonecrosis*, can occur when the blood supply to the bone is disrupted and bone death follows.
  2. *Delayed union* is a fracture that has not healed within 6 months of injury. Some fractures never achieve union; that is, they never completely heal (nonunion). Others heal incorrectly (malunion).

PATIENT-CENTERED COLLABORATIVE CARE
Assessment

- Assess pain level; if the patient is in severe pain, delay the interview until he or she is more comfortable.
- Obtain patient information about:
  1. Cause of the fracture
  2. Events leading to fracture and immediate postinjury care
  3. Drug history, including substance abuse (recreational drug use) and alcohol abuse
  4. Medical history
  5. Occupation and recreational activities
  6. Nutritional history
- Assess for and document:
  1. Life-threatening complications of the respiratory, cardiovascular, and neurologic systems (priority assessment)
  2. Fracture site:
     a. Change in bone alignment
     b. Shortening of change in bone shape
     c. Neurovascular status (circulation, movement, and sensation) to extremity distal to fracture

■NURSING SAFETY PRIORITY: Critical Rescue

If pain occurs when the patient moves the body part or area below the injury, stop the movement immediately.

3. Degree of soft-tissue damage
4. Amount of overt bleeding
5. Muscle spasm
- Special assessment considerations include:
  1. Fractures of the shoulder and upper arm are assessed with the patient in a sitting or standing position, if possible, so that shoulder drooping or other abnormal positioning can be seen.
  2. More distal areas of the arm are assessed with the patient in a supine position so that the extremity can be elevated to reduce swelling.
  3. Place the patient in a supine position for assessment of the lower extremities and pelvis.
  4. Pelvic fractures can cause internal organ damage resulting in hemorrhage. When a pelvic fracture is suspected, assess vital signs, skin color, and the level of consciousness for indications of shock. Check the urine for blood, which indicates damage to the urinary system, often the bladder.
- Psychosocial assessment depends on the extent of the injury and other complications.
- Stresses that result from a chronic condition affect relationships between the patient and family members or friends, body image, sexuality, and financial resources.
- Diagnostic tests for fractures may include:
  1. Standard x-rays and tomograms
  2. Computed tomography (CT) scanning
  3. Magnetic resonance imaging (MRI)

Planning and Implementation

- The patient may experience Acute Pain related to fracture, soft-tissue damage, muscle spasm and edema.
- Perform a head-to-toe assessment (secondary survey).
- Evaluate physiologic stability; provide cardiac monitoring for patients over 50 years because of increased risk for acute coronary events.
- Administer drugs to manage the initial pain, usually an IV opioid such as fentanyl.
- Immobilize the fracture with a splint; maintain the splint to prevent further tissue damage, reduce pain, and increase circulation.
- Place sterile gauze loosely over open areas to prevent further contamination of the wound.

F

- Plan for fracture reduction/realignment; premedicate with opioid drug.
- Administer opioid, nonopioid analgesic, anti-inflammatory drug, and/or muscle relaxants to manage pain that persists for a prolonged time during the healing process.
- Provide adjunctive and distraction therapy.
- See *Pain* in Part One for more interventions.

⚠ NURSING SAFETY PRIORITY: Critical Rescue

For any patient who experiences trauma in the community, first call 911 and assess for airway, breathing, and circulation (ABCs, or primary survey). Then provide lifesaving care if needed before being concerned about the fracture. In the community setting, provide emergency interventions until medical treatment in a hospital is available, or call 911 for the emergency team (first responders).

Nonsurgical Management

- Fracture management begins with reduction (realignment of the bone ends for proper healing) and immobilization of the fracture.
  1. *Closed reduction* is the manipulation of the bone ends for realignment while applying a manual pull, or traction, on the bone.
  2. *Bandages, splints, or commercial immobilizers* may be used to immobilize certain areas of the body, such as the scapula and clavicle.
  3. *Casts* are rigid devices that immobilize the affected body part while allowing other body parts to move. They are used to hold bone fragments in place after reduction for more complex fractures or fractures of the lower extremity. A cast allows early mobility, correction of deformity, prevention of deformity, and reduction of pain.
- Cast materials include:
  1. Plaster of Paris
     a. Requires application of a well-fitted stockinette under the padding material
     b. Takes 24 to 72 hours to dry
     c. Feels warm or hot immediately after application
     d. Is heavy and may have rough edges that require "petaling"
     e. Can become misshapen if handled incorrectly while drying:
        (1) Do not cover casts until dry.
        (2) Handle cast with palms of hands rather than fingers until dry.

(3) Turn patient every 1 to 2 hours to facilitate cast drying.

   f. Can bear more weight than synthetic cast materials

2. Fiberglass, which is lightweight, dries in 10 to 15 minutes, and can bear weight 30 minutes after application, is most often used on upper extremities.

3. Polyester-cotton knit casts, which take 7 minutes to dry and can withstand weight bearing in about 20 minutes, are most often used on upper extremities.

- Types of casts include:
  1. Arm cast:
     a. When a patient is in bed, elevate the arm above the heart to reduce swelling; the hand should be higher than the elbow.
     b. When the patient is out of bed, support the arm with a sling placed around the neck so that the weight is distributed over a large area of the shoulders and trunk, not just the neck.
  2. Leg cast:
     a. Leg casts allow mobility and require the patient to use ambulatory aids such as crutches.
     b. A cast shoe, sandal, or boot that attaches to the foot or a rubber walking pad attached to the sole of the cast assists in ambulation (if weight bearing is allowed) and helps prevent damage to the cast.
     c. Elevate the affected leg on pillows when the patient is in bed or in a chair to reduce swelling.
  3. Cast brace:
     a. This device enables the patient to bend unaffected joints while the fracture is healing. The fracture must show signs of healing and minimal tissue edema before application of this cast.
     b. As healing occurs, the cast may be removed and replaced with a soft brace.
  4. Body and spica cast:
     a. A body cast encircles the trunk of the body, whereas a spica cast encases a portion of the trunk and one or two extremities.
     b. The patient is at risk for skin breakdown, pneumonia or atelectasis, constipation, and joint contractures.
     c. *Cast syndrome* (superior mesenteric artery syndrome) is a serious complication in which partial or complete upper intestinal obstruction can occur and cause abdominal distention, epigastric pain, nausea, and vomiting. Placing a window in the abdominal portion of the cast or bivalving the cast may be sufficient to relieve pressure on the duodenum.

F

- Cast care involves:
    1. Handling a wet cast carefully with the palms of the hands to prevent indentations and resultant pressure areas on the patient's skin
    2. Preventing skin irritation from rough cast edges by petaling the cast with the placement of small strips of tape over the rough edges
    3. Cutting a window (done by the health care provider, orthopedic technician, or specially trained nurse) into the cast over a wound so that the wound can be observed and cared for
    4. Ensuring that the cast is not too tight by inserting a finger between the cast and the skin
    5. Notifying the health care provider when the cast is too tight so that it can be cut with a cast cutter to relieve pressure or allow tissue swelling. The cast may be bivalved (cut lengthwise into two equal pieces) if bone healing is almost complete. Either half of the cast can be removed for inspection or for provision of care. The two halves are then held in place by an elastic bandage wrap.
    6. Protecting the cast in the perineal area from becoming contaminated with urine or feces by encasing the area in plastic before the patient uses the urinal or bedpan
    7. Assisting the patient in a body cast or long-leg cast to use a fracture bedpan
    8. Inspecting the cast daily (after it is dry) for drainage, cracking, crumbling, alignment, and fit:
        a. Describing and documenting any drainage on the cast in the medical record
        b. Notifying the health care provider immediately about any sudden increases in the amount of drainage or change in the integrity of the cast
    9. Smelling the cast for foul odor and palpating it for hot areas every shift
    10. Assessing for and reporting complications from casting:
        a. Infection
        b. Circulation impairment
        c. Peripheral nerve damage
        d. Skin breakdown
        e. Pneumonia or atelectasis
        f. Thromboembolism
        g. Joint contracture
        h. Muscle atrophy
- *Traction* is the application of a pulling force to a part of the body to provide reduction, alignment, and rest. It is also used to

decrease muscle spasm and prevent or correct deformity and
tissue damage.

1. Categories of traction:
   a. *Running traction* provides a pulling force in one
      direction, and the patient's body acts as countertraction.
      Moving the body or bed position can alter the counter-
      traction force.
   b. *Balanced suspension* provides the countertraction so that
      the pulling force of the traction is not altered when the
      bed or patient is moved. This allows for increased move-
      ment and facilitates care.
2. Types of traction:
   a. *Skin traction* involves the use of a Velcro boot (Buck's trac-
      tion), belt, or halter, securely placed around a body part to
      decrease painful muscle spasms. Weight is limited to 5 to
      10 pounds (2.3 to 4.5 kg) to prevent injury to the skin.
   b. *Skeletal traction* uses pins, wires, tongs, or screws that are
      surgically inserted directly into bone to allow the use of
      longer traction time and heavier weights, usually 15 to 30
      pounds (6.8 to 13.6 kg). It aids in bone realignment.
   c. *Plaster traction* combines skeletal traction and a plaster
      cast.
   d. *Brace traction* is a device that exerts a pull for correction
      of alignment deformities.
   e. *Circumferential traction* uses a belt around the body, such
      as pelvic traction for low back problems.
3. Care for the patient in traction includes:
   a. Maintaining correct balance between traction pull and
      countertraction force

⚠ NURSING SAFETY PRIORITY: Action Alert

Weights usually are not removed without a prescription.
They should not be lifted manually or allowed to rest on
the floor. Weights should be freely hanging at all times.

   b. Inspecting the skin at least every 8 hours for signs of ir-
      ritation or inflammation
   c. Removing (when possible) the belt or boot that is used
      for skin traction every 8 hours to inspect under the device
   d. Inspecting the points of entry of pins and wires or pin
      sites for signs of inflammation or infection at least every
      8 hours
   e. Following agency policy for how to clean the pinsite areas
      and ensure that it follows the evidence-based guidelines
      from the National Association of Orthopaedic Nurses

F

    f. Checking traction equipment to ensure its proper functioning and inspecting all ropes, knots, and pulleys at least every 8 to 12 hours for loosening, fraying, and positioning

    g. Checking the weight for consistency with the health care provider's prescription

    h. Replacing the weights if they are not correct and notifying the health care provider or orthopedic technician

    i. Reporting patient complaints of severe pain from muscle spasm to the health care provider when body realignment fails to reduce the discomfort

    j. Assessing neurovascular status of the affected body part at least every 4 hours, or more often if indicated

Surgical Management

- *Open reduction with internal fixation (ORIF)* permits early mobilization. Open reduction allows direct visualization of the fracture site, and internal fixation uses metal pins, screws, rods, plates, or prostheses to immobilize the fracture during healing. An incision is made to gain access to the broken bone and allow implanting one or more devices into bone tissue.

- *External fixation* involves fracture reduction and the percutaneous implantation of pins into the bone. The pins are then held in place by an external metal frame to prevent bone movement.

    1. Advantages of external fixation include:
        a. Minimal blood loss
        b. Early ambulation and exercise of the affected body
        c. Maintaining alignment in closed fractures that will not maintain position in a cast
        d. Stabilization of comminuted fractures that require bone grafting

    2. A disadvantage of external fixation is the increased risk for pinsite infection and osteomyelitis.

- Provide preoperative care, including:

    1. Routine preoperative care, as described in Part One
    2. Teaching the patient about what to expect during and after the surgery
    3. Applying Buck's traction before surgery for a fractured hip
    4. Teaching the patient and family about alterations to clothing that may be required when a large external fixator is in place

- Provide postoperative care, including:

    1. Routine postoperative care, as described in Part One
    2. Monitoring neurovascular status and reporting signs of inadequate perfusion promptly at least every hour for the first 24 hours after surgery and then as often as agency policy, surgeon preference, and patient condition indicate
    3. Assessing for and reporting complications

- Additional procedures may be needed when surgical repairs are not successful and the bone does not heal (nonunion).
    1. *Electrical bone stimulation* may be noninvasive or invasive. It involves using electrical current simulators near or into a fracture site. This procedure, when used for about 6 months, has resulted in bone healing for some patients.
    2. *Bone grafting* is the use of bone chips from the patient, a cadaver donor, or a living donor and packing or wiring the chips between the bone ends to facilitate union.
    3. *Low-intensity pulsed ultrasound (Exogen therapy)* involves the application of ultrasound treatments for about 20 minutes each day to the fracture site.

POTENTIAL FOR NEUROVASCULAR COMPROMISE

- Potential for Neurovascular Compromise is related to tissue edema and/or bleeding.
- Monitor circulation, movement, and sensation every hour from the first hour after cast placement.
- Provide ongoing neurovascular checks until the cast is removed.

POTENTIAL FOR INFECTION

- Potential for Infection is related to a wound caused by an open fracture.
- Monitor the white blood cell (WBC) count with differential for signs of infection.
- Monitor the patient's vital signs every 4 to 8 hours, because increases in temperature and pulse often indicate systemic infection.
- Immediately notify the health care provider if you observe inflammation and purulent drainage. Administer prescribed prophylactic or indicated antibiotics.
- Maintain vacuum-assisted closure (VAC) technique, if prescribed.

■ NURSING SAFETY PRIORITY: Critical Rescue
Older adults may not have a temperature elevation, even in the presence of severe infection. Use other indicators of infection.

IMPAIRED PHYSICAL MOBILITY

- Nursing interventions to prevent complications of impaired mobility focus on assessing for complications in immobilized patients with fractures.
- Nursing interventions to increase mobility include:
    1. Reinforcing the teaching provided by the physical therapist regarding the use of ambulatory aids
    2. Evaluating whether the patient is using the ambulatory aid correctly

- Types of ambulatory aids include:
  1. *Crutches*, which require strong arms, balance, and coordination
     a. To prevent pressure on the axillary nerve, there should be two to three fingerbreadths between the axilla and the top of the crutch when the crutch tip is at least 6 inches (15 cm) diagonally in front of the foot.
     b. The crutch is adjusted so that the elbow is flexed no more than 30 degrees when the palm is on the handle.
     c. The most common gait for crutch walking after musculoskeletal injury is the three-point gait, which allows minimal weight bearing on the affected leg.
  2. *Walkers*, which are most often used by the older patient who needs additional support for balance
  3. *Canes*, which are used when only minimal support is needed for an affected leg
     a. The cane is placed on the unaffected side.
     b. It should create no more than 30 degrees of flexion of the elbow.
     c. The top of the cane should be parallel to the greater trochanter of the femur.

Community-Based Care

- Collaborate with the case manager or the discharge planner in the hospital to plan care for the patient with a fracture who is being discharged.

▼ NATIONAL PATIENT SAFETY GOAL

Be sure to communicate the plan of care to the health care agency receiving the patient.

- Provide continuity of care, including:
  1. Identifying structural barriers to mobility in the home
  2. Ensuring the patient has easy access to the bathroom
  3. Assessing for environmental factors contributing to falls:
     a. Scatter rugs
     b. Waxed floors
     c. Walkway areas
  4. Assessing the patient's ability to safely use a wheelchair or ambulatory aid
  5. Arranging for a home health care nurse to make one or two visits to check that the home is safe and that the patient and family are able to follow the interdisciplinary plan of care
  6. Providing verbal and written instructions on the care of bandages, splints, casts, or external fixators

7. Referring the patient and family for assistance with financial issues, understanding the long-term nature of the recovery period, job counseling, and possible professional counseling
8. Emphasizing the importance of follow-up visits with the health care provider and other therapists
- Teach the patient and family about:
  1. Care of the extremity after removal of the cast:
     a. Remove scaly, dead skin carefully by soaking; do not scrub.
     b. Move the extremity carefully. Expect discomfort, weakness, and decreased range of motion (ROM).
     c. Support the extremity with pillows or an orthotic device until strength and movement return.
     d. Exercise slowly as instructed by the physical therapist.
     e. Wear support stockings or elastic bandages to prevent swelling (for lower extremity).
  2. Wound assessment and dressing
  3. Recognition of complications
  4. When and where to seek professional health care if complications occur

FRACTURES OF SPECIFIC SITES

- *Clavicular, self-healing*: A splint or bandage is used for immobilization.
- *Scapular*: Immobilization with a commercial immobilizer is used until the fracture heals, usually in 2 to 4 weeks.
- *Proximal humerus*: When impacted, the injury is usually treated conservatively with a sling for immobilization; when displaced, the fracture often requires ORIF with pins or a prosthetic device.
- *Humeral shaft*: Correction is achieved by closed reduction and application of a hanging-arm cast or splint.
- *Elbow (olecranon)*: Corrected by closed reduction and application of a cast. ORIF is performed for displaced fractures, and a splint is worn during the healing phase.
- *Forearm*: The ulna without accompanying injury is corrected with closed reduction and casting. If it is displaced, ORIF with intramedullary rods or plates and screws is required.
- *Wrist and hand:* Injury is most commonly to the carpal scaphoid bone, which is corrected by closed reduction and casting for 6 to 12 weeks. If the bone does not heal, ORIF with bone grafting is performed.

- *Colles' (wrist) fracture*: Fracture of the last inch of the distal radius is managed by casting for 6 to 8 weeks.
- *Metacarpals and phalanges (fingers)*: Metacarpal fractures are immobilized for 3 to 4 weeks. Phalangeal fractures are immobilized in finger splints for 10 to 14 days.
- *Hip (intracapsular)*: Involves the upper third of the femur within the joint capsule.
- *Hip (extracapsular)*: Involves the upper third of the femur outside of the joint capsule. Injury is managed by surgical repair, depending on the exact location of the fracture; ORIF may include an intramedullary rod, pins, prostheses (for femoral head or neck fractures), or a compression screw. Buck's traction may be applied before surgery.

Considerations for Older Adults

- Older adults are at risk for hip fracture because of physiologic aging changes, reduced vision, disease processes, drug therapy, and environmental hazards.
- These fractures occur most often in older women with osteoporosis.
- Other disease processes, such as foot disorders and changes in cardiac function, increase the risk for hip fracture.
- Drugs such as diuretics, cardiac drugs, antidepressants, sedatives, opioids, and alcohol are factors that increase the risks for falling in older adults. Use of three or more drugs at the same time drastically increases the risk for falls.
- The older adult is more likely to have complications from the fracture and its management.
- Although older patients recover fully from hip fracture repair and regain their functional ability, many will need rehabilitation and some patients are not able to return to their prefracture ADLs and mobility level.

- *Lower two thirds of the femur:* Usually managed surgically by ORIF with nails, rods, or a compression screw. When extensive bone fragmentation or severe tissue trauma is found, external fixation may be employed.
- *Patellar (knee cap) fracture:* Usually repaired by closed reduction and casting or internal fixation with screws
- *Tibia and fibula*: Corrected with closed reduction with casting for 8 to 10 weeks; internal fixation with nails or a plate and screws, followed by a long leg cast for 4 to 6 weeks; or external fixation for 6 to 10 weeks followed by application of a cast
- *Ankle*: May require a combination of closed and open techniques, depending on the severity and extent of the fracture.

An arthrodesis (fusion) may be needed if the bone does not heal.

- *Foot or phalanges*: Managed with closed or open reduction. Crutches are used for ambulation.
- *Ribs and sternum*: Have the potential to puncture the lungs, heart, or arteries by bone fragments or ends. Fractures of the lower ribs may damage underlying organs, such as the liver, spleen, or kidneys. These fractures tend to heal spontaneously without surgical intervention. Some clinicians may advise splinting or wrapping the chest, but this intervention is somewhat controversial because it also limits chest excursion.
- *Pelvis*: Pelvic fractures are the second most common cause of death from trauma. The major concern related to pelvic injury is venous oozing or arterial bleeding. Loss of blood volume leads to hypovolemic shock. When a non–weight-bearing part of the pelvis is fractured, management can be as minimal as bedrest on a firm mattress or bed board. A weight-bearing pelvis fracture requires external fixation with multiple pins, ORIF, or both. Progression to weight bearing depends on the stability of the fracture after fixation. Some patients can fully bear weight within days of surgery, whereas others managed with traction may not be able to bear weight for as long as 12 weeks.
- *Compression fractures of the vertebrae (spine)*: Are associated with severe pain, deformity (kyphosis), and possible neurologic compromise. Nonsurgical management includes bedrest, analgesics, nerve blocks, and physical therapy to maintain muscle strength. Compression fractures that remain painful and impair mobility may be surgically treated with vertebroplasty or kyphoplasty, in which bone cement is injected through the skin (percutaneously) directly into the fracture site to provide stability and immediate pain relief. Kyphoplasty also includes the insertion of a small balloon into the fracture site and inflating it to contain the cement and to restore height to the vertebra.

FROSTBITE

OVERVIEW

- Frostbite is a significant cold-related injury that occurs as a result of inadequate insulation against cold weather.
- Contributors to frostbite include wearing wet clothing, fatigue, dehydration, poor nutrition, smoking, alcohol consumption, and impaired peripheral circulation.

PATIENT-CENTERED COLLABORATIVE CARE
Assessment
- Severity of frostbite is related to the degree of tissue freezing and the resultant damage it produces.
  1. *Frostnip* is a superficial cold injury with initial pain, numbness, and pallor of the affected area. It is easily remedied with application of warmth and does not induce tissue damage.
  2. *First-degree frostbite* is the least severe type of frostbite, with hyperemia of the involved area and edema formation.
  3. *Second-degree frostbite* has large, fluid-filled blisters that develop with partial-thickness skin necrosis.
  4. *Third-degree frostbite* is a full-thickness injury that appears as small blisters containing dark fluid and an affected body part that is cool, numb, blue, or red and does not blanch.
  5. *Fourth-degree frostbite* is severe, with no blisters or edema; the part is numb, cold, and bloodless. Full-thickness necrosis extends into the muscle and bone.

Interventions: First Aid
- Recognize frostbite by observing for a white, waxy appearance of exposed skin, especially on the nose, cheeks, and ears.
- Seek shelter from the wind and cold.
- Use body heat to warm up superficial frostbite-affected areas by placing warm hands over the affected areas on the face or placing cold hands under the arms in the axillary region.

Interventions: Hospital Care
- Rapidly rewarm in a water bath at a temperature range of 104° to 108° F (40° to 42° C) or by using hot towels.
- Provide analgesic agents, especially IV opiates, and IV rehydration.

■ NURSING SAFETY PRIORITY: Action Alert
Dry heat should never be applied, nor should the frostbitten areas be rubbed or massaged as part of the warming process. These actions produce further tissue injury.

- Handle the injured areas gently, and elevate them above heart level if possible to decrease tissue edema.
- Use splints to immobilize extremities during the healing process.
- Assess the patient at least hourly for the development of compartment syndrome.
- Immunize the patient for tetanus prophylaxis.

- Apply only loose, nonadherent, sterile dressings to the damaged areas.
- Avoid compression of the injured tissues.
- Topical and systemic antibiotics may be prescribed.
- Management of severe, deep frostbite requires the same types of surgical intervention as deep or severe burns.

GASTRITIS

OVERVIEW

- Gastritis is inflammation of the gastric mucosa.
- Mucosal injury occurs and is worsened by histamine release and vagal nerve stimulation.
- Hydrochloric acid diffuses into the mucosa and injures small vessels, resulting in edema, hemorrhage, and erosion of the gastric lining.
- Gastritis can be classified as acute or chronic:
  1. *Acute gastritis,* the inflammation of gastric mucosa or submucosa, may result from the onset of infection (*Helicobacter pylori, Escherichia coli*); after exposure to local irritants such as alcohol or aspirin, NSAIDs, or bacterial endotoxins; after ingestion of corrosive substances; or from the lack of stimulation of normal gastric secretions. While acute gastritis causes mucosal necrosis, complete regeneration and healing usually occurs within a few days without any residual damage.
  2. *Chronic gastritis* is a diffuse chronic inflammatory process involving the mucosal lining of the stomach that usually heals without scarring but can progress to hemorrhage and ulcer formation and is associated with an increased risk for stomach cancer. Chronic gastritis may be caused by chronic local irritation from alcohol, drugs, smoking, radiation, infectious agents (e.g., *H. pylori*), and environmental agents. Of patients with gastric ulcers, 50% have associated chronic gastritis. Three subtypes of chronic gastritis are:
     a. Type A is associated with the presence of antibodies to parietal cells. An autoimmune pathogenesis has been proposed. Type A accompanies pernicious anemia.
     b. Type B usually is caused by *H. pylori* infection.
     c. Atrophic gastritis is found most often in older adults after exposure to toxic substances in the workplace or *H. pylori* infection, or it can be related to autoimmune factors.

G

PATIENT-CENTERED COLLABORATIVE CARE
Assessment
- Acute gastritis, assess for:
  1. Epigastric discomfort, pain, or cramping
  2. Anorexia, dyspepsia, nausea, and vomiting
  3. Hematemesis, melena
  4. Gastric infection, especially *H. pylori*
- Chronic gastritis, assess for:
  1. Nausea, vomiting, or upper GI discomfort.
  2. Anorexia
  3. Infection with *H. pylori*

Interventions
- Acute gastritis is treated symptomatically and supportively. If the patient experienced a GI bleed with severe hemorrhage, a blood transfusion may be needed. Fluid replacement is indicated for severe fluid loss.
- Treatment of chronic gastritis varies with the cause.
- Drug therapy:
  1. Proton pump inhibitors are used to reduce gastric acid secretion.
  2. H_2 histamine blockers may be used instead of proton pump inhibitors.
  3. Antacids are used as buffering agents.
  4. Antibiotics with a proton pump inhibitor and possibly bismuth subsalicylates may be used if the cause is a bacterial infection.
  5. Instruct the patient to avoid using drugs associated with gastric irritation, including steroids, chemotherapeutic agents, and NSAIDs.
- Diet therapy:
  1. Instruct the patient to avoid alcohol and foods that contribute to distress, such as those with caffeine, high levels of acid (e.g., tomatoes), and strong or hot spices.
  2. Instruct the patient to avoid consuming large, heavy meals.
- Teach techniques to reduce discomfort, such as progressive relaxation, cutaneous stimulation, guided imagery, and distraction.
- Advise the patient to stop smoking.

GASTROENTERITIS

OVERVIEW
- Gastroenteritis is an increase in the frequency and water content of stools and vomiting as a result of inflammation of the mucous membranes of the stomach and intestines, primarily affecting the small bowel.

- The disease may be viral or bacterial in origin, causing an inflammatory response in one of three ways:
  1. Release of enterotoxin, causing local inflammation and diarrhea
  2. Penetration of the organism into the intestine, causing cellular destruction, necrosis, and ulceration (Diarrhea occurs with red or white blood cells [WBCs or RBCs].)
  3. Attachment of the organism to the mucosal epithelium, destroying cells of the intestinal villi with resultant malabsorption
- Viral gastroenteritis can be classified as epidemic viral gastroenteritis or rotavirus gastroenteritis.
- Norwalk virus is a common cause of waterborne epidemics of gastroenteritis.
- Common microbes causing bacterial gastroenteritis are *Campylobacter, Escherichia coli,* and *Shigellosis*

PATIENT-CENTERED COLLABORATIVE CARE
Assessment
- Patient's history can provide information about potential cause:
  1. Onset of diarrhea with accompanying abdominal cramping or pain
  2. Nausea and vomiting
  3. Bloody, mucous, or watery, foul-smelling stool
  4. Patient's temperature normal or elevated from 101° to 103° F (38.2° to 39.2° C). When fever is present myalgia, headache, and malaise may also occur.
  5. Dehydration exhibited by poor skin turgor, dry mucous membranes, orthostatic blood pressure changes, hypotension, and oliguria
  6. Positive result of a stool culture

Interventions
- Provide fluid replacement therapy:
  1. Administer oral rehydration therapy with commercially prepared products such as Resol.
  2. Administer hypotonic IV fluids for severe dehydration; add potassium if the patient is hypokalemic.
  3. Check vital signs and orthostatic blood pressure, as clinically indicated.
  4. Check weight daily.
  5. Maintain strict intake and output.
  6. Depending on the type of gastroenteritis, notify the local health department.
- Provide diet therapy:
  1. Advise the patient to take small volumes of clear liquids with electrolytes.

2. Advise the patient not to drink water, because it does not contain any electrolytes to replace those lost.

3. Slowly progress the diet to include small portions of saltine crackers and toast. When this is tolerated, consider adding bland foods (e.g., nonfat soup, custard, yogurt, cottage cheese, baked or mashed potatoes, or cooked vegetables), and then progress to the patient's regular diet.

- Provide drug therapy as ordered:
  1. Drugs that suppress intestinal motility, such as antiemetics or anticholinergics, are not routinely given.
  2. Antimicrobials are given if gastroenteritis is caused by an infecting organism susceptible to therapy. Viral gastroenteritis, which is more likely to have a shorter duration of symptoms (24 to 48 hours), is treated symptomatically.
  3. Diarrhea that continues for 10 days is probably not caused by gastroenteritis, and an investigation for other causes is done.

- Provide skin care:
  1. Teach the patient to avoid toilet paper and harsh soaps and to gently clean the area with warm water and absorbent cotton, followed by thorough drying with absorbent cotton.
  2. Cream, oil, or gel can be applied to a damp, warm washcloth or flushable wipe to remove excrement adhering to excoriated skin.
  3. Hydrocortisone cream or a protective barrier cream should be applied to the skin between stools; witch hazel compresses (e.g., Tucks) and sitz baths can relieve discomfort.

- Teach the patient the following health practices:
  1. Replace lost fluids.
  2. Follow the recommended diet.
  3. Wash hands after each bowel movement to minimize the risk of disease transmission.
  4. Do not share eating utensils, glasses, and dishes, and maintain strict personal hygiene.
  5. Maintain clean bathroom facilities.
  6. Inform the health care provider if symptoms persist beyond 3 days.
  7. Adhere to these precautions for up to 7 weeks after the illness or up to several months if *Shigella* was the causative organism.
  8. Follow written instructions for drugs, if ordered, including the dosage, schedule of administration, and side effects.

GASTROESOPHAGEAL REFLUX DISEASE

OVERVIEW

- Gastroesophageal reflux disease (GERD) occurs as the result of the backward flow (reflux) of GI contents into the esophagus.
- Reflux produces symptoms by exposing the esophageal mucosa to the irritating effects of gastric or duodenal contents, resulting in inflammation.
- A person with acute symptoms of inflammation is often described as having *reflux esophagitis,* which may be mild or severe.
- The degree of inflammation is related to the acid concentration of the refluxed material, the number of reflux episodes, and the length of time that the esophagus is exposed to the irritant.
- *Dyspepsia* (also called *heartburn* or *pyrosis*), the primary symptom, is described as a substernal or retrosternal burning sensation that tends to move up and down the chest in a wavelike fashion; severe heartburn may radiate to the neck or jaw or may be felt in the back. It can resemble angina, the pain associated with *acute coronary syndromes (ACS).*

PATIENT-CENTERED COLLABORATIVE CARE

Assessment

- Record patient information related to heartburn or esophageal pain:
  1. Location, quality, onset, and duration of dyspepsia or esophageal pain
  2. Pain aggravated by bending over, straining, or lying in a recumbent position
- Ask whether he or she has been newly diagnosed with asthma or has experienced morning hoarseness or pneumonia. These symptoms suggest severe reflux reaching the pharynx or mouth or pulmonary aspiration.
- Other symptoms associated with GERD:
  1. Water brash (reflex salivary hypersecretion)
  2. Dysphagia (difficulty swallowing) or odynophagia (painful swallowing)
  3. Chronic cough that occurs mostly at night
  4. Belching and a feeling of flatulence or bloating after eating
  5. Regurgitation not associated with belching or nausea; warm fluid traveling up the throat, resulting in a sour or bitter taste in the mouth
- Assess results of 24-hour pH monitoring, esophageal manometry (motility testing), and scintigraphy (measure of reflux of radioisotope).

Interventions
  Nonsurgical Management
- Explore the patient's meal plan and food preferences, and in collaboration with the nutritionist, meet with the patient and family to plan diet modifications to reduce GERD symptoms. Teach the patient to:
    1. Avoid chocolate, peppermint, fatty (especially fried) foods and carbonated beverages, because they reduce lower esophageal sphincter (LES) pressure or cause local irritation.
    2. Eat small meals.
    3. Avoid eating for 3 hours (or more) before bedtime.
    4. Limit or eliminate alcohol and tobacco.
    5. Remain upright after meals for 1 to 2 hours.
- Teach the patient and family the risk factors that can exacerbate the disease.
- Encourage lifestyle changes:
    1. If the patient is obese, examine approaches to weight reduction with the patient.
    2. Explore the possibility and means of smoking cessation and make appropriate referrals.
    3. Instruct the patient to elevate the head of the bed by 6 inches to prevent nighttime reflux.
    4. Instruct the patient to sleep in the left lateral decubitus (side-lying) position.
    5. Encourage the patient to avoid wearing tight-fitting clothing and working in a bent-over or stooped position.
- Drug therapy:
    1. Proton pump inhibitors are the main treatment for GERD and provide effective, long-acting inhibition of gastric acid secretion.
    2. H_2 histamine receptor blockers are sometimes used instead of proton pump inhibitors to reduce gastric acid production, provide symptom improvement, and support healing of the inflamed esophageal tissue.
    3. Antacids are used to neutralize gastric acids.
    4. Prokinetic drugs are used to accelerate gastric emptying and improve LES pressure and esophageal peristalsis.
- Identify whether the patient uses drugs that may lower LES pressure and cause reflux, such as oral contraceptives, anticholinergic agents, beta-adrenergic agonists, nitrates, and calcium channel blockers.
  Surgical Management
- Noninvasive endoscopic procedures:
    1. The Stretta procedure involves the application of radiofrequency energy near the gastroesophageal junction, which

inhibits the activity of the vagus nerve, reducing discomfort for the patient.

2. The Bard EndoCinch Suturing System (BESS) involves suturing near the LES.

- The major surgical procedure for patients who have not responded to aggressive medical management is the laparoscopic Nissen fundoplication.

⚑NATIONAL PATIENT SAFETY GOAL

Be sure to use two patient identifiers before starting any procedure in any setting. Involve a patient who is alert and cooperative in self-identification before GI diagnostic and treatment procedures.

GLAUCOMA

OVERVIEW

- Glaucoma is a group of ocular diseases resulting in increased intraocular pressure (IOP).
- The normal pressure of fluid in the eye is an IOP of 10 to 21 mm Hg, maintained when there is a balance between production and outflow of aqueous humor.
- If the IOP becomes too high, the extra pressure presses on blood vessels in the eye and prevents blood flow, resulting in poorly oxygenated photoreceptors, which then become ischemic and die. When too many have died, sight is lost, and the person is permanently blind.
- In most types of glaucoma, vision is lost gradually and painlessly from the periphery to the central area, without the person's awareness.
- Types of glaucoma:
  1. *Primary:* The structures involved in circulation and reabsorption of the aqueous humor undergo direct pathologic changes from aging, heredity, and central retinal vessel occlusion.
     a. *Primary open-angle glaucoma (POAG)* has reduced outflow of aqueous humor through the chamber angle. Because the fluid cannot leave the eye at the same rate it is produced, IOP gradually increases.
     b. *Angle-closure glaucoma* (also called *closed-angle glaucoma, narrow-angle glaucoma,* or *acute glaucoma*) has a sudden onset and is an emergency.
  2. *Secondary:* Glaucoma results from other problems within the eye, such as uveitis, iritis, trauma, and ocular surgeries.

G

3. *Associated*: Glaucoma results from systemic disease, such as diabetes mellitus and hypertension.

PATIENT-CENTERED COLLABORATIVE CARE
Assessment
- Assess for manifestations of early POAG:
  1. Increased ocular pressure
  2. Reduced accommodation
- Assess for late manifestations of late POAG:
  1. Peripheral visual field losses
  2. Decreased visual acuity not correctable with glasses
  3. Appearance of halos around lights
  4. Increased cupping and atrophy of the optic disc
  5. IOP tonometry reading between 22 and 32 mm Hg

Interventions
Nonsurgical Management
- Drug therapy for glaucoma focuses on reducing IOP with eyedrops:
  1. Prostaglandin agonists:
     a. Bimatoprost (Lumigan)
     b. Latanoprost (Xalatan)
     c. Travoprost (Travatan)
  2. Adrenergic agonists:
     a. Apraclonidine (Iopidine)
     b. Brimonidine (Alphagan)
     c. Dipivefrin (Propine)
  3. Beta-adrenergic blockers:
     a. Betaxolol (Betoptic)
     b. Carteolol (Cartrol, Ocupress)
     c. Levobunolol (Betagan)
     d. Timolol (Betimol, Timoptic)
     e. Timoptic GFS (gel-forming solution for extended release)
  4. Cholinergic agonists:
     a. Carbachol (Carboptic, Isopto Carbachol, Miostat)
     b. Echothiophate (Phospholine Iodide)
     c. Pilocarpine (Adsorbocarpine, Akarpine, Isopto Carpine, Ocu-Carpine, Ocusert, Piloptic, Pilopine, Pilostat)
  5. Carbonic anhydrase inhibitors:
     a. Brinzolamide (Azopt)
     b. Dorzolamide (Trusopt)
  6. Combination agents
     a. Brimonidine tartrate and timolol maleate (Combigan)

- Teach the patient:
  1. Stress the importance of instilling the drops on time and not skipping doses.
  2. When more than one drug is prescribed, teach the patient to wait 10 to 15 minutes between drug instillations to prevent one drug from "washing out" or diluting another drug.
  3. Teach the technique of punctal occlusion (placing pressure on the corner of the eye near the nose) immediately after eye-drop instillation to prevent systemic absorption of the drug.
  4. Stress the need for good handwashing, keeping the eyedrop container tip clean, and avoiding touching the tip to any part of the eye.

Surgical Management
- Surgery is used when drugs for the patient with open-angle glaucoma are not effective in controlling IOP. The two most common procedures are laser trabeculoplasty and filtering microsurgery.
- *Laser trabeculoplasty* burns the trabecular meshwork, scarring it and causing the meshwork fibers to shrink. Fiber shrinkage increases the size of the spaces between the fibers, improving outflow of aqueous humor and a reduction in IOP.
- *Filtering microsurgery* creates a drainage hole in the iris between the posterior and anterior chambers.
- When surgical therapies fail, other more invasive procedures may be used. These include deep sclerectomy, viscocanalostomy, or an implanted shunt.
- The most serious complication after glaucoma surgery is choroidal hemorrhage. Manifestations include:
  1. Acute pain deep in the eye
  2. Decreased vision
  3. Vital sign changes

GLOMERULONEPHRITIS, ACUTE

OVERVIEW
- Acute glomerulonephritis results from injury to the glomeruli. *Rapidly progressive glomerulonephritis,* a subtype of this condition, develops over several weeks or months and causes a rapid and significant loss of kidney function.
- Glomerular injury is the result of immune complexes deposited in kidney tissue; an immune complex is made up of antigens and antibodies.
- Immune complexes trigger inflammation, which can further damage kidney tissue.

PATIENT-CENTERED COLLABORATIVE CARE
Assessment
- Record patient information:
  1. History of recent infections, particularly skin and upper respiratory infections
  2. Recent travel
  3. Activities with exposure to viruses, bacteria, fungi, or parasites
  4. Recent illnesses, operations, or invasive procedures
  5. Known systemic diseases, especially those associated with inflammation or autoimmunity such as systemic lupus erythematosus
- Assessment findings include:
  1. Skin lesions or incisions, including piercings that could be the source of infection
  2. Presence of symptoms indicating systemic volume overload: extra heart sound (i.e., S_3 gallop), neck vein engorgement, edema, and crackles in the lungs with tachypnea and dyspnea or orthopnea
  3. Changes in urine formation and excretion, including changes in color (typically smoky, reddish brown, or tea-colored urine), clarity, or odor; and altered patterns of urination such as dysuria, urgency, and incontinence
  4. Decreased urine output
  5. Mild to moderate hypertension
  6. Changes in weight
  7. Fatigue, malaise and activity intolerance
  8. Abnormal urinalysis including leukocyte esterase, nitrogen, red blood cells (RBCs), white blood cells (WBCs), and protein
  9. Increased blood urea nitrogen (BUN) and serum creatinine levels
  10. Decreased urine creatinine clearance
  11. Positive cultures from urine, blood, sputum, skin, or throat
  12. Serologic testing for antistreptolysin O titers, C3 complement levels, immunoglobulin G, antinuclear bodies, and circulating immune complexes
- A percutaneous needle biopsy of the kidney may define the pathologic condition, assist in determining prognosis, and help outline treatment.

Interventions
- Appropriate anti-infective agents are given to treat infection.
- Sodium and water restriction, along with diuretics, may be needed for the patient with hypertension, circulatory overload, and edema. The usual fluid allowance is equal to the 24-hour urinary output plus 500 to 600 mL for insensible fluid loss.

- Potassium and protein intake may be restricted to prevent hyperkalemia and additional uremic manifestations.
- Management may include dialysis or plasmapheresis to filter out antigen-antibody complexes and manage uremia or fluid and electrolyte imbalances.
- Health teaching includes:
  1. Reviewing prescribed drug instructions, including purpose, timing, frequency, duration, and side effects
  2. Ensuring that the patient and family understand dietary and fluid modifications. Offer assistance with coping with fluid restrictions, such as a mouth moisturizer or mouth swabs. In some situations ice chips or hard candy may be used to offer relief from a dry mouth.
  3. Advising the patient to measure weight and blood pressure daily and to notify the health care provider of any sudden changes
  4. Instructing the patient about peritoneal or vascular access care if short-term dialysis is required to control excess fluid volume or uremic symptoms

GLOMERULONEPHRITIS, CHRONIC

G

OVERVIEW

- Chronic glomerulonephritis, or *chronic nephritic syndrome,* is the diagnostic name given to known and unknown causes of kidney deterioration or kidney failure that develop over 20 to 30 years.
- The exact cause is unknown. Changes are thought to result from the effects of hypertension, intermittent or recurrent infections and inflammation, and poor blood flow to the kidneys.
- Kidney tissue atrophies, and the functional mass of nephrons decreases, which alters glomerular filtration.
- Glomerular injury results in proteinuria because of increased permeability of the glomerular basement membrane.
- The process eventually results in chronic kidney disease (CKD) and uremia, requiring dialysis or transplantation.

PATIENT-CENTERED COLLABORATIVE CARE
Assessment

- Record the patient's history:
  1. Health problems, including systemic disease, kidney or urologic problems, and infectious diseases, especially streptococcal infections and recent exposure to infection

2. Presence of symptoms indicating systemic volume overload: the cardiac extra sound of an S_3 gallop, neck vein engorgement, edema, and crackles in the lungs with tachypnea
3. Changes in urine and elimination, including amount, frequency of voiding, and changes in urine color, clarity, and odor
4. Changes in activity tolerance and comfort
5. Changes in mental concentration or memory associated with uremia
6. Abnormal urinalysis, especially proteinuria
7. Decreased creatinine clearance
8. Abnormal serum kidney function and electrolyte values
9. Radiographic findings of kidney size (usually small)

- Perform a physical assessment:
  1. Inspect the skin for color, ecchymosis, and rashes.
  2. Inspect for symptoms of fluid overload and electrolyte imbalance.
  3. Measure blood pressure and weight.
  4. Inspect urine and evaluate urinalysis results.
  5. Evaluate laboratory values, especially serum BUN, creatine, and electrolytes and urinalysis.
  6. Assess for uremic symptoms, such as slurred speech, ataxia, tremors, or asterixis (flapping tremor of the fingers or the inability to maintain a fixed posture with the arms extended and wrists hyperextended).

Interventions

- Management of chronic glomerulonephritis is similar to conservative management for CKD, including dialysis when kidneys fail to filter the blood.
- Treatment consists of dietary modification, fluid intake sufficient to prevent reduced blood flow volume to the kidneys, and drug therapy to temporarily control the symptoms of uremia.

GONORRHEA

OVERVIEW

- Gonorrhea is a sexually transmitted bacterial infection caused by *Neisseria gonorrhoeae,* a gram-negative intracellular diplococcus.
- It is transmitted by direct sexual contact with mucosal surfaces (vaginal intercourse, orogenital contact, or anogenital contact).

- The first symptoms of gonorrhea may appear 3 to 10 days after sexual contact with an infected person, or the disease can be present without symptoms and can be transmitted or progress without warning.
- In women, ascending spread of the organism can cause pelvic infection (pelvic inflammatory disease [PID]), endometritis (endometrial infection), salpingitis (fallopian tube infection), and pelvic peritonitis.
- *Neisseria gonorrhoeae* is a multidrug- resistant organism (MDRO) in the United States

PATIENT-CENTERED COLLABORATIVE CARE
Assessment
- Obtain patient information about:
  1. Sexual history that includes sexual orientation and sites of intercourse
  2. Allergies to antibiotics
  3. Symptoms in men:
     a. Dysuria
     b. Penile discharge (profuse, yellowish-green fluid or scant, clear fluid)
     c. Urethritis
     d. Pain or discomfort in the prostate, seminal vesicles, or epididymal regions
  4. Symptoms in women:
     a. Vaginal discharge (yellow, green, profuse, odorous)
     b. Urinary frequency
     c. Dysuria and urethral discharge
  5. Anal manifestations (in men or women):
     a. Itching and irritation
     b. Rectal discharge or bleeding
     c. Diarrhea
     d. Painful defecation
- Assess for and document:
  1. Oral cavity manifestations:
     a. Reddened throat
     b. Ulcerated lips
     c. Tender gingivae
     d. Blisters in the throat
  2. Tenderness of the lower abdomen
  3. Manifestations of disseminated gonococcal infection (DGI):
     a. Fever
     b. Chills
     c. Skin lesions on hands and feet
     d. Joint pain, with or without swelling, heat, or redness

G

- Diagnostic testing may include:
  1. Nucleic acid amplification test (NAAT) using samples from vagina or male urethra
  2. Gram staining and cultures from a smears from penile discharge or from a vaginal swab

▇ NURSING SAFETY PRIORITY: Critical Rescue

All patients with gonorrhea should be tested for syphilis, chlamydia, hepatitis B and C, and HIV infection, because they may have been exposed to multiple sexually transmitted diseases (STDs). Sexual partners who have been exposed in the past 30 days should be examined and specimens for culture should be obtained.

Interventions

- Drug therapy for uncomplicated gonorrhea is a cephalosporin. Treatment of DGI usually requires hospitalization and includes IV or IM ceftriaxone (1 g every 24 hours). If symptoms resolve within 24 to 48 hours, the patient may be discharged to home to continue oral antibiotic therapy for at least a week. In general, antibiotics are started before the culture results are finalized (and are discontinued if there is no evidence of *Neisseria* infection)
- Sexual partners also must be treated.
- A test of cure is not required but the patient should be advised to return for a follow-up examination if symptoms persist after treatment.
- This condition must be reported to the local health department by the health care provider.
- Teach the patient about:
  1. Transmission and treatment of gonorrhea
  2. Prevention of reinfection
  3. Complications of chronic gonorrhea:
     a. PID
     b. Ectopic pregnancy
     c. Infertility
     d. Chronic pelvic pain
  4. Avoiding sexual activity until the antibiotic therapy is completed
  5. Condom use if abstinence is not possible
  6. The need for all sexual contacts to be examined for STDs
- Encourage patients to express their feelings during assessments and teaching sessions.
- Provide privacy for teaching and maintain confidentiality of medical records.

GOUT

OVERVIEW

- Gout, or *gouty arthritis,* is a systemic disease in which urate crystals deposit in the joints and other body tissues, causing inflammation.
- There are two major types of gout:
  1. *Primary gout* results from one of several inborn errors of purine metabolism that allows the production of uric acid to exceed the excretion capability of the kidneys. Urate is deposited in synovium and other tissues, resulting in inflammation. A number of patients have a family history of gout. It is most common in middle-aged and older men and postmenopausal women.
  2. *Secondary gout* results from excessive uric acid crystals that are present in the blood (hyperuricemia) as a result of another disease, condition, or treatment. Causes include renal insufficiency, diuretic therapy, "crash" diets, certain chemotherapeutic agents, and diseases such as multiple myeloma and certain carcinomas. Treatment for secondary gout focuses on management of the underlying disorder.
- There are three clinical stages of primary gout:
  1. *Asymptomatic hyperuricemic stage,* in which these are no symptoms but the serum uric acid level is elevated
  2. *Acute stage,* in which the patient experiences excruciating pain and inflammation in one or more small joints, usually the metatarsophalangeal joint of the great toe, called *podagra*
  3. *Chronic tophaceous stage,* which occurs after repeated episodes of acute gout have caused deposits of urate crystals under the skin and within the major organs, particularly in the kidney system. This stage can begin between 3 and 40 years after the initial gout symptoms occur.

PATIENT-CENTERED COLLABORATIVE CARE
Assessment

- Obtain patient information about:
  1. Age
  2. Gender
  3. Family history of gout
  4. Medical history and drug history to determine whether gout has been caused by another problem
- For acute gout, assess for and document joint inflammation and pain.

G

- For chronic gout, assess for and document:
  1. Presence of tophi (skin deposits of urate crystals):
     a. Outer ear
     b. Arms and fingers near the joints
  2. Infected skin areas
  3. Manifestations of kidney (stones) or kidney dysfunction:
     a. Severe pain
     b. Changes in urine output
- Diagnostic assessment may include:
  1. Serum uric acid level
  2. Urinary uric acid levels
  3. Kidney function tests (in chronic gout)
  4. Synovial fluid aspiration (arthrocentesis)

Interventions

- Drug therapy during acute attacks:
  1. Colchicine (Colsalide, Novocolchicine ✦)
  2. NSAIDs, such as indomethacin (Indocin, Novomethacin ✦) or ibuprofen (Motrin, Amersol ✦)
- Drug therapy for chronic gout
  1. Allopurinol (Zyloprim)
  2. Probenecid (Benemid, Benuryl ✦)
  3. Combination drugs that contain probenecid and colchicine (ColBenemid)

◼ NURSING SAFETY PRIORITY: Action Alert

Aspirin should be avoided, because it inactivates the effects of the drug therapy.

- Nutritional therapy with a low-purine diet by avoidance of:
  1. Organ meats
  2. Red meats
  3. Shellfish
  4. Oily fish with bones (e.g., sardines)
  5. Teaching patients to determine which foods precipitate acute attacks and to try to avoid them
- Other restrictions include:
  1. All forms of aspirin
  2. Diuretics
  3. Excessive physical or emotional stress, which can exacerbate the disease
- Teach the patient to drink plenty of fluids, especially:
  1. Water
  2. Citrus juices
  3. Milk

GUILLAIN-BARRÉ SYNDROME

OVERVIEW

- Guillain-Barré syndrome (GBS) is an *acute inflammatory demyelinating polyneuropathy (AIDP)* that affects the peripheral nervous system, causing motor weakness and sensory abnormalities.
- GBS is the result of a variety of related immune-mediated pathologic processes.
- Three stages make up the acute course:
  1. *Acute phase,* which begins with the onset of the first definitive symptoms and ends when no further deterioration is noted (usually 1 to 4 weeks)
  2. *Plateau phase,* which is a time of little change and lasts several days to 2 weeks
  3. *Recovery phase,* which is thought to coincide with re-myelination and axonal regeneration and occurs gradually over 4 to 6 months (sometimes up to 2 years)
- *Chronic inflammatory demyelinating polyneuropathy (CIDP)* is an unusual type of GBS that progresses over a longer period; complete recovery rarely occurs.
- The patient often relates a history of acute illness, trauma, surgery, or immunization 1 to 8 weeks before the onset of neurologic signs and symptoms.

G

🌐 Cultural Awareness

- GBS has a worldwide distribution and affects people of all races and ages.
- The highest rates have been observed for people 45 years old or older.
- The incidence is higher among whites than African Americans.

PATIENT-CENTERED COLLABORATIVE CARE

Assessment

- Record the patient's medical and surgical history, including:
  1. Occurrence of antecedent illness 1 to 8 weeks before the onset of GBS
  2. Description of symptoms (in chronologic order)
- Assessment findings include:
  1. Paresthesia (numbness or tingling) and pain
  2. Cranial nerve dysfunction resulting in facial weakness, dysphagia, and/or diplopia
  3. Difficulty walking

4. Muscle weakness or flaccid paralysis without muscle wasting in an ascending, distal-to-proximal progression
5. Respiratory compromise or failure:
   a. Dyspnea
   b. Decreased breath sounds from reduced tidal volume or vital capacity
6. Bowel and bladder incontinence
7. Autonomic dysfunction evidenced by:
   a. Labile blood pressure
   b. Cardiac dysrhythmias
   c. Tachycardia
8. Decreased or absent deep tendon reflexes
9. Altered coping manifested by:
   a. Anxiety, fear, and panic
   b Anger and depression
10. Protein in cerebrospinal fluid without leukocytosis
11. Electrophysiologic studies (EPSs) demonstrating demyelinating neuropathy

Planning and Implementation

- Treat with plasma exchange or immunoglobulin:
  1. There is no benefit to combining therapies.
  2. *Plasmapheresis* removes the circulating antibodies thought to be responsible for the disease. Nursing interventions for the patient undergoing plasmapheresis include:
     a. Providing information and reassurance
     b. Monitoring for complications of plasmapheresis: hypovolemia, hypokalemia, hypocalcemia, temporary circumoral and distal extremity paresthesia, muscle twitching, nausea, and vomiting
     c. Monitoring intake and output and weighing the patient after the procedure to detect dehydration or overhydration as a result of treatment
     d. Administering proper care to the shunt, if used

■ NURSING SAFETY PRIORITY: Critical Rescue

If a shunt is used, use these safety interventions:
- Check shunt patency.
- Assess for bruits every 2 to 4 hours.
- Keep double bulldog clamps at the bedside.
- Observe the puncture site for bleeding or ecchymosis (bruising).

- *Intravenous immunoglobulin therapy (IVIG)* is equally effective as plasmapheresis but is safer and immediately available.

- Side effects of immunoglobulin therapy range from minor annoyances (e.g., chills, mild fever, myalgia, headache) to major complications (e.g., anaphylaxis, aseptic meningitis, retinal necrosis, and acute kidney injury and failure).

MANAGING THE AIRWAY AND MONITORING RESPIRATORY STATUS

- Monitor the color, consistency, and amount of secretions obtained.
- Auscultate breath sounds, respiratory rate, rhythm, depth, and chest excursion every 1 to 4 hours.
- Observe for dyspnea, air hunger, adventitious breath sounds, cyanosis, and confusion.
- Administer humidified air or oxygen, as appropriate.
- Administer bronchodilator treatments, as appropriate.
- Keep equipment for suctioning available and equipment for intubation nearby.
- Elevate the head of the bed.
- Encourage the patient to use the incentive spirometer and cough and breathe deeply.
- Monitor peripheral oxygen saturation (SpO_2) and ABG results for hypoxemia, hypercarbia, or disturbances in pH.

IMPROVING MOBILITY AND PREVENTING THE COMPLICATIONS OF IMMOBILITY

- The health care team collaborates with the patient to develop interventions to prevent complications of immobility and address deficits in self-care:
  1. Assess motor function with vital signs.
  2. Assist the patient's hygiene, toileting, and feeding, as needed.
  3. Collaborate with physical therapy and occupational therapy to determine the type and duration of daily exercises or activity, such as transfer to chair, repositioning in bed, ambulation, and ADLs.
  4. Monitor the patient's response to or tolerance of activity and reduce frequency or duration of activity if intolerant.
  5. Provide adequate rest periods between activities.
  6. Collaborate with the nutritionist to develop a nutritional plan, and assist with meals as needed.
  7. Evaluate for dysphagia and implement aspiration precautions if needed
  8. Monitor intake and output for balance, and assess the patient for urinary retention every shift.
  9. Monitor for complications of immobility: atelectasis, pneumonia, pressure ulcers, deep vein thrombosis, and pulmonary emboli.

G

▼ NATIONAL PATIENT SAFETY GOAL

Assess and periodically reassess each patient's risk for developing a pressure ulcer, and take action to address any identified risks. Prevention of hospital-acquired pressure ulcers is a priority for all patients.

MANAGING PAIN

- Assess the severity and nature of the patient's pain, which is typically worse at night.
- Pain is best treated with opiates, which can be administered by a patient-controlled analgesia (PCA) pump or continuous IV drip. Document the patient's response to pain drug.
- Other interventions include frequent positioning, massage, ice, heat, relaxation techniques, guided imagery, and distractions.

PROMOTING COMMUNICATION

- Assist the patient to develop a communication system in collaboration with the speech-language pathologist.
- Develop a communication board that lists common requests.

PROVIDING PSYCHOSOCIAL SUPPORT

- Encourage the patient to verbalize feelings concerning the illness and its effects.
- Provide information regarding the disease process.
- Encourage the patient to participate in his or her care and to make as many choices as possible.
- Provide encouragement and positive reinforcement.
- Identify factors that increase coping abilities by asking the patient and family to describe situations that they have successfully coped with in the past.
- Keep necessary items (call light, radio, or television control) within the patient's reach.
- Use the patient's own personal items, when feasible.

Community-Based Care

- Discharge planning includes:
  1. Providing a detailed plan of care at the time of discharge for patients to be transferred to a long-term care or rehabilitation facility (rehabilitation may be lengthy)
  2. Assessing the patient and family's knowledge and understanding of the disease
  3. Providing oral and written information on therapeutic positioning and mobility
  4. Ensuring that patient and family members understand how to use assistive or adaptive devices
  5. Referring the patient to local or community agencies for assistance in the home setting
  6. Referring the patient to the Guillain-Barré Foundation for information about local resources and educational materials

HEADACHE, CLUSTER

OVERVIEW

- Cluster headaches (also referred to as *trigeminal autonomic cephalalgia*) are manifested by brief (30 minutes to 2 hours), intense unilateral pain that generally occurs in the spring and fall without warning.
- Cluster headaches are classified as the most common type of chronic short-duration headache with pain lasting less than 4 hours.
- The cause and mechanism of cluster headaches are not known but have been attributed to vasoreactivity and neurogenic inflammation.
- Cluster headaches commonly manifest as unilateral (one-sided) oculotemporal or oculofrontal headaches with pain described as excruciating, boring, and nonthrobbing.
- The headaches occur at about the same time of day for about 4 to 12 weeks (hence the term *cluster*), followed by a period of remission for 9 months to a year.

PATIENT-CENTERED COLLABORATIVE CARE
Planning and Implementation

- Management includes:
  1. Administering drugs to treat pain, similar to migraine therapy: triptans, ergotamine preparations, and antiepileptic drug. Additional drugs include calcium channel blockers, especially verapamil (Calan), lithium, and corticosteroids.
  2. Administering 100% oxygen by mask for 15 to 30 minutes with the patient in a sitting position during cluster headache pain
  3. Instructing the patient to wear sunglasses and avoid bright light while the headache is occurring
  4. Helping the patient identify precipitating factors such as bursts of anger, excessive physical activity, and excitement
  5. Teaching the patient the importance of a consistent sleep-wake cycle
  6. Surgical interventions for drug-resistant cluster headaches, such as percutaneous stereotactic rhizotomy and deep brain electrical stimulation at the posterior hypothalamus

H

HEADACHE, MIGRAINE

OVERVIEW

- A migraine headache is a chronic, episodic disorder with multiple subtypes.

- It is characterized by an intense pain in one side of the head (unilateral), worsening with movement, and occurs with either photophobia (sensitive to light) or phonophobia (sensitive to noise). Either moderate to severe nausea or vomiting is also present.
- A migraine is classified as a long-duration headache, because it usually lasts between 4 and 72 hours.
- The cause of migraine headaches is likely a combination of vascular, genetic, neurologic, hormonal, and environmental factors.
- Three categories of migraine headache are migraine with aura (classic migraine), migraine without aura, and atypical migraine.

PATIENT-CENTERED COLLABORATIVE CARE
Planning and Implementation

- Management focuses on the "three R" approach for patients and health care providers:
  1. *R*ecognize migraine symptoms.
  2. *R*espond and see the health care provider.
  3. *R*elieve pain and associated symptoms.

PREVENTIVE THERAPY

- Implement trigger avoidance. Collaborate with the patient to determine factors, if any, that may trigger the development of a headache, such as caffeine, red wine, stress, and monosodium glutamate (MSG).
- Use preventive drug therapy regularly:
  1. NSAIDs
  2. Beta blockers propranolol (Inderal, Apo-Propranolol ✹) and timolol (Blocadren, Apo-Timol ✹) are approved for migraine prevention
  3. Antiepileptics (AEDs)
     a. Topiramate (Topamax) is the most common AED used for migraines, but it should be used in low doses because it can unmask mental health disorders, leading to suicide.

ABORTIVE THERAPY

- Use prescribed drug therapy to treat pain after the headache starts, including:
  1. Acetaminophen (Tylenol, Abenol ✹) or an NSAID such as ibuprofen (Motrin, others), or naproxen (Naprosyn, others) for mild pain
  2. Triptans such as sumatriptan (Imitrex)

NOTE: Triptans are contraindicated in patients with actual or suspected ischemic heart disease, hypertension, or peripheral vascular disease and in pregnant women.

3. Ergotamine derivatives such as dihydroergotamine (D.H.E.), but not within 24 hours of a triptan preparation
4. Isometheptene combinations (Midrin) when ergotamine derivatives are not tolerated
5. Antiemetics if nausea and vomiting occur with the migraine
6. Complementary and alternative therapies that may be used include yoga, meditation, biofeedback, relaxation techniques, and acupuncture. A dark room and rest may mitigate the migraine if used early during onset of the headache pain.
7. If the patient uses herbal or vitamin therapy in alternative treatments, explore the potential for drug-herb or drug-nutraceutical interactions.

HEARING LOSS

OVERVIEW

- Hearing loss, a common handicap worldwide, may be conductive, sensorineural, or a combination of the two.
  1. *Conductive hearing loss* occurs when sound waves are blocked from contact with inner ear nerve fibers because of inflammation or obstruction of the external or middle ear by cerumen or foreign objects, otitis media, tumors, scar tissue buildup, or overgrowth of soft or bony tissue on the ossicles.
  2. *Sensorineural hearing loss* occurs when hair cells or the inner ear sensory nerve fibers from the auditory nerve (cranial nerve VIII) that lead to the cerebral cortex are damaged. Causes include prolonged exposure to loud noise, ototoxic drugs, deficiencies of vitamin B_{12} or folic acid, atherosclerosis, hypertension, infections, prolonged fever, Ménière's disease, diabetes mellitus, and ear surgery. *Presbycusis* is a sensorineural hearing loss that occurs as a result of aging.
  3. *Combined or mixed hearing loss* has components of both conductive and sensorineural loss.
- About one third of people between the ages of 65 and 75 years have a hearing loss. As many as one half of people older than 85 years have some degree of hearing loss.
- The type and cause of hearing loss determine the degree to which loss can be corrected and the amount of hearing that can return.

H

Genetic/Genomic Considerations
- Some hearing loss in adults can have a genetic origin, such as Usher's syndrome and Alport's syndrome. These syndromes usually occur with other physical problems.
- One type of adult onset hearing loss that does not have any other physical problems is associated with a mutation in the *GJB2* gene on chromosome 13. This form of hearing loss has an autosomal dominant pattern of inheritance.

PATIENT-CENTERED COLLABORATIVE CARE
Assessment
- Obtain patient information about:
  1. Any differences in his or her ears or hearing and whether the changes occurred suddenly or gradually, including:
     a. Feeling of ear fullness or congestion
     b. Dizziness or vertigo
     c. Tinnitus
     d. Difficulty understanding conversations, especially in a noisy room
     e. Difficulty hearing sounds
     f. The need to strain to hear
     g. The need to turn the head to favor one ear or the need to lean forward to hear
     h. Pain
  2. Age
  3. Occupational or leisure exposure to loud or continuous noises
  4. Current or previous use of ototoxic drugs
  5. History of external ear or middle ear infection and whether eardrum perforation occurred with the infection
  6. History of ear trauma
  7. Whether any family members are hearing-impaired
  8. Recent upper respiratory infection and allergies affecting the nose and sinuses
  9. Functional hearing
     a. Frequency of asking people to repeat statements
     b. Withdrawal from social interactions or large groups
     c. Shouting in conversation
     d. Failing to respond when not looking in the direction of the sound
     e. Answering questions incorrectly
- Assess for and document:
  1. External ear features (pinna)
     a. Size

     b. Position
2. Otoscopic examination findings
    a. Patency of the external canal; presence of cerumen or foreign bodies, edema, or inflammation
    b. Condition of the tympanic membrane: intact, scars, edema, fluid, inflammation
3. Abnormal Rinne test findings
    a. Air conduction greater than bone conduction in conductive hearing loss
    b. Bone conduction greater than air conduction in sensorineural hearing loss
4. Abnormal Weber test findings
    a. Lateralization to the affected ear in conductive hearing loss
    b. Lateralization to the unaffected ear in sensorineural hearing loss
5. Psychosocial issues
    a. Social isolation
    b. Depression, fear, and despair
- Diagnostic studies include audiometry to determine type and extent of hearing loss and imaging to determine possible causes.

Planning and Implementation
DIFFICULTY HEARING
- Related to obstruction, infection, damage to the middle ear, or damage to the auditory nerve
  Nonsurgical Management
- Early detection helps correct the problem causing the hearing loss.
- Drug therapy is used to correct an underlying pathologic change or to reduce side effects of problems occurring with hearing loss:
  1. Antibiotic therapy
  2. Analgesics
  3. Antiemetics
  4. Antivertiginous drugs
- Hearing-assistive devices:
  1. Telephone amplifiers
  2. Therapy dogs
  3. Portable audio amplifiers
  4. Hearing aids
    a. Teach the patient to start using the hearing aid slowly, at first wearing it only at home and only during part of the day.
    b. Remind him or her that background noise will be amplified along with voices.

H

   c. Teach him or her to care for the hearing aid by:
     (1) Keeping the hearing aid dry
     (2) Cleaning the ear mold with mild soap and water while avoiding excessive wetting
     (3) Cleaning debris from the hole in the middle of the part that goes into the ear with a toothpick or a pipe cleaner
     (4) Turning off the hearing aid and removing the battery when not in use
     (5) Checking and replacing the battery often
     (6) Keeping extra batteries on hand
     (7) Keeping the hearing aid in a safe place
     (8) Avoiding dropping the hearing aid or exposing it to temperature extremes
     (9) Adjusting the volume to the lowest setting that allows hearing to prevent feedback squeaking
    (10) Avoiding using hair spray, cosmetics, oils, or other hair and face products that may come into contact with the receiver
 5. Cochlear implantation

Surgical Management

- The type of operative procedure selected depends on the cause of the hearing loss.
  1. *Tympanoplasty reconstruction* of the middle ear can improve conductive hearing loss. The procedures vary from simple reconstruction of the eardrum (myringoplasty or type I tympanoplasty) to replacement of the ossicles within the middle ear (type II tympanoplasty).
  2. *Stapedectomy* is the removal of the head and neck of the stapes and, less often, the footplate. After removal of the bone, a small hole is drilled or made with a laser in the footplate, and a prosthesis in the shape of a piston is connected between the incus and the footplate.
  3. Placement of a totally implanted device to treat bilateral moderate to severe sensorineural hearing loss
- Provide preoperative care, including:
  1. Adhering to routine preoperative instructions, as described in Part One
  2. Using systemic antibiotics
  3. Irrigating the ear with a solution of equal parts of vinegar and sterile water to restore normal ear pH
  4. Assuring the patient that hearing loss immediately after surgery is normal because of canal packing

    5. Reinforcing the information provided by the surgeon
- Provide postoperative care, including:
  1. Adhering to routine postoperative care, as described in Part One
  2. Keeping the dressing clean and dry, using sterile technique for changes
  3. Keeping the patient flat, with the head turned to the side and the operative ear facing up for at least 12 hours after surgery
  4. Using communication techniques for the hearing-impaired
  5. Giving prescribed antibiotics to prevent infection
  6. Giving prescribed analgesics
  7. Giving prescribed antivertiginous drugs
  8. Assessing for and reporting complications (stapedectomy; implanted devices)
     a. Asymmetric appearance or drooping of features on the affected side of the face
     b. Changes in facial perception of touch and in taste, as reported by patient
  9. Assisting the patient with ambulating
  10. Reminding the patient to move his or her head slowly when changing position to avoid vertigo
  11. Teaching the patient about care and activity restrictions:
      a. Not using small objects, such as cotton-tipped applicators, matches, toothpicks, or hairpins, to clean the external ear canal
      b. Washing the external ear and canal daily in the shower or while washing the hair
      c. Blowing the nose gently
      d. Not occluding one nostril while blowing the nose
      e. Sneezing with the mouth open
      f. Wearing sound protection around loud or continuous noises
      g. Avoiding activities with high risk for head or ear trauma, such as wrestling, boxing, motorcycle riding, and skateboarding; wearing head and ear protection when engaging in these activities
      h. Keeping the volume on head receivers at the lowest setting that allows hearing
      i. Frequently cleaning objects that come into contact with the ear (e.g., headphones, telephone receivers)
      j. Avoiding environmental conditions with rapid changes in air pressure

POTENTIAL FOR REDUCED COMMUNICATION
- Related to difficulty hearing
- Use best practices for communicating with a hearing-impaired patient, including:
    1. Positioning yourself directly in front of the patient
    2. Making sure that the room is well lighted
    3. Getting the patient's attention before you begin to speak
    4. Moving closer to the better hearing ear
    5. Speaking clearly and slowly
    6. Keeping hands and other objects away from your mouth when talking to the patient
    7. Attempting to have conversations in a quiet room with minimal distractions
    8. Having the patient repeat your statements rather than just indicating assent
    9. Rephrasing sentences and repeating information to aid in understanding
    10. Using appropriate hand motions
    11. Writing messages on paper if the patient is able to read

▊ NURSING SAFETY PRIORITY: Action Alert

Do not shout to the patient, because the sound may be projected at a higher frequency, making him or her less able to understand.

- Having the patient use hearing-assistive devices described earlier
- Encouraging the patient to use lip-reading
- Having the patient and family learn a sign language, such as American Sign Language (ASL)
- Managing anxiety and promoting social interaction by:
    1. Enhancing communication, as described earlier
    2. Working with the patient to identify his or her most satisfying activities and social interactions and determine the amount of effort necessary to continue them
    3. Suggesting the use of closed captioning for television programming

Community-Based Care
- Teach patients who have persistent vertigo and their families to determine the best ways to maintain adequate self-care abilities, maintain a safe environment, decide about assistance needs, and provide needed care.
- Give patients written instructions about how to take drugs and when to return for follow-up care.
- Teach patients how to instill eardrops and irrigate the ears, and obtain a return demonstration.

- Refer patients and families to a home care agency if needed for help with meal preparation, cleaning, and personal hygiene.
- Support patients by listening to their concerns and giving additional information when needed.
- Provide information about public and private agencies that offer hearing evaluations and that supply information and counseling for patients with hearing disorders.

HEART FAILURE

OVERVIEW

- Heart failure (HF), sometimes called *pump failure*, is the inadequacy of the heart to pump blood throughout the body.
- HF causes insufficient perfusion of body tissue with vital nutrients and oxygen.
- Basic cardiac physiologic mechanisms such as stroke volume, heart rate, cardiac output, and contractility are altered in HF.
- The American College of Cardiology (ACC) and American Heart Association (AHA) have evidence-based guidelines for staging and managing HF as a chronic progressive disease. These guidelines are combined with the New York Heart Association (NYHA) functional classification system that is used to describe symptoms exhibited by the patient to aid in determining response to interventions and prognostication.
- The major types of HF are:
  1. *Left HF,* characterized by decreased tissue perfusion from poor cardiac output and pulmonary congestion from increased pressure in the pulmonary vessels, and further subdivided into systolic HF and diastolic HF:
     a. *Systolic HF* (systolic ventricular dysfunction, sometimes still referred to as *congestive heart failure*):
        (1) Systolic failure results when the heart is unable to contract forcefully enough during systole to eject adequate amounts of blood into the circulation.
        (2) Preload increases with decreased contractility, and afterload increases as a result of increased peripheral resistance.
        (3) The ejection fraction drops from a normal of 50% to 70% to below 40%.
        (4) Tissue perfusion diminishes and pulmonary edema commonly occur.
     b. *Diastolic HF* (diastolic ventricular function):
        (1) Diastolic failure occurs when the left ventricle is unable to relax adequately during diastole, which prevents the

H

ventricle from filling with sufficient blood to ensure an adequate cardiac output.

(2) The ejection fraction may remain near normal.

2. *Right HF* occurs when the right ventricle is unable to empty completely. Right HF in the absence of left HF is most often the result of pulmonary problems. Increased volume and pressure develop in the systemic veins, and systemic venous congestion develops with peripheral edema.

3. *High-output failure* can occur when cardiac output remains normal or above normal and is caused by increased metabolic needs or hyperkinetic conditions such as septicemia, anemia, and hyperthyroidism.

- When cardiac output is insufficient to meet the demands of the body, compensatory mechanisms operate to improve cardiac output. Although these mechanisms may initially increase cardiac output, they eventually have a damaging effect on pump function. Compensatory mechanisms contribute to increased myocardial oxygen consumption, leading to worsening signs and symptoms of HF. Compensatory mechanisms include:

  1. Sympathetic nervous system stimulation: Increased sympathetic nervous system response causes increased heart rate, increased force of contraction, and arterial vasoconstriction that increases afterload.

  2. Renin-angiotensin aldosterone system (RAAS) activation: Renin, angiotensin, and aldosterone work together to cause sodium and water retention when blood flow to the kidney decreases during HF. Angiotensin also increases arterial constriction or afterload.

  3. Other neurohumoral responses, such as the synthesis and release of B-type natriuretic peptide from the overstretched atrium: This hormone acts on kidneys to promote diuresis and decrease preload. Growth factors are also released.

  4. Myocardial hypertrophy: Growth of existing myocardial cells in size (not numbers of cells) provides more muscle mass.

Considerations for Older Adults

- HF is caused by systemic hypertension in most cases; the next most common reason is myocardial infarctions.
- Long-term NSAIDs and thiazolidinediones used for patients with diabetes can cause fluid and sodium retention, contributing to heart failure.
- Prevalence of HF increases with age.

PATIENT-CENTERED COLLABORATIVE CARE
Assessment
- Assessment findings include:
  1. History of hypertension, acute coronary syndrome, heart valve disease, other myocardial disease such as myocarditis
  2. Dyspnea, orthopnea, breathlessness
  3. Decreased oxygen saturation (SpO_2) or PaO_2
  4. Increased respiratory rate and work of breathing including use of accessory muscles
  5. Crackles or rhonchi on auscultation
  6. Cough
  7. Frothy sputum
  8. Dysrhythmias, especially tachycardia
  9. Weak, thready peripheral pulses
  10. Weight gain, with more than 1 pound per day or 3 pounds per week indicating potential fluid retention (e.g., edema) and a need for consultation with a physician or advanced practice nurse
  11. Decreased mentation, restlessness, or anxiety
  12. Increased vascular or interstitial fluid on chest radiograph
  13. S_3 or S_4 heart sounds
  14. Cardiomegaly by palpation, electrocardiograph (ECG), or chest radiograph
  15. Increased serum B-type natriuretic peptide (BNP)
  16. Peripheral edema
  17. Jugular venous distention
  18. Enlarged liver and spleen, especially with right-sided HF
  19. Reduced kidney function including oliguria and increased blood urea nitrogen (BUN) and serum creatinine
  20. Anxiety and depression or other markers of psychological distress

Interventions
NONSURGICAL MANAGEMENT
Impaired Gas Exchange
- Related to ventilation/perfusion imbalance
- Interventions include:
  1. Monitoring for improving or worsening pulmonary edema by assessing respiratory rate, rhythm, and character every 1 to 4 hours and auscultating breath sounds
  2. Titrating the amount of supplemental oxygen delivered to maintain oxygen saturation at 92% or greater
  3. Placing the patient experiencing respiratory difficulty in a high Fowler's position with pillows under each arm to maximize chest expansion and improve oxygenation

   4. Encouraging the patient to deep-breathe and reposition himself or herself every 2 hours while awake and in bed

Decreased Cardiac Output

- Related to altered contractility, preload, and afterload
- Drug therapy to improve myocardial function:
   1. Angiotensin-converting enzyme (ACE) inhibitors are used to prevent conversion of angiotensin I to angiotensin II, resulting in reduction of arterial constriction. ACE inhibitors also block aldosterone, which prevents sodium and water retention, decreasing fluid overload. Monitor blood pressure, especially orthostatic pressure in older adults. Monitor serum potassium level for hyperkalemia, serum creatinine level for kidney dysfunction, and the patient for development of a cough. Monitor blood pressure to determine the patient's response to effective doses.
   2. Beta blockers reduce the heart rate and interfere with the sympathetic nervous system compensatory mechanisms that promote adverse myocyte remodeling. Monitor for heart rates below 60 beats/min that cause the patient to exhibit symptomatic bradycardia.
   3. Diuretics reduce intravascular volume, especially during an episode of exacerbation of HF. Monitor intake, output, and daily weights to determine fluid balance.
   4. Oxygen therapy can maintain or increase SpO_2 above 92%.
   5. Digoxin (Lanoxin) increases contractility, reduces the heart rate, slows conduction through the arteriovenous node, and inhibits sympathetic activity while enhancing parasympathetic activity. Older patients, particularly those who are hypokalemic, are susceptible to digoxin toxicity.

▮NURSING SAFETY PRIORITY: Drug Alert

Heart failure is managed with polypharmacy; typically, three or more drugs are used. The potential for drug interactions increases when three or more drugs are used regularly. Advise your patient and assist him or her in identifying potential drug interactions, including the use of NSAIDs, which can further cause significant acute kidney injury in the presence of low cardiac output.

- Diet therapy to reduce sodium and promote ideal body weight:
   1. Collaborate with the dietitian and patient to select foods that meet a heart-healthy, sodium-restricted diet and to understand the importance of eliminating table salt and salt used in cooking. Increase the patient's intake of potassium-rich foods if using a loop or thiazide diuretic.

- Fluid restriction and monitoring:
  1. Limit the patients in AHA class 3 or 4 to 2 L/day of fluids, including IV fluids; other HF patients may be restricted to 2.5 to 3 L/day. Weigh the patient every morning before breakfast using the same scale; this is the most reliable indicator of fluid gain or loss (1 kg of weight gain or loss equals 1 L of fluid retained or lost).
  2. Monitor and record intake and output and report or intervene when intake exceeds output by more than 500 mL.
  3. Monitor for and prevent potassium deficiency from diuretic therapy. If the patient's potassium level is below 4 mEq/L, a potassium supplement may be prescribed.
  4. Recognize that patients with kidney problems may develop hyperkalemia, especially with the use of potassium supplements, ACE inhibitors, or potassium-sparing diuretics. Kidney problems are indicated by a creatinine level higher than 1.8 mg/dL.
- Other options to treat HF:
  1. Continuous positive airway pressure (CPAP) improves sleep apnea (oxygen desaturation) and supports cardiac output and ejection fraction.
  2. Cardiac resynchronization therapy (CRT) uses a permanent pacemaker alone or in combination with an implantable cardioverter-defibrillator to provide biventricular pacing.
  3. Investigative stem cell and gene therapy replaces damaged myocytes or genes by a series of injections into the left ventricle.

Fatigue and Weakness Related to Hypoxia

- The most common symptom reported by patients with HF is fatigue. The purpose of collaborative care is to regulate energy, prevent fatigue, and optimize function:
  1. Provide periods of uninterrupted rest.
  2. Assess the patient's response to increased activity. Check for changes in blood pressure, pulse, and oxygen saturation before and after an episode of new or increased activity.

■ NURSING SAFETY PRIORITY: Action Alert

An increase in the heart rate of more than 20 beats/min, a change (increase or decrease) in systolic blood pressure of more than 20 mm Hg, or a decrease in the SpO_2 of more than 5% indicates activity intolerance. The physician should be informed about these findings in case it is necessary to alter drug therapy or initiate a physical therapy consultation to promote rehabilitation.

SURGICAL MANAGEMENT
- Heart transplantation is the ultimate choice for end-stage HF.
- Procedures to improve cardiac output in patients who are not candidates for heart transplant or are awaiting transplantation include:
  1. Left ventricular assist device (LVAD)
  2. Right ventricular assist device (RVAD)
- Surgical therapies to reshape the left ventricle in patients with HF include:
  1. Partial left ventriculectomy
  2. Endoventricular circular patch
  3. Acorn cardiac support device
  4. Myosplint cardiac support device perioperatively
- Care for the HF patient who is receiving a surgical intervention to improve pump failure is similar to patients receiving coronary revascularization or other open heart surgery. Specific monitoring and interventions include:
  1. Assessing the patient with HF for acute pulmonary edema. Clinical manifestations include extreme anxiety; tachycardia; air hunger; moist cough productive of frothy, blood-tinged sputum; cold, clammy, cyanotic skin; crackles in lung bases; disorientation; and confusion.
  2. Administering rapid-acting diuretics, as prescribed
  3. Providing oxygen and maintaining the patient in a high Fowler's position
  4. Administering morphine sulfate intravenously to reduce venous return (preload), decrease anxiety, and reduce the work of breathing
  5. Administering other drugs such as bronchodilators and vasodilators
  6. Monitoring vital signs closely including pulse oximetry
  7. Monitoring intake and output; weighing daily

Community-Based Care
- Collaborate with the case manager or social worker to assess the patient's needs for health care resources (e.g., home care nurse) and social support (family and friends to help with care if needed), and facilitate appropriate placement.
- Discharge preparation includes:
  1. Encouraging the patient to stay as active as possible and developing a regular exercise program; investigating the possibility of a rehabilitation program referral
     a. If the patient experiences chest pain or pronounced dyspnea while exercising or experiences excessive fatigue, he or she is probably advancing the activity too quickly and should be returned to the previous level for 24 to 48 hours.

2. Instructing the patient to watch for and report to the physician
   a. Weight gain of more than 3 pounds in 1 week or 1 to 2 pounds overnight
   b. Decrease in exercise tolerance lasting 2 to 3 days
   c. Cold symptoms (cough) lasting more than 3 to 5 days
   d. Frequent urination at night
   e. Development of dyspnea or angina at rest, or worsening angina
   f. Increased swelling in the feet, ankles, and hands
3. Providing oral and written instructions concerning drugs
4. Teaching the patient and caregiver how to take and record the pulse rate and blood pressure to help monitor response to drug and exercise regimens
5. Instructing the patient to weigh himself or herself each day in the morning
6. Reviewing the signs and symptoms of hypokalemia for patients on diuretics and providing information on foods high in potassium
7. Recommending that the patient restrict dietary sodium, providing written instructions on low-salt diets, and identifying food flavorings to use as a substitute for salt, such as lemon, garlic, and herbs
8. Discussing the importance of advance directives with the patient or family. If resuscitation is desired, the family should know how to activate the Emergency Medical System and how to provide cardiopulmonary resuscitation (CPR) until an ambulance arrives. If CPR is not desired, the patient and family should be given resources on what to do and how to respond.
9. Referring the patient to the AHA for information and support groups

█ NURSING SAFETY PRIORITY: Critical Rescue

A weight gain of 1 kg (2.2 pounds) is equivalent to an additional liter of fluid in the vascular and tissue compartments. Intravascular fluid overload can decrease myocardial recoil, promoting permanent adverse changes in the heart.

HEMOPHILIA

OVERVIEW

- Hemophilia is two different hereditary bleeding disorders resulting from clotting factor deficiencies, which impair the formation of stable fibrin clots and lead to excessive bleeding.

1. *Hemophilia A (classic hemophilia)* is a deficiency of factor VIII and accounts for 80% of cases of hemophilia.
2. *Hemophilia B (Christmas disease)* is a deficiency of factor IX and accounts for 20% of cases.

Genetic/Genomic Considerations

- Hemophilia is an X-linked recessive trait. Women who are carriers (able to pass on the gene without actually having the disorder) have a 50% chance of passing the hemophilia gene to their daughters (who then are carriers) and to their sons (who then have hemophilia). Affected men will pass the gene onto daughters, all of whom will be carriers, but not to their sons.
- About 30% of hemophilia arises from a new gene mutation and has no family history.

- Abnormal bleeding occurs in response to any trauma because of a deficiency of the specific clotting factor. Bleeding may be mild, moderate, or severe, depending on the degree of factor deficiency.

PATIENT-CENTERED COLLABORATIVE CARE

- Assess for and document:
  1. Excessive bleeding from minor cuts, bruises, or abrasions
  2. Joint and muscle hemorrhages that lead to disabling long-term problems
  3. A tendency to bruise easily or experience prolonged nosebleeds
  4. Prolonged and potentially fatal hemorrhage after surgery
  5. Prolonged partial thromboplastin time (PTT), a normal bleeding time, and a normal prothrombin time (PT)
- The bleeding problems of hemophilia A are managed by regularly scheduled infusions of factor VIII (cryoprecipitate) or by intermittent infusions, as needed.
- Similarly, hemophilia B is managed with infusions of factor IX

HEMORRHOIDS

OVERVIEW

- Hemorrhoids are unnaturally swollen or distended veins in the anorectal region that are common and not significant unless they cause pain or bleeding.

- Increased intra-abdominal pressure causes elevated systemic and portal venous pressure, which is transmitted to the anorectal veins.
- Internal hemorrhoids cannot be seen on inspection of the perianal area and lie above the anal sphincter.
- External hemorrhoids can be seen on inspection and lie below the anal sphincter.
- Prolapsed hemorrhoids can become thrombosed or inflamed, or they can bleed.
- Common causes of repeated increased abdominal pressure are straining at stool, pregnancy, and portal hypertension.

PATIENT-CENTERED COLLABORATIVE CARE
Assessment
- Assessment findings include:
  1. Bleeding, which is characteristically bright red and found on toilet tissue or outside the stool
  2. Pain associated with thrombosis
  3. Itching
  4. Mucous discharge
- Diagnosis is made by inspection, digital examination, and proctoscopy, if needed.

Interventions
Nonsurgical Management
- Conservative management focuses on reducing symptoms and includes:
  1. Application of cold packs to the anorectal area followed by tepid sitz baths
  2. Witch hazel soaks and topical anesthetics such as lidocaine (Xylocaine)
  3. OTC remedies such as dibucaine (Nupercainal) ointment used temporarily, because prolonged use can mask worsening symptoms and delay diagnosis of a severe disorder
  4. High-fiber diet and fluids to promote regular bowel movements without straining
  5. Stool softeners
  6. Teaching the patient to cleanse the anal area with moistened cleaning tissues and to gently dab the area rather than wipe

Surgical Management
- Ultrasound, sclerotherapy, circular stapling, or hemorrhoidectomy may be indicated for recurring symptoms.
- Postoperative care
  1. Monitor for bleeding and pain.
  2. Apply moist heat (e.g., sitz baths) three to four times each day after the first 12 hours postoperatively.

H

3. Administer stool softeners such as docusate sodium (Colace).
4. Administer opioid analgesia postoperatively and before the first defecation.

HEMOTHORAX

- Hemothorax is blood loss into the thoracic cavity and is a common result of blunt chest trauma or penetrating injuries.
  1. A simple hemothorax is a blood loss of less than 1500 mL.
  2. A massive hemothorax is a blood loss of more than 1500 mL, usually from heart, great vessels, or intercostals arteries.
- Bleeding can occur with rib and sternal fractures causing lung contusions and lacerations in addition to the hemothorax.
- Physical assessment findings depend on the size of the hemothorax.
  1. A small hemothorax may cause no symptoms.
  2. Symptoms of a hemothorax may include:
     a. Respiratory distress
     b. Reduced breath sounds
     c. Blood in the pleural space (seen on a chest x-ray and confirmed by diagnostic thoracentesis)
- Interventions, aimed at removing the blood in the pleural space to normalize pulmonary function and to prevent infection, include front and back chest tube insertion.
- A hemothorax may require an open thoracotomy to repair torn vessels and to evacuate the chest cavity.
- Nursing interventions include:
  1. Monitoring vital signs and reporting when signs of hypoperfusion or hypotension occur
  2. Carefully monitoring chest tube drainage for excessive blood loss
  3. Measuring intake and output
  4. Assessing the patient's response to the chest tubes
  5. Infusing IV fluids and blood as prescribed
- The blood lost through chest drainage can be autotransfused back into the patient if needed.

HEPATITIS

OVERVIEW

- Hepatitis is the widespread inflammation of liver cells, resulting in enlargement of the liver and congestion with inflammatory cells.
- Viral hepatitis is the most prevalent type and is caused by one of five common viruses. Many patients have multiple infections,

especially the combination of HBV with either HCV, HDV, or HIV infection.

1. Hepatitis A virus (HAV):
   a. HAV is an RNA virus of the enterovirus family. It is a hardy virus and survives on human hands. HAV is spread by the fecal-oral route, consuming contaminated food, or by person-to-person contact (e.g., oral-anal sexual activity). Unsanitary water, shellfish caught in contaminated water, and food contaminated by food handlers infected with the HAV are all potential sources of infection.
   b. It is characterized by a mild course and often goes unrecognized. HAV is the most common type of viral hepatitis.
   c. The incubation period is usually 15 to 50 days.
2. Hepatitis B virus (HBV):
   a. HBV is a double-shelled particle containing DNA composed of a core antigen (HBcAg), a surface antigen (HBsAg), and another antigen found within the core (HBeAg) that circulates in the blood.
   b. HBV is transmitted through broken skin or mucous membranes by infected blood and serous fluids. Lower concentrations of HBV are also found in semen, vaginal fluid, and saliva.
   c. HBV is spread by sexual contact, shared needles, accidental needle sticks or injuries from sharp instruments, blood transfusion, hemodialysis, acupuncture, tattooing, ear or body piercing, mother-fetal route, and close person-to-person contact by open cuts and sores.
   d. The clinical course is varied, with an insidious onset and mild symptoms (anorexia, nausea, vomiting, fever, fatigue, dark urine with light stool).
   e. The incubation period is generally between 25 and 180 days.
3. Hepatitis C virus (HCV):
   a. The causative virus is an enveloped, single-strand RNA virus that is transmitted by exposure of the skin and mucous membrane to infected blood or serum.
   b. HCV is spread by contaminated items such as illicit IV drug needles, blood and blood products and transplanted organs received before 1992, needle stick injury with HCV-contaminated blood, tattoo, and intranasal cocaine use.
   c. It is not transmitted by casual contact or intimate household contacts. However, those infected should not share razors, toothbrushes, or pierced earrings, because there may be microscopic blood on these items.

H

    d. The incubation period is 21 to 140 days, with an average incubation period of 7 weeks.

    e. Chronic liver disease occurs in 85% of those infected. HCV cirrhosis is the leading indicator for liver transplantation.

4. Hepatitis D (delta hepatitis or HDV):

    a. HDV is a defective RNA virus that needs the helper function of HBV for viral replication. HDV co-infects with HBV.

    b. Incubation period is 14 to 56 days.

    c. HDV is transmitted primarily by parenteral routes.

5. Hepatitis E virus (HEV):

    a. HEV was originally identified by its association with epidemics of hepatitis in the Indian subcontinent and has since been found in epidemics in Asia, Africa, Mexico, the Middle East, and Central and South America.

    b. In the United States and Canada, HEV has occurred in people who have visited these endemic areas.

    c. HEV is transmitted by the oral-fecal route and most commonly causes infection from contaminated food or water.

    d. The incubation period is 15 to 64 days.

- Toxic and drug-induced forms of hepatitis result from exposure to hepatotoxins such as industrial toxins, alcohol, or drugs. Treatment is supportive.

- Hepatitis may occur as a secondary infection during the course of other viral infections, such as cytomegalovirus, Epstein-Barr virus, herpes simplex virus, and varicella-zoster virus.

- Fulminant hepatitis is a failure of the liver cells to regenerate, with progression of the necrotic process that is often fatal.

- Liver inflammation persisting longer than 6 months is considered *chronic hepatitis.*

PATIENT-CENTERED COLLABORATIVE CARE
Assessment

- Record patient information:
  1. Known exposure to persons with hepatitis infection
  2. Blood transfusions or organ transplantation
  3. History of hemodialysis
  4. Sexual preferences
  5. Injectable drug use
  6. Recent ear or body piercing
  7. Recent tattooing
  8. Living accommodations, including crowded facilities
  9. Health care employment history

10. Recent travel to foreign countries
11. Recent ingestion of shellfish
12. HIV infection
13. History of alcohol abuse
- Assessment findings for viral hepatitis include:
   1. Abdominal pain
   2. Changes in skin or sclera (icterus)
   3. Arthralgia (joint pain) or myalgia (muscle pain)
   4. Diarrhea or constipation; clay-colored stools
   5. Dark or amber-colored urine
   6. Fever
   7. Lethargy
   8. Malaise
   9. Nausea and vomiting
   10. Pruritus (itching)
   11. Liver tenderness in the right upper quadrant
   12. Elevated serum liver enzymes
   13. Elevated total bilirubin (serum and urine)
   14. Serologic markers for hepatitis A, B, C, or D
- The clinical manifestations of toxic and drug-induced hepatitis depend on the causative agent.
- Patients may be angry about being sick and being fatigued; may feel guilty about having exposed others to the disease; may be embarrassed by the isolation and hygiene precautions that are necessary; and may be worried about the loss of wages, cost of hospitalization, and general financial issues.
- Family members may be afraid of contracting the disease and therefore distance themselves from the patient. Counsel about the value of hepatitis vaccination.

Planning and Implementation
- Promote rest.
   1. Maintain physical rest alternating with periods of activity to promote liver cell regeneration by reducing the liver's metabolic needs.
   2. Individualize the patient's plan of care and change it to reflect the severity of symptoms, fatigue, and results of liver function tests and enzyme determinations.
   3. Promote emotional and psychological rest.
- Provide diet therapy. A special diet is not needed, but diet should be high in carbohydrates and calories with moderate amounts of fat and protein.
   1. Determine food preferences.
   2. Provide small, frequent meals.

H

   3. Provide high-calorie snacks as needed.
- Drug therapy includes:
   1. Supplemental vitamins
   2. Antiemetics, such as trimethobenzamide (Tigan, Tegamide) or dimenhydrinate (Dramamine, Travamine ♣) to relieve nausea
   3. Antiviral drugs and immunomodulators such as tenofovir or entecavir (Baraclude) (as first-line therapy for patients who develop cirrhosis but no co-infection); interferon (as a first-line drug for patients who do *not* have cirrhosis); adefovir dipivoxil (Hepsera) (as second-line therapy); lamivudine (Epivir); and telbivudine (Tyzeka). Ribavirin is used for HCV.
- Liver transplantation may be performed for patients with end-stage liver disease from chronic hepatitis.

Community-Based Care
- Provide health teaching, including:
   1. Give patients information about modes of viral transmission.
   2. Maintain adequate sanitation and personal hygiene. Wash your hands before eating and after using the toilet.
   3. If traveling in underdeveloped or nonindustrialized countries, drink only bottled water. Avoid food washed or prepared with tap water, such as raw vegetables, fruits, and soups. Avoid ice.
   4. Use adequate sanitation practices to prevent the spread of the disease among family members. Do not share bed linens, towels, eating utensils, or drinking glasses.
   5. Do not share needles for injection, body piercing, or tattooing.
   6. Do not share razors, nail clippers, toothbrushes, or Waterpiks.
   7. Use a condom during sexual intercourse, or abstain from this activity.
   8. Cover cuts or sores with bandages.
   9. If ever infected with hepatitis, never donate blood, body organs, or other body tissue.

HERNIA

OVERVIEW
- A hernia is a weakness in the abdominal muscle wall through which a segment of bowel or other abdominal structure protrudes. Increased intra-abdominal pressure can contribute to hernia formation.

- Hernias are labeled by anatomic location, combined with the severity of protrusion:
  1. *Indirect inguinal hernia,* a sac formed from the peritoneum that contains a portion of the intestine or omentum; in men, indirect hernias can become large and descend into the scrotum
  2. *Direct inguinal hernia,* which passes through a weak point in the abdominal wall
  3. *Femoral hernia,* which occurs through the femoral ring as a plug of fat in the femoral canal that enlarges and pulls the peritoneum and the bladder into the sac
  4. *Umbilical hernia,* which is congenital (infancy) or acquired as a result of increased intra-abdominal pressure, most often in obese persons
  5. *Incisional (ventral) hernia,* which occurs at the site of a previous surgical incision as a result of inadequate healing, postoperative wound infection, inadequate nutrition, or obesity
  6. A *reducible hernia* allows the contents of the hernial sac to be reduced or placed back into the abdominal cavity.
  7. An *irreducible,* or *incarcerated, hernia* cannot be reduced or placed back into the abdominal cavity. It requires immediate surgical evaluation.
  8. A *strangulated hernia* results when the blood supply to the herniated segment of the bowel is cut off by pressure from the hernial ring, causing ischemia and obstruction of the bowel loop; this can lead to bowel necrosis and perforation, which are surgical emergencies.

PATIENT-CENTERED COLLABORATIVE CARE
Assessment
- Assess for a hernia when the patient is lying down and again when the patient is standing. If a hernia is reducible, it may disappear when the patient is lying flat.
- Listen for bowel sounds (absence may indicate GI obstruction).
Interventions
  Nonsurgical Management
- A truss (a pad with firm support) may be used for patients who are poor surgical risks.
  Surgical Management
- Herniorrhaphy, the surgical treatment of choice, involves replacing the contents of the hernial sac into the abdominal cavity and closing the opening.
- Hernioplasty reinforces the weakened muscular wall with a mesh patch.

- Postoperative instructions:
  1. Avoid coughing but encourage deep breathing.
  2. Turn frequently and promote early, progressive mobility.
  3. For inguinal hernia repair, wear a scrotal support and apply an ice bag to the scrotum to prevent swelling. Elevate the scrotum with a soft pillow when in bed.
  4. Avoid bladder and bowel distention:
     a. Using techniques to stimulate voiding, such as assisting a man to stand
     b. Catheterizing the patient every 6 to 8 hours if he or she is unable to void
     c. Avoiding constipation and teaching the patient to avoid straining with stool during healing

Community-Based Care
- Teach the patient:
  1. How to care for incision if surgery corrects muscle defect
  2. To limit activity, including avoiding lifting and straining, for several weeks after surgery
  3. To report symptoms such as fever and chills, wound drainage, redness or separation of the incision, and increasing incisional pain to the health care provider

HERNIA, HIATAL

OVERVIEW
- Hiatal hernias, also called *diaphragmatic hernias,* involve the protrusion of the stomach through the esophageal hiatus of the diaphragm into the thorax.
- There are two major types of hiatal hernias:
  1. *Sliding hernia,* which occurs when esophagogastric junction and a portion of the fundus of the stomach slide upward through the esophageal hiatus into the thorax, with the hernia moving freely and sliding into and out of the thorax with changes in position or increases in intra-abdominal pressure
  2. *Paraesophageal,* or *rolling, hernia,* which occurs when the gastroesophageal junction stays below the diaphragm but the fundus and portions of the greater curvature of the stomach roll through the esophageal hiatus and into the thorax beside the esophagus; risk for volvulus, obstruction, and strangulation are high

PATIENT-CENTERED COLLABORATIVE CARE
Assessment
- Assessment findings include:
  1. Symptoms of gastroesophageal reflux (GERD) include heartburn, chest or esophageal pain, belching.

2. Symptoms of rolling hernia include a feeling of fullness after eating or a feeling of breathlessness or suffocation.
3. Increased symptoms occur when the patient is in a recumbent position.
4. Confirmation via a barium swallow study with fluoroscopy is the most specific diagnostic test.

Interventions

Nonsurgical Management

- Drug therapy includes the use of proton pump inhibitors, antacids, and histamine receptor antagonists to control esophageal reflux and its symptoms.
- Teach the patient to avoid fatty foods, coffee, tea, cola, chocolate, alcohol, spicy foods, and acidic foods such as orange juice.
- Encourage the patient to eat small-volume meals and consume liquids between meals to avoid abdominal distention.
- Encourage weight reduction, because obesity increases intra-abdominal pressure.
- Elevate the head of the bed 6 or more inches.
- Instruct the patient to avoid lying down for several hours after eating, straining or excessively vigorous exercise, and wearing tight or constrictive clothing.

Surgical Management

- Elective surgery is indicated when the risk of complications such as aspiration are high and damage from chronic reflux is severe.
- Provide routine preoperative care.
- Inform the patient that he or she will have a nasogastric (NG) tube after surgery.
- Determine whether the patient will have a chest tube after surgery and include this information in preoperative teaching.
- Surgical approaches for sliding hernias involve reinforcement of the lower esophageal sphincter (LES) to restore sphincter competence and prevent reflux through some degree of fundoplication, or the wrapping of a portion of the stomach fundus around the distal esophagus to anchor it and reinforce the LES.
- Provide postoperative care similar to that for any patient with esophageal surgery with a focus on:
    1. Assessing for complications of surgery, such as temporary dysphagia after oral feeding begins, gas bloat syndrome, atelectasis or pneumonia, and obstruction of the NG tube
    2. Preventing aspiration and respiratory complications with positioning, early ambulation, and use of incentive spirometry while providing adequate pain relief

3. Elevating the head of the bed at least 30 degrees
4. Teaching the patient to support the incisional area during coughing and deep breathing
5. Ensuring correct placement and patency of the NG tube
6. Teaching the patient to avoid drinking carbonated beverages, eating gas-producing foods (especially high-fat foods), chewing gum, and drinking with a straw

Community-Based Care

- Advise the patient:
  1. To avoid lifting and restrict stair climbing for 2 to 6 weeks after surgical repair
  2. To inspect the surgical wound daily and report the incidence of swelling, redness, tenderness, or discharge to the physician
  3. About the importance of reporting signs of infection or fever to the physician
  4. To avoid prolonged coughing episodes to prevent dehiscence of the fundoplication
  5. To stop smoking
  6. About diet modifications, including weight loss goals if needed, eating small portions, avoiding irritating foods and liquids, and reporting recurrence of reflux symptoms to the physician
  7. To avoid straining and prevent constipation; stool softeners or bulk laxatives may be needed.

HERPES, GENITAL

OVERVIEW

- Genital herpes (GH) is an acute, recurring, incurable viral disease.
- The two types of herpes simplex virus (HSV) are diagnosed and treated with the same interventions. The two types are:
  1. Type 1 (HSV-1), which causes most nongenital lesions such as cold sores and about one third of genital herpes infections
  2. Type 2 (HSV-2), which causes most of the genital lesions

◆ NURSING SAFETY PRIORITY: Action Alert

Either type of virus can produce oral or genital lesions through oral-genital contact with an infected person.

- The incubation period is 2 to 20 days, with the average period being 1 week, and many people do not have symptoms during this time.

- Recurrences are not caused by re-infection but by reactivation of dormant virus along the sacral ganglia. Additional episodes are usually less severe and of shorter duration than the primary infection. *However, there is viral shedding and the patient is infectious with each outbreak of vesicles.*
- Long-term complications of GH include the risk of neonatal transmission and an increased risk for acquiring HIV infection.

PATIENT-CENTERED COLLABORATIVE CARE
Assessment
- Obtain patient information about:
  1. The sensation of itching or tingling felt in the skin 1 to 2 days before the outbreak
  2. Whether he or she has had headaches or general malaise
  3. Presence of painful urination or urinary retention
  4. Factors that can trigger virus re-activation such as stress, fever, sunburn, poor nutrition, menses, and sexual activity
- Assess for and document:
  1. The presence of *vesicles* (blisters) in a typical cluster on the penis, scrotum, vulva, vagina, cervix, or perianal region
  2. The presence of painful erosions
  3. Swelling of inguinal lymph nodes
- Diagnostic tests for GH include:
  1. Viral culture
  2. Polymerase chain reaction (PCR) assay of the lesions from blister fluid
  3. Serology testing to identify the HSV type, including type specific rapid assays

Interventions
- Antiviral medications such as acyclovir (Zovirax, Avirax ✤); famciclovir (Famvir) or valacyclovir (Valtrex)

◼ NURSING SAFETY PRIORITY: Drug Alert
The drugs do not cure the infection but do decrease the severity, promote healing, and decrease the frequency of recurrent outbreaks while they are being used.

- Emphasize the risk for neonatal infection to all patients, both male and female.

H

- Teach patients to avoid transmission by:
  1. Adhering to suppressive therapy
  2. Abstaining from sexual activity while lesions are present
  3. Using condoms during all sexual exposures

■ NURSING SAFETY PRIORITY: Action Alert

Remind patients to abstain from sexual activity while lesions are present. Urge condom use during all sexual exposures because of the increased risk for HSV transmission. Viral shedding can occur, even when lesions are not present. Teach the patient about how and when to use condoms.

  4. Keeping the skin in the genital region clean and dry
  5. Washing hands thoroughly after contact with lesions and laundering towels that have had direct contact with lesions
  6. Wearing gloves when applying ointments
- Help patients and their partners cope with the diagnosis by:
  1. Assessing the patient's and partner's emotional responses to the diagnosis of genital herpes
  2. Being sensitive and supportive during assessments and interventions
  3. Encouraging social support
  4. Referring them to reliable community or national resources such as those found through the National Institutes of Health (http://www.nlm.nih.gov/medlineplus/genitalherpes.html)

HIV DISEASE (HIV/AIDS)

OVERVIEW

- HIV disease is a continuum of immune deficiency problems that occur as a result of infection with the human immunodeficiency virus (HIV).
- From the onset of HIV infection through progression to acquired immunodeficiency syndrome (AIDS), the late and final stage, HIV disease represents a continuing battle between the virus and the patient's immune system.
- HIV is a retrovirus, with proteins on its surface that allow it to dock onto T4 (CD4+) cells. The virus has *reverse transcriptase (RT)* and *integrase,* which allow it to incorporate its genetic material into the host cell. These features give HIV major advantages for infecting humans by reproducing sufficient viruses to pass the infection along.
- HIV is transmitted in three ways:
  1. *Sexual:* genital, anal, or oral sexual contact with exposure of mucous membranes to infected semen or vaginal secretions

2. *Parenteral:* sharing of needles or equipment contaminated with infected blood or receiving contaminated blood products

3. *Perinatal:* from the placenta, from contact with maternal blood and body fluids during birth, or from breast milk from an infected mother to child

- Needle stick or "sharps" injuries are the main means of occupation-related HIV infection for health care workers. Health care workers also can be infected through exposure of nonintact skin and mucous membranes to blood and body fluids.

- Everyone who has AIDS has HIV infection; however, not everyone who has HIV infection has AIDS.

- A diagnosis of AIDS requires that the person is HIV positive and has one of the following:
  1. A CD4+ T-cell count of less than 200 cells/mm^3.
  2. An opportunistic infection

- Immune system abnormalities resulting from HIV disease include:
  1. Lymphocytopenia (decreased numbers of lymphocytes, especially CD4+ T-cell levels)
  2. Increased production of incomplete and nonfunctional antibodies
  3. Abnormally functioning macrophages

- *The person with HIV infection can transmit the virus to others at all stages of disease.*

- As a result of these abnormalities, the patient is at risk for bacterial, fungal, and viral infections, as well as for some opportunistic cancers.

- *Opportunistic infections* are those caused by organisms that are present as part of the normal environment and are kept in check by normal immune function.

- Once AIDS is diagnosed, even if the patient's cell count goes higher than 200 cells/mm^3 or if the infection is successfully treated, the AIDS diagnosis remains and the patient never reverts to being just HIV positive.

- The time from the beginning of HIV infection to development of AIDS ranges from months to years, depending on:
  1. How HIV was acquired
  2. Personal factors, such as frequency of re-exposure to HIV, presence of other sexually transmitted diseases (STDs), nutritional status, and stress
  3. Interventions used

Genetic/Genomic Considerations

- About 1% of people with HIV infection are *long-term nonprogressors (LTNPs),* sometimes called *elite controllers.* These people have been infected with HIV (as measured by enzyme-linked

H

immunosorbent assay [ELISA]) for at least 10 years and have remained asymptomatic, with CD4+ T-cell counts within the normal range and a viral load that is either undetectable or very low.
- A genetic difference for this population is that their CCR5/CXCR4 co-receptors on the CD4+ T-cells are abnormal and nonfunctional. This mutation creates a defective receptor that does not bind to the HIV docking proteins.
- Cells with this defective receptor successfully resist the entrance of HIV.

🌐 Cultural Awareness
- More than 72% of new HIV infections reported in the United States occur in racial and ethnic minority groups, particularly among African Americans and Hispanics.
- Factors that may increase the incidence of HIV infection and progression to AIDS among minority groups include:
  1. Fear of or lack of faith in the U.S. health care system
  2. Poverty and limited access to high-cost drugs
  3. Health beliefs about HIV treatment

Considerations for Older Adults
- Infection with HIV can occur at any age, and older patients should be assessed for risk behaviors, including a sexual and drug use history.
- Age-related decline in immune function increases the likelihood that the older adult will develop the infection after an HIV exposure.
- In the older woman, thinning of vaginal tissue as a result of decreased estrogen may increase susceptibility to all STDs, including HIV infection.

Women's Health Considerations
- Women are the fastest growing group with HIV infection and AIDS in North America.
- In less affluent countries, 50% of cases occur among women.
- Risk factors are sexual exposure (75%) and injection drug use (25%).
- Women with HIV infection have a poorer outcome with a shorter mean survival time than men. This outcome may be the result of late diagnosis and social or economic factors that reduce access to medical care.
- Gynecologic problems, especially persistent or recurrent vaginal candidiasis, may be the first signs of HIV infection in women. Other common problems include genital herpes, pelvic inflammatory disease, and cervical dysplasia or cancer.

- The effect of HIV on pregnancy outcomes includes a higher incidence of premature delivery, low–birth-weight infants, and transmission of the disease to the infant.

PATIENT-CENTERED COLLABORATIVE CARE
Assessment
- Obtain patient information about:
  1. Age and gender
  2. Occupation
  3. Current illness:
     a. Nature of the illness
     b. When it started
     c. Severity of symptoms
     d. Associated problems
     e. Interventions to date
  4. When HIV infection was diagnosed
  5. Chronologic history of infections and clinical problems since the diagnosis
  6. Health history, including transfusion history
  7. Sexual practices, STDs, and any major infectious diseases, including tuberculosis and hepatitis
  8. Injection drug use, including needle exposure and needle sharing
  9. Level of knowledge regarding the diagnosis, symptom management, diagnostic tests, treatments, community resources, and modes of HIV transmission
  10. Understanding and use of safer sex practices
- Assess for and document:
  1. Immune system changes:
     a. White blood cell (WBC) count and differential
     b. Hypergammaglobulinemia
     c. Opportunistic infections
     d. Lymphadenopathy
     e. Fatigue
  2. Skin changes:
     a. Dry, itchy, irritated skin
     b. Rashes
     c. Folliculitis
     d. Eczema
     e. Psoriasis
     f. Poor wound healing
     g. Purple lesions
  3. Respiratory changes:
     a. Shortness of breath
     b. Cough

H

4. Central nervous system (CNS) changes:
   a. Confusion
   b. AIDS dementia complex
   c. Fever
   d. Headache
   e. Visual changes
   f. Memory loss
   g. Personality changes
   h. Pain
   i. Peripheral neuropathies
   j. Gait changes, ataxia
   k. Seizures
5. GI changes:
   a. Diarrhea
   b. Nausea
   c. Weight loss
6. Opportunistic infections:
   a. Protozoal infections:
      (1) *Pneumocystis jiroveci* pneumonia
      (2) *Toxoplasma gondii*
      (3) *Cryptosporidium*
   b. Fungal infections:
      (1) *Candida albicans*
      (2) *Cryptococcus neoformans*
      (3) *Histoplasma capsulatum*
   c. Bacterial infections:
      (1) *Mycobacterium avium*
      (2) *Mycobacterium intracellulare*
      (3) *Mycobacterium tuberculosis*
   d. Viral infection:
      (1) Cytomegalovirus (CMV)
      (2) Herpes simplex virus (HSV)
      (3) Varicella-zoster virus (VZV)
7. Malignancies:
   a. Kaposi's sarcoma (KS)
   b. Hodgkin's lymphoma
   c. Non-Hodgkin's lymphoma
   d. Invasive cervical cancer
8. Endocrine changes:
   a. Gonadal dysfunction
   b. Adrenal insufficiency
   c. Diabetes mellitus
   d. Hyperlipidemia
9. Abnormal laboratory findings:
   a. WBC count of less than 3500 cells/mm^3

        b. CD4+ T-cell numbers decreased
        c. Low ratio of CD4+ to CD8+ T-cells
- Assess psychosocial issues, such as:
    1. Availability of a support system, such as family and significant others:
        a. Learn who in this support system is aware of the patient's diagnosis.
        b. Identify whether a health care proxy or durable power-of-attorney document has been signed.
    2. Employment status and occupation
    3. Changes in performance of ADLs
    4. Living arrangements
    5. Financial resources, including health insurance
    6. Alcohol or recreational drug use
    7. Anxiety level, mood, cognitive ability, and level of energy
    8. Self-esteem and changes in body image
    9. Suicidal ideation, depression
    10. Use of support groups or other community resources
    11. Energy level
- Diagnostic testing includes:
    1. Antibody tests:
        a. ELISA
        b. Western blot analysis
        c. Genomic viral testing
    2. Viral load testing (also called viral burden testing) by quantitative RNA assays:
        a. Reverse transcriptase-polymerase chain reaction (RT-PCR)
        b. Branched deoxyribonucleic acid method (bDNA)
        c. Nucleic acid sequence-based assay (NASBA)
    3. Other laboratory tests to monitor for abnormal values or changes affect the overall health of the patient:
        a. Blood chemistries
        b. Complete blood count (CBC) with differential
        c. Toxoplasmosis antibody titer
        d. Liver function tests
        e. Serologic test for syphilis (STS)
        f. Antigens to hepatitis A, hepatitis B, and hepatitis C

Planning and Implementation
POTENTIAL FOR INFECTION
- Potential for Infection is related to immune deficiency.
- Patients with AIDS are at high risk for opportunistic infections.
- Drug therapy for HIV/AIDS prolongs immune function and prevents opportunistic infections.
- Antiretroviral therapy only inhibits viral replication and does not kill the virus.

H

- Multiple drugs are used together in regimens popularly called *cocktails,* consisting of combinations of different types of antiretroviral agents, an approach called *highly active antiretroviral therapy (HAART).*

◼ NURSING SAFETY PRIORITY: Critical Rescue

Ensure that HAART drugs are not missed, delayed, or administered in doses lower than prescribed in the inpatient setting to prevent the development of drug resistance in the virus.

1. *Nucleoside analogue reverse transcriptase inhibitors (NARTI)* suppress production of reverse transcriptase (RT) and inhibit viral DNA synthesis and replication. Drugs in this class include zidovudine (Retrovir), didanosine (ddI, Videx), lamivudine (Epivir), stavudine (d4T, Zerit), tenofovir (Viread), emtricitabine (Emtriva), and abacavir (Ziagen).
2. *Non-nucleoside reverse transcriptase inhibitors (NNRTI)* inhibit synthesis of reverse transcriptase to suppress viral replication. These drugs include nevirapine (Viramune), delavirdine (Rescriptor), efavirenz (Sustiva), and etravirine (Intelence).
3. *Protease inhibitors* block the HIV protease enzyme, preventing release of viral particles from the infected T4 cell. These drugs include ritonavir (Norvir), indinavir (Crixivan), saquinavir (Invirase), nelfinavir (Viracept), lopinavir (Kaletra), atazanavir (Reyataz), fosamprenavir (Lexiva), and darunavir (Prezista), and tipranavir (Aptivus).
4. *Fusion inhibitors* work by blocking the fusion of HIV with a host cell; without fusion, infection of new cells does not occur. The major drug in this category is enfuvirtide (Fuzeon).
5. *Entry inhibitors* work to prevent infection by blocking the CCR5 receptor on CD4+ T-cells. Because this drug prevents only one type of receptor-virus interaction, the HIV virus must be tested to be sure it uses this receptor before adopting this drug. The major drug in this category is maraviroc (Selzentry).
6. *Integrase inhibitors* work to prevent infection by inhibiting the enzyme integrase, which is needed to insert the viral RNA into the host cell's human DNA. The major drug in this category is raltegravir (Isentress).
- Nursing measures to prevent infection in the patient with HIV/AIDS include:
   1. Placing the patient in a private room whenever possible

2. Using good handwashing technique or using alcohol-based hand rubs before touching the patient or any of his or her belongings

3. Ensuring that the patient's room and bathroom are cleaned at least once daily

4. Not using supplies from common areas (e.g., keeping a sleeve or box of paper cups in the patient's room and not sharing this box with any other patient; other articles to avoid sharing are drinking straws, plastic knives and forks, dressing materials, gloves, and bandages).

5. Limiting the number of health care personnel entering the patient's room

6. Monitoring vital signs and temperature every 4 hours to detect significant changes

7. Inspecting the patient's mouth at least every 8 hours for open lesions or white patches

8. Inspecting the patient's skin and mucous membranes (especially the anal area) for the presence of fissures and abscesses at least every 8 hours

9. Inspecting open areas, such as IV sites, every 4 hours for manifestations of infection

10. Changing wound dressings daily

11. Obtaining specimens of all suspicious areas for culture (as specified by the agency), and promptly notifying the physician

12. Assisting the patient in performing coughing and deep-breathing exercises

13. Encouraging activity at a level appropriate for the patient's current health status

14. Keeping frequently used equipment in the room for use with this patient only (e.g., blood pressure cuff, stethoscope, thermometer)

15. Limiting visitors to healthy adults

16. Using strict aseptic technique for all invasive procedures

17. Avoiding the use of indwelling urinary catheters

18. Keeping fresh flowers and potted plants out of the patient's room

19. Teaching the patient to eat a low-bacteria diet (e.g., avoiding raw fruits or vegetables; undercooked meat, eggs, or fish; and pepper and paprika as seasonings sprinkled on food right before eating)

INADEQUATE GAS EXCHANGE

- Inadequate Gas Exchange is related to anemia, respiratory infection, or lung cancer.
- Drug therapy is a mainstay for gas exchange problems resulting from *Pneumocystis carinii* pneumonia (PCP).

1. Trimethoprim/sulfamethoxazole (Apo-Sulfatrim ✤, Bactrim, Cotrim, Septra)
2. Pentamidine (Pentacarinat ✤, Pentam), given IV, IM, or by aerosol
3. Dapsone (Avlosulfon)
4. Atovaquone (Mepron)
- Nursing interventions include:
  1. Respiratory support and maintenance:
     a. Assessing the respiratory rate, rhythm, and depth; breath sounds; and vital signs and monitoring for cyanosis at least every 8 hours
     b. Applying oxygen and humidifying the room as prescribed
     c. Monitoring mechanical ventilation to ensure safe, effective respiratory support
     d. Performing suctioning as needed
     e. Performing chest physical therapy as needed
     f. Evaluating blood gas results
  2. Comfort:
     a. Assessing the patient's comfort
     b. Elevating the head of the bed
     c. Pacing activities to reduce shortness of breath and fatigue
  3. Rest and activity changes:
     a. Pacing activities to conserve energy
     b. Guiding the patient in active and passive ROM exercises
     c. Scheduling non–time-critical activities, such as bathing, so that he or she is not fatigued at mealtime

MANAGING PAIN
- Pain with HIV/AIDS has many origins, including enlarged organs stretching the viscera or compressing nerves, tumor invasion of bone and other tissues, peripheral neuropathy, and generalized joint and muscle pain.
- Drug therapy with different classes of drugs is used to manage pain from different causes:
  1. Arthralgia and myalgia respond to NSAIDs.
  2. Neuropathic pain of peripheral neuropathy:
     a. Tricyclic antidepressants, such as amitriptyline (Elavil)
     b. Anticonvulsant drugs, such as phenytoin (Dilantin) or carbamazepine (Tegretol)
  3. General pain can be managed with opioids:
     a. Weaker opioids, such as oxycodone or codeine
     b. Stronger opioids, such as morphine, hydromorphone (Dilaudid), or transdermal fentanyl (Duragesic)
- Comfort measures:
  1. Pressure-relieving mattress pads

  2. Warm baths or other forms of hydrotherapy
  3. Massage
  4. Application of heat or cold to painful areas
  5. Use of lift sheets to avoid pulling or grasping the patient with joint pain
  6. Frequent position changes
- Complementary and alternative therapies:
  1. Guided imagery
  2. Distraction
  3. Progressive relaxation
  4. Body-talk
  5. Biofeedback

ENHANCING NUTRITION
- Poor nutrition has many causes and requires an interdisciplinary team to determine the exact cause or causes.
  1. Drug therapy:
     a. Administering antifungal agents for esophagitis, such as ketoconazole (Nizoral) or fluconazole (Diflucan)
     b. Administering antiemetics for nausea and vomiting
  2. Comfort measures:
     a. Providing frequent mouth care
     b. Keeping the environment pleasant and free from offensive odors
  3. Nutritional therapy:
     a. Assessing food preferences and any dietary cultural or religious practices
     b. Monitoring weight, intake and output, and calorie count to detect weight gain/loss
     c. Teaching the patient about a high-calorie, high-protein, nutritionally sound diet
     d. Encouraging him or her to avoid dietary fat
     e. Collaborating with the dietitian
     f. Providing small, frequent meals
     g. Administering prescribed supplemental vitamins
     h. Providing prescribed tube feedings or total parenteral nutrition

MINIMIZING DIARRHEA
- Nursing interventions include:
  1. Administering antidiarrheals, such as diphenoxylate (Diarsed ♣, Lomotil) or loperamide (Imodium), as prescribed
  2. Consulting with the dietitian to offer less roughage; less fatty, spicy, and sweet food; and no alcohol or caffeine
  3. Assessing the perineal skin every 8 to 12 hours
  4. Providing a bedside commode or a bedpan if needed

H

RESTORING SKIN INTEGRITY
- KS is the most common skin lesion:
  1. Lesions may be localized or widespread; monitor for progression.
  2. Lesions are managed with local radiation, intralesional chemotherapy, or cryotherapy.
  3. Lesions respond well to antiretroviral therapy. For rapidly progressive disease or with major involvement of the intestinal tract, lungs, or other organs, therapy may include:
     a. Anti-neoplastic agents (chemotherapy)
     b. Interferon-alpha
     c. Zidovudine
  4. Clean and dress open, weeping KS lesions.
  5. To disguise the lesions, teach patients to:
     a. Use makeup over intact lesions.
     b. Wear long-sleeved shirts.
     c. Wear hats.
- HSV lesions or shingles may occur and form abscesses.
  1. Provide good skin care to keep the area clean and dry.
  2. Clean abscesses at least once per shift with normal saline and allow them to air-dry.
  3. Provide aluminum acetate (Burow's solution, Domeboro) soaks.
  4. Administer prescribed antiviral drugs, including acyclovir (Zovirax) or valacyclovir (Valtrex).

MINIMIZING CONFUSION
- Nursing interventions include:
  1. Assessing baseline neurologic and mental status
  2. Evaluating the patient for subtle changes in memory, ability to concentrate, affect, and behavior
  3. Reorienting the confused patient to person, time, and place
  4. Reminding the patient of your identity and explain what is to be done at any given time
  5. Giving simple directions:
     a. Using short, uncomplicated sentences
     b. Explaining activities in simple language
     c. Involving the patient in planning the daily schedule
  6. Asking relatives or significant others to bring in familiar items from home
  7. Arranging all items in the patient's environment in the same location as at home
  8. Making the environment safe and comfortable
  9. Administering prescribed psychotropic drugs, antidepressants, or anxiolytics
  10. Assessing the patient with neurologic manifestations for increased intracranial pressure

⬛ NURSING SAFETY PRIORITY: Critical Rescue

Report immediately any seizure activity or changes in level of consciousness (one of the earliest signs of increased intracranial pressure), vital signs, pupil size or reactivity, or limb strength to the physician for appropriate intervention.

SUPPORTING SELF-ESTEEM
- Self-esteem is affected by dramatic changes in appearance that alter the person's body image; abrupt, significant changes in their relationships with others; and changes in day-to-day activities, employment, or other productive activities.
- Nursing interventions include:
  1. Provide a climate of acceptance for patients with AIDS by promoting a trusting relationship.
  2. Help patients to express feelings and identify positive aspects of themselves.
  3. Allow for privacy, but do not avoid or isolate the patient.
  4. Encourage self-care, independence, control, and decision making by helping him or her set short-term, attainable goals and offering praise when goals are achieved.

MAINTAIN SOCIAL CONTACT
- Nursing interventions include:
  1. Promote patient interaction first by establishing a therapeutic nurse-patient relationship, and do not isolate the patient. Spend time with him or her, even when not performing a procedure or assessment, just to be present. Reduce barriers to social contact. Assess his or her social support resources.
  2. Teach family and significant others about HIV transmission and the use of Standard Precautions to reduce anxiety and increase contact with the patient.
  3. Encourage the patient to state feelings about self, coping skills, and a sense of control over the situation.
  4. Help him or her identify support systems, including those already in place and those that need to be arranged.

Community-Based Care
- *Teaching about HIV transmission is the most important aspect for prevention of HIV.* All people, regardless of age, gender, ethnicity, or sexual orientation, are susceptible to HIV infection. HIV infection is preventable because of the mode of viral transmission and the fragile nature of the virus.
- Collaborate with the health care team members, patient, and family to plan for self-management:
  1. Assess the patient's status, ability to perform self-care activities, and identify the potential need for care, such as:
     a. Assistance with ADLs
     b. Around-the-clock nursing care

      c. Drug administration

      d. Nutritional support

2. Assess available resources, including family members and significant others willing and able to be caregivers.

3. Help the family make arrangements for outside caregivers or respite care, if needed.

4. Refer the patient to support groups, a financial counselor, a social worker, legal services, and a spiritual counselor.

5. Determine the need for assistance with funeral arrangements.

- Teach the patient, family, and significant others about:

  1. Modes of HIV transmission and preventive behaviors

  2. Guidelines for safer sex

  3. Not sharing toothbrushes, razors, and other potentially blood-contaminated articles

  4. Manifestations of infection:

     a. Temperature higher than 100° F (38° C)

     b. Persistent cough (with or without sputum)

     c. Pus or foul-smelling drainage from any open skin area or normal body opening

     d. Presence of a boil or abscess

     e. Urine that is cloudy or foul-smelling or that causes burning on urination

  5. Good infection control practices, such as:

     a. Avoiding crowds and other large gatherings of people where someone may be ill

     b. Not sharing personal toilet articles, such as toothbrushes, toothpaste, washcloths, or deodorant sticks, with others

     c. Bathing daily, using an antimicrobial soap; if total bathing is not possible, washing the armpits, groin, genitals, and anal area twice daily with an antimicrobial soap

     d. Cleaning the toothbrush daily by running it through the dishwasher or rinsing it in liquid laundry bleach

     e. Washing hands thoroughly with an antimicrobial soap before eating or drinking, after touching a pet, after shaking hands with anyone, returning home from any outing, and after using the toilet

     f. Washing dishes between uses with hot sudsy water or using a dishwasher

     g. Not drinking water, milk, juice, or other cold liquids that have been standing for longer than an hour

     h. Not reusing cups and glasses without washing

     i. Not changing pet litter boxes; if unavoidable, using gloves and washing hands immediately

      j. Avoiding turtles and reptiles as pets
      k. Not feeding pets raw or undercooked meat
6. Teaching good dietary habits, including:
      a. Proper nutrition
      b. Eating a low-bacteria diet
      c. Avoiding salads; raw fruit and vegetables; undercooked meat, fish, or eggs; pepper; and paprika
      d. Thoroughly washing fruit and vegetables
      e. Refrigerating perishable foods
7. Psychosocial preparation:
      a. Helping identify ways to avoid problems with social stigma and rejection
      b. Identifying coping strategies for difficult situations
      c. Supporting family members and friends in efforts to help the patient and provide protection from discrimination
      d. Encouraging patients to continue as many usual activities as possible
      e. Supporting patients in their selection of friends and relatives with whom to discuss the diagnosis
      f. Reminding the patient that sexual partners and care providers should be informed of the diagnosis
      g. Making referrals to community resources, mental health professionals, behavioral health professionals, and support groups

HUNTINGTON'S DISEASE

- Huntington's disease is a hereditary disorder transmitted as an autosomal dominant trait at the time of conception.
- It is most prevalent in people of western European ancestry.
- The two main symptoms of the disease are progressive mental status changes leading to dementia and choreiform involuntary movements.
- Other clinical manifestations of Huntington's disease include poor balance, hesitant or explosive speech, dysphagia, impaired respirations, and bowel and bladder incontinence. Mental status changes include decreased attention span, poor judgment, memory loss, personality changes, and later, dementia.
- The first drug to be approved to decrease chorea associated with Huntington's disease is tetrabenazine (Xenazine). It is thought to work by depleting the monoamines (e.g., dopamine, serotonin) from nerve terminals.
- There is no known cure for the disease.
- Genetic testing can determine risk for Huntington's disease; it is an autosomal dominant trait with high penetrance on

chromosome 4. This means that a person who inherits just one mutated allele has nearly a 100% chance of developing the disease.

- Management of the disease is symptomatic. Physical and occupational therapy and social support can promote function and engagement.

HYDROCELE

- A hydrocele usually is a painless cystic mass filled with a straw-colored fluid that forms around the testis.
- It is caused by impaired lymphatic drainage of the scrotum, leading to swelling of the tissue surrounding the testes.
- Unless the swelling becomes large and uncomfortable or begins to impair blood flow to the testis, no treatment is necessary.
- When a hydrocele is large, uncomfortable, or cosmetically unacceptable, intervention is done by one of the following two methods:
    1. Drainage through a needle and syringe
    2. Surgical removal
- Provide postoperative care, including:
    1. Explaining the importance of wearing a scrotal support (jock strap) for the first 24 to 48 hours after surgery to keep the dressing in place and to prevent edema
    2. Assessing for pain and wound complications (infection or bleeding)
    3. Instructing the patient to schedule a follow-up visit with the surgeon
    4. Instructing the patient to stay off his feet for several days and to limit physical activity for a week
    5. Reassuring him that this swelling is normal and eventually subsides

HYDRONEPHROSIS, HYDROURETER, AND URETHRAL STRICTURE

- Several disorders obstruct the outflow of urine.
- In *hydronephrosis,* the kidney becomes enlarged as urine accumulates in the renal pelvis and the calyces. Obstruction within the pelvis or ureteropelvic junction results in renal pelvic distention, and extensive damage to the vasculature and renal tubules can result.
- *Hydroureter* is the obstruction of the ureter at the point of the iliac vessel crossing or the ureterovesical entry. Dilation of

the ureter occurs at the point proximal to the obstruction as urine accumulates.

- A *urethral stricture* is the most distal point of obstruction, with bladder distention occurring before hydroureter and hydronephrosis.
- Urinary tract obstruction results in direct pressure buildup on the tissue, causing structural damage with potential for subsequent infection and kidney failure.
- Causes of hydronephrosis and hydroureter include tumors, stones, trauma, congenital structural defects, and retroperitoneal fibrosis.
- Urethral stricture occurs from chronic inflammation.
- Management includes:
  1. Recording history of kidney or urologic disorders
  2. Documenting pattern of urination, including amount and frequency
  3. Describing urine, including color, clarity, and odor
  4. Reporting new symptoms, including flank or abdominal pain, chills, fever, and malaise
  5. Treating the cause and re-establishing urine flow to prevent kidney failure
  6. Managing flank, abdominal, or ureteral pain
  7. Intervening and communicating early when urine flow decreases or stops postprocedure to restore urologic integrity
  8. Monitoring urinalysis for bacteria or white blood cells (WBCs) to determine if infection is present
  9. Anticipating an enlarged ureter or kidney on x-ray, computed tomography (CT) and IV urography

HYPERALDOSTERONISM

OVERVIEW

- Hyperaldosteronism is increased secretion of aldosterone by the adrenal glands that results in mineralocorticoid excess.
- Primary hyperaldosteronism (Conn's syndrome), which results from excessive secretion of aldosterone from one or both adrenal glands, is most often caused by a benign adrenal tumor (adrenal adenoma).
- Secondary hyperaldosteronism is excessive secretion of aldosterone because of high levels of angiotensin II that are stimulated by high plasma renin levels. Causes include kidney hypoxemia and the use of thiazide diuretics.
- Regardless of the cause, hyperaldosteronism is manifested by hypernatremia, hypokalemia, metabolic alkalosis, and hypertension.

PATIENT-CENTERED COLLABORATIVE CARE
Assessment
- Obtain patient information about:
  1. Headache
  2. Fatigue
  3. Muscle weakness
  4. Nocturia (excessive urination at night)
  5. Polydipsia (excessive fluid intake)
  6. Polyuria (excessive urine output)
  7. Paresthesias (sensations of numbness and tingling)
- Assess for and document:
  1. Hypertension
  2. Elevated serum levels of sodium
  3. Low serum levels of potassium
- Diagnostic assessment includes:
  1. Serum electrolyte levels
  2. Serum renin levels (low)
  3. Serum aldosterone levels (high)
  4. X-rays
  5. Imaging with computed tomography (CT) scans or magnetic resonance imaging (MRI)

Interventions
- Adrenalectomy of one or both adrenal glands is the most common treatment for early-stage hyperaldosteronism.
- Provide preoperative care, including:
  1. Implementing routine preoperative care, as described in Part One
  2. Correcting the serum potassium levels by administering prescribed potassium supplements, potassium-sparing diuretics, or aldosterone antagonists
  3. Providing a low-sodium diet
- Provide postoperative care, including:
  1. Implementing routine postoperative care, as described in Part One
  2. Teaching the patient about glucocorticoid replacement (replacement is lifelong if both adrenal glands are removed)
  3. Instructing him or her to wear a medical alert bracelet while taking glucocorticoids
- For patients who do not have surgery and must remain on spironolactone therapy to control hypokalemia and hypertension, teach them about:
  1. Avoiding potassium supplements and foods rich in potassium
  2. Increasing dietary sodium
  3. Reporting symptoms of hyponatremia:
     a. Mouth dryness

    b. Thirst
    c. Lethargy or drowsiness
  4. Side effects of spironolactone therapy:
    a. Gynecomastia
    b. Diarrhea
    c. Drowsiness
    d. Headache
    e. Rash, urticaria (hives)
    f. Confusion
    g. Erectile dysfunction
    h. Hirsutism
    i. Amenorrhea

HYPERCALCEMIA

OVERVIEW

- Hypercalcemia is a total serum calcium level above 10.5 mg/dL or 2.75 mmol/L.
- Because the normal range for serum calcium is so narrow, even small increases have severe effects.
- The effects of hypercalcemia occur first in excitable tissues.
- Common causes of hypercalcemia include:
  1. Increased absorption of calcium:
     a. Excessive oral intake of calcium
     b. Excessive oral intake of vitamin D
  2. Decreased excretion of calcium:
     a. Kidney failure
     b. Use of thiazide diuretics
  3. Increased bone resorption of calcium:
     a. Hyperparathyroidism
     b. Malignancy
     c. Hyperthyroidism
     d. Immobility
     e. Use of glucocorticoids
  4. Dehydration

PATIENT-CENTERED COLLABORATIVE CARE
Assessment

- Assess for and document:
  1. Cardiovascular changes, which are the most serious and life threatening:
     a. Increased heart rate and blood pressure (early)
     b. Slow heart rate (late or severe)

    c. Cyanosis and pallor

    d. Dysrhythmias on electrocardiograph (ECG), especially a shortened QT interval

    e. Slowed or impaired blood flow:

      (1) Measure calf circumferences.

      (2) Assess foot temperature, color, and capillary refill.

2. Neuromuscular changes, which include:

    a. Severe muscle weakness

    b. Decreased deep tendon reflexes without paresthesia

    c. Altered level of consciousness (confusion, lethargy, coma)

3. Intestinal changes, which include:

    a. Constipation, anorexia, nausea, vomiting, and abdominal pain

    b. Hypoactive or absent bowel sounds

    c. Increased abdominal size

Interventions

- Measures to prevent increases in calcium:
  1. Discontinuing IV solutions containing calcium (lactated Ringer's solution)
  2. Discontinuing oral drugs containing calcium or vitamin D (e.g., calcium-based antacids, over-the-counter [OTC] vitamin supplements)
  3. Discontinuing thiazide diuretics that increase kidney calcium resorption
- Drug therapy:
  1. Dilute serum calcium with IV normal saline (0.9% sodium chloride)
  2. Administer diuretics that enhance calcium excretion, such as furosemide (Lasix, Furoside ♦)
  3. Administer calcium chelators (calcium binders):
     a. Plicamycin (Mithracin)
     b. Penicillamine (Cuprimine, Pendramine ♦).
  4. Administer and monitor effects of drugs that inhibit calcium resorption from bone:
     a. Calcitonin (Calcimar)
     b. Bisphosphonates (etidronate)
     c. Prostaglandin synthesis inhibitors (aspirin, NSAIDs)
- Dialysis by hemodialysis or blood ultrafiltration may be needed for rapid calcium reduction when levels are life threatening.
- Continuous cardiac monitoring may be requested:
  1. Compare recent ECG tracings with the patient's baseline tracings (when calcium was normal).
  2. Examine for changes in the T waves, QT interval, and heart rate and rhythm.

- Additional nursing actions include:
  1. Monitoring intake and output to detect imbalances and report imbalances in a timely manner
  2. Assessing for fluid overload
  3. Encouraging weight-bearing exercise to slow bone resorption in chronic conditions of hypercalcemia

HYPERCORTISOLISM (CUSHING'S SYNDROME)
OVERVIEW
- Excess cortisol (i.e., hypercortisolism) results in *Cushing's syndrome.*
- Excess cortisol secretion can be a result of a problem in the adrenal cortex, the anterior pituitary gland, or the hypothalamus. Glucocorticoid therapy also can lead to hypercortisolism.
- *Cushing's disease* is a condition in which the pituitary gland releases too much adrenocorticotropic hormone (ACTH). Oversecretion of ACTH can result from a pituitary adenoma, an adrenal adenoma, or drug therapy with corticosteroids (also known as glucocorticoids) for another health problem. Cushing's disease is a form of Cushing's syndrome.
- Regardless of cause, excess cortisol or cortisol-like drugs affect metabolism and all body systems to some degree.

PATIENT-CENTERED COLLABORATIVE CARE
Assessment
- Obtain patient information about:
  1. History of other health problems and drug therapies
  2. Age, gender, and usual weight
  3. Weight gain
  4. Increased appetite
  5. Change in activity or sleep patterns, fatigue, and muscle weakness
  6. Bone pain or a history of fractures
  7. Frequent infections
  8. Easy bruising
  9. Cessation of menses
  10. GI ulcers
- Assess for and document:
  1. General appearance:
     a. Buffalo hump on shoulder
     b. Enlarged trunk
     c. Moon face

H

      d. Thin arms and legs

      e. Generalized muscle wasting and weakness

  2. Skin changes:

      a. Bruises

      b. Thin, translucent skin

      c. Wounds that have not healed

      d. Reddish purple striae ("stretch marks") on the abdomen, thighs, and upper arms

      e. Acne

      f. Fine coating of hair over the face and body

  3. Cardiac changes:

      a. Tachycardia

      b. Hypertension

      c. Edema and evidence of hypervolemia

  4. Emotional lability, mood swings, irritability, confusion, depression

  5. Hyperglycemia

  6. Hypernatremia

- Diagnostic assessment includes:

  1. Elevated blood, salivary, and urine cortisol levels

  2. Dexamethasone suppression testing

  3. Abnormal serum electrolyte values (increased sodium, decreased calcium, decreased potassium)

  4. X-rays, computed tomography (CT) scans or magnetic resonance imaging (MRI) to identify lesions of the adrenal or pituitary glands, lung, GI tract, or pancreas.

Planning and Implementation

FLUID OVERLOAD

  Nonsurgical Management

- Restore fluid volume balance. Prevent fluid overload leading to pulmonary edema and heart failure:

  1. Monitor for indicators of increased fluid overload (increased pulse quality, increasing neck vein distention, presence of crackles in lungs, increasing peripheral edema, reduced urine output) at least every 2 hours.

◼ NURSING SAFETY PRIORITY: Critical Rescue

Notify the health care provider of any change that indicates the fluid overload is not responding to therapy or is becoming worse.

  2. Prevent skin breakdown by:

      a. Using a pressure-reducing or pressure-relieving overlay on the mattress

      b. Assessing skin pressure areas every 2 to 4 hours for signs of redness or open areas

      c. Assisting the patient to change position every 2 hours

- Drug therapy
  1. Administer prescribed drugs to interfere with adrenocorticotropic hormone (ACTH) production or adrenal hormone synthesis:
     a. Aminoglutethimide (Elipten, Cytadren)
     b. Metyrapone (Metopirone)
     c. Cyproheptadine (Periactin)
     d. Mitotane (Lysodren)
  2. Monitor the patient for response to drug therapy:
     a. Weight loss
     b. Increased urine output
  3. Assess laboratory findings, especially sodium and potassium values.
- Nutrition therapy:
  1. Restriction of sodium
  2. Restriction of fluids
- Radiation therapy for hypercortisolism caused by pituitary adenomas:
  1. Observe for any changes in the patient's neurologic status, such as headache, elevated blood pressure or pulse, disorientation, or changes in pupil size or reaction.
  2. Assess for skin dryness, redness, flushing, or alopecia at the radiation site.

Surgical Management

- The surgical treatment of adrenocortical hypersecretion depends on the cause of the condition.
- When adrenal hyperfunction results from increased pituitary secretion of ACTH, removal of a pituitary adenoma may be attempted.
- When hypercortisolism is caused by adrenal tumors, a partial or complete adrenalectomy (removal of the adrenal gland) may be performed by open abdominal procedures or laparoscopic procedures.
- Provide preoperative care, including:
  1. Implementing routine preoperative care (see Part One)
  2. Implementing prescribed drug and diet therapy to correct electrolyte imbalances
  3. Monitoring blood potassium, sodium, and chloride levels for abnormal values
  4. Monitoring ECG for dysrhythmias
  5. Monitoring blood glucose levels and managing hyperglycemia
  6. Preventing infection with handwashing and aseptic technique
  7. Implementing fall prevention measures with changes in mental status
  8. Teaching the patient about the care needs after surgery and the need for long-term drug therapy

H

- Provide postoperative care, including:
  1. Implementing routine postoperative care as described in Part One
  2. Assessing the patient every 15 minutes for shock (e.g., hypotension, a rapid and weak pulse, decreasing urine output) during the first 6 hours
  3. Monitoring vital signs and other hemodynamic variables to detect hypervolemia/hypovolemia:
     a. Central venous pressure
     b. Pulmonary wedge pressure
     c. Intake and output
     d. Daily weights
     e. Serum electrolyte levels
  4. Teaching about the need (after bilateral adrenalectomy) for lifelong glucocorticoid replacement

RISK FOR INJURY

- Risk for Injury is related to skin thinning, poor wound healing, and bone density loss
- Prevent skin injury by:
  1. Assessing the patient's skin for reddened areas, excoriation, breakdown, and edema.
  2. Turning or assisting him or her to turn every 2 hours
  3. Padding bony prominences
  4. Teaching the patient activities to avoid trauma:
     a. Use a soft toothbrush.
     b. Use an electric shaver.
     c. Keep the skin clean and dry it thoroughly after washing.
     d. Use a moisturizing lotion.
  5. Using tape sparingly and taking care when removing it
  6. Exerting pressure over an injection or venipuncture site
- Prevent pathologic fractures by:
  1. Using a lift sheet to move the patient instead of grasping him or her
  2. Reminding the patient to call for help when ambulating
  3. Reviewing the use of ambulatory aids (walkers or canes), if needed
  4. Keeping rooms free of extraneous objects that may cause a fall
  5. Teaching unlicensed assistive personnel (UAP) to use a gait belt when ambulating the patient
  6. Teaching the patient about safety issues and dietary needs
- Prevent GI bleeding by:
  1. Implementing prescribed drug therapy
     a. Antacids

     b. H2 histamine receptor blockers:
       (1) Cimetidine (Tagamet, Peptol ✿, Novo-Cimetine ✿)
       (2) Ranitidine (Zantac, Apo-Ranitidine ✿)
       (3) Famotidine (Pepcid)
       (4) Nizatidine (Axid)
     c. Proton pump inhibitors:
       (1) Omeprazole (Losec ✿, Prilosec)
       (2) Esomeprazole (Nexium)
2. Encouraging the patient to reduce or eliminate habits that contribute to gastric irritation, such as:
     a. Consuming alcohol or caffeine
     b. Smoking
     c. Fasting
     d. Taking NSAIDs and drugs that contain aspirin or other salicylates

RISK FOR INFECTION
- Protect the patient from infection by:
  1. Using aseptic technique when performing any invasive procedure
  2. Performing frequent, thorough handwashing
  3. Ensuring that anyone with an upper respiratory tract infection who must enter the patient's room wears a mask
  4. Continually assessing the patient for the presence of infection:
     a. Monitoring the daily complete blood count (CBC) with differential white blood cell (WBC) count and absolute neutrophil count (ANC) to detect and report abnormal values
     b. Inspecting the mouth during every shift for mucosal integrity
     c. Assessing the lungs every 8 hours for crackles, wheezes, or reduced breath sounds
     d. Assessing all urine for odor and cloudiness
     e. Asking the patient about any urgency, burning, or pain present on urination
     f. Taking vital signs at least every 4 hours to assess for fever
  5. Providing skin care and daily hygiene
  6. Turning the immobile patient every 2 hours and applying skin lubricants
  7. Assessing the lungs for crackles, wheezes, or reduced breath sounds
  8. Urging the patient to cough and deep breathe or to perform sustained maximal inhalations every 1 to 2 hours while awake

H

POTENTIAL FOR ACUTE ADRENAL INSUFFICIENCY
- Teach the patient who must take glucocorticoids to:
  1. Take the drug in divided doses, with the first dose in the morning and the second dose between 4 and 6 PM.
  2. Take the drug with meals or snacks.
  3. Weigh himself or herself daily, record it, and compare it with previous weights.
  4. Increase the dosage as directed for increased physical stress or severe emotional stress, including surgery, dental work, influenza, fever, pregnancy, and family problems.
  5. *Never skip a dose of drug.* If the patient has persistent vomiting or severe diarrhea and cannot take the drug by mouth for 24 to 36 hours, he or she must call the physician. If the patient cannot reach the physician, he or she must go to the nearest emergency department, because an injection may be needed in place of the usual oral drug.
  6. Always wear his or her medical alert bracelet or necklace.
  7. Make regular visits for health care follow-up.
  8. Learn how to give himself or herself an IM injection of hydrocortisone.

Community-Based Care
- Instruct the patient taking exogenous glucocorticoids to call his or her health care provider if more than 3 pounds are gained in a week or more than 1 to 2 pounds is gained within 24 hours.
- Urge him or her to use proper hygiene and to avoid crowds or others with infections.
- Encourage the patient and all people living in the same home with him or her to have yearly influenza vaccinations.

HYPERKALEMIA

OVERVIEW
- Hyperkalemia is a serum potassium level greater than 5 mEq/L (5 mmol/L).
- The normal range for serum potassium values is narrow, so even slight increases above normal values can affect excitable tissues, especially the heart.
- The consequences of hyperkalemia can be life threatening, and the imbalance usually is not seen in people with normally functioning kidneys.

- Causes include:
  1. Intake of potassium-containing foods or drugs:
     a. Salt substitutes
     b. Potassium chloride
     c. Potassium-sparing diuretics
  2. Rapid infusion of potassium-containing IV solution
  3. Transfusions of whole blood or packed cells
  4. Adrenal insufficiency (Addison's disease, adrenalectomy)
  5. Tissue damage (crushing injuries, burns)
  6. Acidosis
  7. Hyperuricemia
  8. Chronic or acute kidney disease
- The problems that occur with hyperkalemia are related to how rapidly extracellular fluid (ECF) potassium levels increase. Sudden rises in serum potassium cause severe problems at potassium levels between 6 and 7 mEq/L. When serum potassium rises slowly, problems may not occur until potassium levels reach 8 mEq/L or higher.

PATIENT-CENTERED COLLABORATIVE CARE
Assessment
- Obtain patient information about:
  1. Age
  2. Chronic illnesses (particularly kidney disease and diabetes mellitus)
  3. Recent medical or surgical treatment
  4. Urine output, including the frequency and amount of voiding
  5. Drug use, particularly potassium-sparing diuretics and angiotensin-converting enzyme (ACE) inhibitors
  6. Nutrition history to determine the intake of potassium-rich foods or the use of salt substitutes that contain potassium
  7. Palpitations, skipped heartbeats, and other cardiac irregularities
  8. Muscle twitching and weakness in the leg muscles
  9. Unusual tingling or numbness in the hands, feet, or face
  10. Recent changes in bowel habits, especially diarrhea
- Assess for and document:
  1. Cardiovascular changes:
     a. Bradycardia
     b. Hypotension
     c. Electrocardiographic (ECG) changes:
        (1) Tall, peaked T waves

  (2) Prolonged PR intervals
  (3) Flat or absent P waves
  (4) Wide QRS complexes
2. Neuromuscular changes, early:
   a. Skeletal muscle twitches
   b. Tingling and burning sensations followed by numbness in the hands and feet and around the mouth
3. Neuromuscular changes, late:
   a. Muscle weakness
   b. Flaccid paralysis first in hands and feet, then moving higher
4. Intestinal changes
   a. Increased motility
   b. Hyperactive bowel sounds
   c. Frequent watery bowel movements
5. Laboratory data: serum potassium level greater than 5 mEq/L

Interventions

- Interventions for hyperkalemia are aimed at rapidly reducing the serum potassium level, preventing recurrences, and ensuring patient safety during the electrolyte imbalance.
- Drug therapy:
  1. IV therapy:
     a. Discontinuing potassium-containing infusions
     b. Keeping the IV catheter open
     c. Administering IV preparation of 100 mL of 10% to 20% glucose with 10 to 20 units of regular insulin
  2. Withholding oral potassium supplements
  3. Potassium-excreting diuretics, such as furosemide
  4. Sodium polystyrene sulfonate (Kayexalate) exchange resins
- Hemodialysis or ultrafiltration
- Nursing care priorities include:
  1. Cardiac monitoring for early recognition of dysrhythmias and other manifestations of hyperkalemia on cardiac function

---

⊞ NURSING SAFETY PRIORITY: Critical Rescue

Notify the health care provider or Rapid Response Team if the patient's heart rate falls below 60 beats/min or if the T waves become spiked.

---

  2. Collaborating with the dietitian to reduce dietary potassium intake by reading product packages and avoiding foods high in potassium including many salt substitute products, preserved meats, dried fruit, and large volumes of dark green vegetables or beans

HYPERNATREMIA

OVERVIEW

- Hypernatremia is a serum sodium level greater than 145 mEq/L and is often accompanied by changes in fluid volumes.
- It makes excitable tissues more easily excited, a condition known as irritability, and leads to cellular dehydration.
- Common causes include:
  1. NPO status
  2. Dehydration
  3. Watery diarrhea
  4. Excessive diaphoresis
  5. Excessive oral sodium ingestion
  6. Excessive administration of sodium-containing IV fluids
  7. Fever
  8. Increased rate of metabolism
  9. Hyperventilation
  10. Infection
  11. Hyperaldosteronism
  12. Kidney failure
  13. Corticosteroids
  14. Cushing's syndrome or disease

PATIENT-CENTERED COLLABORATIVE CARE

Assessment

- Assess for and document:
  1. Nervous system changes:
     a. Decreased attention span and recall of recent events
     b. Agitation or confusion
     c. Lethargy, drowsiness, stupor, or coma (when accompanied by fluid overload)
  2. Skeletal muscles changes:
     a. Muscle twitching and irregular muscle contractions (mild hypernatremia)
     b. Muscle weakness
     c. Reduced or absent deep tendon reflexes
  3. Cardiovascular changes that differ with fluid status:
     a. Hypovolemia leads to increased pulse rate, hypotension, and reduced quality of peripheral pulses.
     b. Hypervolemia leads to slow to normal bounding pulses, full peripheral pulses, neck veins distention, and elevated diastolic blood pressure.
  4. Respiratory changes occur with hypervolemia:
     a. Pulmonary edema
     b. Decreased oxygen saturation

H

Interventions

- Restore fluid balance when hypernatremia is caused by fluid loss with hypotonic IV infusions, usually 0.25% or 0.45% sodium chloride.
- Restoring fluid balance when hypernatremia is caused by fluid and sodium losses requires fluid replacement with IV infusions of isotonic sodium chloride (NaCl) solutions.
- Drug therapy includes diuretics that promote sodium loss, such as furosemide (Lasix, Furoside ✤) or bumetanide (Bumex).
- Assess the patient hourly for symptoms of excessive fluid and sodium or potassium losses.
- Dietary sodium restriction may be needed to prevent sodium excess when kidney problems are present.
- Fluid restriction may also be needed.
- Priorities for nursing care of the patient with hypernatremia include monitoring the patient's response to therapy and preventing hyponatremia and dehydration:
  1. Prevent fluid overload from becoming worse, leading to pulmonary edema and heart failure:
     a. Monitor for indicators of increased fluid overload at least every 2 hours.

■ NURSING SAFETY PRIORITY: Critical Rescue

Pulmonary edema can occur very quickly and can lead to death. Notify the health care provider about any change that indicates the fluid overload is not responding to therapy or is becoming worse.

  2. Reduce risk for pressure ulcer formation:
     a. Use a pressure-reducing or pressure-relieving overlay on the mattress.
     b. Assess skin pressure areas, especially the coccyx, elbows, hips, and heels, daily for signs of redness or open areas.
     c. Assist the patient to change positions at least every 2 hours.
  3. Monitor for patient response to drug therapy:
     a. Weigh the patient daily.
     b. Anticipate increased urine output; document intake and output.
  4. Observe for manifestations of electrolyte imbalance:
     a. Changes in nerve, muscles or cardiac excitability including electrocardiographic (ECG) patterns of hyperacute T waves
     b. Changes in sodium and potassium values

5. Nutrition therapy, teach patients and families about:
   a. Sodium restriction
   b. Fluid restriction

HYPERPARATHYROIDISM

OVERVIEW

- Hyperparathyroidism results from increased levels of parathyroid hormone (PTH) that act directly on the kidney, causing increased kidney resorption of calcium and increased phosphate excretion. These processes cause hypercalcemia (excessive calcium) and hypophosphatemia (inadequate phosphate).
- Primary hyperparathyroidism results when one or more parathyroid glands do not respond to the normal feedback mechanisms for serum calcium levels. The most common cause is a benign tumor in one parathyroid gland.
- Secondary hyperparathyroidism is a response to the hypocalcemia associated with chronic kidney disease and vitamin D deficiency, which leads to hyperplasia of the parathyroid glands.

PATIENT-CENTERED COLLABORATIVE CARE

Assessment

- Obtain patient information about:
  1. Bone fractures
  2. Recent weight loss
  3. Arthritis
  4. Psychological distress
  5. History of radiation treatment to the head or neck
  6. History of kidney stones
- Assess for and document:
  1. Waxy pallor of the skin
  2. Bone deformities in the extremities and back
  3. GI manifestations:
     a. Anorexia, nausea, vomiting
     b. Epigastric pain
     c. Constipation
  4. Fatigue and lethargy
  5. Confusion, coma (severe hyperparathyroidism)
  6. Laboratory values:
     a. High serum calcium levels
     b. High serum PTH levels
     c. Low serum phosphorus levels
- Diagnostic studies include:
  1. Serum electrolyte levels

H

2. Serum PTH and urine cyclic adenosine monophosphate (cAMP) levels
3. X-rays that show calcium deposits, renal stones, or bone lesions and loss of bone density
4. Computed tomography (CT) with or without arteriography

Interventions

Nonsurgical Management

- Diuretic and hydration therapies are used most often for reducing serum calcium levels in patients who are not candidates for surgery.
- Nursing management includes:
  1. Evaluating cardiac rate, rhythm, and waveforms with continuous electrocardiographic [ECG] monitoring
  2. Measuring intake and output 2 to 4 hours during hydration therapy
  3. Closely monitoring serum calcium levels for return to safe range

◼ NURSING SAFETY PRIORITY: Critical Rescue

Immediately report any sudden drop in the calcium level to the health care provider.

  4. Assessing for tingling and numbness in the hands, feet, and around the mouth
  5. Preventing injury by:
     a. Teaching all members of the health care team to handle the patient carefully
     b. Using a lift sheet to reposition the patient rather than pulling him or her
     c. Ensuring that the patient is accompanied when ambulating to prevent falls

- Drug therapy when hydration and furosemide (Lasix) do not correct hypercalcemia:
  1. Oral phosphates
  2. Calcium chelators:
     a. Plicamycin (Mithracin)
     b. Penicillamine (Cuprimine, Pendramine ♣)
  3. Drugs that inhibit calcium resorption from bone:
     a. Calcitonin (Calcimar)
     b. Bisphosphonates (etidronate)
     c. Prostaglandin synthesis inhibitors (aspirin, NSAIDs)

Surgical Management

- Surgical management of hyperparathyroidism is parathyroidectomy. It involves a transverse incision in the lower neck. All four parathyroid glands are examined for enlargement. If a tumor is present on one side but the other side is normal, the surgeon removes the glands containing tumor and leaves the remaining glands on the opposite side intact. If all four glands are diseased, they are all removed.

- Provide preoperative care, including:
  1. Implementing routine preoperative care as described in Part One
  2. Teaching about neck support by having the patient place both hands behind his or her neck to assist in elevating the head
- Provide postoperative care, including:
  1. Implementing routine postoperative care as described in Part One
  2. Closely observing the patient for respiratory distress, which may occur from calcium gluconate, compression of the trachea by hemorrhage, or swelling of neck tissues
  3. Ensuring that emergency equipment, including suction, oxygen, and tracheostomy equipment, is at the bedside

■ NURSING SAFETY PRIORITY: Critical Rescue

If severe swelling occurs and the airway begins to be obstructed, notify the Rapid Response Team to remove the clips from the incision to preserve the airway.

  4. Monitoring vital signs and identifying/reporting significant changes in status
  5. Checking the neck dressing for abnormal amounts of drainage or bleeding
  6. Checking serum calcium levels immediately after surgery and every 4 hours thereafter until calcium levels stabilize
  7. Monitoring for manifestations of hypocalcemia:
     a. Tingling and twitching in the extremities and face
     b. Positive Trousseau's sign
     c. Positive Chvostek's sign (see *Hypocalcemia*)
  8. Assess for damage to the recurrent laryngeal nerve:
     a. Changes in voice patterns
     b. Hoarseness
- If all four parathyroid glands are removed, the patient will need lifelong treatment with calcium and vitamin D, because the resulting hypoparathyroidism is permanent.

HYPERPITUITARISM

OVERVIEW

- Hyperpituitarism is a condition of hormone oversecretion that occurs with pituitary tumors or hyperplasia.

- Tumors occur most often in the anterior pituitary cells that produce growth hormone (GH), prolactin (PRL), and adrenocorticotropic hormone (ACTH).
- Overproduction of GH results in acromegaly, manifested by increased skeletal thickness, hypertrophy of the skin, and enlargement of all visceral organs.
- Excess ACTH overstimulates the adrenal cortex, resulting in excessive production of glucocorticoids, mineralocorticoids, and androgens, which leads to the development of Cushing's disease.

Genetic/Genomic Considerations

- An uncommon cause of hyperpituitarism is type 1 multiple endocrine neoplasia (MEN1), in which there is inactivation of a suppressor gene. This problem has an autosomal dominant inheritance pattern and is usually expressed as a benign tumor that affects the pituitary gland, parathyroid glands, and pancreas.
- In pituitary function, MEN1 leads to excessive production of GH and acromegaly.

PATIENT-CENTERED COLLABORATIVE CARE
Assessment

- Obtain patient information about:
  1. Age and gender
  2. Family history of endocrine problems
  3. Any change in hat, glove, ring, or shoe size
  4. Fatigue and lethargy
  5. Backache
  6. Arthralgias (joint pain)
  7. Headaches and changes in vision
  8. Menstrual changes (e.g., amenorrhea, irregular menses, difficulty in becoming pregnant)
  9. Changes in sexual functioning (e.g., decreased libido, painful intercourse, impotence)
  10. Loss of or change in secondary sexual characteristics
  11. Weight gain or loss (unplanned)
- Assess for and document:
  1. Changes in the facial features (e.g., increases in lip and nose sizes; prominent brow ridge; increases in head, hand, and foot sizes)
  2. Moon face
  3. Extremity muscle wasting
  4. Acne
  5. Hirsutism
  6. Striae
  7. Hypertension

    8. Areas of uneven pigmentation or hyperpigmentation
    9. Tachycardia or bradycardia
   10. Dysrhythmias
- Diagnostic testing may include:
    1. Blood test for hormone levels (any or all may be elevated)
    2. Skull x-rays
    3. Computed tomography (CT)
    4. Magnetic resonance imaging (MRI)
    5. Angiography (brain)
    6. Hormone suppression tests

Interventions

Surgical Management

- Surgical removal of the pituitary gland and tumor (hypophysectomy) is the most common treatment for hyperpituitarism.
- A minimally invasive transnasal or a trans-sphenoidal hypophysectomy is the most commonly used surgical approach. With a trans-sphenoidal approach, the surgeon makes an incision just above the upper lip and reaches the pituitary gland through the sphenoid sinus.
- A craniotomy may be needed if the tumor cannot be reached by a trans-sphenoidal approach.
- Provide preoperative care, including:
    1. Implementing routine preoperative care as described in Part One
    2. Explaining that hypophysectomy decreases hormone levels, relieves headaches, and may reverse changes in sexual functioning
    3. Reminding the patient that body changes, organ enlargement, and visual changes are not usually reversible
    4. Explaining that because nasal packing is present for 2 to 3 days after surgery, it will be necessary to breathe through the mouth, and a "mustache dressing" ("drip pad") will be placed under the nose
    5. Instructing the patient not to brush teeth, cough, sneeze, blow the nose, or bend forward after surgery
- Provide postoperative care, including:
    1. Implementing routine postoperative care as described in Part One
    2. Monitoring neurologic responses hourly for the first 24 hours and then every 4 hours and documenting any changes in vision, mental status, altered level of consciousness, or decreased strength of the extremities
    3. Observing for complications such as transient diabetes insipidus, cerebrospinal fluid (CSF) leakage, infection, and increased intracranial pressure (ICP):
       a. Excess output may indicate onset of diabetes insipidus.

H

     b. Any postnasal drip may indicate leakage of CSF.

     c. Assess nasal drainage for quantity, quality and odor; send a sample to the laboratory for testing as the presence of glucose may confirm CSF drainage.

4. Keeping the head of the bed elevated

5. Instructing the patient to avoid coughing early after surgery and reminding him or her to perform deep-breathing exercises hourly while awake

6. Instructing the patient to avoid bending at the waist for any reason, because this position increases ICP

7. Performing frequent oral rinses and applying water-soluble jelly to dry lips

8. Assessing for manifestations of meningitis:

     a. Headache

     b. Fever

     c. Nuchal (neck) rigidity

9. Teaching the patient self-administration of the prescribed hormones

Nonsurgical Management

- The goals of therapy for the patient who has hyperpituitarism are to return hormone levels to normal or near-normal, reduce or eliminate headache and visual disturbances, prevent complications, and reverse as many of the body changes as possible.
- Encourage the patient to express concerns and fears about his or her altered physical appearance.
- Help him or her identify personal strengths and positive characteristics.
- Drug therapy may be used alone or in combination with surgery or radiation:
  1. Dopamine agonists to stimulate dopamine receptors in the brain and inhibit the release of many pituitary hormones, especially prolactin and GH:
     a. Bromocriptine (Parlodel)
     b. Cabergoline (Dostinex)
     c. Pergolide (Permax)
  2. Somatostatin analogs and GH receptor blockers (for GH-secreting tumors)
     a. Octreotide (Sandostatin)
     b. Pegvisomant (Somavert)
- Radiation therapy regimens take a long time to complete, and several years may pass before a therapeutic effect can be seen. Side effects of radiation therapy include hypopituitarism, optic nerve damage, and other eye and vision problems.

HYPERTENSION

OVERVIEW

- Hypertension is a systolic blood pressure (SBP) at or above 140 mm Hg and/or a diastolic blood pressure (DBP) at or above 90 mm Hg in people who do not have diabetes mellitus. Patients with diabetes and heart disease should have a blood pressure (BP) below 130/90.
- *Prehypertension* is defined as an SBP of 120 to 139 mm Hg or a DBP of 80 to 89 mm Hg.
- Hypertension is the major risk factor for coronary, cerebral, kidney, retinal (vision), and peripheral vascular disease.
- There are two major classifications of hypertension:
  1. Primary, with no known cause and associated with risk factors such as a family history of hypertension, age older than 60 years, hyperlipidemia, stress, and smoking
  2. Secondary hypertension, which results from specific diseases such as kidney vascular and kidney disease, primary aldosteronism, Cushing's disease, coarctation of the aorta, brain tumors and encephalitis, psychiatric disorders, and some drugs, such as estrogen-containing oral contraceptives, glucocorticoids, mineralocorticoids, cyclosporine, and erythropoietin
- The process of *vascular autoregulation*, which keeps perfusion of tissues in the body relatively constant, appears to be important in causing hypertension. This mechanism is poorly understood.

⊕ Cultural Awareness

The prevalence of hypertension in African Americans in the United States is among the highest in the world and is constantly increasing. When compared with Euro-Americans, they develop high BP earlier in life, making them much more likely to die from strokes, heart disease, and kidney disease. The reason for these differences is not known, but genetics and environmental factors may play a role.

PATIENT-CENTERED COLLABORATIVE CARE

Assessment

- Record patient information:
  1. Age
  2. Race or ethnic origin
  3. Family history of hypertension
  4. Average daily intake of calories, sodium, and potassium-containing foods
  5. Alcohol intake

6. Smoking history
7. Exercise habits
8. Past and present history of kidney or cardiovascular disease
9. Drug use (prescribed, over-the-counter [OTC], and illicit)
10. Blood pressure readings in both arms
11. Blood pressure readings in supine and erect positions
12. Peripheral pulse rate, rhythm, and force
13. Psychosocial stressors

✓ NATIONAL PATIENT SAFETY GOAL

Accurately and completely reconcile medications from home used to treat hypertension so that home drugs can be continued in the hospital.

- Assess for hypertensive symptoms:
  1. Headache, dizziness, facial flushing or fainting
  2. Edema
  3. Nocturia
  4. Lethargy
  5. Nosebleeds
  6. Vision changes or retinal changes on funduscopic examination
  7. Signs of kidney injury, such as elevated blood urea nitrogen (BUN) or creatinine levels or low urine output
  8. Physical findings related to vascular damage, including atherosclerosis, acute coronary syndrome, and heart failure:
     a. Abdominal, carotid, or femoral bruits
     b. Tachycardia, sweating, and pallor
     c. Decreased or absent femoral pulses
     d. Cardiomegaly or left ventricular hypertrophy
  9. Diagnostic tests that indicate severity of primary or secondary causes of hypertension:
     a. Kidney disease can be diagnosed by the presence of protein, red blood cells, pus cells, and casts in the urine; elevated levels of BUN; and elevated serum creatinine levels.
     b. Urinary test results are positive for the presence of catecholamines in patients with a pheochromocytoma (tumor of the adrenal medulla).
     c. An elevation in levels of serum corticoids and 17-ketosteroids in the urine is diagnostic of Cushing's disease.
     d. An electrocardiogram (ECG) determines the degree of cardiac involvement. Left atrial and ventricular hypertrophy is the first ECG sign of heart disease resulting from hypertension. Left ventricular remodeling can be detected on the 12-lead ECG.

NOTE: When a diagnosis of hypertension is made, most people have no symptoms.

Planning and Implementation

- Assist with planning and implementing lifestyle changes, including the regular evaluation of BP outside of office visits:
  1. In collaboration with the dietitian:
     a. Advise the patient to restrict sodium intake to less than 2 g daily by not adding table salt to food, not cooking with salt, and not adding seasonings that contain sodium and to limit eating canned, frozen, and other processed foods.
     b. Suggest that the patient use spices, herbs, fruits, and other non–salt-containing substances such as powdered garlic and onion or a salt substitute to enhance the flavor of food.
     c. Advise the patient to consider strategies to promote ideal body weight.
     d. Develop a plan to reduce saturated fat and cholesterol in the diet.
  2. Advise the patient to restrict alcohol intake and smoking.
  3. Collaborate with the physician and physical therapist to assist the patient in developing a regular exercise program.
  4. Teach or refer the patient to stress management programs including yoga, massage, biofeedback, and hypnosis programs.
  5. In collaboration with the pharmacist, provide drug therapy as prescribed and support adherence to prescribed drugs at home. Most patients require two drugs from different classes to control hypertension:
     a. Diuretics:
        (1) Thiazide diuretics prevent sodium and water resorption in the distal tubules of the kidneys and may improve endothelial health.
        (2) Loop diuretics depress sodium resorption in the ascending loop of Henle and promote potassium excretion.
        (3) Potassium-sparing diuretics act on the distal tubules of the kidneys to inhibit resorption of sodium in exchange for potassium ions, retaining potassium. Aldosterone inhibitors also interfere with the renin-angiotensin-aldosterone system, promoting vascular health.
     b. Angiotensin blockers:
        (1) Angiotensin-converting enzyme (ACE) inhibitors convert angiotensin I to angiotensin II, resulting in vasorelaxation and diuresis.

H

(2) Angiotensin receptor blockers (ARBs) selectively block the binding of angiotensin II in the vascular and adrenal tissue.

(3) Beta-adrenergic blockers lower blood pressure by blocking beta receptors in the heart and kidneys, reducing the cardiac rate and blocking renin release.

(4) Central alpha agonists act on the central nervous system, preventing reuptake of norepinephrine, resulting in lower peripheral vascular resistance and blood pressure.

(5) Calcium channel blockers lower blood pressure by interfering with transmembrane influx of calcium ions, resulting in vasoconstriction.

(6) A newer class of drugs, *renin inhibitors,* is effective for mild to moderate hypertension.

(7) *Alpha-adrenergic antagonists,* such as prazosin (Minipress), doxazosin (Cardura), and terazosin (Hytrin), dilate the arterioles and veins. These drugs can lower blood pressure quickly, but their use is limited because of frequent and bothersome side effects.

✅ NATIONAL PATIENT SAFETY GOAL

Improve the safety of using drugs to treat hypertension by standardizing the drug concentrations used within the organization and identifying look-alike and sound-alike drugs to determine how to prevent errors involving the interchange of these drugs.

⬛ NURSING SAFETY PRIORITY: Action Alert

Monitor the patient's serum potassium level for abnormal values when administering a diuretic, ACE inhibitor, or ARB.

- Monitor risk for and actual end-organ damage from chronic hypertension, particularly kidney function, cardiac function, and vascular perfusion to the brain and periphery. Evaluate for noncompliance related to knowledge and behaviors needed to implement lifestyle changes, medication use and self-monitoring of BP.

Community-Based Care

- Provide educational information for hypertension control, especially:
  1. Salt restriction
  2. Weight maintenance or reduction
  3. Possibly a diet intake record to increase self-awareness of food selections
  4. Stress reduction or coping strategies

    5. Alcohol restriction

    6. Exercise program

    7. Taking prescribed antihypertensive drugs even in the absence of symptoms

    8. Regular ongoing follow-up with health care provider

- Give oral and written information on drug therapy, including:
  1. Rationale for use, dose, and time of administration
  2. Side effects and vigilance for drug interactions
  3. The importance of taking the drugs even when there are no symptoms
- Instruct the patient and family members in the technique of blood pressure monitoring at home.
- Teach the patient or family member to obtain heart rate and record blood pressure readings in a logbook or diary.
- Refer the patient to home care agency, if necessary.
- Provide written and visual education materials from authoritative sources such as the American Heart Association (AHA).

HYPERTHYROIDISM

OVERVIEW

- Hyperthyroidism is excessive thyroid hormone secretion from the thyroid gland. It is one of the most common endocrine disorders and affects women 5 to 10 times more often than men.
- The manifestations of hyperthyroidism are called *thyrotoxicosis,* regardless of the origin of the thyroid hormones.
- Thyroid hormones affect metabolism in all body organs and excesses produce many different manifestations.
- The most common cause is Graves' disease, an autoimmune disorder in which antibodies are made and attach to the thyroid-stimulating hormone (TSH) receptor sites on the thyroid tissue. The thyroid-stimulating immunoglobulins (TSIs) bind to the thyroid gland, increasing its size and overproducing thyroid hormones.

Genetic/Genomic Considerations

- Graves' disease appears to have a strong association with other autoimmune disorders, such as diabetes mellitus, vitiligo, and rheumatoid arthritis.
- It often occurs in both members of identical twins, with an inheritance pattern of familial clustering or complex polygenic inheritance.

- Other causes include benign or malignant tumors and excessive use of thyroid replacement drugs.

H

- *Thyroid storm*, or *thyroid crisis*, is a life-threatening condition of an extreme state of hyperthyroidism that can occur when the condition is uncontrolled or can be triggered by stressors such as trauma, infection, diabetic ketoacidosis, and pregnancy. Key manifestations include fever, tachycardia, and systolic hypertension.

PATIENT-CENTERED COLLABORATIVE CARE
Assessment
- Obtain patient information about:
  1. Age and gender
  2. Usual weight and any unplanned weight loss
  3. Increased appetite
  4. Increased number of daily bowel movements
  5. Heat intolerance
  6. Diaphoresis (increased sweating) even when environmental temperatures are comfortable for others
  7. Palpitations or chest pain
  8. Dyspnea (with or without exertion)
  9. Visual changes, especially exophthalmos (specific to Graves' disease)
  10. Fatigue, weakness
  11. Insomnia (common)
  12. Irritability, depression
  13. Amenorrhea or a decreased menstrual flow (common)
  14. Changes in libido
  15. Previous thyroid surgery or radiation therapy to the neck
  16. Past and current drugs, especially the use of thyroid hormone replacement or antithyroid drugs
- Assess for and document:
  1. Exophthalmos (Graves' disease)
  2. Photophobia
  3. General appearance:
     a. Eyelid retraction (Graves' disease)
     b. Eyeball lag (the upper eyelid pulls back faster than the eyeball when the patient gazes upward) (Graves' disease)
  4. Presence or absence of a goiter (enlarged thyroid gland)
  5. Hypertension
  6. Tachycardia
  7. Dysrhythmias
  8. Fine, soft, silky hair
  9. Warm, moist skin
  10. Tremors
  11. Hyperactive deep tendon reflexes

- Psychosocial issues or changes may include:
  1. Wide mood swings
  2. Irritability
  3. Decreased attention span
  4. Mild to severe hyperactivity
- Diagnostic assessment may include:
  1. Blood tests for:
     a. Triiodothyronine (T_3)
     b. Thyroxine (T_4)
     c. T_3 resin uptake (T_3RU)
     d. TSH
     e. Antibodies to TSH (TSH-rAb) (Graves' disease)
  2. Thyroid scan:
  3. Ultrasonography of the thyroid gland
  4. Electrocardiograph (ECG)
     a. Tachycardia
     b. Atrial fibrillation
     c. Dysrhythmias
     d. Changes in P and T waveforms

Interventions

- Interventions are described for Graves' disease, because it is the most common form of hyperthyroidism. The goals of management are to decrease the effect of thyroid hormone on cardiac function and to reduce thyroid hormone secretion.

  Nonsurgical Management
- Monitoring, including:
  1. Measuring apical pulse and blood pressure at least every 4 hours and reporting status changes in a timely manner
  2. Checking temperature at least every 4 hours and reporting fever in a timely manner

⬛ NURSING SAFETY PRIORITY: Critical Rescue

Immediately report a temperature increase of even 1° F (.3° C), because it may indicate impending thyroid crisis.

  3. Instructing the patient to immediately report:
     a. Palpitations
     b. Dyspnea
     c. Vertigo
     d. Chest pain
- Drug therapy:
  1. Antithyroid drugs:
     a. Propylthiouracil (PTU)
     b. Methimazole (Tapazole)
  2. Iodine preparations

   3. Lithium
   4. Supportive drug therapy with propranolol (Inderal, Detensol ✦) to relieve diaphoresis, anxiety, tachycardia, and palpitations
- Radioactive iodine (RAI) therapy:
   1. Is not used in pregnant women because ^{131}I crosses the placenta and can damage the fetal thyroid gland
   2. Can be delivered as an oral drug or IV
   3. Is dependent on the thyroid gland's size and sensitivity to radiation for dosage
   4. Destroys some of the cells that produce thyroid hormone
   5. Is performed on an outpatient basis
   6. May be sufficient with one dose, although a second or third dose may be needed
   7. Is at a low enough dosage of radiation that radiation precautions are not needed
   8. May take 4 to 8 weeks for results
   9. May cause some patients to experience hypothyroidism as a result of the treatment

   Surgical Management
- Surgery to remove all (total thyroidectomy) or part of the thyroid gland (subtotal thyroidectomy) may be needed for patients who have a large goiter causing tracheal or esophageal compression or who do not have a good response to antithyroid drugs.
- A thyroidectomy is performed with the patient under general anesthesia. The surgeon makes a "collar incision" just above the clavicle.
- After a total thyroidectomy, patients must take lifelong thyroid hormone replacement.
- Provide preoperative care, including:
   1. Implementing routine preoperative care as described in Part One
   2. Administering antithyroid drugs and iodine preparations to decrease the secretion of thyroid hormones and reduce thyroid size and vascularity
   3. Ensuring that hypertension, dysrhythmias, and tachycardia are controlled before surgery
   4. Teaching patient to support the neck when coughing or moving by placing both hands behind the neck when moving
   5. Explaining that hoarseness may be present for a few days as a result of endotracheal tube placement during surgery
   6. Reassuring the patient by calmly explaining the surgery and the care after surgery

7. Reminding him or her that a drain and dressing may be in place after surgery
8. Answering any questions the patient and family have
- Providing postoperative care, including:
   1. Implementing routine postoperative care as described in Part One
   2. Using sandbags or pillows to support the head and neck
   3. Placing the patient, while he or she is awake, in a semi-Fowler's position
   4. Decreasing tension on the suture line by avoiding neck extension
   5. Humidifying the air
   6. Suctioning oral and tracheal secretions when necessary
   7. Preventing complications:
      a. Respiratory distress:
         (1) Listening for laryngeal stridor (harsh, high-pitched respiratory sounds)
         (2) Keeping emergency tracheostomy equipment in the patient's room
         (3) Ensuring that oxygen and suctioning equipment are nearby and in working order

■ NURSING SAFETY PRIORITY: Critical Rescue

If symptoms of obstruction occur, notify the Rapid Response Team. In some agencies, the nurse can remove clips or sutures when medical assistance is not immediately available and swelling at the surgical site is obstructing the airway.

      b. Hemorrhage:
         (1) Inspecting the neck dressing and behind the patient's neck for blood at least every 2 hours for the first 24 hours
         (2) Assessing drainage for amount, color, and character
      c. Hypocalcemia and tetany:
         (1) Asking the patient hourly about any tingling around the mouth or of the toes and fingers
         (2) Assessing for muscle twitching
         (3) Ensuring calcium gluconate or calcium chloride is available
      d. Laryngeal nerve damage:
         (1) Assessing the patient's voice at 2-hour intervals
         (2) Reassuring the patient that hoarseness is usually temporary

H

- Emergency management of thyroid storm or thyroid crisis:
  1. Thyroid storm or crisis is a life-threatening event that occurs in patients with uncontrolled hyperthyroidism and occurs most often with Graves' disease.
  2. Key manifestations include fever, tachycardia, and systolic hypertension.
  3. Even with treatment, thyroid storm may lead to death:
     a. Maintain a patent airway and adequate ventilation.
     b. Give antithyroid drugs as prescribed: propylthiouracil (PTU, Propyl-Thyracil ✤), 300 to 900 mg daily, and methimazole (Tapazole), up to 60 mg daily.
     c. Administer sodium iodide solution, 2 g IV daily, as prescribed.
     d. Give propranolol (Inderal, Detensol ✤), 1 to 3 mg IV, as prescribed. Give slowly over 3 minutes; the patient should be connected to a cardiac monitor, and a central venous pressure catheter should be in place.
     e. Give glucocorticoids as prescribed: hydrocortisone, 100 to 500 mg IV daily; prednisone, 4 to 60 mg orally daily; or dexamethasone, 2 mg IM or IV every 6 hours.
     f. Monitor continually for cardiac dysrhythmias.
     g. Monitor vital signs every 30 minutes for early detection of status change.
     h. Provide comfort measures, including a cooling blanket.
     i. Give nonsalicylate antipyretics, as prescribed.
     j. Correct dehydration with normal saline infusions.
     k. Apply cooling blanket or ice packs to reduce fever.

Community-Based Care

- Teach the patient and family about:
  1. The manifestations of hyperthyroidism and instructing them to report an increase or recurrence of symptoms
  2. The manifestations of hypothyroidism and the need for thyroid hormone replacement
  3. The need for regular follow-up, because hypothyroidism can occur several years after radioactive iodine (RAI) therapy
  4. Pertinent information about any prescribed drugs, including side effects
  5. Inspecting the incision area and reporting redness, tenderness, drainage, or swelling to the surgeon
  6. Possible continued mood changes, reassuring the patient and family that these effects will decrease with continued treatment

HYPOCALCEMIA

OVERVIEW

- Hypocalcemia is a total serum calcium (Ca^{2+}) level less than 9 mg/dL or 2.25 mmol/L.
- Because the normal blood level of calcium is so low, any change in calcium levels has major effects on function.
- Common causes of hypocalcemia include:
  1. Decreased calcium absorption from the GI tract:
     a. Inadequate oral intake of calcium
     b. Lactose intolerance
     c. Malabsorption syndromes (celiac disease [sprue], Crohn's disease)
     d. Inadequate intake of vitamin D
  2. Increased calcium excretion:
     a. End-stage kidney disease
     b. Kidney failure (polyuric phase)
     c. Diarrhea
     d. Steatorrhea
     e. Wound drainage (especially GI)
  3. Conditions that reduce calcium in the blood:
     a. Hyperproteinemia
     b. Alkalosis
     c. Calcium chelators or binders (citrate, mithramycin, penicillamine, cellulose sodium phosphate [Calcibind], pamidronate [Aredia])
     d. Acute pancreatitis
     e. Hyperphosphatemia
     f. Immobility
     g. Removal or destruction of parathyroid glands
- Low serum calcium levels increase sodium movement across excitable membranes, allowing depolarization to occur more easily and at inappropriate times.
- The more rapidly hypocalcemia occurs and the more severe it is, the more likely life-threatening manifestations will occur.

Cultural Awareness

- Lactose intolerance caused by a deficiency of the enzyme lactase occurs in 75% to 90% of all Asians, African Americans, and American Indians.
- People with lactose intolerance cannot use the nutrients in milk and have cramping, diarrhea, and abdominal pain after ingesting dairy products. Dairy products, especially milk, are common and rich sources of calcium and vitamin D.

H

- People with lactose intolerance may have difficulty obtaining enough calcium and vitamin D from other sources to maintain normal calcium levels in the blood and bones.

Women's Health Considerations
- Postmenopausal women are at risk for chronic calcium loss as a result of decreased estrogen levels.
- Reduced weight-bearing exercise can contribute to hypocalcemia and accelerate osteoporosis; older women particularly need to maintain weight-bearing activities such as walking and running.

PATIENT-CENTERED COLLABORATIVE CARE
Assessment
- Assess for and document:
  1. Neuromuscular changes (most common):
     a. Paresthesias with sensations of tingling and numbness
     b. Muscle twitches, painful cramps, and spasms
     c. Anxiety, irritability
     d. Hyperactive deep tendon reflexes
     e. Positive Trousseau's sign: Place a blood pressure cuff around the upper arm, inflate the cuff to greater than the patient's systolic pressure, and keep the cuff inflated for 1 to 4 minutes. Under these hypoxic conditions, a positive Trousseau's sign occurs when the hand and fingers go into spasm in palmar flexion.
     f. Positive Chvostek's sign: Tap the face just below and in front of the ear (over the facial nerve) to trigger facial twitching of one side of the mouth, nose, and cheek.
  2. Cardiovascular changes:
     a. Bradycardia
     b. Weak, thready pulse
     c. Hypotension
     d. Electrocardiographic (ECG) changes (prolonged ST interval, prolonged QT interval)
  3. GI changes:
     a. Hyperactive bowel sounds
     b. Abdominal cramping
     c. Diarrhea
  4. Skeletal changes (thin, brittle, and fragile bones):
     a. Overall loss of height
     b. Presence of spinal curvatures
     c. Unexplained bone pain

Interventions

- Drug therapy with:
  1. Direct calcium replacement (oral and IV)
  2. Drugs that enhance the absorption of calcium, such as aluminum hydroxide and vitamin D
  3. Drugs that decrease nerve and muscle responses (magnesium sulfate and various muscle relaxants)
- Nutrition therapy with a high-calcium diet (collaborate with a dietitian to teach patients about foods high in calcium)
- Additional interventions include:
  1. Environmental management to reduce stimulation:
     a. Keeping the room quiet
     b. Limiting visitors
     c. Adjusting the lighting
     d. Using a soft but reassuring voice
  2. Keeping emergency equipment (e.g., oxygen, suction, emergency drugs, endotracheal tray) readily available
  3. Injury prevention strategies:
     a. Using a lift sheet when lifting or moving a patient with fragile bones
     b. Observing for normal range of joint motion and for any unusual surface bumps or depressions over bony areas

HYPOKALEMIA

OVERVIEW

- Hypokalemia is a serum potassium level less than 3.5 mEq/L (3.5 mmol/L).
- It can be life threatening, because every body system is affected.
- With hypokalemia, the cell membranes of all excitable tissues, such as nerve and muscle, are less responsive to normal stimuli.
- Rapid reduction of serum potassium levels causes dramatic changes in function, whereas gradual reductions may not show changes in function until the level is very low.
- Common causes include:
  1. Inappropriate or excessive use of drugs:
     a. Diuretics
     b. Digitalis
     c. Corticosteroids
  2. Increased secretion of aldosterone
  3. Cushing's syndrome/disease
  4. Diarrhea
  5. Vomiting
  6. Wound drainage (especially GI)

   7. Prolonged nasogastric suction
   8. Excessive diaphoresis
   9. Kidney disease impairing resorption of potassium
  10. NPO status
  11. Alkalosis
  12. Hyperinsulinism
  13. Total parenteral nutrition
  14. Water intoxication
  15. IV therapy with potassium-poor solutions
  16. Age; kidneys may have reduced ability to concentrate
       urine

PATIENT-CENTERED COLLABORATIVE CARE
Assessment
- Obtain patient information about:
  1. Age
  2. Drugs, especially diuretics, corticosteroids, digoxin, beta-adrenergic agonists or antagonists, and potassium supplements
  3. Presence of any acute or chronic disease
  4. Diet history
- Assess for and document:
  1. Respiratory changes:

■ NURSING SAFETY PRIORITY: Critical Rescue

Skeletal muscle weakness results in shallow respirations. Respiratory status should be assessed first in any patient who may have hypokalemia.

---

   a. Breath sounds
   b. Ease of respiratory effort
   c. Color of nail beds and mucous membranes
   d. Rate and depth of respiration
   e. Oxygen saturation
  2. Musculoskeletal changes for weakness:
   a. Weak hand grasps
   b. Decreased deep tendon reflexes
   c. Flaccid paralysis
  3. Cardiovascular changes:
   a. Rapid, thready pulse
   b. Peripheral pulses difficult to palpate
   c. Dysrhythmias and electrocardiographic (ECG) changes:
       (1) ST-segment depression
       (2) Flat or inverted T waves
       (3) Increased U waves

◼ NURSING SAFETY PRIORITY: Critical Rescue

Dysrhythmias can lead to death, particularly in older adults. Report ECG changes consistent with hypokalemia to the physician or Rapid Response Team.

    d. Orthostatic hypotension
4. Neurologic changes:
    a. Altered mental status
    b. Irritability and anxiety
    c. Lethargy, acute confusion, coma
5. GI changes:
    a. Hypoactive bowel sounds
    b. Nausea, vomiting
    c. Constipation
    d. Abdominal distention
    e. Paralytic ileus
6. Serum potassium value below 3.5 mEq/L (3.5 mmol/L)

Interventions

- Interventions for hypokalemia aim to prevent potassium loss, increase serum potassium levels, and provide a safe environment for the patient.
- Medical interventions include:
  1. Drug therapy:
     a. Oral potassium supplements
     b. IV potassium for severe hypokalemia
     c. In the presence of persistent hypokalemia despite replacement therapy, evaluate and consider replacing magnesium.

H

▽ NATIONAL PATIENT SAFETY GOAL

Potassium is available in different concentrations, and this drug carries a high alert warning as a concentrated electrolyte solution. Although the drug is usually added to the IV solution in the pharmacy, it may be added on the nursing unit. Check and re-check the concentration of the drug in the vial with another registered nurse, a pharmacist, or a physician, and carefully calculate the required dilution before adding it to the IV solution. A dilution of no more than 1 mEq/10 mL of solution is recommended. The maximum recommended infusion rate is 5 to 10 mEq/hr; this rate is never to exceed 20 mEq/hr under any circumstances. Cardiac monitoring may be necessary during IV potassium administration. Because rapid infusion of potassium can cause cardiac arrest, potassium is not given by IV push.

⚠ NURSING SAFETY PRIORITY: Drug Alert

Potassium is a severe tissue irritant and is never given by IM or subcutaneous injection.

   d. Potassium-sparing diuretics:
      (1) Spironolactone (Aldactone, Novo-Spiroton ✦)
      (2) Triamterene (Dyrenium)
      (3) Amiloride (Midamor)
   2. Nutrition therapy to increase dietary potassium intake
- The priorities for nursing care of the patient with hypokalemia are ensuring adequate oxygenation, preventing patient falls, preventing injury from potassium administration, and monitoring the patient's response to therapy.
   1. Implementing safety measures:
      a. Instituting falls precautions
      b. Eliminating hazards in the ambulation path
      c. Assisting with ambulation
   2. Performing respiratory monitoring at least hourly for severe hypokalemia:
      a. Rate and depth (checking for increasing rate and decreasing depth)
      b. Oxygen saturation by pulse oximetry
      c. Patient's ability to cough
      d. Evaluation of arterial blood gas values (when available).

HYPONATREMIA

OVERVIEW

- Hyponatremia is a serum sodium (Na^+) level less than 136 mEq/L (136 mmol/L), and it often occurs with fluid volume imbalances.
- The problems caused by hyponatremia involve reduced excitable membrane depolarization and cellular swelling.
- Common causes of hyponatremia include:
   1. Poor intake of sodium or excessive sodium loss:
      a. Excessive diaphoresis
      b. Diuretics (high-ceiling diuretics)
      c. Wound drainage (especially GI)
      d. Decreased secretion of aldosterone
      e. Hyperlipidemia
      f. Kidney disease (scarred distal convoluted tubule)
      g. NPO status
      h. Low-salt diet

2. Dilution of serum sodium:
   a. Excessive ingestion of hypotonic fluids
   b. Freshwater submersion accident
   c. Kidney failure (nephrotic syndrome)
   d. Irrigation with hypotonic fluids
   e. Syndrome of inappropriate antidiuretic hormone (SIADH)
   f. Hyperglycemia
   g. Heart failure

PATIENT-CENTERED COLLABORATIVE CARE
Assessment
- Assess for and document:
   1. Cerebral changes:
      a. Acute confusion
      b. Reduced level of cognition
      c. Seizure activity
   2. Neuromuscular changes:
      a. General muscle weakness, especially in arms and legs
      b. Diminished deep tendon reflexes

◼ NURSING SAFETY PRIORITY: Critical Rescue

If the patient has muscle weakness, immediately check respiratory effectiveness, because ventilation depends on adequate strength of respiratory muscles.

H

   3. GI changes:
      a. Increased motility
      b. Diarrhea
      c. Abdominal cramping
      d. Hyperactive bowel sounds
   4. Cardiovascular changes:
      a. Hyponatremia with hypovolemia:
         (1) Rapid, weak, thready pulse
         (2) Reduced peripheral pulses
         (3) Hypotension
      b. Hyponatremia with hypervolemia:
         (1) Full, bounding pulse
         (2) Normal or high blood pressure
         (3) Edema

Interventions
- Drug therapy:
   1. Discontinuing or reducing drugs that increase sodium loss, such as loop diuretics and thiazide diuretics

2. Hyponatremia with a fluid deficit: prescribing IV saline infusion to restore both sodium and fluid volume. Severe hyponatremia may be treated with small-volume infusions of hypertonic (2% to 3%) saline.

3. Hyponatremia with fluid excess: using osmotic diuretics that promote the excretion of water rather than sodium, such as mannitol (Osmitrol), or conivaptan (Vaprisol)

4. Hyponatremia caused by inappropriate secretion of antidiuretic hormone (ADH): therapy that includes agents that antagonize ADH, such as lithium and demeclocycline (Declomycin)

- Nutrition therapy:
  1. Increased oral sodium intake
  2. Fluid restriction when hyponatremia occurs with fluid excess

- Priorities for nursing care of the patient with hyponatremia include monitoring the patient's response to therapy and preventing hypernatremia and fluid overload:
  1. Prevent fluid overload from becoming worse, leading to pulmonary edema and heart failure:
     a. Monitor for indicators of increased fluid overload at least every 2 hours.

■ NURSING SAFETY PRIORITY: Critical Rescue

Pulmonary edema can occur very quickly and can lead to death. Notify the health care provider or Rapid Response Team about any change that indicates the fluid overload is not responding to therapy or is becoming worse.

  2. Reduce risk for pressure ulcer formation in the presence of reduced consciousness, sweating, or peripheral edema:
     a. Use a pressure-reducing or pressure-relieving overlay on the mattress.
     b. Assess skin pressure areas, especially the coccyx, elbows, hips, and heels, daily for signs of redness or open areas.
     c. Assist the patient to change positions at least every 2 hours.
  3. Monitor for patient response to drug therapy:
     a. Weigh daily
     b. Monitor amount and quality of urine output
  4. Observe for manifestations of electrolyte imbalance:
     a. Changes in neurologic, muscular, GI and cardiovascular health, including ECG patterns
     b. Changes in serum and urine sodium and potassium values

5. Nutritional therapy; teach patients and families about:
   a. Sodium intake
   b. Fluid restriction

HYPOPARATHYROIDISM

OVERVIEW

- Hypoparathyroidism is a rare endocrine disorder in which parathyroid function is decreased, resulting in a deficiency of circulating parathyroid hormone (PTH) levels.
- The main result is hypocalcemia.
- There are two forms:
  1. *Iatrogenic hypoparathyroidism,* the most common form, which is caused by the removal of all parathyroid tissue during total thyroidectomy or by deliberate surgical removal of the parathyroid glands
  2. *Idiopathic hypoparathyroidism,* which is rare and probably caused by an autoimmune problem

PATIENT-CENTERED COLLABORATIVE CARE
Assessment

- Obtain patient information about:
  1. Any head or neck surgery
  2. History of head or neck radiation therapy
  3. History of serious neck injury from a car crash or strangulation
  4. Presence of mild tingling and numbness around the mouth or in the hands and feet
  5. Presence of severe muscle cramps and spasms of the hands and feet
- Assess for and document:
  1. Irritability
  2. Psychosis
  3. Excessive or inappropriate muscle contractions that cause finger, hand, and elbow flexion
  4. Positive Chvostek's sign (see *Hypocalcemia*)
  5. Positive Trousseau's sign (see *Hypocalcemia*)
  6. Bands or pits encircling the crowns of the teeth
- Diagnostic tests for hypoparathyroidism include:
  1. Electroencephalography (EEG)
  2. Serum electrolyte tests, PTH levels
  3. Computed tomography (CT) of the brain (may show calcium deposits) and neck
  4. Urine cyclic adenosine monophosphate (cAMP) levels

H

Interventions

- Medical management focuses on correcting hypocalcemia, vitamin D deficiency, and hypomagnesemia.
  1. IV calcium is given as a 10% solution of calcium chloride or calcium gluconate over 10 to 15 minutes.
  2. Calcitriol (Rocaltrol), 0.5 to 2 mg daily for vitamin D deficiency
  3. For hypomagnesemia, magnesium sulfate is typically given orally at 3 g/dose to a maximum of 12 g/24 hr, or IV as 1 g/100 mL over 2 or more hours, repeated as needed to a maximum of 5 g/24 hr
  4. Long-term oral therapy of calcium, 0.5 to 2 g daily, in divided doses
  5. Long-term therapy with 50,000 to 400,000 units of ergocalciferol daily
- Nursing management includes:
  1. Teaching about the drug regimen and interventions to reduce anxiety
  2. Teaching the patient to eat foods high in calcium but low in phosphorus (milk, yogurt, and processed cheeses are avoided because of their high phosphorus content)
  3. Stressing that therapy for hypocalcemia is lifelong
  4. Advising the patient to wear a medical alert bracelet

HYPOPITUITARISM

OVERVIEW

- Hypopituitarism is a deficiency of one or more anterior pituitary hormones, resulting in metabolic problems and sexual dysfunction.
- Decreased production of all anterior pituitary hormones is a rare condition known as *panhypopituitarism.*
- Usually, there is a decrease in the secretion of one hormone and a lesser decrease in the other hormones.
- Clinical features will depend on which hormone is undersecreted.
- Deficiencies of adrenocorticotropic hormone (ACTH) and thyroid-stimulating hormone (TSH) are the most life threatening, because they result in a corresponding decrease in the secretion of vital hormones from the adrenal and thyroid glands.
- Causes of hypopituitarism include pituitary tumors, severe malnutrition or rapid loss of body fat, shock or severe hypotension, head trauma, brain tumors or infection, radiation or surgery of the head and brain, and AIDS.

PATIENT-CENTERED COLLABORATIVE CARE
Assessment
- Assess for and document:
  1. Loss of secondary sexual characteristics (men):
     a. Facial and body hair loss
     b. Impotence
     c. Decreased libido
  2. Loss of secondary sexual characteristics (women):
     a. Absence of menstrual periods
     b. Painful intercourse
     c. Infertility
     d. Decreased libido
     e. Breast atrophy
     f. Decreased amount or absence of auxiliary and pubic hair
  3. Changes in vision:
     a. Loss of visual acuity, especially peripheral vision
     b. Temporal headaches
     c. Diplopia (double vision)
     d. Ocular muscle paralysis, limiting eye movement
- Diagnostic assessment may include:
  1. Blood levels of pituitary hormones
  2. Hormone stimulation testing
  3. Skull x-rays
  4. Computed tomography (CT) scans
  5. Magnetic resonance imaging (MRI)
  6. Angiography (brain)

Interventions
- Management of the patient with hypopituitarism focuses on replacement of deficient hormones.
- Instruct the patient about the hormone replacement method and regimen:
  1. Men with gonadotropin deficiency receive sex steroid replacement therapy with androgens (testosterone) by IM injections or transdermal testosterone patches:
     a. High doses are used until virilization (presence of male secondary sex characteristics) occurs, and then maintenance doses are used.
     b. Side effects may include gynecomastia (development of breast tissue in men), acne, baldness, and prostate enlargement.
     c. Fertility is difficult and requires additional therapy.
  2. Women who have gonadotropin deficiency receive hormone replacement with a combination of estrogen and progesterone:
     a. Drugs are taken orally or by transdermal patch.

H

    b. Complications include hypertension and deep vein thrombosis.

    c. Additional therapy is needed for fertility.

3. Adult patients with growth hormone (GH) deficiency may be treated with injections of GH.

HYPOTHYROIDISM

OVERVIEW

- Hypothyroidism is the underproduction of thyroid hormones by the thyroid gland, resulting in decreased whole-body metabolism.
- Most cases of hypothyroidism in the United States occur as a result of thyroid surgery and radioactive iodine (RAI) treatment of hyperthyroidism.
- Worldwide, hypothyroidism is common in areas where the soil and water have little natural iodide, causing endemic goiter.
- Other causes of hypothyroidism include autoimmune thyroid destruction; infection of thyroid tissue; congenital absence or hypoplasia of thyroid tissues; neck surgery, irradiation, or trauma; and a wide variety of drugs.
- Women are affected much more often than men.
- Myxedema coma is a rare, serious complication of untreated or poorly treated hypothyroidism.

PATIENT-CENTERED COLLABORATIVE CARE

Assessment

- Obtain patient information about:
  1. Activity levels now compared with those a year earlier
  2. Amount of time spent sleeping
  3. Generalized weakness, anorexia, muscle aches, and paresthesias
  4. Constipation
  5. Cold intolerance (use of more blankets at night or sweaters and extra clothing, even in warm weather)
  6. Change in libido
  7. Heavy, prolonged menses or amenorrhea
  8. Impotence and infertility
  9. Current or previous use of drugs known to interfere with thyroid function, such as lithium, amiodarone, aminoglutethimide, sodium or potassium perchlorate, thiocyanates, or cobalt

10. Medical history, including whether the patient has ever been treated for hyperthyroidism and what specific treatment was used
11. Recent weight gain
- Assess for and document:
  1. Overall appearance:
     a. Coarse features
     b. Edema around the eyes and face
     c. Blank expression
     d. Thick tongue
  2. Slow muscle movement
  3. Slurred or unclear speech
  4. Slow response to questions
  5. Bradycardia
  6. Hypotension
  7. Slow respiratory rate
  8. Low core body temperature
  9. Presence or absence of a goiter

⚠ NURSING SAFETY PRIORITY: Action Alert

A goiter may or may not be present with hypothyroidism and can be present with some types of hyperthyroidism. Therefore do not use the presence of a goiter to determine whether the thyroid problem is excessive hormone secretion or too little hormone secretion.

- Psychosocial assessment and issues may include:
  1. Depression
  2. Lethargy, apathy, drowsiness
  3. Reduced attention span and memory
- Diagnostic assessment may include blood tests for:
  1. Triiodothyronine (T_3)
  2. Thyroxine (T_4)
  3. Thyroid-stimulating hormone (TSH) levels

Interventions

- Drug therapy is the mainstay of management for hypothyroidism.
- The patient requires lifelong thyroid hormone replacement; the most commonly used drug is levothyroxine (Synthroid, Levothroid, Levoxyl, Unithroid, generic)
  1. Therapy is started with a low dose that is gradually increased over a period of weeks.
  2. The patient with more severe symptoms of hypothyroidism is started on the lowest dose of thyroid hormone replacement, because starting at too high a dose or increasing the

dose too rapidly can cause severe hypertension, heart failure, and myocardial infarction:

- a. Teach patients and the families of patients who are beginning thyroid replacement hormone therapy to take the drug exactly as prescribed and not to change the dose or schedule without consulting the health care provider.
- b. Assess the patient for chest pain and dyspnea during initiation of therapy.

3. The final dosage is determined by blood levels of TSH and the patient's physical responses.

4. Monitor for and teach the patient and family about the manifestations of hyperthyroidism/excess treatment, including:
   - a. Tachycardia
   - b. Intolerance to heat
   - c. Difficulty sleeping
   - d. Diarrhea
   - e. Excessive weight loss
   - f. Fine tremors of the hands

- Management of myxedema coma:
  1. *Myxedema coma* is a severe and life-threatening form of hypothyroidism in which the patient's overall metabolism slows to the point that cardiac and respiratory arrest can occur.
  2. Factors leading to myxedema coma include acute illness, surgery, chemotherapy, discontinuing thyroid replacement therapy, and the use of sedatives or opioids.
  3. Manifestations include:
     - a. Coma
     - b. Respiratory failure
     - c. Hypotension
     - d. Hyponatremia
     - e. Hypothermia
     - f. Hypoglycemia
  4. Untreated myxedema coma leads to shock, organ damage, and death.
  5. Treatment is instituted quickly according to the patient's manifestations and without waiting for laboratory confirmation.
  6. Best practices for emergency care of the patient with myxedema coma are:
     - a. Maintaining a patent airway
     - b. Replacing fluids with IV normal or hypertonic saline
     - c. Giving levothyroxine IV as prescribed
     - d. Giving glucose IV as prescribed
     - e. Giving corticosteroids as prescribed

    f. Checking the patient's temperature hourly

    g. Monitoring blood pressure hourly and reporting significant or symptomatic changes

    h. Covering the patient with warm blankets

    i. Monitoring for changes in mental status, reporting decreased consciousness in a timely manner

    j. Turning every 2 hours

    k. Instituting aspiration precautions

Community-Based Care

- Hypothyroidism is usually a chronic condition, and the patient may live in any type of environment. Ensure that whoever is responsible for overseeing the patient's daily care is aware of the condition and understands its treatment.
- Discuss the need for extra heat or clothing because of cold intolerance.
- The patient who has a decreased attention span may need help from family, friends, or a home care aide with the drug regimen.
- Develop a plan for drug therapy, and be sure that one person is clearly designated as responsible for drug preparation and delivery so that doses are neither missed nor duplicated.
- Teach the patient and family about hormone replacement therapy and it side effects:
  1. Emphasize the need for lifelong drugs.
  2. Review the manifestations of both hyperthyroidism and hypothyroidism.
  3. Teach the patient to wear a medical alert bracelet.
  4. Instruct the patient to carefully evaluate over-the-counter (OTC) drugs, because thyroid hormone preparations interact with many other drugs.
  5. Advise the patient to eat a well-balanced diet with adequate fiber and fluid intake to prevent constipation.
  6. Caution patients that the use of fiber supplements may interfere with the absorption of thyroid hormone and to not take these supplements within 4 hours of taking the hormone.
- Teach the family to orient the patient often and to explain everything clearly, simply, and as often as needed.
- Teach the patient to monitor himself or herself for therapy effectiveness by assessing the need for sleep and the frequency of bowel elimination.
  1. When the patient requires more sleep and is constipated, the dose of replacement hormone may need to be increased.
  2. When the patient has difficulty getting to sleep and has more bowel movements than normal for him or her, the dose may need to be decreased.

IMMUNODEFICIENCIES

OVERVIEW

- Immunodeficiency is a failure of the immune system to recognize infectious agents or foreign proteins as a result of a missing or damaged immune component.
- A *primary (congenital) immunodeficiency* is a condition in which one or more parts of the system are not functioning properly from birth.
- A *secondary immunodeficiency* is acquired after birth as the result of viral infection, contact with a toxin, or drug therapy.
- The immunodeficient patient is at increased risk for infection, cancer, and other diseases.
- Types of congenital or primary antibody-mediated immunodeficiencies that adults may have include:
  1. Bruton's agammaglobulinemia:
     a. This is a classic congenital antibody-mediated immune deficiency that has an X-linked pattern of inheritance.
     b. Boys born with this disease usually start to have problems at about age 6 months with manifestations of recurrent otitis, sinusitis, pneumonia, furunculosis, meningitis, and septicemia.
     c. Laboratory assessment shows an absence of circulating immunoglobulin (antibodies).
     d. The overall prognosis is good if antibody replacement is started early.
     e. Antibiotics are used for specific infections, and long-term prophylactic antibiotic therapy may also be used.
  2. Common variable immune deficiency:
     a. Common variable immune deficiency affects men and women.
     b. Patients have low levels of circulating antibodies (immunoglobulins) of all classes.
     c. It usually first appears later (in adolescence or young adulthood), and the infections are less severe than those seen in patients with Bruton's agammaglobulinemia.
     d. Common problems include giardiasis (intestinal infection with *Giardia lamblia*), pneumonia, sinusitis, gastric cancer, bronchiectasis, and gallstones.
     e. Management requires regular infusions of immune serum globulin and regular or intermittent use of antibiotics to protect the affected person against infection.

3. Selective immunoglobulin A (IgA) deficiency:
   a. This is the most common congenital immunodeficiency seen in adults.
   b. The person may be asymptomatic or have chronic or recurrent upper respiratory tract infections, skin infections, urinary tract infections, vaginal infections, and diarrhea.
   c. It does not reduce the person's life span.
   d. Management is limited to vigorous treatment of infections.

⚠ NURSING SAFETY PRIORITY: Action Alert

Unlike other immunoglobulin deficiencies, IgA deficiency should never be treated with exogenous immune globulin. Because patients with IgA deficiency make normal amounts of all other antibodies, they are at high risk for severe allergic reactions to exogenous immune globulin.

- Types of iatrogenic or therapy-induced immunodeficiencies include:
  1. Drug-induced immune deficiencies caused by:
     a. Cytotoxic drugs used in the treatment of cancer and autoimmune disorders
     b. Corticosteroids used to treat many autoimmune diseases, neoplasms, and endocrine disorders
     c. Cyclosporine (Sandimmune, Neoral), a specific immunosuppressant that is used to prevent organ transplant rejection and graft-versus-host disease and is occasionally used for other disorders, such as uveitis, rheumatoid arthritis, and other autoimmune disorders
     d. Biologics or disease-modifying immune suppressive drugs specifically slow the damage caused by a variety of autoimmune diseases.
  2. Radiation-induced immunodeficiency when the iliac and femur in adults are exposed to high doses of radiation (these are the blood cell-producing sites of adults)
- Management of treatment-induced immune deficiency aims to improve immune function and protect the patient from infection.
- Usually, treatment-related immunedeficiencies resolve after the suppressive drug or radiation therapy is stopped and the hematopoietic cells recover.
- Teach the patient how to protect himself or herself from infection by:
  1. Avoiding crowds and other large gatherings of people where someone might be ill

2. Not sharing personal toilet articles, such as toothbrushes, toothpaste, washcloths, or deodorant sticks, with others
3. Bathing daily, using an antimicrobial soap, and, if total bathing is not possible, washing the armpits, groin, genitals, and anal area twice daily with an antimicrobial soap
4. Cleaning the toothbrush daily by running it through the dishwasher or rinsing it in liquid laundry bleach
5. Cleaning hands thoroughly with an antimicrobial soap or solution before eating or drinking, after touching a pet, after shaking hands with anyone, returning home from any outing, and after using the toilet
6. Washing dishes between uses with hot, sudsy water, or using a dishwasher
7. Not drinking water, milk, juice, or other cold liquids that have been standing for longer than an hour
8. Not reusing cups and glasses without washing
9. Not changing pet litter boxes or, if unavoidable, using gloves and washing hands immediately
10. Avoiding birds, turtles, and other reptiles as pets
11. Avoiding raw or undercooked meat, even if served as pet food
12. Avoiding salads; raw fruit and vegetables; undercooked meat, fish, or eggs; pepper; and paprika
13. Thoroughly washing fruit and vegetables
14. Refrigerating perishable foods such as prepared or cooked meats or meals

INFLUENZA, SEASONAL AND PANDEMIC

OVERVIEW

- Influenza, or "flu," is a highly contagious, acute viral respiratory infection that can occur in adults of all ages.
- Epidemics are common and lead to complications of pneumonia or death, especially in older adults or debilitated or immunocompromised patients.
- Seasonal influenza may be caused by one of several virus families, referred to as A, B, and C.
- Pandemic influenza usually refers to respiratory viral infection that is transmitted after mutating from animal or bird viruses with the potential to infect global populations.
- The H1N1 strain, also known as swine flu, mutated and became highly infectious to humans in 2009, infecting an estimated 61 million people, resulting in more than 12,000 deaths.

- The H5N1 strain, known as Avian influenza or bird flu, has infected millions of birds, especially in Asia and now has started to spread by human-to-human contact with potential to become a pandemic, because humans have essentially no naturally occurring immunity to this virus.

PATIENT-CENTERED COLLABORATIVE CARE

- The prioritized care reduces risk of infection through hand-washing, avoiding droplet spread of the virus, and vaccination. Adults are contagious from 24 hours before symptoms occur and up to 5 days after they begin.

Assessment

- Assess for:
  1. Fever
  2. Severe headache
  3. Muscle aches
  4. Chill
  5. Fatigue and weakness

Interventions

- Vaccination for everyone older than 3 months of age:
  1. Seasonal vaccination, usually in late fall with a vaccine containing three antigens for the three expected viral strains (trivalent influenza vaccine [TIV]).
  2. Influenza vaccinations can be taken as an IM injection (Fluvirin, Fluzone) or as a live attenuated influenza vaccine (LAIV) by intranasal spray (FluMist). The attenuated virus is recommended only for healthy adults 18 to 49 years of age.
  3. Pandemic vaccination is recommended when the risk is increased, as in 2009 or 2010 with the H1NI strain.
- For infected patients:
  1. Bedrest
  2. Fluids
  3. Saline gargles to ease sore throat pain
  4. Antihistamines that may reduce the rhinorrhea
  5. Antiviral agents given within 12 to 24 hours of symptom onset that may reduce the severity or duration of influenza; these agents include amantadine (Symmetrel) and rimantadine (Flumadine) for influenza A strains and zanamivir (Relenza), which is used as an oral inhalant, and oseltamivir (Tamiflu) for any strain of influenza
- For frail or immunocompromised patients, infants, and older adults, hospitalization may be required for close monitoring to detect organ impairment or provide respiratory support.

IRRITABLE BOWEL SYNDROME

OVERVIEW

- In patients with irritable bowel syndrome (IBS), bowel motility changes and increased or decreased bowel transit times result in changes in the normal *bowel elimination* pattern to one of these classifications: diarrhea (IBS-D), constipation (IBS-C), alternating diarrhea and constipation.
- In most patients, no actual pathophysiologic bowel changes occur with IBS. However, microscopic inflammatory changes have recently been found in some patients with the disease as a result of bacterial overgrowth and subsequent infection.

PATIENT-CENTERED COLLABORATIVE CARE

Assessment

- Assess for and document:
  1. Weight change
  2. Fatigue, malaise
  3. Abdominal pain
  4. Changes in the bowel pattern (constipation, diarrhea, or an alternating pattern of both) or consistency of stools and the passage of mucus
  5. Gastrointestinal infections
  6. Food intolerance
  7. Serum albumin, complete blood count (CBC), erythrocyte sedimentation rate

Interventions

- Diet therapy includes:
  1. Suggesting a symptom diary to help identify triggers and bowel habits
  2. Helping the patient identify and eliminate foods associated with exacerbations
  3. Consulting with the dietitian
  5. Teaching the patient to ingest 30 to 40 g of fiber daily
  6. Teaching the patient to drink 8 to 10 cups of liquid per day
- Drug therapy includes:
  1. Bulk-forming laxatives, such as psyllium hydrophilic mucilloid (Metamucil), may be taken at mealtimes with a glass of water to prevent dry, hard, or liquid stools.
  2. Lubiprostone (Amitiza) is a new oral drug available for women with IBS-C. The drug is not effective for men. Lubiprostone is classified as a locally acting chloride channel activator that increases intestinal chloride without affecting intestinal sodium and potassium concentrations. Teach the patient to take the drug with food and water.

3. Antidiarrheal agents may be used to decrease cramping and frequency of stools such as loperamide (Imodium).

4. Muscarinic-blocking agents (anticholinergic drugs specific to GI receptors) may be used.

5. Serotonin (5-HT4) drugs may be used for women with diarrhea-predominant IBS.

6. Many patients with IBS who have bloating and abdominal distention without constipation have success with rifaximin (Xifaxan), an antibiotic that works locally with little systemic absorption.

7. For IBS in which pain is the predominant symptom, tricyclic antidepressants, such as amitriptyline (Elavil), have also been successfully used.

8. Probiotics have been shown to be effective for reducing bacteria and successfully alleviating GI symptoms of IBS.

9. Acupuncture and moxibustion (Acumoxa) treatment has helped some patients by reducing flatulence and bloating, and improving stool consistency

10. Stress management is also an important part of holistic care. Suggest relaxation techniques, meditation, imagery, and/or yoga to help the patient decrease GI symptoms.

KIDNEY DISEASE, POLYCYSTIC

OVERVIEW

- Polycystic kidney disease (PKD) is an inherited kidney disorder in which fluid-filled cysts develop in nephrons.
- Growing cysts damage the nephron (i.e., glomerular and tubular membranes), reducing kidney function.
- Kidney tissue is eventually replaced by nonfunctioning cysts; each cystic kidney may enlarge to two to three times its normal size, causing discomfort and abdominal organ displacement. The fluid-filled cysts are at increased risk for infection, rupture, and bleeding.
- Most patients with PKD have high blood pressure and heart problems.
- Cysts may occur in other tissues, such as the liver or blood vessels.

PATIENT-CENTERED COLLABORATIVE CARE
Assessment

- Obtain patient information about:
  1. Family history and genetic testing, because PKD can be autosomal dominant (most common form of PKD with several

K

different subtypes) or autosomal recessive (which is more severe, with death typically occurring in early childhood)
2. Current health status
3. Family history of sudden death from a stroke
4. Changes in urine or pattern of urination
5. Hypertension
- Assess for and document:
  1. Pain (flank or abdominal)
  2. Distended abdomen
  3. Enlarged, tender kidney on palpation
  4. Changes in urine including, hematuria, clarity, odor
  5. Changes in pattern of urination including nocturia
  6. Dysuria
  7. Hypertension
  8. Edema
  9. Uremic symptoms: nausea, vomiting, pruritus, and fatigue
  10. Emotional responses such as anger, resentment, futility, sadness, or anxiety related to chronicity or inheritable condition
- Diagnostic studies may include:
  1. Urinalysis with findings of proteinuria and hematuria
  2. Urine culture and sensitivity if infection is suspected
  3. Serum creatinine and blood urea nitrogen (BUN) to assess kidney function
  4. Renal sonography, computed tomography (CT) scan, or magnetic resonance imaging (MRI) to assess presence and size of cysts

Interventions

- Manage pain:
  1. Provide drug therapy:
     a. Administer analgesics for comfort; use NSAIDs cautiously, and avoid aspirin-containing products.
     b. Administer antibiotics such as trimethoprim/sulfamethoxazole (Bactrim, Septra) or ciprofloxacin (Cipro) if a cyst infection is causing discomfort.
  2. Provide other interventions:
     a. Apply dry heat to the abdomen or flank.
     b. Teach relaxation or distraction techniques to self-manage pain and discomfort.
- Provide hypertension and fluid management:
  1. Administer antihypertensive agents, including angiotensin-converting enzyme (ACE) inhibitors, vasodilators, beta blockers, and calcium channel blockers, as ordered.
  2. Administer diuretics, as ordered, to eliminate fluid overload.
  3. Monitor daily weight to detect fluid-related weight gain

- Implement diet therapy with dietitian consultation to slow progression of kidney injury with salt and protein restriction.
- Prevent constipation associated with fluid restriction and intestinal tract displacement from cysts.
- Provide counseling, support, and teaching about health maintenance to promote self-management.
- Teach the patient and family:
  1. How to measure and monitor blood pressure and weight
  2. Diet considerations to promote health; salt, protein, and fiber intake may need special attention or dietitian consultation
  3. Self-administration of drugs and potential adverse effects of prescribed drugs, including antihypertensive drugs and diuretics
  4. Resources that are available for research and education, such as the Polycystic Kidney Research Foundation and the National Kidney and Urologic Disease division of the National Institutes of Health

KIDNEY INJURY, ACUTE (ACUTE KIDNEY FAILURE)

OVERVIEW

- Acute kidney injury (AKI), formerly known as acute renal failure, is a rapid decrease in kidney function leading to the accumulation of metabolic wastes in the body.
- AKI can result from conditions that reduce blood flow or oxygen to the kidneys (prerenal failure); damage to the glomeruli, interstitial tissue, or tubules (intrarenal or intrinsic renal failure); or obstruction of urine flow (postrenal failure).
- When kidney decline is sudden, the functioning nephrons are overworked and kidney failure may develop with the loss of only 50% of functioning nephrons. When acute kidney injury occurs in the presence of chronic kidney disease (acute on chronic injury), rapid progression to kidney failure can occur more.
- AKI is associated with acute and severe illnesses; the most common etiology is volume depletion. Recognizing and treating hypovolemia promptly can prevent AKI and progression of the condition.
- AKI is classified by the extent of changes in serum creatinine, decreases in urine output, and persistence of symptoms. There are five classes, ranging from risk to end-stage disease:

K

Risk, Injury, Failure, Loss, and End-Stage Kidney (RIFLE) Classification

Class	Glomerular Filtration Rate Criteria	Urine Output Criteria
Risk	Serum creatinine × 1.5	<0.5 mL/kg/hr × 6 hr
Injury	Serum creatinine × 2	<0.5 mL/kg/hr × 12 hr
Failure	Serum creatinine × 3 or serum creatinine ≥4 mg/dL with an acute rise >0.5 mg/dL	<0.3 mL/kg/hr × 24 hr or anuria × 12 hr
Loss	Persistent acute kidney failure: complete loss of kidney function >4 weeks	
End-stage kidney disease	Loss of kidney function >3 months	

PATIENT-CENTERED COLLABORATIVE CARE
Assessment
- Obtain patient information about:
  1. Exposure to nephrotoxins, including:
     a. Contrast dye used in imaging procedures
     b. Drugs, especially antibiotics, ACE inhibitors, and NSAIDs
  2. History of diseases that contribute to impaired kidney function such as diabetes mellitus, systemic lupus erythematosus, and hypertension
  3. History of acute infections, including influenza, colds, gastroenteritis, and sore throat or pharyngitis
  4. History of intravascular volume depletion (from surgery or trauma) or the need for transfusion
  5. History of urinary obstructive disease, such as prostatic hypertrophy or kidney stones
- Assess for and document:
  1. Symptoms of low tissue perfusion, including hypotension with tachycardia, low cardiac output (ejection fraction)
  2. Decreased or absent urine output
  3. Abnormal values for blood urea nitrogen (BUN), serum creatinine, serum electrolytes, and urinalysis or reduced creatinine clearance

   4. Symptoms of fluid overload including pulmonary edema (dyspnea, crackles, reduced SpO_2) and peripheral edema
   5. Electrocardiographic (ECG) changes indicating electrolyte abnormalities
   6. Symptoms of electrolyte derangements including nausea and vomiting, anorexia, impaired cognitions, and acute abnormalities in neuromuscular function
   7. Flank pain
- Diagnostic studies may include:
   1. Urinalysis
   2. Urine and serum electrolytes, creatinine, and BUN
   3. Abdominal or pelvic x-ray to assess the size of the kidneys and computed tomography (CT) without contrast dye to identify obstruction
   4. Renal biopsy to determine uncertain cause of AKI or if immunologic disease is suspected

Interventions

- Monitor fluid and electrolyte status to detect imbalance and abnormal values. The patient may move from an oliguric phase (fluids and electrolytes are retained) to a diuretic phase, in which hypovolemia and electrolyte loss are the main problems.
- Asses patient response to renoprotective and other drugs to manage fluid and electrolytes:
   1. As kidney function changes, drug dosages are modified.
   2. Monitor for drug side effects and interactions.
- Fluid challenges and diuretics are commonly used to promote fluid balance and kidney perfusion.
   1. Monitor for fluid overload and dehydration.
- Hypercatabolism during illness, surgery, or trauma results in the breakdown of muscle for protein, which leads to increased azotemia. Patients require increased calories.
- Indications for hemodialysis or peritoneal dialysis in patients with AKI are symptomatic uremia, persistent hyperkalemia, uncompensated metabolic acidosis, fluid overload, uremic pericarditis, and uremic encephalopathy (see *Kidney Disease, Chronic,* for a discussion of dialysis).
- Continuous hemofiltration, an alternative to dialysis, may be used in the intensive care unit (ICU).

Community-Based Care

- The needs of the patient depend on the status of the disease on discharge (see *Community-Based Care* under *Kidney Disease, Chronic*).
- Follow-up care may include medical visits, laboratory tests, consultation with a nutritionist, temporary dialysis, home nursing care, and social work assistance.

K

KIDNEY DISEASE, CHRONIC

OVERVIEW

- Chronic kidney failure (CKD) is a progressive, irreversible kidney injury; kidney function does not recover.
- The progression toward CKD occurs in five stages:
  1. *Stage 1:* At risk for CKD. Normal kidney function with an estimated glomerular filtration rate (GFR) greater than 90 mL/min. Kidney function is normal, but the patient has sufficient risk factors to require screening and ongoing monitoring of kidney function.
  2. *Stage 2:* Mild CKD. GFR is reduced to 60 to 89 mL/min. The focus of care is to be vigilant about reducing risk factors for kidney disease.
  3. *Stage 3:* Moderate CKD. GFR 30 to 59 mL/min. The focus of care is to slow progression of the disease through diet and increase vigilance to avoid hypoperfusion, toxins, and other risk factors.
  4. *Stage 4:* Severe CKD. GFR 15 to 29 mL/min. Care intensity increases to manage complications (anemia, hypertension) and prepare for eventual renal replacement therapy
  5. *Stage 5:* End-stage kidney disease (ESKD); renal replacement therapy is started. Alternatively, kidney transplantation is performed.
- Pathologic alterations as kidney disease progresses include abnormal urine production, poor water excretion, electrolyte imbalance, and metabolic (e.g., loss of erythropoietin synthesis) anomalies.
- When less than 20% of nephrons are functional, hyposthenuria (loss of urine concentrating ability) and polyuria occur; left untreated, severe dehydration occurs.
- Urea is the primary product of protein metabolism and is normally excreted by the kidney; blood urea nitrogen (BUN) varies with dietary intake of protein.
- Creatinine is derived from creatine and phosphocreatine; the normal rate of excretion depends on muscle mass, physical activity, and diet.
- Azotemia is increased accumulation of nitrogenous waste (BUN) in the blood and is a classic indicator of kidney failure.
- Variations in sodium excretion occur and depend on the stage of CKD:
  1. There is increased risk for hyponatremia, or sodium depletion, in early CKD.
  2. Hyponatremia occurs because the reduced number of functional nephrons is insufficient to reabsorb sodium, and sodium is lost in the urine.

- Hyperkalemia results from an increase in potassium load, including ingestion of potassium in drugs, failure to restrict potassium in the diet, blood transfusions, and excess bleeding.
- Other metabolic derangements in CKD include changes in pH (metabolic acidosis), calcium (hypocalcemia) and phosphorus (hyperphosphatemia) imbalances, and vitamin D insufficiency.
    1. Renal osteodystrophy caused by hypocalcemia and phosphorus retention results in skeletal demineralization manifested by bone pain, pseudofractures, sclerosis of the spine, skull demineralization, osteomalacia, reabsorption of bone, and loss of tooth lamina.
- Cardiovascular alterations include anemia, hypertension, hyperlipidemia, heart failure, and pericarditis.
- GI alterations include uremic stomatitis, anorexia, peptic ulcer disease, nausea, and vomiting.

PATIENT-CENTERED COLLABORATIVE CARE
Assessment
- Obtain patient information about:
    1. Age (because a reduction in the number and function of nephrons occurs with age)
    2. Height and weight, including recent weight gain or loss
    3. Current and past medical conditions
    4. Drugs, prescription and nonprescription
    5. Family history of kidney disease
    6. Dietary and nutritional habits, including food preferences
    7. History of GI problems, such as nausea, vomiting, anorexia, diarrhea, or constipation
    8. Recent injuries and abnormal bruising or bleeding
    9. Activity intolerance, weakness and fatigue
    10. Detailed urinary elimination history
- Assess for and document:
    1. Neurologic manifestations:
        a. Changes in mentation or new lethargy
        b. Changes in sensation or weakness in extremities indicating uremic neuropathy
    2. Cardiovascular manifestations of CKD from fluid overload, hypertension, or cardiac disease:
        a. Systolic blood pressure (SBP) higher than 130 mm Hg or diastolic blood pressure (DBP) higher than 80 mm Hg (lower tolerance for elevations in blood pressure with CKD)
        b. Cardiomyopathy

K

   c. Uremic pericarditis
   d. Peripheral edema
   e. Heart failure
   f. Pericardial friction rub or effusion
3. Respiratory manifestations:
   a. Breath that smells like urine (uremic fetor or halitosis)
   b. Deep sighing or yawning
   c. Tachypnea or shortness of breath
   d. Pulmonary edema or pleural effusion
   e. Kussmaul respiration with acidemia
   f. Uremic lung or hilar pneumonitis
4. Hematologic manifestations:
   a. Anemia
   b. Abnormal bleeding: bruising petechiae, abnormal vaginal bleeding, GI bleeding
5. GI disruptions:
   a. Mouth ulceration
   b. Abdominal pain or cramping
   c. Nausea or vomiting
6. Urinary findings:
   a. Change in urinary amount, frequency, and appearance of urine
   b. Proteinuria or hematuria
7. Integumentary or dermatologic manifestations:
   a. Yellow coloration from pigment deposition; darkening of skin for some African Americans
   b. Severe itching (pruritus)
   c. Uremic frost, a layer of uremic crystals from evaporated sweat on the face, eyebrows, axilla, and groin (rare)
   d. Bruises or purple patches and rashes
8. Immunologic considerations:
   a. Increased susceptibility to infections
- Diagnostic testing may include:
   1. Serum creatinine, BUN, sodium, potassium, calcium, phosphorus, bicarbonate, hemoglobin, and hematocrit
   2. Urinalysis
   3. A 24-hour urinalysis for creatinine and creatine clearance
   4. Ultrasound, computed tomography (CT) scan, or x-ray to observe progression, which manifests as small and fibrotic kidneys

Planning and Implementation

Priority problems for patients with CKD are:

FLUID OVERLOAD

- Fluid Overload is related to the inability of diseased kidneys to maintain body fluid balance.

- The goal is to achieve and maintain acceptable fluid balance. Indicators include:
  1. Blood pressure
  2. Heart rate
  3. Body weight
  4. Central venous pressure
  5. Serum electrolytes
- Diuretic drugs may be used in patients with CKD in stages 1 through 4.

POTENTIAL FOR PULMONARY EDEMA

- Potential for Pulmonary Edema is related to fluid overload.
- The goal is to remain free of pulmonary edema and maintain optimal fluid balance.
- Interventions include:
  1. Assessing for early signs of pulmonary edema, such as restlessness, dyspnea, and crackles
  2. If the patient is dyspneic, placing the patient in a high Fowler's position and giving oxygen to maximize lung expansion and improve gas exchange
  3. Measuring and recording intake and output
  4. Assessing cardiovascular system for fluid overload: S_3 heart sounds, peripheral edema, jugular venous distention, tachycardia, hypotension, or hypertension
  5. Monitoring serum chemistry results for electrolyte imbalance
  6. Monitoring peripheral oxygenation (Spo_2) to detect hypoxemia
  7. Providing drug therapy:
     a. Diuretics for stages 1 through 4 CKD; monitor for ototoxicity with loop diuretics
     b. Morphine to reduce myocardial oxygen demands; monitor for respiratory depression
     c. Vasodilators such as nitroglycerin

REDUCED CARDIAC OUTPUT

- Reduced Cardiac Output is related to reduced stroke volume, dysrhythmias, fluid overload, and increased peripheral vascular resistance.
- The goal is to attain and maintain adequate cardiac output. Indicators include:
  1. Systolic and diastolic blood pressures
  2. Ejection fraction
  3. Peripheral pulses
  4. Cognitive status
- Interventions include:
  1. Administering calcium channel blockers, angiotensin-converting enzyme (ACE) inhibitors, alpha- and beta-adrenergic blockers, and vasodilators

K

2. Teaching the family to measure the patient's blood pressure and weight daily and to bring these records when visiting the physician, nurse, or nutritionist
3. Monitoring the patient for decreased cardiac output, heart failure, congestive heart failure, and dysrhythmias

INADEQUATE NUTRITION

- Inadequate Nutrition is related to inability to ingest and digest food or to absorb nutrients as a result of physiologic factors. Provide food and fluids to prevent malnutrition.
- The nutritional need and diet restrictions for the patient with CKD vary according to the degree of remaining kidney function and the type of renal replacement therapy used.
- Common changes include control of protein intake; fluid intake limitation; restriction of potassium, sodium, and phosphorus intake; taking vitamin and mineral supplements; and eating enough calories to meet metabolic demand.
- Consult with the nutritionist to provide nutritional teaching and planning and to assist the patient in adapting the diet to food preferences, ethnic background, and budget.

POTENTIAL FOR INFECTION

- Potential for Infection is related to skin breakdown, chronic disease, or malnutrition.
- The goals are to prevent infection and detect infection early by monitoring for:
  1. Fever
  2. Lymph node enlargement
  3. Positive urine or other culture
  4. Tenderness, redness, or drainage at dialysis access site
  5. Abnormal white blood cell (WBC) count and differential
  6. Skin integrity

POTENTIAL FOR INJURY

- Potential for Injury is related to effects of kidney disease on bone density, blood clotting, and drug elimination.
- The goals are to prevent the following problems: falls, pathologic fractures, bleeding, and toxic effects of prescribed drugs. Interventions include:
  1. Monitoring the patient closely for drug-related complications
  2. Teaching the patient to avoid certain drugs that can increase kidney damage, such as NSAIDs, antibiotics, antihypertensives, and diuretics in the presence of hypovolemia
  3. Anticipating dosage adjustment as kidney function decreases
  4. Administering agents to control phosphorus excess, such as calcium acetate, calcium carbonate, and aluminum hydroxide

5. Instructing the patient to avoid compounds containing magnesium
6. Administering opioid analgesics cautiously, because the effects may last longer and uremic patients are sensitive to the respiratory depressant effects

FATIGUE

- Fatigue is related to kidney disease, anemia, and reduced energy production.
- The goal is to conserve energy and preserve the ability to perform self-care, retain interest in surroundings, and sustain mental concentration. Interventions include:
  1. Providing vitamin and mineral supplementation
  2. Administering erythropoietin to maintain hemoglobin 7 to 9 g/dL3. Administer iron supplements to maintain safe level of hemoglobin and hematocrit (hematocrit goals is usually 27% to 28%)
  3. Monitoring dietary intake (improved appetite challenges patients in their attempts to maintain protein and potassium) and fluid restriction

ANXIETY

- Anxiety is related to threat to or change in health status, economic status, relationships, role function, systems, or self-concept; situational crisis; threat of death; lack of knowledge about diagnostic tests, disease process, treatment; loss of control; or disrupted family life
- The goal is to reduce feelings of apprehension and tension. Interventions include:
  1. Observing the patient's behavior for signs of anxiety
  2. Evaluating the patient's support system
  3. Explaining all procedures, tests, and treatments
  4. Providing instruction on kidney function and kidney failure
  5. Encouraging the patient to discuss current problems, fears, or concerns and to ask questions
  6. Facilitating discussion with family members concerning the patient's prognosis and potential impacts on the patient's lifestyle

RENAL REPLACEMENT THERAPY

- Renal replacement therapy is required when the clinical and laboratory manifestations of kidney failure present complications that are potentially life threatening or that pose continuing discomfort to the patient.
- *Hemodialysis* removes excess fluid and waste products and restores chemical and electrolyte balance. It is based on the principle of diffusion, in which the patient's blood is circulated through a semipermeable membrane that acts as an artificial kidney.

1. Dialysis settings include the acute care facility, free-standing centers, and the home.
2. Total dialysis time is usually 12 hours per week, which usually is divided into three 4-hour treatments.
3. Vascular access route is needed to perform hemodialysis.
4. Long-term vascular access for hemodialysis is accomplished by:
   a. Arteriovenous (AV) fistula
   b. AV graft
5. Complications of vascular access include:
   a. Thrombosis or stenosis
   b. Infection
   c. Ischemia
   d. Aneurysm formation

- Temporary vascular access for hemodialysis is accomplished by a specially designed catheter inserted into the subclavian, internal jugular, or femoral vein.
- Nurses are specially trained to perform hemodialysis.
- Postdialysis care includes:
  1. Closely monitoring for side effects: hypotension, headache, nausea, malaise, vomiting, dizziness, and muscle cramps
  2. Obtaining the patient's weight and vital signs
  3. Avoiding invasive procedures for 4 to 6 hours because of heparinization of the dialysate
  4. Monitoring for signs of bleeding
  5. Monitoring laboratory results for abnormal values
- Complications of hemodialysis include:
  1. Dialysis disequilibrium
  2. Infectious disease
  3. Hepatitis infection
  4. Human immunodeficiency virus (HIV) infection

Considerations for Older Adults

- ESKD occurs most often in people between 65 and 69 years old.
- Patients older than 65 years who are receiving dialysis are more at risk than younger patients for dialysis-induced hypotension. Older adults require more frequent monitoring of vital signs and level of consciousness during and after dialysis.

- Peritoneal dialysis (PD), an alternative and slower dialysis method, is accomplished by the surgical insertion of a silicone rubber catheter (Tenckhoff catheter) into the abdominal cavity to instill dialysis solution into the abdominal cavity.
- Candidates for PD include:
  1. Patients who are unable to tolerate anticoagulation

2. Patients who lack vascular access
3. Patients without peritoneal adhesions and without extensive abdominal surgery
- The PD process occurs by means of a transfer of fluid and solutes from the bloodstream through the peritoneum.
- The types of PD include intermittent, continuous ambulatory (CAPD), automated, and others; the type is selected based on patient ability and lifestyle.
- Complications of PD include:
  1. Peritonitis
  2. Pain
  3. Poor dialysate flow
  4. Leakage of the dialysate
  5. Exit site and tunnel infection
- Nursing interventions include:
  1. Implementing and monitoring PD therapy and instilling, dwelling, and draining the solution, as ordered
  2. Maintaining PD flow data and monitoring for negative or positive fluid balances
  3. Obtaining baseline and daily weights
  4. Monitoring laboratory results to measure the effectiveness of the treatment
  5. Maintaining accurate intake and output records
  6. Taking vital signs every 15 to 30 minutes during initiation of PD
  7. Performing an ongoing assessment for signs of respiratory distress or pain
- Kidney transplantation is appropriate for selected patients with ESKD (see *Transplantation*).

Community-Based Care
- Case manager helps plan, coordinate, and evaluate care.
  1. The physical and occupational therapist collaborates with the patient and family to evaluate the home environment and to obtain needed equipment before discharge.
  2. Refer the patient to home health nursing as needed.
- Provide in-depth health teaching about diet and pathophysiology of kidney disease and drug therapy:
  1. Provide information and emotional support to assist the patient with decisions about treatment course, personal lifestyle, support systems, and coping.
  2. Teach the patient about the hemodialysis treatment.
  3. Teach the patient about care of the vascular access.
  4. Provide patients with home-based renal replacement therapy with extensive teaching and assist the patient to obtain the needed equipment and supplies. Emphasize

K

the importance of strict sterile technique and of reporting manifestations of infection at any dialysis access site.

5. Assist the patient and family to identify coping strategies to adjust to the diagnosis and treatment regimen.

6. Instruct patients and family members in all aspects of diet therapy, drug therapy, and complications. Assist patients to schedule drugs so that drugs will not be unintentionally eliminated by dialysis.

7. Teach patients and family members to report complications, such as fluid overload, bleeding, and infection.

8. Stress that although uremic symptoms are reduced as a result of dialysis procedures, the patient will not return completely to his or her previous state of well-being.

9. Instruct the family to monitor the patient for any behaviors that may contribute to nonadherence to the treatment plan and to report such to the health care provider.

10. Refer the patient to a home health nurse and to local and state support groups and agencies such as the National Kidney Foundation.

LABYRINTHITIS

- Labyrinthitis is an infection, usually viral, of the labyrinth of the inner ear.
- Causes include complications of acute or chronic otitis media, cholesteatoma, complications of middle ear or inner ear surgery, and aftermath of an upper respiratory infection or mononucleosis.
- Manifestations include hearing loss, tinnitus, nystagmus on the affected side, and vertigo with nausea and vomiting.
- The most common complication is meningitis.
- Management includes:
  1. Supportive care with bedrest in a darkened room, antiemetics and antivertiginous drugs
  2. Systemic antibiotic therapy if symptoms do not resolve
  3. Psychosocial support for persistent balance problems and possible hearing loss
  4. Gait training and physical therapy for persistent balance problems

LACERATIONS, EYE

- Lacerations are wounds caused by sharp objects and projectiles.
- The most commonly injured areas involved in eye lacerations are the eyelids and the cornea.

1. Eyelid lacerations:
   a. Bleed heavily and look more severe than they are
   b. Are managed by closing the eye and applying a small ice-pack, checking visual acuity, and cleaning and suturing the eyelid
   c. Should be managed by an ophthalmologist if they involve the eyelid margin, affect the lacrimal system, involve a large area, or have jagged edges
2. Corneal lacerations:
   a. Are an emergency because eye contents may prolapse through the laceration
   b. Are manifested by severe eye pain, photophobia, tearing, decreased visual acuity, and inability to open the eyelid

⚠ NURSING SAFETY PRIORITY: Action Alert

If an object is seen protruding from the eye, do not remove it. The object should be removed only by the ophthalmologist, because it may be holding eye structures in place.

   c. Are managed with surgical repair and antibiotic therapy
   d. May require a corneal transplant if scarring alters vision
   e. May need *enucleation* (surgical eye removal) if the eye contents have prolapsed through the laceration or if the injury is severe

LEIOMYOMAS (UTERINE FIBROIDS)

OVERVIEW

- Uterine leiomyomas, also called *fibroids* or *myomas,* are the most commonly occurring benign pelvic tumors.
- Leiomyomas develop from excessive local growth of smooth muscle cells.
- These tumors are classified according to their position in the layers of the uterus and anatomic position. The most common types are:
  1. *Intramural tumors,* contained in the uterine wall in the myometrium
  2. *Submucosal tumors,* which protrude into the cavity of the uterus
  3. *Subserosal tumors,* which protrude through the outer uterine surface and may extend into the broad ligament

PATIENT-CENTERED COLLABORATIVE CARE
Assessment

- Assessment findings include:
  1. No symptoms

2. Abnormal uterine bleeding
3. Reports of a feeling of pelvic pressure
4. Constipation
5. Urinary frequency or retention
6. Increased abdominal size
7. Dyspareunia (painful intercourse)
8. Infertility
9. Abdominal pain occurring with torsion of the fibroid around a connecting stalk or pedicle
10. Uterine enlargement on abdominal, vaginal, or rectal examination

Planning and Implementation
POTENTIAL FOR HEMORRHAGE
Nonsurgical Management

- The patient who has no symptoms or who desires childbearing is observed and examined for changes in the size of the leiomyoma every 4 to 6 months.
- Many fibroids spontaneously shrink after menopause and require no treatment.
- Mild leiomyoma symptoms can be managed with NSAIDs, hormonal contraceptives, or a levonorgestrel intrauterine device (IUD).
- Artificial menopause and fibroid shrinkage can be induced with agonists to gonadotropin-releasing hormone (GnRH).
- Magnetic resonance imaging (MRI) focused ultrasound pulsed into the uterus can destroy the fibroid.
- Uterine artery embolization or uterine fibroid embolization (UFE) involves the injection of embolic particles into the blood supply of the tumors, occluding the blood supply to the tumor and thereby causing its shrinkage and resorption.

Surgical Management

- Surgical management depends on whether future childbearing is desired, the age of the woman, the size of the fibroid, and the degree of symptoms.
- A *myomectomy* (removal of the leiomyomas with preservation of the uterus) is performed to preserve childbearing capabilities and relieve the symptoms. This procedure can be done by a laparoscopic approach or by more traditional open abdominal and vaginal approaches.
- A *transcervical endometrial resection (TCER)* involves destroying the endometrium with a diathermy rectoscope or with radioablation. This procedure manages submucosal fibroids and menorrhagia.

⚠NURSING SAFETY PRIORITY: Critical Rescue

Monitor for rare, but potential complications of hysteroscopic surgery, which include:

- Fluid overload (fluid used to distend the uterine cavity can be absorbed)
- Embolism
- Hemorrhage
- Perforation of the uterus, bowel, or bladder and ureter injury
- Persistent increased menstrual bleeding
- Incomplete suppression of menstruation

Monitor for any indications of these problems, and report signs and symptoms, such as severe pain and heavy bleeding, to the surgeon immediately. Scarring may cause a small risk for complications in future pregnancies.

- *Hysterectomy,* surgical removal of the uterine body, is the usual surgical management in the older woman who has multiple leiomyomas and unacceptable symptoms.
  1. A *total hysterectomy* involves removal of the uterus by a vaginal approach (total vaginal hysterectomy [TVH]), an open abdominal approach, or minimally invasive surgery by laparoscopy.
  2. *Total abdominal hysterectomy* (TAH), includes the removal of the uterus, ovaries, and fallopian tubes.
  3. A *radical hysterectomy* involves removal of the uterus, lymph nodes, upper one third of the vagina, and the surrounding tissues.
- Provide preoperative nursing care, including:
  1. Routine preoperative care as described in Part One
  2. Listening to patient's concerns about her sexuality
  3. Identifying the patient's support system
- Provide postoperative care for the patient after abdominal hysterectomy, including:
  1. Routine postoperative care as described in Part One
  2. Provide specific attention to:
     a. Vaginal bleeding (there should be less than one saturated perineal pad in 4 hours)
     b. Abdominal bleeding at the incision site(s) (a small amount is normal)
     c. Intactness of the incision(s)
     d. Urine output per urinary catheter for 24 hours or less (for open surgery)
     e. Pain management

L

- Specific postoperative interventions for a vaginal hysterectomy include:
  a. Assessment of vaginal bleeding (there should be less than one saturated pad in 4 hours)
  b. Urinary catheter care
  c. Perineal care

Considerations for Older Adults
- Older women are more at risk for all complications, especially pulmonary complications, than are younger women.
- Obese women are more at risk for all complications than are women who are not obese.

LEUKEMIA

OVERVIEW
- The leukemias are a type of cancer with uncontrolled production of immature white blood cells (WBCs) in the bone marrow. This results in bone marrow overcrowding with immature, nonfunctional cells and in decreased production of normal blood cells.
- Leukemia may be *acute,* with a sudden onset and short duration, or *chronic,* with a slow onset and symptoms that persist for a period of years.
- The two major types of leukemia are:
  1. *Lymphocytic (lymphoblastic) leukemia,* in which the abnormal cells are lymphoid in origin and which can be acute or chronic:
     a. Acute lymphocytic leukemia makes up about 10% of adult leukemias but is more common in children. Chronic lymphocytic leukemia (CLL) occurs rarely (less than 5% of adult leukemias).
  2. *Myelocytic* (myelogenous), in which the abnormal cells are myeloid in origin and which can be acute or chronic
- Acute myelogenous leukemia (AML) is the most common form of adult-onset leukemia and has eight subtypes. Chronic myelogenous leukemia (CML) occurs in about 20% of adult leukemia diagnoses.
- Possible causes of leukemia include exposure to ionizing radiation, exposure to chemicals and drugs, bone marrow hypoplasia (reduced production of blood cells), genetic factors, immunologic factors, environmental factors, and the interaction of these factors.

- The basic pathologic defect is damage to the genes of early precursor leukocyte cells, causing excessive growth of a specific type of immature leukocyte. These cells are abnormal, and their excessive production in the bone marrow stops normal bone marrow production of red blood cells (RBCs), platelets, and mature leukocytes. Anemia, thrombocytopenia, and leukopenia result. Without treatment, the patient will die of infection or hemorrhage. In acute leukemia, these changes occur rapidly and, without intervention, progress to death. Chronic leukemia may be present for years before changes appear.
- Leukemic cells can invade all tissues and organs.

PATIENT-CENTERED COLLABORATIVE CARE
Assessment
- Obtain patient information about:
  1. Age
  2. Environmental exposure to agents that increase the risk for leukemia
  3. Previous illnesses and exposure to ionizing radiation or drugs
  4. History of infections, such as colds, influenza, pneumonia, bronchitis, or unexplained fevers
  5. Any excessive bleeding episodes, because platelet function is often decreased with leukemic disorders. Bleeding can manifest as:
     a. Tendency to bruise easily
     b. Nosebleeds
     c. Increased menstrual flow
     d. Bleeding from the gums
     e. Rectal bleeding
     f. Hematuria
     g. Prolonged bleeding after minor abrasions or cuts
  6. Weakness and fatigue
  7. Associated symptoms (headaches, behavior changes, increased somnolence, decreased attention span, lethargy, muscle weakness, loss of appetite, or weight loss)
- Assess for and document:
  1. Cardiovascular changes
     a. Anemia
     b. Tachycardia
     c. Hypotension
     d. Murmurs and bruits
     e. Slow capillary refill
     f. Bleeding from the gums

L

   2. Respiratory changes:
     a. Increased respiratory rate
     b. Coughing and shortness of breath
     c. Abnormal breath sounds
   3. Skin changes:
     a. Pallor on the face, around the mouth, and in the nail beds
     b. Coolness to the touch
     c. Pale conjunctiva and palmar creases
     d. Petechiae
     e. Ecchymosis
     f. Mouth sores that do not heal
   4. GI changes:
     a. Nausea and anorexia
     b. Weight loss
     c. Rectal fissures
     d. Bloody stools
     e. Reduced bowel sounds
     f. Constipation
     g. Enlarged liver and spleen
     h. Abdominal tenderness
   5. Central nervous system (CNS) changes (in advanced disease):
     a. Papilledema
     b. Seizures
     c. Coma
   6. Miscellaneous changes:
     a. Bone and joint tenderness
     b. Lymph node enlargement
   7. Psychosocial issues and concerns, especially anxiety and fear about the diagnosis, treatment, and outcome
   8. Laboratory abnormalities
     a. Decreased hemoglobin and hematocrit levels
     b. Low platelet count
     c. WBC count (low, normal, or elevated)
- Diagnosis of leukemia is based on findings from bone marrow aspiration and biopsy. The bone marrow is full of leukemic *blast phase cells* (immature cells that are dividing). The leukemia type is diagnosed by cell surface antigens and chromosomal or gene markers.

Planning and Implementation
POTENTIAL FOR INFECTION
- Potential for Infection is related to decreased immune response.
- Infection is a major cause of death in the patient with leukemia, because the WBCs are immature and unable to function, and sepsis is a common complication.
- Infection occurs through *autocontamination* (normal flora overgrows and penetrates the internal environment) and

cross-contamination (organisms from another person or the environment are transmitted to the patient).

- The three most common sites of infection are the skin, respiratory tract, and intestinal tract.
- Implement infection control and patient protection measures:
    1. Use frequent, thorough handwashing before any patient contact
    2. Wear a mask when entering the patient's room if there is a chance of transmitting an upper respiratory tract infection.
    3. Observe strict aseptic procedures when performing dressing changes or accessing a central venous catheter.
    4. Place the patient in a private room, if possible.
    5. Reduce environmental sources of contamination:
        a. Do not leave standing collections of water in vases, denture cups, or humidifiers in the patient's room.
        b. Use of a minimal bacteria diet (no raw fruits and vegetables, undercooked meat, pepper, or paprika)
        c. Use of high-efficiency particulate air (HEPA) filtration or laminar airflow systems
    6. Monitor for infection:
        a. Monitor the daily complete blood count (CBC) with differential WBC count and absolute neutrophil count (ANC).
        b. Inspect the mouth during every shift for lesions and mucosa breakdown.
        c. Assess the lungs every 8 hours for crackles, wheezes, or reduced breath sounds.
        d. Assess all urine for odor and cloudiness.
        e. Ask the patient about any urgency, burning, or pain present on urination.
        f. Take vital signs, including temperature, at least every 4 hours.

◼ NURSING SAFETY PRIORITY: Critical Rescue

A temperature elevation of even 1 °F (or 0.5 °C) above baseline is significant for a patient with leukopenia and indicates infection until it has been proved otherwise.

    7. Provide meticulous skin care to maintain skin integrity.
    8. Implement pulmonary hygiene to prevent pulmonary infection.
    9. Implement agency neutropenia protocols for cultures, infection identification, and initiation of anti-infective therapy when infection is suspected.
- Drug therapy for acute leukemia (for patients with AML) is divided into three distinctive phases:

L

1. *Induction therapy* is intense and consists of combination chemotherapy started at the time of diagnosis. The goal of this therapy is to achieve a rapid, complete remission of all manifestations of disease. These agents cause extreme side effects and toxicities. Care issues for chemotherapy are described under *Cancer Treatment, General,* in Part One.

2. *Consolidation therapy* often consists of another course of the same drugs used for induction at a different dosage or a different combination of chemotherapy drugs. This treatment occurs early in remission, and its intent is to cure.

3. *Maintenance therapy* may be used after successful induction and consolidation therapies for patients with acute lymphoblastic leukemia (ALL) and acute promyelocytic leukemia (APL). The purpose is to maintain the remission achieved through induction and consolidation. Drugs are milder and are often given orally for 2 to 5 years.

- Targeted therapy with imatinib mesylate (Gleevec) may be used for CML that is Philadelphia chromosome positive. Rituximab (Rituxan) may be used as targeted therapy for CLL. Care issues for targeted therapies are listed under *Cancer Treatment, General,* in Part One.
- Drug therapy for infection may include:
  1. Antibiotic and antibacterial drugs:
     a. Aminoglycoside antibiotics
     b. Penicillin or a third-generation cephalosporin
  2. Systemic antifungal drugs:
     a. Amphotericin B
     b. Ketoconazole (Nizoral)
     c. Voriconazole (Vfend)
     d. Fluconazole (Diflucan)
     e. Nystatin (Mycostatin, Nadostine ✦, Nilstat)
  3. Antiviral drugs, most commonly, acyclovir
- The definitive treatment for cure of leukemia after remission is achieved is a hematopoietic stem cell transplantation (HSCT). Care issues for this procedure are discussed under *Hematopoietic Stem Cell Transplantation (Bone Marrow Transplantation).*

POTENTIAL FOR INJURY

- Potential for Injury is related to thrombocytopenia and chemotherapy.
- Normal bone marrow production of platelets is severely limited as a result of the disease or its treatment, leading to thrombocytopenia and increasing the risk for excessive bleeding in response to minimal trauma.
- Nursing interventions

1. Institute bleeding precautions:
   a. Handle the patient gently.
   b. Use and teach unlicensed assistive personnel (UAP) to use a lift sheet when moving and positioning the patient in bed.
   c. Avoid IM injections and venipunctures.
   d. When injections or venipunctures are necessary, use the smallest-gauge needle for the task.
   e. Apply firm pressure to the needle stick site for 10 minutes or until the site no longer oozes blood.
   f. Apply ice to areas of trauma.
   g. Test all urine and stool for the presence of occult blood.
   h. Observe IV sites every 4 hours for bleeding.
   i. Instruct alert patients to notify nursing personnel immediately if any trauma occurs or if bleeding or bruising is noticed.
   j. Avoid trauma to rectal tissues.
   k. Instruct the patient to use an electric shaver rather than a razor.
   l. Provide mouth care using a soft-bristled toothbrush or tooth sponges, and do not floss.
   m. Instruct the patient not to blow the nose or insert objects into the nose.
   n. Ensure that the patient wears shoes with firm soles when ambulating.
2. Monitoring laboratory values daily, especially platelets, and reporting abnormal values
3. Assessing the patient for bleeding
4. Administering prescribed erythropoietic growth factors

FATIGUE
- Fatigue is related to decreased tissue oxygenation and increased energy demands.
- Normal production of RBCs is limited in leukemia, causing anemia, which results in fatigue.
- Interventions aim to reduce fatigue through energy management and improving RBC counts:
  1. Nutrition therapy:
     a. Collaborate with a nutritionist.
     b. Provide small, frequent meals high in protein and carbohydrates.
  2. Transfusion therapy
  3. Drug therapy with colony-stimulating factors:
     a. Epoetin alfa (Epogen or Procrit)
     b. Darbepoetin alfa (Aranesp)
  4. Energy management by eliminating or postponing activities that do not have a direct positive effect on the patient's condition

L

Community-Based Care
- Teach the patient and family about:
  1. Measures to prevent infection
  2. The importance of continuing therapy and medical follow-up
  3. The need to report manifestations of infection or bleeding immediately to the health care provider
  4. Assessing for petechiae, avoiding trauma and sharp objects, applying pressure to wounds for 10 minutes, and reporting blood in the stool or urine or headache that does not respond to acetaminophen
  5. The importance of eating a healthy diet
  6. Resources for psychological and financial support and for role and self-esteem adjustment
  7. Care of the central catheter if in place at discharge
- Assess the patient's need for a home care nurse, aide, or equipment.

LIVER, FATTY

- Fatty liver is caused by the accumulation of triglycerides and other fats in the hepatic cells.
- The most common cause is chronic alcoholism.
- Other causes include malnutrition, diabetes mellitus, obesity, pregnancy, prolonged parenteral nutrition, and exposure to toxic drugs.
- The patient usually has no symptoms; the typical finding is hepatomegaly (an enlarged liver).
- Assess for:
  1. Right upper abdominal pain
  2. Ascites
  3. Edema
  4. Jaundice
  5. Fever
  6. Signs of cirrhosis (see *Cirrhosis*)
- Liver biopsy confirms the diagnosis.
- Interventions are aimed at removing the underlying cause of the infiltration and dietary restrictions.

LYME DISEASE

- Lyme disease is transmitted by infected deer ticks.
- The disease can be prevented by avoiding heavily wooded areas or areas with thick underbrush; by wearing long-sleeved tops, long pants, and socks; and by using an insect repellent on skin

and clothing when in an area where infected ticks are likely to be found.

- Symptoms appear in three stages:
  1. Stage I symptoms appear in 3 to 32 days after the tick bite:
     a. Fever and chills
     b. Swollen glands
     c. Headache
     d. Joint and muscle aches
     e. Spreading, oval or circular rash (erythema migrans)
     f. Drug therapy, including doxycycline, amoxicillin, or cefuroxime
  2. Stage II symptoms appear 2 to 12 weeks after the tick bite:
     a. Cardiac symptoms (dysrhythmia, dizziness, palpitations, dyspnea)
     b. Neurologic symptoms (meningitis, cranial neuropathy, peripheral neuritis)
     c. Drug therapy, including ceftriaxone or cefotaxime
  3. Stage III, chronic persistent Lyme disease, occurs weeks to years after the tick bite and may lead to chronic complications:
     a. Arthralgia and arthritis (may be the only symptom of Lyme disease)
     b. Memory and thinking problems
     c. Fatigue
     d. Enlarged lymph nodes
     e. Drug therapy, including oral tetracycline or IV cephalosporins (for severe disease)
- Testing for Lyme disease is not accurate until 4 to 6 weeks after the initial tick bite.
- Vaccination against Lyme disease is available and should be encouraged for adults living in high-risk areas.
- Refer patients to the Lyme Disease Foundation.

LYMPHOMA, HODGKIN'S AND NON-HODGKIN'S
OVERVIEW
- *Hodgkin's lymphoma (HL)* is a cancer of the lymphoid tissues with abnormal overgrowth of one type of leukocyte, the lymphocyte. It usually starts in a single lymph node or a single chain of nodes and contains a specific cancer cell type, the Reed-Sternberg cell. HL usually spreads from one group of lymph nodes to the next in an orderly fashion.
- *Non-Hodgkin's lymphoma (NHL)* includes all lymphoid cancers that do not have the Reed-Sternberg cell. There are more than

L

602 subtypes of NHL, and they usually spread through the lymphatic system in a less orderly way than HL.
- The exact cause of either type of lymphoma is unknown.
- HL affects any age group, but it is most common among teens and young adults and among adults in their 50s and 60s. NHL is more common in older white men.
- The most common manifestation of either lymphoma type is lymphadenopathy, a large but painless lymph node or nodes.
- Other manifestations of either type may include fever, drenching night sweats, and unexplained weight loss.
- Diagnosis is made on the basis of findings from lymph node biopsy. After diagnosis, lymphoma is classified by subtype and staged to determine extent of disease (which determines exact therapy).

PATIENT-CENTERED COLLABORATIVE CARE
- HL is one of the most treatable types of cancer. Generally, for stage I and stage II disease, the treatment is external irradiation of involved lymph node regions. With more extensive disease, irradiation and combination chemotherapy are used to achieve remission.
- Treatment options for patients with NHL vary based the subtype of the tumor, international prognostic index (IPI) score, stage of the disease, performance status, and overall tumor burden. Options include combinations of chemotherapy drugs, targeted therapies, localized radiation therapy, radiolabeled antibodies, hematopoietic stem cell transplantation, and newer investigational agents.
- Nursing management of the patient undergoing chemotherapy treatment for HL or NHL focuses on the side effects of therapy, especially:
  1. Drug-induced pancytopenia, which increases the risk for infection, anemia, and bleeding
  2. Severe nausea and vomiting
  3. Constipation or diarrhea
  4. Impaired hepatic function
  5. Additional interventions listed under *Cancer Treatment, General,* in Part One
- Nursing management of the patient undergoing radiation therapy for HL or NHL focuses on side effects of therapy, especially:
  1. Skin problems at the site of radiation
  2. Fatigue and taste changes
  3. Permanent sterility for men receiving radiation to the abdominopelvic region in the pattern of an inverted Y in combination with specific chemotherapy drugs
  4. Specific interventions listed under *Cancer Treatment, General,* in Part One

MACULAR DEGENERATION

OVERVIEW

- Macular degeneration is the deterioration of the macula (the area of central vision), and it can be age-related (atrophic) or exudative.
- Age-related macular degeneration (AMD) has two types:
  1. Dry AMD, caused by gradual blockage of retinal capillaries, allows retinal cells in the macula to become ischemic and necrotic. Central vision declines first, but eventually, the person loses all central vision. It is more common and progresses at a faster rate among smokers.
  2. Wet AMD is caused by the growth of new blood vessels in the macula, which have thin walls and leak blood and fluid.
- Exudative macular degeneration is also wet, but it can occur at any age. The condition may occur only in one eye or in both eyes. Patients have a sudden decrease in vision after a serous detachment of pigment epithelium in the macula.

PATIENT-CENTERED COLLABORATIVE CARE

- Management of dry AMD aims to slow disease progression and maximize remaining vision, because there is no cure.
- The loss of central vision reduces the ability to read, write, recognize safety hazards, and drive.
- Suggest alternative strategies (e.g., large-print books, public transportation) and referrals to community organizations that provide a wide range of adaptive equipment.
- See *Visual Impairment (Reduced Vision)* for more discussion of patients' care needs.
- Management of wet macular degeneration focuses on slowing the process and identifying further changes in visual perception.
- Laser therapy to seal the leaking blood vessels in or near the macula can limit the extent of the damage.
- Vascular endothelial growth factor inhibitors (VEGFIs) injected monthly into the vitreous can also slow disease progression
- Photodynamic therapy (PDT) can also seal leaking retinal blood vessels. The patient is given an IV agent to increase photosensitivity. After the agent is absorbed, a special laser light is applied in the specific area to activate the agent, occluding the leaking vessels and preventing excessive formation of new vessels.
  1. The photosensitizer used in PDT increases the sensitivity of the eye and the skin to sunlight and other bright lights for weeks. During this time, the patient is at high risk for skin and retinal burns and must take steps to stay out of the sun and avoid bright lights.

M

MALABSORPTION SYNDROME

- Malabsorption syndrome is associated with a variety of disorders and intestinal surgical procedures and interferes with the ability to absorb nutrients as a result of altered mucosa of the small intestine.
- Physiologic mechanisms limit absorption because of one or more abnormalities, including:
  1. Bile salt deficiencies
  2. Enzyme deficiencies
  3. Presence of bacteria
  4. Disruption of the mucosal lining of the small intestine
  5. Alteration in lymphatic or vascular circulation
  6. Decreased gastric or intestinal surface area
- Clinical manifestations of malabsorption include diarrhea, steatorrhea, weight loss, fatigue, bloating and flatus, decreased libido, easy bruising, anemia, bone pain, and edema.
- Interventions focus on avoiding dietary substances that aggravate malabsorption, supplementing nutrients, and surgical or nonsurgical management of the primary causative disease.

MALNUTRITION

OVERVIEW

- Malnutrition, also known as *undernutrition*, results from inadequate nutrient intake, increased nutrient loss, and increased nutrient requirements; it is a multinutrient problem.
- A weight loss of 5% or more in 30 days, a weight loss of 10% in 6 months, or a weight that is below ideal may indicate malnutrition.
- *Protein-calorie malnutrition (PCM)* affects all aspects of immune function; it causes reduced energy and protein synthesis and increases the risk for infection. There are three forms of PCM:
  1. *Marasmus* is a calorie malnutrition in which body fat and protein are wasted. Serum proteins are often preserved.
  2. *Kwashiorkor* is a lack of protein quantity and quality in the presence of adequate calories. Body weight is normal, and serum levels of proteins are low.
  3. Marasmic-kwashiorkor is a combined protein and energy malnutrition.
- Unrecognized dysphagia is a common problem in older patients and can cause malnutrition.

- Anorexia nervosa (self-induced starvation) and bulimia nervosa (binge eating followed by purging behavior such as self-induced vomiting) also lead to malnutrition.
- Clinical manifestations include:
  1. Leanness and cachexia
  2. Decreased effort tolerance and lethargy
  3. Intolerance to cold
  4. Edema
  5. Dry, flaking skin; dermatitis; or other skin impairment
  6. Poor wound healing
  7. Infections, particularly postoperative

Considerations for Older Adults

Body weight and the body mass index (BMI) usually increase throughout adulthood until about 60 years of age. As people get older, they become less hungry and eat less, even if they are healthy. Older adults should have a BMI between 23 and 27.

PATIENT-CENTERED COLLABORATIVE CARE

- Initiate safety precautions to prevent potential injury from falls due to weakness
- Evaluate skin and initiate interventions to prevent pressure ulcer formation related to nutritional deficits
- Treatment
  1. Identify and treat the precipitating cause.
  2. Examine and treat oral conditions (e.g., caries, pain, ill-fitting dentures) that may contribute to impaired oral intake.
  3. Determine the patient's height and weight, and calculate a BMI.
  4. Provide a high-calorie, high-protein diet and consider fortified nutritional supplements.
  5. Monitor the patient's ability to eat the ordered diet and the amount eaten.
  6. Obtain a dietician consultation.
  7. Provide an environment conducive to eating.
  8. Multivitamins and minerals may be used to supplement intake. Anabolic hormones or steroids such as megestrol (Megace) may be given to stimulate appetite.
  9. Maintain a daily calorie count, and weigh the patient daily. Evaluate whether nutrients consumed are sufficient to meet basal and stress-related energy needs.
  10. Monitor laboratory results for abnormal serum values, especially electrolytes, protein, albumin, prealbumin, hematocrit, hemoglobin, and white blood cell count.

M

- Ensure best practices with enteral feeding:
  1. Prevent tube clogging by rinsing with at least 60 mL of water whenever feeding is interrupted (when giving a drug or stopping feeding).
  2. Mark the tube at the nares or lip, and evaluate tube placement by noting migration of the mark every 4 hours.
  3. Monitor intake and output to determine fluid excess or dehydration.
  4. Prevent aspiration by maintaining back rest elevation greater than 35 degrees unless contraindicated by the patient's condition.
  5. Prevent contamination of the enteral solution and equipment; replace every 24 hours.
- If patient cannot meet caloric and protein goals with oral or combined oral and enteral intake, add specialized nutrition support (parenteral nutrition).
- Evaluate nutritional indices at least weekly: skin intactness, weight, serum albumin, electrolytes, renal function, hemoglobin and hematocrit, and white blood cell count.

⬛ NURSING SAFETY PRIORITY: Action Alert

Undernutrition is a risk factor for development of iatrogenic pressure ulcers. Implement nutritional consultation and skin pressure-relieving interventions for patients with a BMI less than 18.

MASTOIDITIS

- Mastoiditis is an infection of the mastoid air cells that are embedded in the temporal bone.
- It is caused by untreated or inadequately treated otitis media and can be acute or chronic.
- Manifestations include swelling behind the ear and pain with minimal movement of the tragus, the pinna, or the head. Cellulitis develops on the skin or external scalp over the mastoid process, and the ear is pushed sideways and down.
- Otoscopic examination shows a red, dull, thick, immobile eardrum with or without perforation.
- Other manifestations include low-grade fever, malaise, ear drainage, loss of appetite, and enlarged lymph nodes.
- Hearing loss is common.
- Management involves IV antibiotics and surgical removal of the infected tissue if the infection does not respond to antibiotic

therapy. A simple or modified radical mastoidectomy with tympanoplasty is the most common treatment.
- Complications of surgery include damage to cranial nerves VI
  and VII, decreasing the patient's ability to look sideways (cranial
  nerve VI) and causing a drooping of the mouth on the affected
  side (cranial nerve VII). Other complications include vertigo,
  meningitis, brain abscess, chronic purulent otitis media, and
  wound infection.

MELANOMA

OVERVIEW
- Melanomas are pigmented cancers arising in the melanin-
  producing epidermal cells.
- Melanoma is highly metastatic, and a person's survival depends
  on early diagnosis and treatment.
- Risk factors include genetic predisposition, excessive exposure
  to UV light, and the presence of one or more precursor lesions
  that resemble unusual moles.
- It occurs most often among light-skinned races and people older
  than 60 years.

PATIENT-CENTERED COLLABORATIVE CARE
Assessment
- Obtain patient information about:
  1. Age and ethnicity/race
  2. Family history of skin cancer
  3. Any past surgery for removal of skin growths
  4. Recent changes in the size, color, or sensation of any mole,
     birthmark, wart, or scar
  5. Geographic regions where the patient has lived or currently
     lives
  6. Sun exposure
  7. Exposure to arsenic, coal tar, pitch, radioactive waste, or
     radium
- Assess for and document all lesions for:
  1. Location, size, and color
  2. Surface features (ABCDE):
     a. *A*symmetry of shape
     b. *B*order irregularity
     c. *C*olor variation within one lesion
     d. *D*iameter greater than 6 mm
     e. *E*xudate presence and quality
- Diagnosis is made on the bases of biopsy findings.

M

Interventions

Surgical Management

- Surgical intervention is the management of choice for melanoma.
  1. *Excision* is used for the biopsy of small lesions, and a sentinel node biopsy can determine whether tumor spread has started.
  2. *Wide excision* for deeper melanoma often involves removing full-thickness skin in the area of the lesion. Subcutaneous tissues and lymph nodes may also be removed, and grafting may be needed for wound closure.

Nonsurgical Management

- Drug therapy may involve systemic chemotherapy, biotherapy, or targeted therapy.
  1. Systemic chemotherapy with a combination of agents. The general management issues for care of patients undergoing chemotherapy are presented in Part One under *Cancer Therapy.*
  2. Biotherapy with interferon
  3. Targeted therapy with experimental drugs such as a CTLA4 receptor blocker
- Radiation therapy for melanoma may be helpful for patients with metastatic disease when used in combination with systemic corticosteroids. General management issues for care of patients undergoing radiation therapy are presented in Part One under *Cancer Therapy.*

MELANOMA, OCULAR

- Melanoma is the most common malignant eye tumor in adults and is associated with exposure to UV light. Because of its rich blood supply, a melanoma can spread easily into nearby tissue and the brain.
- Manifestations may not be readily apparent, and the tumor may be discovered during a routine examination.
- Manifestations vary with the exact location and may include blurred vision, reduced visual acuity, increased intraocular pressure (IOP), change in iris color, and visual field loss.
- Diagnostic tests usually include ultrasonography or magnetic resonance imaging (MRI).
- Management depends on the tumor's size and growth rate and on the condition of the other eye:
  1. *Enucleation* (surgical removal of the entire eyeball) with insertion of a ball implant to provide a base for fitting the socket prosthesis (in about 1 month)

2. *Radiation therapy* using an implanted radioactive disk to reduce the size and thickness of melanoma:
   a. Complications include vascular changes, retinopathy, glaucoma, necrosis of the sclera, cataract formation, and vitreous hemorrhage.
   b. Cycloplegic eyedrops and an antibiotic-steroid combination are used during the therapy period.

MÉNIÈRE'S DISEASE

OVERVIEW

- Ménière's disease is an excess of endolymphatic fluid that distorts the entire inner-ear canal system.
- This fluid excess leads to tinnitus, one-sided sensorineural hearing loss, and vertigo, occurring in intermittent attacks that can last for several days.
- At first, hearing loss is reversible, but repeated damage to the cochlea from increased fluid pressure leads to permanent hearing loss.
- The disease usually begins in people between the ages of 20 and 50 years and is more common in men and in white people.

PATIENT-CENTERED COLLABORATIVE CARE

Assessment

- Assess patients for:
  1. Sensation of a feeling of fullness in one ear before an attack
  2. Tinnitus, a continuous, low-pitched roar or a humming sound, which worsens just before and during a severe attack
  3. Hearing loss that occurs first with the low-frequency tones but worsens to include all levels after repeated episodes
  4. Vertigo, periods of a whirling sensation that may cause patients to fall. The vertigo is severe and usually lasts 3 to 4 hours.
  5. Nausea and vomiting
  6. Rapid eye movements (nystagmus)
  7. Severe headaches

Interventions

Nonsurgical Management

- Teach patients about attack prevention strategies, including:
  1. Making slow head movements to prevent worsening of the vertigo
  2. Stopping smoking, because nicotine constricts blood vessels
  3. Participating in the hydrops diet to reduce endolymphatic fluid excess; the diet includes:

M

   a. Distributing food and fluid intake evenly throughout the
      day and from day to day
   b. Avoiding foods or fluids that have a high salt content
   c. Drinking adequate amounts of fluids (low in sugar) daily
   d. Avoiding caffeine-containing fluids and foods
   e. Limiting alcohol intake to one glass of beer or wine
      each day
   f. Avoiding foods containing monosodium glutamate (MSG)
- Drug therapy to control the vertigo and vomiting and restore
  normal balance:
  1. Mild diuretics
  2. Nicotinic acid
  3. Antihistamines (just before and during an acute attack)
     a. Diphenhydramine hydrochloride (Benadryl, Allerdryl ✦)
     b. Dimenhydrinate (Dramamine, Gravol ✦)
  4. Antiemetics
  5. Intratympanic therapy with gentamycin and steroids
- Use of the Meniett device, which applies low-pressure micro-
  pulses to the inner ear for 5 minutes three times daily
  Surgical Management
- Surgical treatment of Ménière's disease is a last resort,
  because the hearing in the affected ear is often lost from the
  procedure.
- The specific surgical procedure depends on the degree of ser-
  viceable hearing, the severity of the spells, and the condition
  of the opposite ear.
- A labyrinthectomy is performed through the ear canal.
- Endolymphatic decompression is performed with drainage and
  a shunt.

MENINGITIS

OVERVIEW
- Meningitis is inflammation of the meninges that surround the
  brain and spinal cord.
- The infecting organism produces an inflammatory response in
  the pia mater, the arachnoid, the cerebral spinal fluid (CSF), and
  the ventricles.
- Bacterial meningitis is potentially life threatening; viral meningitis is usually self-limiting; and cryptococcal meningitis is the
  most common fungal meningitis.
- Vaccinations can prevent meningitis from meningococcal and
  Haemophilus influenzae microorganisms.

PATIENT CENTERED COLLABORATIVE CARE

Assessment

- Obtain patient information about:
  1. Recent viral or respiratory diseases and exposure to communicable disease
  2. Shared utensils, cups, or water bottles
  3. Head or spine surgery or trauma or ear, nose, or sinus infection
  4. Heart disease, diabetes mellitus, cancer, immunosuppressive therapy, and neurologic procedures that increase risk for infection or invading organisms
- Assess for and document:
  1. Fever, neck stiffness, headache, and altered mental status
  2. Rash, especially on trunk or abdomen
  3. Photophobia
  4. Nuchal rigidity and Kernig's and Brudzinski's signs, which are present in only a small percentage of patients with definite meningitis
  5. Seizure and focal neurologic deficits, especially with bacterial meningitis
  6. Change in level of consciousness
  7. Possible syndrome of inappropriate antidiuretic hormone (SIADH)
  8. Complications of meningitis, including coagulopathy resulting in emboli that compromise peripheral circulation
- Diagnostic studies may include:
  1. Lumbar puncture to obtain cerebrospinal fluid for cell count, differential, protein, and culture. Although antibiotic administration should NOT be delayed for this procedure, it is desirable to complete the spinal fluid collection before the first dose of antibiotics.
  2. Serum levels of white blood cells (WBCs) and electrolytes, especially to detect low sodium levels associated with diuresis
  3. Computed tomography (CT) scan to detect inflamed meninges, abscess (encapsulated pus), and intracranial hypertension

Interventions

- Assess and record the patient's neurologic status with vital signs and peripheral circulation at least every 4 hours. Level of consciousness is the most sensitive indicator of change in patient status.
- Assess and record with particular attention to cranial nerves III, IV, VI, VII, and VIII (pupillary response to light and ability to move eyes through four quadrants promotes early detection, concerning deterioration of patient condition).

M

- Administer drugs such as antibiotics and analgesics as ordered.
- Maintain isolation precautions according to hospital policy.
- Implement institutional seizure precautions when indicated.
- Monitor for complications such as vascular compromise from emboli, shock, coagulation disorders, prolonged fever, and septic complications.
- Encourage vaccinations, especially if travelling or living in shared residential spaces (e.g., group homes, dormitories, or skilled nursing facilities).

METABOLIC SYNDROME

- Metabolic syndrome, also called *syndrome X*, is classified as the simultaneous presence of metabolic factors known to increase risk for developing type 2 diabetes and cardiovascular disease.
- A diagnosis is made based on the presence of three or more of the following features:
  1. Abdominal obesity, with waist circumference of at least 40 inches (100 cm) for men and 35 inches (88 cm) for women
  2. Hyperglycemia, with an elevated fasting blood glucose level of 100 mg/dL or more or receiving drug treatment for elevated glucose
  3. Hypertension, with a systolic blood pressure of 130 mm Hg or more, diastolic blood pressure of 85 mg Hg or more, or receiving drug treatment for hypertension
  4. Dyslipidemia, with a total cholesterol level > 200 mg/dL or receiving drug therapy for hypercholesterolemia; triglyceride level 150 mg/dL or more or receiving drug treatment for elevated triglycerides; high-density lipoprotein (HDL) cholesterol less than 40 mg/dL for men or less than 50 mg/dL for women
- Any one of these health problems increases the rate of atherosclerosis and the risk for stroke, coronary heart disease, and early death.
- Teach patients about the lifestyle changes that can improve health, including:
  1. Reducing weight to within 20% of ideal or body mass index (BMI) to 18 to 25 kg/m^2
  2. Increasing physical activity to a moderate intensity most days of the week
  3. Adhering to drug therapy to achieve desired glycemic, lipid, blood pressure, and weight goals

METHICILLIN-RESISTANT *STAPHYLOCOCCUS AUREUS*

OVERVIEW

- *Staphylococcus aureus* is a common skin bacterium that does not cause infection unless it invades the body. Methicillin-resistant *Staphylococcus aureus* (MRSA) is a variation of this common skin bacterium.
- MRSA manifests as an infection that is not responsive to penicillin and penicillin-like drugs.
- MRSA further varies by site of infection acquisition. One strain is characteristic of hospital-acquired infections and a separate strain is associated with community-acquired infections.
- MRSA is easily spread to other body areas and to other people through direct contact with infected skin and by contact with articles of clothing, bed linens, athletic equipment, towels, and other objects used by a person with MRSA.
- If MRSA infects a wound or gains access into the blood, deep wound infection, sepsis, organ damage, and death can occur.
- The incidence of the problem is highest among adults living in communal environments, such as dormitories or prisons, and among patients in hospitals or other residential health care settings.

PATIENT-CENTERED COLLABORATIVE CARE

- Drug therapy for patients infected with MRSA may include vancomycin (IV only), linezolid, doxycycline, or clindamycin.
- Nursing care focuses on teaching the patient and family techniques to prevent the spread of MRSA, including the use of contact precautions when the infected patient is in a hospital setting:
  1. Avoiding contact with others, including participation in contact sports, until the infection has cleared
  2. Taking all prescribed antibiotics exactly as prescribed for the entire time prescribed
  3. Keeping the infected skin area covered with clean, dry bandages
  4. Changing the bandage whenever drainage seeps through it
  5. Placing soiled bandages in a plastic bag and sealing it closed before placing it in the regular trash
  6. Washing hands with soap and warm water before and after touching the infected area or handling the bandages

M

7. Showering (rather than bathing) daily using an antibacterial soap or chlorhexidine. Daily dilute bleach baths for several weeks may also be prescribed.
8. Washing all uninfected skin areas before washing the infected area or using a fresh washcloth to wash the uninfected areas
9. Using each washcloth only once before laundering and avoiding using bath sponges or puffs
10. Sleeping in a separate bed from others until the infection is cleared
11. Avoiding sitting on or using upholstered furniture
12. Not sharing clothing, washcloths, towels, athletic equipment, shavers or razors, or any other personal items
13. Cleaning surfaces that may have come into contact with infected skin, drainage, or used bandages (e.g., bathroom counters, shower or bath stalls, toilet seats) with household disinfectant or bleach water mixed daily (1 tablespoon of liquid bleach to 1 quart water)
14. Washing all soiled clothing and linens with hot water and laundry detergent; drying clothing in a hot dryer or outside on a clothesline in the sun
15. Urging family members and close friends to shower daily with an antibacterial soap
16. Ensuring that anyone who assists changing the bandages uses disposable gloves, pulls them off inside out when finished, places them with the soiled bandages in a sealed bag, and washes his or her hands thoroughly

MULTIPLE SCLEROSIS

OVERVIEW
- Multiple sclerosis (MS) is a chronic autoimmune disease that affects the myelin sheath and conduction pathway of the central nervous system (CNS).
- Women are affected twice as often as men.
- MS often mimics other neurologic diseases, which makes the diagnosis difficult and prolonged.
- The major types of MS are:
  1. Relapsing-remitting MS (RRMS), which is characterized as mild or moderate, depending on the degree of disability. Symptoms develop and resolve in a few weeks to months, after which the patient may return to baseline.
  2. Primary progressive MS (PPMS), which is characterized by a steady and gradual neurologic deterioration without

remission of symptoms. The patient has progressive disability with no acute attacks. Patients with this type of MS tend to be between 40 and 60 years old at onset of the disease.

3. Secondary progressive MS (SPMS) begins with a relapsing-remitting course that later becomes steadily progressive. About half of all people with RRMS develop SPMS within 10 years. The current addition of disease-modifying drugs as part of disease management may decrease the development of SPMS.

4. Progressive-relapsing MS (PRMS) is characterized by frequent relapses with partial recovery, but not a return to baseline. This type of MS is seen in only a small percentage of patients. Progressive, cumulative symptoms and deterioration occur over several years.

PATIENT-CENTERED COLLABORATIVE CARE
Assessment
- Assess for and document:
  1. Progression of symptoms (the patient often reports that symptoms were noticed several years earlier but disappeared, and medical attention was not sought)
  2. Factors that aggravate symptoms:
     a. Stress
     b. Fatigue
     c. Overexertion
     d. Temperature extremes
     e. Hot shower or bath
  3. Motor function:
     a. Fatigue
     b. Stiffness of legs
     c. Flexor spasms
     d. Increased deep tendon reflexes
     e. Clonus
     f. Positive Babinski's reflex
     g. Absent abdominal reflexes
  4. Cerebellar function:
     a. Ataxic gait
     b. Intention tremor (tremor when performing activity)
     c. Dysmetria (inability to direct or limit movement)
     d. Clumsy motor movements
  5. Cranial nerve function:
     a. Hearing loss
     b. Facial weakness
     c. Swallowing difficulties (dysphagia)
     d. Tinnitus

M

  e. Vertigo
6. Vision:
    a. Decreased visual acuity
    b. Blurred vision
    c. Diplopia
    d. Scotoma (changes in peripheral vision)
    e. Nystagmus
7. Sensation:
    a. Hypalgesia
    b. Paresthesia
    c. Facial pain
    d. Change in bowel and bladder function
    e. Impotence, difficulty sustaining an erection
    f. Decreased vaginal secretion
8. Cognitive changes seen late in the course of the disease:
    a. Memory loss
    b. Decreased ability to perform calculations
    c. Inattention
    d. Impaired judgment
9. Psychosocial function:
    a. Apathy, emotional lability, and depression
    b. Disturbed body image
- Diagnostic testing may include:
  1. Magnetic resonance imaging (MRI) to determine the presence of plaques in the CNS
  2. Lumbar puncture for analysis of cerebral spinal fluid (CSF)

Interventions

- Provide sufficient time to complete ADLs; as a result of weakness and fatigue, the patient requires more time or assistance.
- Collaborate with physical and occupational therapists and vocational rehabilitation specialists to assist the patient with:
  1. Implementing an exercise program to strengthen and stretch muscles
  2. Using assistive devices for ambulation, such as a cane, walker, or electric (Amigo) cart
  3. Using assistive-adaptive devices to remain independent in ADLs
  4. Valuing the importance of avoiding rigorous activities that lead to an increase in body temperature, which may lead to fatigue, decreased motor ability, and decreased visual acuity
- Drug therapy includes:

1. Current therapies are designed to treat the dysfunctional immune system that is associated with MS:
   a. Interferon-beta (Avonex, Betaseron, Rebif), immunomodulators that modify the course of the disease and have antiviral effects
   b. Glatiramer acetate (Copaxone), a synthetic protein that is similar to myelin-based protein
   c. Natalizumab (Tysabri), the first monoclonal antibody approved for MS that binds to white blood cells (WBCs) to prevent further damage to the myelin; its use is controversial due to serious adverse drug reactions
   d. Mitoxantrone (Novantrone), a chemotherapy drug, reduces disability and the frequency of clinical relapses in patients with secondary progressive, progressive-relapsing, or worsening relapsing-remitting MS.
   e. Fingolimod (Gilenya) is the first oral immunomodulator approved for the management of MS. Monitor heart rate (HR) as the drug can cause bradycardia, especially within the first 6 hours after taking it.
   f. A combination of cyclophosphamide (Cytoxan) and methylprednisolone (Solu-Medrol) may be used for some patients to stabilize the disease process and decrease inflammation. IV adrenocorticotropic hormone (ACTH) may be given instead of methylprednisolone and tapered gradually over 2 to 4 weeks.
2. Steroid therapy (glucocorticoid)
3. Adjunctive therapy to treat muscle spasticity and paresthesia
4. Adjunctive therapy for bladder and bowel dysfunction. Urine and fecal incontinence can be debilitating for this population.
5. Antispasmodics, antiepileptic drugs (AEDs), analgesics, NSAIDs, tranquilizers, or antidepressants to treat pain, paresthesia, and mood disorder
- Other interventions include:
  1. Strategies to maintain or modify mobility and independence in ADLs
  2. Managing cognitive problems in the areas of attention, memory, problem solving, visual perception, and use of speech
  3. Applying an eye patch to relieve diplopia and switching the eye patch every few hours
  4. Teaching scanning techniques to compensate for peripheral vision deficits

M

5. Teaching the patient to test the temperature of the bath water at home before placing his or her hands in hot water
6. Referring the patient to a therapist or nurse educated in issues surrounding sexuality

- Patients using complementary therapies, such as nutritional supplements, acupressure, and bee stings, report improvement in their condition, but these modalities have not been scientifically tested.

Community-Based Care
- Home care management includes:
  1. Explaining the development of MS and the factors that may exacerbate the symptoms
  2. Stressing the importance of avoiding overexertion, extremes of temperatures (fever, hot baths, overheating, excessive chilling), humidity, and exposure to infection
  3. Providing drug information, as needed
  4. Encouraging the patient to follow the exercise program developed by the physical therapist and to remain independent in all activities for as long as possible
  5. Encouraging the patient to engage in regular social activities, obtain adequate rest, and manage stress
  6. Teaching the family strategies to cope with personality changes
  7. Reviewing the established bowel and bladder, skin care, and nutrition programs
  8. Referring the patient to local and national support groups as needed

MYASTHENIA GRAVIS

OVERVIEW
- Myasthenia gravis (MG) is an acquired autoimmune disease characterized by fatigue and weakness primarily in muscles innervated by the cranial nerves, as well as in skeletal and respiratory muscles.
- MG is caused by an autoantibody attack on the acetylcholine receptors (AChRs) in the muscle end plate membranes. As a result, nerve impulses are not transmitted to the skeletal muscle at the neuromuscular junction.
- The thymus gland is often abnormal.
- In *Eaton-Lambert syndrome,* a form of myasthenia often observed in combination with small cell carcinoma of the lung, the muscles of the trunk and the pelvic and shoulder girdles are most commonly affected.

PATIENT-CENTERED COLLABORATIVE CARE

Assessment

- Obtain patient information about:
  1. Muscular weakness that increases on exertion or as the day wears on and improves with rest (with a temporary increase in weakness sometimes noted after vaccination, menstruation, and exposure to extremes in environmental temperature)
  2. Rapid, temporary onset of fatigue or weakness associated with infection, pregnancy, or anesthesia and after vaccination, menstruation, and exposure to extremes in environmental temperature
  3. Inability to perform ADLs
  4. Ptosis, diplopia or weakness in facial muscles
  5. Difficulty swallowing (dysphagia), choking
  6. Respiratory distress
  7. Family history of MG or thymic disorder
  8. Weakness of voice
  9. Decreased sensation (paresthesia) or aching in weakened muscles
- Assess for and document:
  1. Progressive paresis of affected muscle groups that is resolved by rest, at least in part
  2. Symptoms related to involvement of the levator palpebrae or extraocular muscles:
     a. Ocular palsies
     b. Ptosis
     c. Diplopia
     d. Weak or incomplete eye closure
  3. Involvement of muscles for facial expression, chewing, and speech:
     a. The patient's smile may turn into a snarl.
     b. The jaw hangs.
     c. Difficulty chewing and swallowing may lead to severe nutritional deficits.
  4. Because of proximal limb weakness, difficulty climbing stairs, lifting heavy objects, or raising arms overhead
  5. Mild or severe neck weakness
  6. Difficulty sustaining a sitting or walking posture
  7. Respiratory distress
  8. Bowel and bladder incontinence
  9. Weakness of the pelvic and shoulder girdles (seen in Eaton-Lambert syndrome, a special form of MG often observed in combination with small cell carcinoma of the lung)
  10. Disturbed body image

M

11. Feelings of loss, fear, helplessness, and grief
12. Usual coping methods
13. Positive AChR antibodies
14. Significant improvement after Tensilon testing
- Diagnostic studies may include:
  1. Serum thyroid function tests
  2. Serum protein electrophoresis tests to evaluate presence of autoantibodies
  3. Serum AChR antibodies
  4. Chest x-ray and computed tomography (CT) scan to evaluate the thymus gland in the mediastinum
  5. Pharmacologic tests with the cholinesterase inhibitors edrophonium (Tensilon) and neostigmine (Prostigmin); anticipate a marked improvement of muscle tone that lasts 4 to 5 minutes.
  6. Repetitive nerve stimulation of proximal nerves, the most common electrodiagnostic test performed to detect MG; alternatively, electromyography to test muscle contraction or single fiber contraction after electrical stimulation is used.

Interventions

Nonsurgical Management

- Administer drugs to reduce the symptoms of MG without influencing the actual course of the disease (anticholinesterases or cholinergic drugs). Give these drugs for MG on time to avoid respiratory compromise and muscular weakness:
  1. Cholinesterase inhibitor drugs, also referred to as *anticholinesterase drugs,* typically pyridostigmine (Mestinon, Regonol) to prevent the breakdown of acetylcholine by enzymes in the neuromuscular junction, thereby increasing the response of muscles to nerve impulses and improving strength:
      a. The drug is given with a small amount of food to minimize GI side effects; meals are provided 45 minutes to 1 hour after taking the drug.
      b. Drugs containing magnesium, morphine or its derivatives, curare, quinine, quinidine, procainamide, hypnotics, or sedatives are avoided, because they may increase weakness.
      c. Antibiotics such as neomycin, kanamycin, streptomycin, polymyxin B, and certain tetracyclines increase myasthenic symptoms by impairing transmitter release.
  2. Implement interventions to induce remission, such as the administration of immunosuppressive drugs or corticosteroids, plasmapheresis, and thymectomy (removal of the thymus gland)

- Observe for myasthenic crisis, an exacerbation of the myasthenic symptoms caused by underdosing with anticholinergic drugs or by infection.
  1. Maintain adequate respiratory functioning (ABCs [airway, breathing, circulation] of emergency care); intubation and mechanical ventilation may be needed.
  2. Withhold cholinesterase-inhibiting drugs, because they increase respiratory secretion and are usually ineffective for the first few days after the crisis begins.
  3. Anticipate restarting drugs gradually at lower doses.
- Observe for cholinergic crisis, an acute exacerbation of muscle weakness caused by overdosing with cholinergic (anticholinesterase) drugs.
  1. Withhold cholinesterase-inhibiting drugs until symptoms resolve.
  2. Anticipate administration of atropine to treat excess acetylcholine. Atropine may thicken secretions, causing more difficulty with airway clearance and possible development of mucous plugs.
- Monitor the patient's responses to and vascular access for plasmapheresis. Plasmapheresis is a method by which autoantibodies are removed from the plasma.
- Provide respiratory support and frequent assessment of airway and breathing, including:
  1. Performing a respiratory assessment at least every 4 hours
  2. Reporting respiratory distress: dyspnea, shortness of breath, air hunger, and confusion
  3. Encouraging the patient to turn, cough, and deep breathe every 2 hours
  4. Performing chest physiotherapy, including postural drainage, percussion, and vibration to aid in removal of secretions
  5. Keeping an Ambu bag, equipment for oxygen administration, and endotracheal intubation equipment at the bedside in case of respiratory distress
- Promote mobility and in-bed positioning to maintain function
- Enhance self-care, including:
  1. Assessing the patient's ability to perform ADLs to establish his or her abilities and limitations
  2. Encouraging the patient to perform activities as independently as possible
  3. Planning activities to follow the administration of drug to maximize independence and successful attempts at self-care
  4. Collaborating with physical and occupational therapists to identify the need for assistive devices

M

- Assist with communication:
    1. Collaborate with the speech-language pathologist to develop communication strategies as needed.
    2. Instruct the patient to speak slowly and repeat information to verify that it is correct.
    3. Develop alternative communication systems such as flash cards.
- Ensure adequate nutritional support:
    1. Provide small, frequent meals and high-calorie snacks. Record calorie counts.
    2. Measure intake and output, serum albumin levels, and daily weight.
    3. Assess for the onset of dysphagia. Implement aspiration precautions as needed.
    4. Promote or provide oral hygiene.
    5. Obtain a dietary consultation to optimize nutritional strategies.
- Maintain eye protection:
    1. Apply artificial tears to keep corneas moist and free from abrasion.
    2. Consider a lubricant gel and eye shield at bedtime.
    3. To help relieve diplopia, cover alternate eyes with a patch for 2 to 3 hours at a time.

Surgical Management

- Thymectomy may be performed early in the disease. Remission may not occur even with a thymectomy or may take up to 2 years to show effect.
- Provide routine preoperative care as outlined in Part One, including:
    1. Administering pyridostigmine (Mestinon), as ordered, to keep the patient stable throughout surgery
    2. If steroids have been used, administering before surgery but tapering postoperatively
    3. Giving antibiotics before and after surgery
- Provide routine postoperative care as outlined in Part One, including:
    1. Observing for signs of pneumothorax or hemothorax such as chest pain, sudden shortness of breath, diminished or absent breath sounds, and restlessness or a change in vital signs
    2. Focusing on respiratory health, including using spirometry, coughing, deep breathing, and frequent monitoring for respiratory distress
    3. Observing for signs and symptoms of wound infection
    4. Providing chest tube care if indicated

Community-Based Care

- Emphasize specific points concerning the disease process:
  1. MG is characterized by episodic exacerbations (worsening of symptoms). If rest does not relieve symptoms or respiratory distress occurs, contacting your health care provider is indicated.
  2. Avoid factors that predispose the patient to exacerbation, such as infection, stress, surgery, and hard physical exercise.
  3. Teach the patient and family to monitor for these two types of crises:
     a. Myasthenic crisis: an exacerbation (flare-up or worsening) of the myasthenic symptoms caused by not enough anticholinesterase drugs
     b. Cholinergic crisis: an acute exacerbation of muscle weakness caused by too many anticholinesterase drugs
  4. Promote lifestyle adaptations, such as avoiding heat (sauna, sunbathing), crowds, overeating, and erratic changes in sleep habits.
- Provide information concerning the drug regimen, and include the name, effects, side effects, and the importance of taking drugs on time and not missing doses.
- Encourage the patient's family to become certified in cardiopulmonary resuscitation (CPR).
- Refer the patient to community agencies and support groups such as the Myasthenia Gravis Foundation.

NEPHROSCLEROSIS

- Nephrosclerosis is a problem of thickening in the nephron blood vessel, resulting in narrowing of the lumen, decreased renal blood flow, and chronically hypoxic kidney tissue.
- Ischemia and fibrosis develop over time.
- Nephrosclerosis is associated with hypertension, atherosclerosis, and diabetes mellitus.
- Prevention and reduction of kidney damage includes control of lipidemia, glycemia, and hypertension.

NEPHROTIC SYNDROME

- Nephrotic syndrome is a condition of increased glomerular permeability that allows larger molecules to pass through the membrane into the urine and be removed from the blood.
- Nephrotic syndrome is commonly caused by changes in an immune or inflammatory process.

- The main features are severe proteinuria, hypoalbuminemia, hyperlipidemia, lipiduria, facial and periorbital edema, and derangements in blood pressure.
- Treatment depends on what is causing the disorder (identified by renal biopsy) and may include:
    1. Angiotensin-converting enzyme inhibitors to preserve kidney function in early stages
    2. Cholesterol-lowering drugs and drugs to control glycemia
    3. Anti-inflammatory and immunosuppressive agents such as glucocorticoids
    4. Heparin to reduce clot formation and extension (clots form as part of the inflammatory response)
    5. Diuretics
    6. Diet changes, including fluid and sodium restriction
- Assess the patient's hydration status, and monitor for dehydration. If the plasma volume is depleted, kidney problems worsen.
- Assess laboratory values for changes in kidney function including serum blood urea nitrogen (BUN), creatinine, electrolytes, and urinalysis

NEUROMA, ACOUSTIC

- An acoustic neuroma is a nonmalignant tumor of cranial nerve VIII (vestibulocochlear nerve, also known as the *auditory* or *acoustic* nerve). Damage to hearing, facial movements, and sensation can occur as the tumor grows.
- Manifestations begin with tinnitus and progress to gradual sensorineural hearing loss in most patients. Constant, mild vertigo occurs later.
- Diagnosis is made by computed tomography (CT) scanning, magnetic resonance imaging (MRI), audiograms, and cerebrospinal fluid assays.
- Surgical removal is achieved by a craniotomy, and the remaining hearing is lost. Extreme care is taken to preserve the function of the facial nerve (cranial nerve VII). For care of the patient having a craniotomy, see *Surgical Management* under *Tumors, Brain.* See *Hearing Loss* for a review of care needs for the patient whose hearing is reduced.

OBESITY

OVERVIEW

- *Obesity* refers to an excess amount of body fat compared with lean body mass.

- An obese person weighs at least 20% above the upper limit of the normal range for ideal body weight (IBW) and has a body mass index (BMI) of 30 cm/kg^2 or more.
- *Morbid obesity,* also called *extreme obesity,* refers to a weight that has a severely negative effect on health, usually more than 100% above IBW or a BMI of 40 cm/kg^2 or more.
- More than one third of the U.S. population is obese, and another third is overweight. At least 10% of adults are morbidly obese. This problem is the second leading cause of preventable deaths in the United States.
- Obesity involves complex interrelationships among genetic, environmental, psychological, social, cultural, pathologic, behavioral, and physiologic factors.
- Causes of obesity include high-fat and high-cholesterol diets, physical inactivity, drug treatment (corticosteroids, NSAIDs), and familial and genetic factors.
- Complications include diabetes mellitus, hypertension, hyperlipidemia, cardiac disease, sleep apnea, cholelithiasis, chronic back pain, early degenerative arthritis, susceptibility to infections, and certain cancers.
- Bariatrics is a branch of medicine that manages obesity and its related diseases.

◤NATIONAL PATIENT SAFETY GOAL

The Joint Commission's Patient Care Standards require that a nutritional screening occur within 24 hours after the patient's admission to the intensive care unit. If indicated, an in-depth nutritional assessment should be performed. When patients are in the hospital for more than 1 week, nutritional assessment should be part of the daily plan of care.

PATIENT-CENTERED COLLABORATIVE CARE
- Obtain patient information about:
  1. Economic status
  2. Usual food intake
  3. Eating behaviors
  4. Cultural background
  5. Attitude toward food and current weight
  6. Appetite
  7. Drugs
  8. Physical activity
  9. Height and weight
  10. Chronic diseases
  11. Family history of obesity
  12. 24-hour diet history recall

- Management includes:
  1. Diet programs managed through close interaction among the patient, dietitian, nutritionist, and health care provider
  2. Exercise program
  3. Drug therapy:
     a. Anorectic drugs suppress appetite, which reduces food intake and over time may result in weight loss.
     b. Orlistat (Xenical) inhibits lipase and leads to partial hydrolysis of triglycerides. Because fats are only partially digested and absorbed, calorie intake is decreased.
  4. Behavioral treatment to change habits around eating and weight management
- Surgery is indicated for the patient who is morbidly obese or who has a BMI greater than 35 with comorbidities that contribute to poor health.
  1. Bariatric surgical procedures include three types: gastric restrictive, malabsorption, or both. *Restrictive surgeries* decrease the volume capacity of the stomach to limit the amount of food that can be eaten at one time. As the name implies, *malabsorption procedures* interfere with the absorption of food and nutrients from the GI tract.
     a. Most patients have laparoscopic adjustable gastric band (LAGB) surgery or the laparoscopic sleeve gastrectomy (LSG). Both procedures are classified as restrictive surgeries.
     b. Malabsorptive procedures are no longer common or preferred.
- Provide routine postoperative care after bariatric surgery:
  1. Attention to airway management, because a thick neck may lead to a compromised airway.
  2. Focus on patient and staff safety, using specialized bariatric equipment to promote mobility and reduce skin complications.
  3. Monitor the patency of the nasogastric tube (NGT) and record the amount of drainage.
  4. Monitor for manifestations of anastomotic leak if this process was part of the surgical approach. Manifestations of leak are increasing back, shoulder, or abdominal pain; restlessness; unexplained tachycardia; and oliguria (scant urine). Report any of these findings to the surgeon immediately.
  5. Apply an abdominal binder to prevent wound dehiscence.
  6. Place the patient in a semi-Fowler's position.
  7. Use continuous positive airway pressure (CPAP) ventilation at night to improve ventilation and decrease risk for sleep apnea.
  8. Implement best practices for maintaining skin integrity and observe skin folds for redness, excoriation, or breakdown.

9. Observe for dumping syndrome, manifested by frequent, liquid stools.

Community-Based Care

- Give the patient a list of community resources, such as Weight Watchers, Overeaters Anonymous, and Take Off Pounds Sensibly (TOPS).
- In collaboration with the nutritionist, provide health teaching regarding the diet and the importance of maintaining a healthy eating pattern.
- Encourage the patient to increase physical activity, decrease fat intake and reliance on drug use, establish a normal eating pattern in response to physiologic hunger, and address medical and psychological problems.
- Emphasize the necessity for follow-up after bariatric surgery to avoid complications and ensure safe weight loss.

OBSTRUCTION, INTESTINAL

OVERVIEW

- Intestinal obstruction can be partial or complete; intestinal contents accumulate at or above the obstruction.
- Intestinal obstruction can occur in the small intestine or large intestine (bowel). It can be either mechanical or nonmechanical (paralytic):
  1. *Mechanical obstruction* occurs when the bowel is physically obstructed by disorders outside the intestine (adhesions or hernias) or blockages in the lumen of the intestine (tumors, fecal impactions, and strictures).
  2. *Nonmechanical obstruction (paralytic or adynamic ileus)* occurs when peristalsis is decreased or absent, resulting in a slowing of the movement or a backup of intestinal content caused by physiologic, neurogenic, or chemical imbalances:
     a. Paralytic ileus is associated with trauma, abdominal surgery, hypokalemia, myocardial infarction, or vascular insufficiency.
- Distention results from the inability of the intestine to absorb and mobilize intestinal contents. Edema of the bowel and increased capillary permeability occur with intestinal distention. Absorption of fluid and electrolytes into the vascular space is compromised and can lead to reduced circulatory blood volume and electrolyte imbalances. Hypovolemia ranges from mild to extreme.
- Strangulated obstruction results when there is obstruction with compromised blood flow. This is a surgical emergency.

PATIENT-CENTERED COLLABORATIVE CARE
Assessment
- Obtain patient information about:
  1. Medical history, including abdominal surgical procedures, radiation therapy, and bowel diseases such as Crohn's disease, ulcerative colitis, diverticular disease, gallstones, hernias, trauma, and peritonitis
  2. Diet history
  3. Bowel elimination patterns, including the presence of blood in the stool
  4. Familial history of colorectal cancer
  5. Nausea and vomiting, including color of emesis
- Assess for and document:
  1. Quality of abdominal pain, onset, and aggravating and alleviating factors associated with pain
  2. Bowel sounds: High-pitched bowel sounds (borborygmi) may be heard early in an obstructive process and absent bowel sounds in later stages.
  3. Abdominal distention (hallmark sign)
  4. Nausea, vomiting, and character of emesis:
     a. Obstruction above the ileum causes early and profuse vomiting of partially digested food and chyme, changing to watery contents containing bile and mucus.
     b. Obstruction in the large intestine produces vomitus with an orange-brown color and a foul odor caused by bacterial overgrowth, which may be fecal contamination.
  5. No passage of stool (obstipation), which is characteristic of total small- and large-bowel mechanical obstruction
  6. Hiccups (singultus), which is common with all types of intestinal obstruction
- Diagnostic studies may include:
  1. Flat-plate and upright abdominal x-rays
  2. Abdominal ultrasound or computed tomography (CT) scan to further pinpoint the location and cause of the obstruction

■ NURSING SAFETY PRIORITY: Critical Rescue
The sudden change in abdominal pain from dull to sharp or local to generalized may indicate a perforation after obstruction. Inform the physician immediately of this change in patient pain, along with current vital signs and oxygen status. A perforation is a surgical emergency.

Interventions
- Interventions are aimed at uncovering the cause and relieving the obstruction.

Nonsurgical Management
- Decompress the GI tract by inserting or maintaining a gastric or intestinal tube, which can be inserted nasally or orally.
  1. Ensure that the patient receives nothing by mouth or decompressive tube.
  2. Maintain patency of decompressive tube:
     a. The Salem sump or Anderson suction tube sits distally in the stomach and is connected to low continuous suction.
     b. Levine tubes are connected to low intermittent suction.

🚹 NURSING SAFETY PRIORITY: Action Alert

At least every 4 hours, assess for proper placement of the tube, tube patency, and output (quality and quantity). Monitor the nasal skin around the tube and opening where the nasogastric tube (NGT) is inserted for irritation. Use a device that secures the tube to the nose to prevent accidental removal. Clean the nose with the same type of skin protectant used for ostomy skin care before applying the NGT-securing device. Assess for peristalsis by auscultating for bowel sounds with the suction disconnected (suction masks peristaltic sounds).

  3. Monitor and record quantity and character of nasogastric (NG) or nasointestinal tube output every 4 hours.
  4. Assess the nares for integrity at the site of tube insertion.
  5. Mark the tube at the nares to provide ongoing confirmation of placement.
  6. Record the passage of flatus and the amount and character of bowel movements.
  7. Measure the patient's abdominal girth daily.
  8. Inform the health care provider if gastric or intestinal outflow stops or becomes bloody.
- Obstruction caused by fecal impaction resolves after disimpaction and enema.
- Intussusception (telescoping of bowel) may resolve with hydrostatic pressure changes during a barium enema or with manipulation under fluoroscopy.
- Administer fluid and electrolyte replacement:
  1. Administer IV fluid because of vascular fluid losses from lack of normal reabsorption in the intestine, increased intestinal secretions, NG suction, and NPO status (normal saline solutions with potassium replacement are used according to electrolyte results).
  2. Provide blood products in case of strangulated obstruction because of blood loss into the bowel or peritoneal cavity.

3. Provide oral care.

   NOTE: The oral and gastrointestinal tract continue to secrete secretions, adding to the luminal contents that are not being passed.

4. Monitor vital signs and other measures of fluid status, such as adequacy of urine output, skin turgor, and moistness of the mucous membranes.

5. Measure intake and output.

6. Assess the patient for edema and ascites.

7. Weigh the patient daily.

8. Administer parenteral nutrition, as ordered.

- Provide pain management:
  1. Report changes in pain to the physician, including pain that significantly increases or changes from a colicky, intermittent type to constant discomfort (changes could indicate perforation or peritonitis).
  2. Opioid analgesics can be given in the diagnostic period while waiting for a surgical consultation.
  3. Provide a position of comfort, including the semi-Fowler's position, to relieve the pressure of abdominal distention and facilitate thoracic excursion and normal breathing patterns.
- Broad-spectrum antibiotics are given if strangulation is suspected.

Surgical Management
- Surgical management is required for complete mechanical obstruction and for many cases of incomplete mechanical obstruction.
- An exploratory laparotomy is performed to locate the obstruction and determine the nature of the problem.
- The specific surgical procedure performed depends on the cause and location of the obstruction. Examples of procedures include lysis of adhesions, colon resection with anastomosis for obstruction resulting from tumor or diverticulitis, and embolectomy or thrombectomy for intestinal infarction. A colon resection and colostomy may be necessary.
- Nursing care for abdominal surgery is similar to that described under *Cancer, Colorectal.*

Community-Based Care
- Patient and family education depend on the specific cause and treatment of the obstruction.
  1. Report signs that may indicate recurrent obstruction, including abdominal pain or distention, nausea, vomiting, or constipation (for nonmechanical obstruction after surgery or trauma).

   2. Develop a structured bowel regimen, such as a high-fiber diet or fiber supplements and daily exercise with sufficient oral water for prevention of recurrences of fecal impaction.
- Information about incision care (if surgery was performed), drug therapy, and activity restriction is given to the patient and family.

O

OBSTRUCTION, UPPER AIRWAY

OVERVIEW

- Upper airway obstruction, a life-threatening emergency, is an interruption in airflow through the nose, mouth, pharynx, or larynx.
- Causes include:
  1. Tongue edema (surgery, trauma, angioedema as an allergic response to a drug)
  2. Tongue occlusion (e.g., loss of gag reflex, loss of muscle tone, unconsciousness, and coma)
  3. Laryngeal edema
  4. Peritonsillar and pharyngeal abscess
  5. Head and neck cancer
  6. Thick secretions
  7. Stroke and cerebral edema
  8. Smoke inhalation edema
  9. Facial, tracheal, or laryngeal trauma
  10. Foreign body aspiration
  11. Burns of the head or neck area
  12. Anaphylaxis
  13. Inspissated oral and nasopharyngeal secretions or poor oral hygiene leading to thickening and hardening of secretions that can completely block the airway
- Partial obstruction may have only subtle or general manifestations such as diaphoresis, tachycardia, and elevated blood pressure. To rule out a tumor, foreign body, or infection, diagnostic procedures, such as a chest x-ray, neck films, laryngoscopic examination, and computed tomography (CT) scan, are performed.
- Observe for hypoxia and hypercarbia, restlessness, increasing anxiety, sternal retractions, a "seesawing" chest, abdominal movements, or a feeling of impending doom related to actual air hunger.
- Use pulse oximetry for ongoing monitoring of oxygen saturation to maintain values above 92%. Continually assess for stridor, cyanosis, and changes in level of consciousness.

⊞ NURSING SAFETY PRIORITY: Critical Rescue

Early recognition is essential to prevent further complications, including respiratory arrest. Unexplained or persistent recurrent symptoms warrant evaluation even if the symptoms are vague.

PATIENT-CENTERED COLLABORATIVE CARE

* Management depends on the cause of the obstruction:
    1. Prevent airway obstruction with regular oral hygiene and adequate hydration.
    2. For tongue occlusion or excessive secretions, slightly extend the patient's head and neck and insert a nasal or oral airway, suctioning to remove secretions.
    3. For a foreign body, perform abdominal thrusts.
    4. For complete obstruction from edema, cancer, or abscesses:
        a. Direct laryngoscopy
        b. Cricoidectomy
        c. Endotracheal intubation
        d. Tracheotomy

OSTEOARTHRITIS

OVERVIEW

* Osteoarthritis (OA), sometimes called *osteoarthrosis* or *degenerative joint disease (DJD)*, is the most common arthritis, with joint pain and loss of function leading to disability.
* The disease course includes progressive deterioration and loss of cartilage in one or more joints (articular cartilage), especially the hips and knees, the vertebral column, and the hands.
* The major pathologic problems are thinning and deteriorating joint cartilage, narrowing of the joint space, bone spur formation, inflammation, and joint deformity leading to immobility, pain, muscle spasm, and muscle atrophy.
* Known risk factors for OA include obesity, joint trauma, and smoking.

Considerations for Older Adults

Age is the biggest risk factor for OA, because the production of proteoglycans and synovial fluid in the joint decrease with age, reducing cartilage strength and function.

Genetic/Genomic Considerations

Some patients report a family history of OA, which supports a possible genetic cause, especially for women who have hand involvement. Inheritance may contribute to cartilage destruction, osteophyte formation, or the inability of the cartilage to repair itself.

O

PATIENT-CENTERED COLLABORATIVE CARE
Assessment
- Obtain patient information about:
  1. The course of the disease:
     a. Nature and location of joint pain
     b. Location and duration of joint stiffness
     c. When and where any joint swelling has occurred
     d. What relieves or controls pain or stiffness
     e. Any loss of function or difficulty in performing ADLs
  2. Age and gender
  3. Trauma or recurrent stress to joints for occupational or recreational activity or sports
  4. Weight history
  5. Smoking history
  6. Family history of arthritis
  7. Any medical condition that may cause joint manifestations
- Assess for and document:
  1. Chronic joint pain and stiffness that diminishes after rest and intensifies after activity or that occurs with slight motion or even when at rest
  2. Joint pain or tenderness by palpation or by putting the joint through its range of motion (ROM)
  3. Crepitus (a continuous grating sensation felt or heard as the joint goes through its ROM)
  4. Joint enlarged from bony hypertrophy
  5. Any joint warmth or inflammation (indicates a secondary synovitis)
  6. Hand changes with Heberden's nodes (at the distal interphalangeal [DIP] joints) and Bouchard's nodes (at the proximal interphalangeal [PIP] joints)
  7. Joint effusions (excess joint fluid), especially in the knee
  8. Atrophy of skeletal muscle from disuse
  9. Loss of range of joint motion
  10. Compression of spinal nerve roots that produces radiating pain, stiffness, and muscle spasms in one or both extremities with vertebral involvement
  11. Reduced level of mobility and function
- Assess for psychosocial issues:
  1. Change in role and self-esteem
  2. Depression, anger, stress

- Laboratory changes may include:
  1. Elevated erythrocyte sedimentation rate (ESR)
  2. Elevated high-sensitivity C-reactive protein (hsCRP)
- Imaging assessment may include x-rays or magnetic resonance imaging (MRI).

Planning and Implementation
CHRONIC PAIN
Nonsurgical Management
- Drug therapy:
  1. Analgesic drugs:
     a. Acetaminophen (Tylenol, Exdol, Datril), because OA is not primarily an inflammatory process
  2. Topical drug applications:
     a. Lidocaine 5% patches
     b. Topical salicylates (trolamine salicylate [Aspercreme], 1% diclofenac [Voltaren])
  3. NSAIDs:
     a. Celecoxib (Celebrex)
     b. Ibuprofen (Advil)
  4. Joint injection (typically no more than three times per year):
     a. Cortisone
     b. Hyaluronan (Hyalgan)
     c. Hylan G-F 20 (Synvisc)
  5. Muscle relaxants (cyclobenzaprine [Flexeril])
- Nonpharmacologic measures:
  1. Joint rest, using a joint immobilizer
  2. Balancing rest and activity to promote 8 to 10 hours of nighttime sleep and avoid prolonged inactivity.
  3. Position joint to avoid excessive flexion of involved joint and maintain normal extension
  4. Heat or cold applications (hot showers and baths, hot packs or compresses, moist heating pads)
  5. Weight control
  6. Complementary and alternative therapies (topical capsaicin products, acupuncture, acupressure, tai chi, music therapy)
  7. Cognitive-behavioral therapies (imagery, prayer, meditation)
Surgical Management
- Surgery may be indicated when conservative measures no longer provide pain control, when mobility becomes so restricted that the patient cannot participate in enjoyable activities, or when he or she is unable to maintain the desired quality of life:
  1. *Total joint arthroplasty (TJA)* (surgical creation of a joint), also known as *total joint replacement (TJR)*, is the most common type of surgery for OA. Almost any synovial joint of the

body can be replaced with a prosthetic system that consists of at least two parts, one for each joint surface.

2. An *osteotomy (bone resection)* may be performed to correct joint deformity, but this procedure is less common because of the success rate of TJR.

- *Total hip arthroplasty (THA)* with a replacement prosthesis can be done by a traditional open hip incision or, for select patients, by minimally invasive surgery (MIS) using one or two smaller 2- to 4-inch incisions with special instruments to reduce muscle cutting. The replacement joint consists of two parts, the acetabular component and the femoral component.
  1. Provide preoperative care:
     a. Performing routine preoperative care as described in Part One
     b. Assessing the patient's level of understanding about the surgery
     c. Reinforcing the surgeon's explanations about the procedure and postoperative expectations
     d. Explaining about transfers, positioning, ambulation, and postoperative exercises
     e. Demonstrating assistive/adaptive devices for ADLs
     f. Teaching patients having MIS how to perform muscle-strengthening exercises at home before the procedure
     g. Explaining the importance of having any necessary dental procedures done before the surgery to decrease risk of oral bacterial infection resulting in prosthetic site infection
     h. Assessing the patient's risk factors for clotting problems and administering any prescribed anticoagulants
     i. Determining whether the patient needs preoperative supplementation to treat anemia or has made an autologous blood donation for perioperative blood loss
     j. Administering any prescribed antibiotic therapy before the initial surgical incision is made
  2. Provide postoperative care:
     a. Performing routine postoperative care as described in Part One
     b. Preventing operative joint dislocation by:
        (1) Maintaining correct positioning (supine position with the head slightly elevated)
        (2) Placing a trapezoid-shaped abduction pillow, wedge, sling, or splint (with or without straps) between the legs to prevent adduction beyond the midline of the body

(3) Placing and supporting the affected leg in neutral rotation
(4) Following agency policy or surgeon preference for postoperative turning
(5) Observing for signs of possible hip dislocation (increased hip pain, shortening of the affected leg, and leg rotation)

■ NURSING SAFETY PRIORITY: Critical Rescue

If manifestations of hip dislocation occur, keep the patient in bed and notify the surgeon immediately.

c. Preventing thromboembolic complications by:
   (1) Administering prescribed anticoagulants, such as subcutaneous heparin or low–molecular-weight heparin
   (2) Assessing for manifestations of venous thromboembolism (VTE) (swelling, pain)
   (3) Teaching leg exercises (plantar flexion and dorsiflexion, circles of the feet, gluteal and quadriceps muscle setting, straight-leg raises)
   (4) Applying prescribed antiembolic stockings or devices
d. Preventing infection:
   (1) Monitoring the surgical incision for drainage and signs of poor healing with vital signs for signs of fever or infection. Do this every 4 hours for the first 24 hours and every 8 hours thereafter.
   (2) Observing for signs of infection (elevated temperature and excessive or foul-smelling drainage from the incision)

■ NURSING SAFETY PRIORITY: Critical Rescue

An older patient may not have a fever with infection but instead may experience an altered mental state. Consider infection in any older patient with new-onset confusion or inability to rouse.

e. Preventing anemia:
   (1) Observing the surgical hip dressing for bleeding or other type of drainage at least every 4 hours or when vital signs are taken
   (2) Emptying and measuring the bloody fluid in the surgical drains every shift
   (3) Checking the results of the periodic hemoglobin and hematocrit (H&H) tests

  f. Preventing neurovascular complications:
    (1) Checking and documenting color, temperature, distal pulses, capillary refill, movement, and sensation
    (2) Comparing these parameters with those of the non-operative leg
    (3) Reporting any changes to the surgeon
  g. Managing pain by:
    (1) Assessing the patient's pain level
    (2) Ensuring proper use of pain control devices such as epidural analgesia, intraspinal analgesia, patient-controlled analgesia (PCA), and IV opioid analgesia
    (3) Administering prescribed analgesics as needed
  h. Progressing activity by assisting the patient with getting out of bed by:
    (1) Standing on the same side of the bed as the affected leg
    (2) Teaching the patient to stand on the unaffected leg and pivot to the chair
    (3) Assisting the patient to a sitting position
    (4) Ensuring that the patient does not flex the hips beyond 90 degrees
    (5) Preventing hyperflexion of the replaced joint with the use of raised toilet seats, straight-back chairs, and reclining wheelchairs
3. Weight bearing on the affected leg depends on the surgeon, type of prosthesis, and surgical procedure.
4. Work with the physical therapist (PT) to teach the patient how to follow weight-bearing restrictions and progress to full weight–bearing (FWB) status.
5. The occupational therapist (OT) may recommend assistive-adaptive devices to help with ADLs, especially for those patients having traditional surgery.
6. For patients who have traditional surgery, the length of stay in the acute care hospital is typically 3 days; those who have MIS procedures may be discharged on the second postoperative day or, in a few cases, on the day of surgery.
7. The interdisciplinary team provides written instructions for posthospital care and reviews them with patients and their family members.
8. Complete recovery may take 6 weeks or more.
- *Total knee arthroplasty (TKA)* can be performed by traditional open surgery or by MIS procedures for some patients:
  1. Provide preoperative care:
    a. Routine preoperative care described in Part One
    b. Care as described for THA

    c. Explanation and demonstration of a continuous passive motion (CPM) machine (if prescribed)

2. Provide postoperative care:
   a. Routine postoperative care as described in Part One
   b. Care to prevent complications as described for THA
   c. Implementing the CPM machine as prescribed for ROM and cycles per minute:
      (1) Checking the cycle and ROM settings at least once every 8 hours
      (2) Ensuring that the joint being moved is properly positioned on the machine
      (3) Placing the controls to the machine out of reach of a confused patient
      (4) Assessing the patient's response to the machine
      (5) Turning off the machine while the patient is having a meal
      (6) Storing the machine off the floor when it is not in use
   d. Applying ice packs or a Hot/Ice device to decrease surgical site swelling
   e. Ensuring safe use of continuous peripheral nerve blockade (CPNB) for pain control:
      (1) Performing neurovascular assessments every 2 to 4 hours or according to hospital protocol
      (2) Assessing that the patient can plantar flex and dorsiflex the affected foot but does not feel pain in the extremity
      (3) Checking for movement, sensation, warmth, color, pulses, and capillary refill
      (4) Monitoring for symptoms of systemic infusion of the nerve-blocking drug (a metallic taste, tinnitus, restlessness, nervousness, slurred speech, bradycardia, hypotension, decreased respirations)
   f. Maintaining the knee in a neutral position and not rotated internally or externally
   g. Ensuring that the surgical knee is not hyperextended
   h. Monitoring neurovascular status frequently to check for compromise to the distal operative leg every time vital signs are taken

- *Total shoulder arthroplasty (TSA)* can be performed either as a total joint replacement or as a hemiarthroplasty (replacement of part of the joint, typically the humeral component). These surgeries are most commonly performed using traditional open incisions, but minimally invasive shoulder arthroplasty can be used instead for some patients:
   1. Preoperative care and postoperative care are similar to those for other joint replacement surgeries.

2. A sling is applied to immobilize the joint and prevent dislocation until therapy begins.
3. The hospital stay for TSA is usually 1 to 2 days, until pain is controlled.
4. Rehabilitation with an OT usually takes 2 to 3 months.

- Other joints that can be replaced include:
    1. Elbow (total elbow arthroplasty [TEA])
    2. Hand or foot joints (phalangeal joint, metacarpal, or metatarsal arthroplasty)
    3. Any bone of the wrist
    4. Ankle (total ankle arthroplasty [TAA]), which has more postoperative complications than other arthroplasties

IMPAIRED PHYSICAL MOBILITY

- Reinforce the techniques and principles of exercise, ambulation, promotion of ADLs, and use of assistive devices developed by the PT and OT to meet the goal of independent function.
- The ideal time for exercise is immediately after the application of heat.
- Teach the patient to follow these instructions:
    1. Follow the exercise instructions that have been specifically prescribed. There are no universal exercises; exercises have been specifically tailored to each individual's needs.
    2. Do exercises on both "good" and "bad" days. Consistency is important.
    3. Respect pain. If pain increases with exercise, stop and report this to the health care provider.
    4. Use active rather than active-assist or passive exercise whenever possible.
    5. Reduce the number of repetitions if the inflammation is severe and there is more pain.
    6. Do not substitute normal activities or household tasks for the prescribed exercises.
    7. Avoid resistive exercises if joints are severely inflamed.

Community-Based Care

- Collaborate with the discharge planner and the health care provider to determine the best placement for the patient with OA at discharge.
- Provide health teaching:
    1. Explaining the general principles of joint protection:
        a. Use large joints instead of small ones; for example, place a purse strap over the shoulder instead of grasping the purse with a hand.
        b. Turn doorknobs toward the thumb (rather than toward the little finger) to avoid twisting the arm and promoting ulnar deviation.

    c. Use two hands instead of one to hold objects.

    d. Sit in a chair that has a high, straight back.

    e. When getting out of bed, do not push off with the fingers; use the entire palm of both hands.

    f. Do not bend at the waist; instead, bend the knees while keeping the back straight.

    g. Use long-handled devices, such as a hairbrush with an extended handle.

    h. Use assistive-adaptive devices, such as Velcro closures and built-up utensil handles, to protect joints.

    i. Do not use pillows in bed, except a small one under the head.

    j. Avoid twisting or wringing the hands.

2. Explaining the drug protocol, desired and potential side effects, and toxic effects

3. Emphasizing the importance of reducing weight and eating a well-balanced diet to promote tissue healing

4. Referring the patient to the Arthritis Foundation for up-to-date information about new treatments and helpful complementary and alternative practices

5. Providing written instructions about the required care, regardless of whether the patient goes home or to another inpatient facility

6. Referring the patient to the nutritionist, counselor, home health nurse, rehabilitation therapist, financial counselor, and local and state support groups as needed

OSTEOMALACIA

OVERVIEW

- Osteomalacia is a softening of the bone tissue related to vitamin D deficiency, causing inadequate deposits of calcium and phosphorus in the bone matrix.
- Vitamin D deficiency can occur as a result of inadequate exposure to sunlight, poor dietary intake, abnormal metabolism, chronic use of many drugs, or the presence of chronic disease.
- Older adults are most at risk for osteomalacia.

PATIENT-CENTERED COLLABORATIVE CARE

- Obtain patient information about:
  1. Age
  2. Exposure to sunlight and skin pigmentation (darker skin reduces vitamin D activation)
  3. Dietary habits

4. Current prescribed and over-the-counter (OTC) drug use
5. Chronic disease processes of the GI tract:
   a. Inflammatory bowel disease
   b. Gastric or intestinal bypass surgery
6. Renal or liver dysfunction
7. History of bone fracture

- Assess for and document:
  1. Muscle weakness (causing a waddling and unsteady gait) and cramping
  2. Bone pain (aggravated by activity and worse at night)
  3. Bone tenderness to palpation (especially tibia or rib cage)
  4. Skeletal misalignment (long-bone bowing or spinal deformity)
  5. Hypocalcemia or hypophosphatemia
  6. Presence of radiolucent bands (Looser's lines or zones) on x-ray
- The major intervention for osteomalacia is vitamin D:
  1. Teach patients to take the amount of vitamin D supplementation prescribed by their health care provider.
  2. Remind patients, especially those who are homebound, about the importance of daily sun exposure (at least 15 minutes each day) to activate the vitamin.
  3. Teach patients to choose foods that are fortified with vitamin D (milk and dairy products) or are rich in vitamin D (eggs, swordfish, chicken, and liver), as well as enriched cereals and bread products.

OSTEOMYELITIS

OVERVIEW
- Osteomyelitis is an infection in bony tissue caused by bacteria, viruses, or fungi.
- Osteomyelitis is difficult to treat and can result in chronic recurrence of infection, loss of function, amputation, and even death.
- The pathologic processes that occur in infected bone tissue include inflammation, blood vessel thromboses, and necrosis.
- Categories of osteomyelitis include:
  1. *Exogenous osteomyelitis,* in which infectious organisms enter from outside the body, as in an open fracture
  2. *Endogenous osteomyelitis,* also called *hematogenous osteomyelitis,* in which organisms are carried by the bloodstream from other areas of infection in the body
  3. *Contiguous osteomyelitis,* in which bone infection results from skin infection of adjacent tissues
- The two major types of osteomyelitis are acute and chronic.

- Common causes include bacteremia, pre-existing conditions that interfere with immune health or wound healing such as diabetes, penetrating and nonpenetrating trauma, long-term IV therapy, hemodialysis, *Salmonella* infection of the GI tract, sickle cell disease, poor dental hygiene and periodontal (gum) infection, and skin infection with methicillin-resistant *Staphylococcus aureus* (MRSA).

Considerations for Older Adults

- The most common cause of contiguous spread in older adults is slow-healing foot ulcers in patients with diabetes or peripheral vascular disease.
- Multiple organisms tend to be responsible for osteomyelitis in these patients.

PATIENT-CENTERED COLLABORATIVE CARE
Assessment
- Assess for and document:
  1. Bone pain described as a constant, localized, pulsating sensation that worsens with movement
  2. Fever, usually greater than 101° F (38° C) (in acute disease)
  3. Swelling, tenderness, erythema, and heat around the site of infection
  4. Ulcerations on the feet or hands (if circulation is poor)
  5. Sinus tract formation and drainage (with chronic infection)
  6. Elevated white blood cell (WBC) count and erythrocyte sedimentation rate (ESR)
  7. Positive blood cultures

Interventions
Nonsurgical Management
- Nonsurgical interventions include:
  1. Administering IV antibiotic therapy for several weeks, followed by oral antibiotic therapy for weeks or months

■ NURSING SAFETY PRIORITY: Action Alert
Even if symptoms of the disease appear to be improved, the full course of IV and oral antibiotics must be completed. Teach patients the importance of completing the full course of therapy.

  2. Irrigating the wound either continuously or intermittently, with one or more antibiotic solutions
  3. Packing the wound with beads made of bone cement that have been impregnated with an antibiotic
  4. Administering drugs for pain control

5. Covering the wound to prevent infection spread
6. Implementing Contact Precautions for severe infections, particularly if the purulent material cannot be adequately contained by a dressing
7. Administering hyperbaric oxygen (HBO) therapy for patients with chronic, unremitting osteomyelitis

Surgical Management

- Surgery is reserved for patients with chronic osteomyelitis and may include:
  1. Sequestrectomy with excision of dead and infected bone to allow revascularization of tissue
  2. Application of bone grafts to repair bone defects
  3. Reconstruction with microvascular bone transfers if excision is extensive
  4. Closure of the defect with muscle flaps and skin grafts
  5. Amputation of the affected limb if the infection cannot be controlled or revascularization is not successful
- Provide postoperative care:
  1. Implementing routine postoperative care described in Part One
  2. Performing frequent neurovascular (NV) assessments:
     a. Pain
     b. Movement
     c. Sensation
     d. Warmth
     e. Temperature
     f. Distal pulses
     g. Capillary refill

NURSING SAFETY PRIORITY: Critical Rescue

Immediately report to the surgeon any of these signs of neurovascular compromise: pain that cannot be controlled, paresis or paralysis (weakness or inability to move), paresthesias (abnormal tingling sensation), pallor, and pulselessness.

3. Elevating the affected extremity to increase venous return and control swelling

OSTEOPOROSIS

OVERVIEW

- Osteoporosis is a chronic metabolic disease in which bone loss causes decreased density and possible fracture, most often of the spine, hip, and wrist.

- The main mechanism of osteoporosis is an imbalance in the continuous bone remodeling processes such that osteoclastic (bone resorption) activity is greater than osteoblastic (bone building) activity.
- Generalized osteoporosis involves many structures in the skeleton and is further divided into two categories:
  1. *Primary osteoporosis,* which is more common and occurs in postmenopausal women and in men in their sixth or seventh decade of life
  2. *Secondary osteoporosis,* which results from other medical conditions, such as hyperparathyroidism, long-term drug therapy (such as with corticosteroids) or prolonged immobility
- Regional osteoporosis occurs when a limb is immobilized related to a fracture, injury, or paralysis for longer than 8 to 12 weeks.
- Risk factors include menopause; lean and thin body build; Euro-American or Asian ancestry; sedentary lifestyle; diet deficient in calcium and vitamin D; malabsorption syndromes; high intake of caffeine and carbonated beverages; excessive alcohol and tobacco use; family history; and long-term use of certain drugs, especially corticosteroids.

⊕ Cultural Awareness
- Although there is some advantage of increased bone density in dark-skinned women, lifestyle and health beliefs about prevention may put all women at equal risk for osteoporosis.
- Many African Americans and Asians have lactose intolerance and cannot drink milk or eat other dairy-based foods, which are good sources of calcium; African Americans may experience vitamin D deficiency.

PATIENT-CENTERED COLLABORATIVE CARE
Assessment
- Obtain patient information about:
  1. Age, gender, race, body build, weight
  2. Change in height
  3. Back pain after bending, lifting, or stooping (worse with activity, relieved with rest)
  4. Mobility
  5. Muscular weakness
  6. History of falls
  7. Current drugs
- Assess for and document:
  1. Features of the spinal column (presence of classic "dowager's hump," or kyphosis of the dorsal spine)

2. Location of all painful areas
3. Manifestations of fractures (swelling and malalignment)
4. Constipation, abdominal distention
5. Respiratory compromise
6. Fear of falling
7. Body image disturbance
8. Changes in quality of life and sexuality
- Diagnostic tests may include:
  1. Biochemical markers (commonly used to determine response to therapy)
     a. Bone-specific alkaline phosphatase (BSAP)
     b. Osteocalcin
     c. Pyridinium (PYD)
     d. N-telopeptide (NTX)
     e. C-telopeptide (CTX)
     f. Levels of serum calcium, vitamin D, phosphorus, and protein
  2. Imaging (to determine bone density):
     a. Dual-energy x-ray absorptiometry (DXA or DEXA)
     b. Quantitative computed tomography (QCT)
     c. Quantitative ultrasound (QUS)

Interventions
Nonsurgical Management
- Nutrition therapy:
  1. Coordinate health teaching and nutrition planning with the nutritionist.
  2. Teach patients to eat a diet that includes:
     a. Calcium and vitamin D
     b. Low-fat protein sources
     c. Moderation in alcohol and caffeine intake
     d. Adequate amounts of protein, magnesium, vitamin K, and trace minerals
     e. Low soda intake; phosphorus in diet soda can reduce calcium absorption
  3. Work with patients who are lactose intolerant to choose from a variety of soy and rice products, fruit juices, bread, and cereal products that are fortified with or have additional calcium and vitamin D.
- Exercise, which is important in both prevention and management of osteoporosis:
  1. Coordinate health teaching with the physical therapist (PT) for exercises to improve posture, support, and pulmonary capacity; strengthen extremity muscles; and improve ROM:
     a. Abdominal muscle tightening
     b. Deep breathing

   c. Pectoral stretching
   d. Extremity muscle tightening, resistive, and ROM exercises
   e. Swimming
   f. Walking for 30 minutes three to five times a week
2. Teach patients to avoid high-impact recreational activities, such as running, bowling, and horseback riding.
- Teach about other lifestyle changes:
   1. Avoiding tobacco in any form, especially cigarette smoking
   2. Preventing falls
   3. Maintaining a hazard-free environment by avoiding scatter rugs, cluttered rooms, and wet floor areas
- Drug therapy for prevention and management:
   1. Bisphosphonates:
      a. Alendronate (Fosamax) (oral drug)
      b. Ibandronate (Boniva) (oral and IV)
      c. Risedronate (Actonel) (oral drug)
      d. Pamidronate (Aredia) (IV drug)
      e. Zoledronic acid (Reclast) (IV drug)
   2. Estrogen and hormone therapy in low doses for short durations
   3. Calcium and vitamin D supplementation

▌NURSING SAFETY PRIORITY: Drug Alert

Osteonecrosis of the jaw is a rare but serious complication of zoledronic acid and pamidronate bisphosphonate therapy. Teach the patient to have an oral assessment and preventive dentistry before beginning therapy and to inform any dentist who is planning invasive treatment, such as a tooth extraction or implant, that he or she is taking a bisphosphonate.

   4. Selective estrogen receptor modulators (SERMs) (raloxifene [Evista])
   5. Other drugs:
      a. Parathyroid hormone
      b. Calcitonin
      c. Androgens (testosterone propionate [Testex, Malogen ✦])
   Surgical Management
- *Vertebroplasty* is the injection of bone cement into the vertebral body to reduce a fracture or fill the space created by osteoporosis.
- *Kyphoplasty* includes the use of a balloon in the vertebral body to contain the bone cement.

Community-Based Care
- Ensure that the patient and family understand drug and exercise regimens.

- Help the patient and family identify and correct hazards in the home before discharge.
- Refer the patient to a home health agency.
- Refer the patient and family to community resources, such as the National Osteoporosis Foundation and local osteoporosis specialty clinics.

OTITIS MEDIA

OVERVIEW

- Otitis media is an infection of the middle ear that causes an inflammatory process within the mucosa. Most infections of the middle ear are bacterial.
- The inflammation leads to swelling and irritation of the small bones (ossicles) within the middle ear, a purulent exudate, pain, and temporary hearing loss.
- If otitis media progresses or recurs without treatment, permanent conductive hearing loss may occur.
- Otitis media can be acute, chronic, or serous.

PATIENT-CENTERED COLLABORATIVE CARE

Assessment

- Assess for manifestations of acute or chronic otitis media:
  1. Ear pain with or without movement of the external ear (which is relieved when the ear drum ruptures)
  2. Sensation of fullness in the ear
  3. Reduced or distorted hearing
  4. Tinnitus
  5. Headaches
  6. Dizziness or vertigo
  7. Systemic symptoms:
     a. Malaise
     b. Fever
     c. Nausea and vomiting
  8. Otoscopic examination findings:
     a. Dilated and red eardrum blood vessels
     b. Red, thickened, or bulging eardrum
     c. Decreased eardrum mobility
     d. Eardrum perforation with pus present in the canal

Interventions

- Nonsurgical management:
  1. Bedrest to limit head movements that intensify the pain
  2. Application of heat or cold
  3. Systemic antibiotic therapy

  4. Analgesics:
      a. Mild, such as aspirin, ibuprofen (Advil), and acetamino-
         phen (Tylenol, Abenol 🍁)
      b. Opioids such as codeine and meperidine (Demerol) for
         severe pain
  5. Antihistamines and decongestants
- Surgical management with a myringotomy (surgical opening of
  the pars tensa of the eardrum) may be needed:
  1. Preoperative care:
      a. Providing reassurance
      b. Administering systemic antibiotic therapy
      c. Cleaning the external canal
  2. Postoperative care:
      a. Teach the patient to keep the external ear and canal free of
         other substances.
      b. Instruct him or her to avoid washing the hair or shower-
         ing for 48 hours.

OVARIAN CYSTS

OVERVIEW
- There are several types of ovarian cysts:
  1. Follicular cysts, which usually occur in young, menstruating
     women, are not malignant, and do not grow without hor-
     monal influences
      a. A follicular cyst can develop when a mature follicle fails to
         rupture or an immature follicle fails to reabsorb follicular
         fluid during the second half of the menstrual cycle.
      b. The cyst is usually small (2.4 to 3.2 inches [6 to 8 cm])
         and may be asymptomatic unless it ruptures.
      c. Rupture of a follicular cyst or torsion (twisting)
         may cause acute, severe pelvic pain that usually
         resolves after several days of bedrest and use of mild
         analgesics.
      d. If the cyst does not rupture, it usually disappears within
         two or three menstrual cycles without intervention.
      e. For cysts that persist, oral contraceptives may be prescribed
         for one or two menstrual cycles to suppress ovulation.
      f. Surgery is recommended only after menopause or for
         cysts that are larger than 3.2 inches (4 cm).
  2. Corpus luteum cysts:
      a. These cysts occur after ovulation and often occur with
         increased secretion of progesterone.
      b. The cysts are usually small, averaging 1.5 inches (4 cm),
         and are purplish red as a result of hemorrhage within the
         corpus luteum.

   c. They are associated with a delay in the onset of menses, irregular or prolonged flow, and low abdominal or pelvic pain on one side.

   d. Cyst rupture can cause intraperitoneal hemorrhage.

   e. Cysts may disappear in one or two menstrual cycles or with suppression of ovulation.

   f. Management is the same as for follicular cysts.

3. Theca-lutein cysts:

   a. These cysts are uncommon and are associated with hydatidiform mole pregnancies. They develop as a result of prolonged stimulation of the ovaries by excessive amounts of human chorionic gonadotropin (hCG).

   b. These cysts regress spontaneously within 3 months after removal of the molar pregnancy or the source of excessive hCG.

- Polycystic ovary syndrome (PCOS) (Stein-Leventhal syndrome) results when high levels of luteinizing hormone (LH) overstimulate the ovaries, producing multiple cysts on one or both ovaries. High levels of estrogen are produced by these cysts and are unopposed by postovulatory progesterone, resulting in endometrial hyperplasia (tissue overgrowth) or even carcinoma. Patients are usually obese, are hirsute, have irregular menses, and may be infertile because of lack of ovulation.

PATIENT-CENTERED COLLABORATIVE CARE

- Management of the patient with PCOS depends on which problem is of greatest concern to the woman:

1. Conservative management includes the use of oral contraceptives to inhibit LH production and prevent excessive ovarian stimulation.

2. For a woman who is older than 35 years and no longer desires childbearing, management may involve a bilateral salpingo-oophorectomy (BSO) (removal of both tubes and ovaries) and hysterectomy (removal of the uterus and cervix).

3. In women who desire fertility, PCOS can be managed with drugs such as clomiphene (Clomid) to stimulate ovulation.

PAGET'S DISEASE OF THE BONE

OVERVIEW

- Paget's disease, or osteitis deformans, is a chronic metabolic disorder in which bone is excessively broken down (osteoclastic activity) and reformed (osteoblastic activity). The result is structurally disorganized bone that is weak with increased risk of bowing of long bones and fractures.

- There are three phases of the disorder:
  1. *Active*, in which there is a rapid increase in osteoclasts (cells that break down bone), causing massive bone destruction and deformity
  2. *Mixed*, in which the osteoblasts (bone-forming cells) react to compensate in forming new but structurally weak bone
  3. *Inactive*, in which the osteoblastic activity exceeds the osteoclastic activity, resulting in hard, sclerotic bone
- The most common areas of disease involvement are the vertebrae, femur, skull, clavicle, humerus, and pelvis.
- The risk for developing Paget's disease increases as a person ages and is particularly high for those 80 years old or older.
- Most patients with Paget's disease are asymptomatic and have disease confined to one bone. In more severe disease, the manifestations are diverse and potentially fatal.

Genetic/Genomic Considerations

- Two types of Paget's disease can occur: familial and sporadic. Possible mutation areas for the familial form include the *RANKL/RANK/OPG* gene system, the gene for the valosin-containing protein *(VCP)* that controls complement, and the gene for sequestosome 1 *(SQSTM1)*.
- Teach patients the importance of genetics in familial Paget's disease, and refer them to the appropriate genetic counseling resource.
- Ask the patient whether genetic testing is desired.

PATIENT-CENTERED COLLABORATIVE CARE
Assessment
- Obtain patient information about:
  1. History of fracture
  2. Bone pain (mild to moderate aching, deep, worsened by pressure and weight bearing), especially of the hip and pelvis
  3. Redness and warmth at affected sites
  4. Arthritis at the joints (cartilage) of the affected bones
  5. Nerve impingement in the lumbosacral area of the vertebral column (back pain that radiates along one or both legs)
  6. Any changes in hearing, vision, swallowing, balance, or speech
  7. Loose teeth or difficulty chewing
- Assess for and document:
  1. Posture, stance, and gait for gross bony deformities
  2. Loss of normal spinal curvature, lower extremity malalignment, and decreased height

3. Kyphosis or scoliosis of the spinal column
4. Long-bone bowing in the legs or arms
5. Flexion contracture in the hip joint
6. Soft, thick, and enlarged skull
7. Deafness and vertigo
8. Problems with vision, swallowing, or speech
9. Hydrocephalus
10. Bone fractures, especially of the femur or tibia, after minimal trauma
11. Apathy, lethargy, and fatigue
12. Hyperparathyroidism and gout (along with an increase in serum and urinary calcium levels and serum uric acid levels)
13. Kidney stones (renal calculi)
14. Cardiac complications (heart failure)

- Diagnosis is made on the basis of physical findings, increases in serum alkaline phosphatase (ALP) and urinary hydroxyproline levels, x-ray findings, and radionuclide bone scanning.

Interventions

- Drug therapy for pain management includes:
  1. Aspirin or NSAIDs such as ibuprofen (Motrin, Apo-Ibuprofen ✤) for mild to moderate pain
  2. More potent analgesics for severe pain
- Drug therapy to decrease bone resorption includes:
  1. Bisphosphonates:
     a. Alendronate (Fosamax) (oral drug)
     b. Risedronate (Actonel) (oral drug)
     c. Etidronate (Didronel) (oral drug)
     d. Tiludronate (Skelid) (oral drug)
     e. Pamidronate (Aredia) (IV drug)
     f. Zoledronic acid (Reclast) (IV drug)
  2. Calcium: 1500 mg daily
  3. Vitamin D: 800 IU daily
  4. Calcitonin (subcutaneous injection or nasal spray)
  5. Plicamycin (Mithracin) (potent antineoplastic agent with many side effects)
- Non-impact exercises
- Use of orthotic device to immobilize and provide support for the vertebrae or long bones
- Nutrition therapy with a diet rich in calcium

PAIN, BACK

OVERVIEW

- The areas of the back most commonly affected by back pain are the cervical and lumbar vertebrae.

- *Acute lumbosacral (low back) pain (LBP)* is typically caused by a muscle strain, spasm, ligament sprain, disk degeneration, or herniated nucleus pulposus (usually between the fourth and fifth lumbar vertebrae). Osteoporosis can cause vertebral fractures and back pain. Over time, these injuries can contribute to spinal stenosis, a narrowing of the spinal canal, nerve root canals or intervertebral foramina.
- Back pain may also be caused by *spondylolysis,* a defect in one of the vertebrae—usually in the lumbar spine. Spondylolisthesis occurs when one vertebra slips forward on the one below it, often as a result of spondylolysis. This problem causes pressure on the nerve roots, leading to pain in the lower back and into the buttocks. Pain or numbness may also occur in the leg and foot.
- If back pain continues for 3 months or if repeated episodes occur, back pain is classified as chronic.
- Risk factors for acute back pain include:
  1. Trauma (twisting or hyperflexion during lifting)
  2. Obesity
  3. Congenital spinal problems, such as scoliosis
  4. Smoking (causes premature disk degeneration)
- Risk factors for chronic back pain include:
  1. Age-related disk disease
  2. Sedentary lifestyle
  3. Prior injury to back
  4. Obesity
  5. Structural and postural abnormalities
  6. Systemic diseases, especially when they are inflammatory or activity-limiting

Considerations for Older Adults

- In older adult patients, osteoarthritis and osteoporosis contribute to back pain.
- Cervical pain is also common in patients with advanced rheumatoid arthritis who experience cervical disk subluxation, most often at the C1-2 level (first and second cervical vertebrae).
- Physiologic changes associated with aging, such as spinal stenosis, vertebral malalignment, and vascular changes, contribute to back pain in the older adult.

PATIENT-CENTERED COLLABORATIVE CARE
Assessment

- Assess and document:
  1. Pain location, quality, radiation, severity, alleviating and aggravating factors

  2. Posture and gait
  3. Vertebral alignment and swelling
  4. Muscle spasm
  5. Tenderness of the back and involved extremity
  6. Sensory changes: paresthesia and numbness
  7. Muscle tone and strength
  8. Limitations in movement
  9. Psychosocial reaction to illness
  10. Vertebral changes seen on an x-ray, computed tomography (CT) scan, or magnetic resonance imaging (MRI) scan
  11. Abnormal electromyography and nerve conduction studies
  12. Medication and other interventions to treat pain, including over-the-counter drugs and homeopathic treatments

Interventions

Nonsurgical Management

- To treat acute LBP:
  1. Have the patient use the Williams position when in bed (semi-Fowler's bed position with the knees flexed). A bed board or firm mattress may be useful for patients with a muscle injury. For patients with a herniated disk, a flat position may aggravate the pain. In a sidelying position, a pillow between the knees may be helpful.
  2. Collaborate with the physical therapist to develop an individualized exercise program.
  3. Drug therapy includes muscle relaxants and NSAIDs.
  4. Epidural or local steroid injection may be helpful in some cases.
  5. Apply ice and heat therapy:
     a. Apply moist heat in the form of heat packs or hot towels for 20 to 30 minutes four times daily; hot showers or baths also are beneficial for some patients.
     b. Apply ice therapy using ice packs or ice massage over the affected area for 10 to 15 minutes every 1 to 2 hours.
     c. Some patients prefer alternating ice and heat therapy.
     d. Deep heat therapy such as ultrasound treatments and diathermy may be administered by the physical therapist (PT).
- Approaches for treating chronic back pain:
  1. Collaborate with the dietitian to implement a weight loss program if appropriate.
  2. Facilitate evaluation and use of a custom-fitted lumbosacral brace.
  3. Collaborate with the occupational therapist for ergonomic and adaptive furniture and aids.

   4. Administer drugs to relieve neuropathic pain such as gabapentin (Neurontin) or oxcarbazepine (Trileptal).
   5. Local electrical stimulation may provide significant pain relief.
   6. Adjunctive therapy such as spinal manipulative therapy, distraction, imagery, and music therapy can reduce maladaptive responses to chronic pain.

   Surgical Management
- Conventional open operative procedures include:
   1. *Diskectomy,* in which a portion of the disk is removed
   2. *Laminectomy,* which is the removal of one or more vertebral laminae, plus osteophytes, and the herniated nucleus pulposus through a 3-inch (7.5-cm) incision
   3. *Spinal fusion,* which stabilizes the spine if repeated laminectomies are performed
   4. *Disk prosthesis,* involving insertion of an artificial compound or a hard plastic prosthesis that replaces the patient's natural disk and is shaped to allow full spinal movement
- Minimally invasive operative procedures include *microscopic (or surgical) endoscopic diskectomy (MED)* and *percutaneous endoscopic diskectomy (PED),* a procedure that may be used with *laser thermodiskectomy* to shrink the herniated disk before removal.
- Provide preoperative care as described in Part One and additional care:
   1. Explain to the patient that various sensations may be experienced in the affected leg or both legs (for lumbar surgery) because of manipulation of nerves and muscles during surgery.
   2. Address the need for a postoperative brace and bone grafting if the patient is having a spinal fusion.
- Provide routine postoperative care as described in Part One and additional care:
   1. Perform neurologic assessment with vital signs every 4 hours during the first 24 hours.
   2. Check the patient's ability to void. An inability to void may indicate damage to sacral spinal nerves. Opioid analgesics have been associated with difficulty voiding and constipation.
   3. Log roll the patient if bedrest is prescribed immediately after surgery.
   4. Ensure that a brace or other type of thoracolumbar support is worn when the patient is out of bed (for spinal fusion).
   5. Implement venothromboembolism (VTE) prophylaxis per institutional guidelines

Community-Based Care

- Health teaching includes:
  1. The prescribed exercise program, including daily walking (patient mastery is ensured by observing correct performance on return demonstration, in collaboration with physical therapy)
  2. Restrictions on climbing stairs, lifting, bending, and activities such as driving
  3. The use of a firm mattress or bed board, if appropriate
  4. Drug information, using the medication reconciliation form and including over the counter drugs
  5. A weight-reduction diet, if needed
  6. The importance of smoking cessation
  7. For unresolved pain, referral to a pain specialist or clinic

PAIN, CERVICAL SPINE

OVERVIEW

- Cervical spine or neck pain is usually related to herniation of the nucleus pulposus in an intervertebral disk (ruptured disk) between the fifth and sixth vertebrae or to nerve compression caused by osteophyte formation.
- Pain also may result from muscle strain or ligament sprain, repetitive motion, poor posture, or past history of trauma.

PATIENT-CENTERED COLLABORATIVE CARE

Assessment

- Assess for:
  1. Pain, numbness, and tingling that radiates to the scapula and down the arm
  2. Sleep disturbances caused by pain
  3. Headache
  4. Vertebral changes seen on computed tomography (CT) scan or magnetic resonance imaging (MRI)

Interventions

Nonsurgical Management

- Nonsurgical management of cervical spine pain is the same as for back pain, except that the exercises focus on the neck and shoulder.
- A cervical collar may be prescribed for the patient for no more than 10 days; prolonged used can lead to increased pain and decreased muscle strength and range of motion (ROM).
- Cervical traction can be done intermittently at home, guided by a physical therapist (PT) initially.

Surgical Management
- Depending on the causative factors, an anterior or a posterior approach may be used.
- Provide routine postoperative care as described in Part One.
  1. Anticipate that the patient will wear some type of cervical collar for several weeks.
  2. Assess the patient's ability to void.
  3. Assist the patient with ambulation, usually on the evening of surgery unless a multilevel fusion was performed.
  4. Monitor for complications:
     a. Hoarseness resulting from laryngeal injury
     b. Dysphagia
     c. Esophageal, tracheal, or vertebral artery injury
     d. Graft extrusion and screw loosening if a fusion was performed

PANCREATITIS, ACUTE

OVERVIEW
- Acute pancreatitis is a serious and, at times, life-threatening inflammatory process of the pancreas caused by premature activation of pancreatic enzymes and resulting in autodigestion and fibrosis of the pancreas.
- The extent of the inflammation and tissue destruction ranges from mild involvement, characterized by edema and inflammation, to severe, necrotizing hemorrhagic damage leading to diffusely bleeding pancreatic tissue with fibrosis and tissue death.
- Many factors can cause injury to the pancreas:
  1. Biliary tract disease with gallstones
  2. Excessive alcohol ingestion
  3. Postoperative trauma from surgical manipulation after biliary tract, pancreatic, gastric, and duodenal procedures
  4. External blunt trauma
  5. Metabolic disturbances
  6. Kidney failure or kidney transplant
  7. Drug toxicities, including opiates, sulfonamides, thiazides, steroids, and oral contraceptives
  8. Other medical diseases
- Complications include transient hyperglycemia, pleural effusions, atelectasis, pneumonia, multisystem organ failure, acute lung injury progressing to acute respiratory distress syndrome (ARDS), shock, and coagulation defects.

PATIENT-CENTERED COLLABORATIVE CARE
Assessment
- Obtain patient information about:
  1. History of abdominal pain, especially if related to alcohol ingestion or high intake of fat
  2. Individual and family history of alcoholism, pancreatitis, or biliary tract disease
  3. Previous abdominal surgeries or diagnostic procedures
  4. Medical history, including peptic ulcer disease, kidney failure, vascular disorders, hyperparathyroidism, and hyperlipidemia
  5. Recent viral infection
  6. Use of prescription and OTC drugs
- Assess for and document:
  1. Abdominal pain (the most frequent symptom), including sudden-onset pain in a midepigastric or left upper quadrant location with radiation to the back, aggravated by a fatty meal, ingestion of a large amount of alcohol, or lying in the recumbent position
  2. Weight loss, with nausea and vomiting
  3. Jaundice
  4. Gray-blue discoloration of the abdomen and periumbilical area (Cullen's sign)
  5. Gray-blue discoloration of the flanks (Turner's sign)
  6. Absent or decreased bowel sounds
  7. Abdominal tenderness, rigidity, and guarding
  8. Dull sound on abdominal percussion, indicating ascites
  9. Elevated temperature with tachycardia and decreased blood pressure
  10. Adventitious breath sounds, dyspnea, or orthopnea
  11. Elevated serum amylase and lipase levels

■ NURSING SAFETY PRIORITY: Critical Rescue
Monitor for significant changes in vital signs that may indicate the life-threatening complication of shock. Hypotension and tachycardia may result from pancreatic hemorrhage, excessive fluid volume shifting, or the toxic effects of abdominal sepsis from enzyme damage. Observe the patient for changes in behavior and level of consciousness (LOC) that may be related to alcohol withdrawal, hypoxia, or impending sepsis with shock.

- Diagnostic studies may include:
  1. Serum lipase, amylase, alkaline phosphatase, alanine aminotransferase (ALT), bilirubin, white blood cell (WBC),

hemoglobin, hematocrit, coagulation factors, sodium, potassium, calcium, magnesium, triglycerides, and albumin
2. Imaging of the pancreas and gallbladder with ultrasound or computed tomography (CT) scan

Planning and Implementation

- The priority for patient care is to provide supportive care by relieving symptoms, decreasing inflammation, and anticipating or treating complications. As for any patient, continually assess for and support the ABCs (airway, breathing, and circulation).

ACUTE PAIN

Nonsurgical Management

- Diet therapy includes:
  1. Withholding food and fluids in the acute period; maintaining hydration with IV fluids
  2. Maintaining nasogastric (NG) intubation to decrease gastric distention and suppress pancreatic secretion
  3. Initiating nasojejunal enteral nutrition
  4. Assessing frequently for the presence of bowel sounds
- Drug therapy may include:
  1. Opioids such as morphine or hydromorphone, often with a patient-controlled analgesia (PCA) device
  2. Proton pump inhibitors or H_2-histamine receptor blockers to decrease gastric hydrochloric acid production during fasting
  3. Antibiotics for patients with acute necrotizing pancreatitis
- Comfort measures include:
  1. Helping the patient assume a side-lying position to decrease abdominal pain
  2. Avoiding oral stimulation while providing measures to keep mucous membranes from drying
  3. Encouraging the patient to express the emotions and responses he or she is feeling
  4. Providing reassurance and diversional activities to reduce anxiety

Surgical Management

- Surgical management usually is not indicated for acute pancreatitis.
- Patients with complications such as pancreatic pseudocyst or abscess may require surgical drainage.

IMBALANCED NUTRITION

- Interventions include:
  1. Withholding oral food and fluids in the early stages of the disease
  2. Providing jejunal enteral or parenteral nutrition early, within 72 hours of admission to the hospital for treatment of pancreatitis

3. When food is tolerated, providing small-volume, high-carbohydrate and high-protein feedings with limited fats

4. Providing supplemental dietary agents, vitamins, and minerals as needed

Community-Based Care

- Patient and family health teaching is aimed at preventing future episodes and preventing disease progression to chronic pancreatitis:

1. Encourage alcohol abstinence to prevent further pain and extension of the inflammation and insufficiency.

2. Teach the patient to notify the physician if he or she is experiencing acute abdominal pain or symptoms of biliary tract disease such as jaundice, clay-colored stools, and dark urine.

3. Emphasize the importance of follow-up visits with the health care provider.

4. Refer the patient with an alcohol abuse problem to support groups such as Alcoholics Anonymous.

5. Refer the patient to home health nursing as needed.

PANCREATITIS, CHRONIC

OVERVIEW

- Chronic pancreatitis is a progressive, destructive disease of the pancreas with remissions and exacerbations.
- Inflammation and fibrosis of the tissue contribute to pancreatic insufficiency and diminished exocrine and endocrine function.
- Pancreatic insufficiency is characterized by the loss of exocrine function, which causes a decreased output of enzymes and bicarbonate; loss of endocrine function results in diabetes mellitus.

PATIENT-CENTERED COLLABORATIVE CARE

Assessment

- Assess for and document:

1. Abdominal pain (major clinical manifestation): continuous, burning, or gnawing dullness with intense and relentless exacerbations

2. Left upper quadrant mass, indicating a pseudocyst or abscess

3. Dullness on abdominal percussion, indicating pancreatic ascites

4. Steatorrhea, foul-smelling stools that may increase in volume as pancreatic insufficiency progresses

5. Weight changes

6. Jaundice and dark urine
7. Signs and symptoms of diabetes mellitus
8. Elevated serum amylase, bilirubin, and alkaline phosphatase levels
9. Identification of calcification of pancreatic tissue in biopsy specimen
10. Fatigue and muscle wasting

Interventions

Nonsurgical Management

- Drug therapy includes:
    1. Opioid analgesia (The patient may become dependent on opioids with long-term use.)
    2. Non-opioid analgesics
    3. Pancreatic-enzyme replacement therapy (PERT) is the standard of care to prevent malnutrition, malabsorption, and excessive weight loss

---

⚠ NURSING SAFETY PRIORITY: Drug Alert

Teach the patient to take these drugs with meals and snacks and a glass of water. If needed, open the capsules and spread their contents over applesauce, mashed fruit, or rice cereal. Enzyme preparations should not be mixed with foods containing proteins, because the enzymatic action dissolves the food into a watery substance. Be sure that patients drink a full glass of water after taking the drug to ensure than none of the enzymes remain in the mouth. Advise the patient to wipe his or her lips with a wet towel to prevent the skin irritation and breakdown that residual enzymes can cause.

---

4. Insulin or oral hypoglycemic agents to control diabetes
5. H_2-histamine receptor antagonist or proton pump inhibitor to decrease gastric acid

- Record daily weight and the number and consistency of stools per day to monitor the effectiveness of drug therapy.
- Diet therapy includes:
    1. Fasting to avoid recurrent pain exacerbated by eating
    2. Providing jejunal or total parenteral nutrition (TPN)
    3. Consult with the dietician to provide sufficient calories and protein to maintain health

Surgical Management

- Surgical management is not the primary intervention for chronic pancreatitis. Surgery may be indicated for intractable pain, incapacitating pain relapses, or complications such as pseudocyst and abscess.

- Surgical procedures include:
  1. Incision and drainage for abscesses or pseudocysts
  2. Laparoscopic cholecystectomy or choledochotomy for underlying biliary tract disease
  3. Sphincterotomy (incision of the sphincter) for fibrosis
  4. Pancreatojejunostomy (the pancreatic duct is opened and anastomosed to the jejunum, relieving obstruction) to relieve pain and preserve pancreatic tissue and function
  5. Partial pancreatectomy, which may be performed for advanced pancreatitis or disabling pain
  6. Vagotomy with gastric antrectomy to alter nerve stimulation and decrease pancreatic secretion
- For preoperative and postoperative care, see care of the patient undergoing a Whipple procedure under *Cancer, Pancreatic.*

Community-Based Care
- Health teaching is aimed at preventing further exacerbations:
  1. Avoid known precipitating factors, such as alcohol and foods with a high-fat content.
  2. Comply with diet instructions: high protein, high carbohydrate, low or no fat.
  3. Follow written instructions and prescriptions for pancreatic enzyme therapy:
     a. How and when to take enzymes
     b. The importance of maintaining therapy
     c. The importance of notifying the physician of increased steatorrhea, abdominal distention, cramping, and skin breakdown
  4. Comply with elevated glucose management, including oral hypoglycemic drugs or insulin injections and monitoring of blood glucose levels.
  5. Keep follow-up visits with the physicians.
- Refer the patient to financial counseling, social services, vocational rehabilitation, home health services, and Alcoholics Anonymous, as needed.

PARALYSIS, FACIAL

- Facial paralysis, or Bell's palsy, is an acute paralysis of cranial nerve VII, with maximal paralysis reached within 2 to 5 days of onset.
- The disorder is characterized by an inability to close the eye, wrinkle the forehead, smile, whistle, or grimace; the face appears masklike and sags.

- This syndrome is thought to be caused by inflammation from herpes simplex virus-1 (HSV-1).
- Treatment includes:
  1. Administering antiviral agents early in the syndrome
  2. Administering mild analgesics for pain
  3. Protecting the eye from corneal abrasion or ulceration by patching and administering artificial tears
  4. Teaching the patient to use warm, moist heat; massage; and facial exercises such as whistling, grimacing, and blowing air out of the cheeks three or four times a day

PARKINSON DISEASE

OVERVIEW

- Parkinson disease is a common, debilitating neurologic disorder involving the basal ganglia and substantia nigra. Loss of dopamine in the affected central nervous system (CNS) structures results in difficulty with initiation and coordination of voluntary movement. Loss of other neurotransmitters can contribute to mood disorders and autonomic dysfunction.
- The disease is characterized by muscle rigidity, akinesia (slow movements), postural instability, and tremors.
- The disease involves five stages:
  1. *Stage 1*: Mild disease with unilateral limb involvement
  2. *Stage 2*: Bilateral limb involvement
  3. *Stage 3*: Significant gait disturbances and moderate generalized disability
  4. *Stage 4*: Severe disability, akinesia, and muscle rigidity
  5. *Stage 5*: Complete dependency in all aspects of ADLs

PATIENT-CENTERED COLLABORATIVE CARE

Assessment

- Obtain patient information about:
  1. Time and progression of symptoms such as resting tremors, bradykinesia, and difficulty in completing fine motor tasks such as handwriting
  2. Family history related to neurologic disorders
  3. History of head injury, which can damage CNS structures
  4. Use of drugs to treat serious mental illness; some antipsychotic medications can have Parkinson-like adverse effects
- Assess for and document:
  1. Rigidity, which is present early in the disease process and progresses over time:
     a. Cogwheel rigidity, manifested by a rhythmic interruption of the muscles of movement

    b. Plastic rigidity, or mildly restrictive movements

    c. Lead-pipe rigidity, which is total resistance to movement

2. Posture:
   a. Stooped posture
   b. Flexed trunk
   c. Fingers adducted and flexed at the metacarpophalangeal joint
   d. Wrists slightly dorsiflexed

3. Gait:
   a. Slow and shuffling
   b. Short, hesitant steps
   c. Propulsive gait
   d. Difficulty stopping quickly

4. Speech:
   a. Soft, low-pitched voice
   b. Dysarthria
   c. Echolalia, or automatic repetition of what another person says
   d. Repetition of sentences
   e. Change in voice volume, phonation, or articulation

5. Motor dysfunction:
   a. Bradykinesia or difficulty completing two tasks simultaneously
   b. Akinesia
   c. Tremors, especially at rest
   d. "Pill-rolling" movement
   e. Masklike face
   f. Difficulty chewing and swallowing
   g. Uncontrolled drooling, especially at night
   h. Difficulty getting into and out of bed
   i. Little arm swinging when walking
   j. Change in handwriting, micrographia

6. Autonomic dysfunction:
   a. Orthostatic hypotension
   b. Excessive perspiration and oily skin
   c. Flushing, changes in skin texture
   d. Blepharospasm

7. Psychosocial effects:
   a. Emotional lability
   b. Depression
   c. Paranoia
   d. Easily upset
   e. Rapid mood swings
   f. Cognitive impairments
   g. Delayed reaction time
   h. Sleep disturbances

Interventions
- Provide drug therapy:
  1. Administer drug therapy on time to maintain continuous therapeutic drug levels:
     a. Levodopa combinations
     b. Dopamine agonists
     c. Catechol O-methyltransferase (COMT) inhibitors to interfere with the breakdown of dopamine in the CNS
     d. Anticholinergic drugs, if the patient's primary symptom is tremor
     e. Monoamine oxidase inhibitors
     f. Variety of investigational drugs
  2. Monitor the patient for drug toxicity and side effects such as delirium, cognitive impairment, decreased effectiveness of the drug, postural hypotension, and hallucination.
  3. Treatment of drug toxicity or intolerance includes:
     a. Reduction in drug dosage
     b. Change in drugs or in the frequency of administration
     c. Drug holiday (particularly with levodopa therapy) for up to 10 days with close surveillance
- Other interventions include:
  1. Physical therapy (PT) and occupational therapy (OT) consultations to plan and maintain a mobility and muscle-stretching program (e.g., traditional exercise, yoga, tai chi) and exercises for the muscles of the face and tongue to facilitate swallowing and speech
  2. Providing assistive devices for participation in ADLs; PT and OT consultation to provide training in ADLs and the use of adaptive devices
  3. Teaching the patient and family to monitor the patient's sleeping pattern and to discuss whether it is safe for the patient to operate machinery or perform other potentially dangerous tasks
  4. Monitoring the patient's ability to eat and swallow; monitoring food and fluid intake; collaborating with the registered dietitian for caloric calculation and diet planning
  5. Assessing the need for a speech-language pathologist consultation for evaluation of swallowing dysfunction and communication problems
  6. Teaching the patient to speak slowly and clearly; using alternative communication methods such as a communication board
  7. Referring the patient and family to a social worker to help with financial and health insurance agencies and to state and social agencies and support groups

8. Instructing the patient with orthostatic hypotension to wear elastic stockings and to change position slowly, especially when moving from a sitting to a standing position

9. Allowing sufficient time for the patient to complete activities; scheduling appointments and activities for late in the morning to prevent rushing the patient, or scheduling them at the time of the patient's optimal level of functioning

10. Implementing interventions to prevent complications of immobility such as constipation, pressure ulcers, contractures, and atelectasis

- Surgical interventions may be used to treat severe or early onset of Parkinson disease:

1. Stereotactic pallidotomy can be a very effective treatment for Parkinson disease. Through a probe, the target area in the brain receives a mild electrical stimulation to decrease tremor and rigidity. The probe is placed in the ideal location, and a temporary lesion is made. If this is successful, a permanent lesion is made.

2. Unilateral thalamotomy treats the tremor through thermocoagulation of brain cells.

3. Deep brain stimulation involves placing a thin electrode in the thalamus or subthalamus and connecting it to a "pacemaker" that delivers electrical current to interfere with "tremor cells." The electrodes are connected to an implantable pulse generator that is placed underneath the skin in the patient's chest, something like a cardiac pacemaker.

PELVIC INFLAMMATORY DISEASE

OVERVIEW

- Pelvic inflammatory disease (PID) is a complex infectious process in which organisms from the lower genital tract migrate from the endocervix upward through the uterine cavity into the fallopian tubes.
- It is a major cause of infertility and ectopic pregnancies.
- It is most often caused by sexually transmitted organisms, especially *Chlamydia trachomatis* and *Neisseria gonorrhoeae*. Other organisms may include *Gardnerella vaginalis*, *Haemophilus influenzae*, *Staphylococcus*, *Streptococcus*, and *Escherichia coli*.
- The infection may spread to other organs and tissues. Resultant infections include:
  1. Endometritis (infection of the endometrial cavity)
  2. Salpingitis (inflammation of the fallopian tubes)

    3. Oophoritis (ovarian infection)
    4. Parametritis (infection of the parametrium)
    5. Peritonitis (infection of the peritoneal cavity)
    6. Tubal or tubo-ovarian abscess
- Sepsis and death can occur, especially if treatment is delayed or inadequate.
- Although common manifestations include tenderness in the tubes and ovaries (adnexa) and low, dull abdominal pain, some patients have only mild discomfort or menstrual irregularity, and others experience no symptoms at all. These variations can make the diagnosis of PID challenging.

PATIENT-CENTERED COLLABORATIVE CARE
Assessment
- Obtain patient information about:
  1. Medical history
  2. Menstrual history
  3. Obstetric and sexual history, including whether unprotected sex occurred
  4. Results of cultures or serum analysis congruent with infection or infecting organism
  5. Results of pelvic examination, particularly presences of purulent cervical discharge or friable cervical tissue
  6. Previous reproductive surgery
  7. Abnormal vaginal bleeding
  8. Dysuria (painful urination)
  9. Increase or change in vaginal discharge
  10. Dyspareunia (painful sexual intercourse)
  11. Risk factors, including:
      a. Age younger than 26 years
      b. Multiple sexual partners
      c. Intrauterine device (IUD) in place within the previous 3 weeks
      d. Smoking
      e. Previous episodes of sexually transmitted diseases or PID
- Assess for and document:
  1. Pain, especially lower abdominal pain
  2. Fever, chills, generalized aches
  3. Hunched-over gait
  4. Abdominal tenderness, rigidity, or rebound tenderness
- Assess for psychosocial issues, such as:
  1. Anxiety and fear
  2. Need for reassurance and support during the physical examination
  3. Embarrassment
  4. Discomfort when discussing symptoms or sexual history

- Diagnosis is made on the basis of history, physical symptoms and signs, cervical or vaginal mucopurulent discharge, presence of white blood cells (WBCs) on saline microscopy of vaginal secretions, and positive culture (e.g., laboratory documentation of cervical infection with *N. gonorrhoeae* or *Chlamydia*). Other tests that may be helpful include ultrasonography, MRI, and endometrial biopsy.

Planning and Implementation

INFECTION

- Uncomplicated PID is usually treated on an ambulatory care basis.
- Hospitalization for PID is recommended if the patient has a complicated history, does not respond to oral antibiotic therapy, or has severe illness.
- Drug therapy includes oral or parenteral antibiotics, or both, for 14 days.
- Teach the patient about the need to:
  1. Abstain from sexual intercourse during treatment.
  2. Check her temperature twice a day.
  3. Be seen by the health care provider within 72 hours after starting the antibiotics and then at 1 and 2 weeks from the time of the initial diagnosis.
- In a small number of patients, a laparotomy may be needed to remove an abscess.

PERICARDITIS

OVERVIEW

- Pericarditis is an inflammation or alteration of the pericardium, the membranous sac enclosing the heart.
- There are two types of pericarditis:
  1. *Acute pericarditis,* which is most commonly associated with infective organisms (bacteria, viruses, fungi), malignant neoplasms, postmyocardial infarction syndrome, postpericardiotomy syndrome, systemic connective tissue diseases, kidney failure, and idiopathic causes
  2. *Chronic constrictive pericarditis,* which is caused by tuberculosis, radiation therapy, trauma, kidney failure, and metastatic cancer, with the pericardium becoming rigid, preventing adequate ventricular filling and resulting in cardiac failure

PATIENT-CENTERED COLLABORATIVE CARE

- Obtain patient information about:
  1. History of cardiac disease, cardiac surgery, chest trauma, or recent systemic infections
  2. History of chest radiation, connective tissue diseases, or cancer

- Assess for and document:
  1. Substernal precordial pain that can radiate to the left neck, shoulder, and back and is aggravated by breathing, coughing, and swallowing
  2. Pericardial friction rub
  3. Acute pericarditis:
     a. Elevated white blood cell (WBC) count
     b. Nonspecific ST-T wave elevation on electrocardiogram (ECG)
     c. Fever (infectious cause)
  4. Chronic constrictive pericarditis:
     a. Right-sided heart failure, including dyspnea, exertional fatigue, and orthopnea
     b. Pericardial thickening on echocardiogram and computed tomography (CT) scan
     c. Inverted or flat T waves on ECG
     d. Atrial fibrillation
- Treatment depends on the type of pericarditis.
- Acute pericarditis is treated by:
  1. Administering NSAIDs
  2. Administering corticosteroid therapy
  3. Administering antibiotics
  4. Encouraging rest
- For chronic constrictive pericarditis, the definitive treatment is surgical excision of the pericardium (pericardiectomy).
- Complications of pericarditis include pericardial effusions and cardiac tamponade, which is manifested by jugular venous distention, paradoxical pulse (systolic blood pressure at least 10 mm Hg higher on expiration than on inspiration), decreased cardiac output, muffled heart sounds, and circulatory collapse.
  1. Treatment of cardiac tamponade includes pericardiocentesis, in which a needle is inserted into the pericardial space. After the needle is properly positioned, a catheter is inserted and the pericardial fluid is withdrawn. IV fluids are administered to improve cardiac output.
  2. For recurrent tamponade or effusions or adhesions resulting from chronic pericarditis, a partial or complete pericardiectomy is done to allow adequate ventricular filling and contraction.

PERIPHERAL ARTERIAL DISEASE

OVERVIEW

- Peripheral arterial disease (PAD) is a condition in which partial or total arterial occlusion deprives the tissue of oxygen and nutrients, resulting in damage.

- Obstruction is commonly the result of atherosclerosis.
- Patients with PAD have an increased risk for developing chronic angina, myocardial infarction (MI), or stroke and are much more likely to die within 10 years compared with those who do not have the disease.
- The most common sites of PAD are the vessels of the lower extremities ("outflow disease"), and the most common symptom is pain. Characteristic PAD leg pain is known as *intermittent claudication.*
- Inflow PAD obstructions involve the distal end of the aorta and the common, internal, and external iliac arteries, manifested by discomfort in the lower back, buttocks, or thighs.
- Acute peripheral vascular disease occurs when there is an acute obstruction by a thrombus or embolus, causing severe, acute pain below the level of the obstruction.

PATIENT-CENTERED COLLABORATIVE CARE
Assessment
- Assessment findings include:
  1. Abnormal ankle-brachial index (ABI): The value can be derived by dividing the ankle blood pressure by the brachial blood pressure. A value of less than 0.9 indicates outflow disease. With inflow disease, pressures taken at the thigh level indicate the severity of disease. Mild inflow disease may cause a difference of only 10 to 30 mm Hg in pressure on the affected side compared with the brachial pressure.
  2. Leg pain (burning, cramping in calves, ankles, feet, and toes with exercise or rest) or discomfort in the lower back, buttocks, or thighs
  3. Ischemic changes of the extremity:
     a. Loss of hair on the lower calf, ankle, and foot
     b. Dry, scaly skin
     c. Thickened toenails
     d. Color changes (elevation pallor or dependent rubor)
     e. Mottled and cool or cold extremity
  4. Presence or absence of pulses: The most sensitive and specific indicator of arterial function is the quality of the posterior tibial pulse, because the pedal pulse is not palpable in a small percentage of people.
  5. Ulcer formation
  6. Painful arterial ulcers that develop on the toes, between the toes, or on the upper aspect of the foot: PAD ulcers differ from diabetic and venous ulcers:
     a. Diabetic ulcers develop on the plantar surface of the foot, over metatarsal heads, on the heel, or on pressure areas; they may not be painful.

   b. Venous stasis ulcers occur at the ankles, with discol-
      oration of the lower extremity at the ulcer; they cause
      minimal pain.
- Diagnostic assessment includes:
   1. Segmental systolic blood pressure measurement using a
      Doppler probe
   2. Exercise tolerance test
   3. Plethysmography

Planning and Implementation

Nonsurgical Management

- Teach the following methods of increasing arterial blood flow in
  chronic arterial disease:
   1. Exercising to promote collateral circulation
   2. Positioning to promote circulation and decrease swelling:
      a. Legs should be elevated at rest but not above the level of
         the heart.
      b. Avoid crossing legs and wearing restrictive clothing.
   3. Avoiding cold exposure to the affected extremity:
      a. Teach the patient to wear socks or insulated bedroom
         shoes and maintain a warm home environment.
      b. Caution the patient not to apply direct heat to the lower
         limbs, which may cause burns because of decreased
         sensitivity.
   4. Avoiding nicotine, caffeine, and emotional stress
   5. Complying with drug therapy, including antiplatelet therapy
   6. Controlling blood pressure
- Endovascular procedures may be used to restore arterial circulation. Treat the patient with typical preoperative interventions.
  The procedural approach is one of the following:
   1. Percutaneous transluminal angioplasty (PTA) dilates arter-
      ies that are occluded or stenosed with a balloon catheter;
      a stent may be placed.
   2. Laser-assisted angioplasty may be used to open an occluded
      artery.
   3. Mechanical rotational abrasive atherectomy is used to im-
      prove blood flow to ischemic limbs for scraping plaque while
      minimizing danger to the vessel wall.
- After PTA, care of the patient includes:
   1. Observing the puncture site for bleeding
   2. Closely monitoring vital signs
   3. Checking the distal pulses of both limbs
   4. Encouraging the patient to maintain bedrest for 6 to 8 hours,
      as ordered, with the limb straight
   5. Administering anticoagulation therapy, which may continue
      for 3 to 6 months after the procedure

6. Encouraging the patient to take aspirin on a permanent basis, as ordered

Surgical Management

- An emergency surgical embolectomy is performed on patients who experience an acute peripheral artery occlusion by an embolus.
- Acute arterial insufficiency often presents with the "6 *P*s" of ischemia:
  1. Pain
  2. Pallor
  3. Pulselessness
  4. Paresthesia
  5. Paralysis
  6. Poikilothermia (coolness)
- Arterial revascularization surgery is used to increase arterial blood flow in an affected limb and includes inflow procedures such as aortoiliac bypass, aortofemoral bypass, and axillofemoral bypass and outflow procedures, including femoropopliteal bypass and femorotibial bypass.
- Grafting materials for bypass surgeries include the autogenous saphenous vein and synthetic graft material such as polytetrafluoroethylene.
- Provide postoperative care:
  1. Monitor for the patency of the graft by checking for changes in the extremity:
     a. Color
     b. Temperature
     c. Pulse intensity
     d. Pain intensity (Typical pain is described as throbbing pain, which occurs from increased blood flow to the affected limb.)
  2. Mark the site of the distal pulses, located by palpation or auscultated with Doppler ultrasonography.
  3. Monitor the patient's blood pressure, notifying the physician about increases and decreases beyond desired ranges.
  4. Avoid bending the knee and hip of the affected limb.
  5. Monitor for signs and symptoms at or around the graft and incision sites, such as hardness, tenderness, redness, or warmth.
- Thrombectomy (removal of the clot) is the most common treatment for acute graft occlusion; thrombolytic therapy may be used.
- Compartment syndrome occurs when tissue pressure within a confined body space becomes elevated and restricts blood flow.

- Use sterile technique when in contact with the incision and observe for symptoms of infection.

❗NURSING SAFETY PRIORITY: Critical Rescue

Immediately inform the vascular surgeon if assessment of the operative extremity includes worsening pain, swelling or tenseness, absent pulse, demarcations of color or temperature distal to revascularization, or loss of sensation.

Community-Based Care

- The patient benefits from a case manager who can follow the patient across the continuum of care.
- Patient and family education includes:
    1. Reinforcing the need for individualized positioning and an exercise plan
    2. Teaching the patient to avoid raising the legs above the level of the heart unless he or she also has venous stasis
    3. Providing written and oral foot care instructions, instructing the patient to:
        a. Keep the feet clean by washing with a mild soap in room-temperature water.
        b. Keep the feet dry, especially between the toes and ankles.
        c. Avoid injury or extended pressure to the feet and ankles.
        d. Always wear comfortable, well-fitting shoes.
        e. Keep the toenails clean, and cut the nails straight across.
        f. Prevent dry, cracked skin.
        g. Prevent exposure to extreme heat or cold.
        h. Avoid heating pads.
        i. Avoid constricting garments.
    4. Providing dressing change and incision care instructions, if necessary
    5. Providing instructions concerning discharge medications
    6. Encouraging the patient to avoid smoking and to limit daily intake of fat to less than 30% of total calories
- Identify the need for a home care nurse or home health aide.
- Home care assessment of the patient includes:
    1. Assessing tissue perfusion to affected extremity:
        a. Distal circulation, sensation, and motion
        b. Presence of pain, pallor, paresthesias, pulselessness, paralysis, coolness
    2. Assessing adherence to therapeutic regimen:
        a. Following foot care instructions
        b. Quitting smoking

   c. Maintaining dietary restrictions

   d. Participating in exercise regimen

   e. Avoiding both exposure to cold and constrictive clothing

3. Assessing patient's ability to manage wound care and prevent further injury

4. Assessing coping ability of patient and family members

5. Assessing home environment for safety hazards

PERIPHERAL VENOUS DISEASE

OVERVIEW

- Peripheral venous disease (PVD) is a group of diseases that alter the natural flow of blood through the veins of the peripheral circulation.
- Venous blood flow may be altered by thrombus formation and defective valves.
- Thrombus formation is associated with stasis of blood flow, endothelial injury, and hypercoagulability.
- Phlebitis occurs when inflammation in superficial veins occurs, often in conjunction with thrombus (i.e., thrombophlebitis).
- Deep vein thrombophlebitis, commonly referred to as *deep vein thrombosis (DVT),* is the most common type of thrombophlebitis. Deep vein thrombophlebitis (thrombosis) is more serious than superficial thrombophlebitis because it presents a greater risk for pulmonary embolism (PE). In PE, a dislodged blood clot travels to the pulmonary artery. DVT develops most often in the legs but can occur also in the upper arms as a result of increased use of central venous devices.
- Venous insufficiency results from prolonged venous hypertension and phlebitis, which stretch the veins and damage valves, resulting in swelling, venous stasis ulcers, and cellulitis.

PATIENT-CENTERED COLLABORATIVE CARE

- For the patient with DVT, assess for:
  1. Calf or groin tenderness and pain
  2. Unilateral swelling of the leg
  3. Warmth and edema of the extremity
  4. Induration along the blood vessel
  5. Size comparison with the contralateral limb
  6. Localized pitting edema
  7. Results of ultrasonography or Doppler flow studies identifying the location of thrombosis
  8. Serum markers of inflammation and coagulation

- For recovery from thrombosis, phlebitis syndromes, and venous insufficiency, interventions include:
  1. Informing patient of increased risk for future venothrombophlebotic events and to monitor for symptoms.
  2. Having the patient wear elastic or compression stockings during the day and evening
  3. Teaching the patient to elevate his or her legs for 20 minutes four or five times a day
  4. Continuing activity and avoiding bedrest or prolonged periods of inactivity such as standing still or sitting for more than 2 hours
  5. Teaching the patient to use a sequential gradient compression device, if ordered
  6. Treating open venous ulcers with occlusive dressings and topical agents, with or without antibiotics to chemically débride the ulcer
  7. If the patient is ambulatory, using an Unna boot to promote ulcer healing by relieving pressure
  8. Adhering to anticoagulation drug regimens for 3 to 6 months after diagnosis and monitoring serum factors to avoid unintended bleeding
  9. Teaching the patient to meet follow-up care appointments.

PERITONITIS

OVERVIEW

- Peritonitis is an acute inflammation of the viscera/parietal and endothelial peritoneum (lining of the abdominal cavity).
- Primary peritonitis is an acute bacterial infection that develops as a result of contamination of the peritoneum through the vascular system and is rare.
- Secondary peritonitis is caused by bacterial invasion as a result of perforation or a penetrating wound, such as appendicitis, diverticulitis, peptic ulcer, ascending genital infection, or a gunshot injury to the abdomen. Chemical peritonitis is the result of leakage of bile, pancreatic enzymes, and gastric acid.
- Peritonitis can be life-threatening with accompanying shock, respiratory problems, and paralytic ileus.

PATIENT-CENTERED COLLABORATIVE CARE
Assessment

- Obtain patient information about:
  1. History of abdominal trauma or surgery
  2. Character of abdominal pain, onset, duration, location, quality, aggravating and alleviating factors. The cardinal

signs of peritonitis are abdominal pain and tenderness. Often, pain is aggravated by coughing or movement and relieved by knee flexion

3. Abdominal distention and presence/absence of bowel sounds
4. Tachypnea with low peripheral saturation (decreased SpO_2)
5. Low-grade fever or recent spikes in temperature

■ NURSING SAFETY PRIORITY: Action Alert

With generalized peritonitis, tenderness is widespread. Assess for abdominal wall rigidity, which is a classic finding that is sometimes referred to as a "boardlike" abdomen. Monitor the patient for a high fever because of the infectious process. Assess for tachycardia occurring in response to the fever and decreased circulating blood volume. Observe whether he or she has dry mucous membranes and a low urine output seen with third spacing. Nausea and vomiting may also be present. Hiccups may occur as a result of diaphragmatic irritation. Be sure to document all assessment findings.

- Diagnostic tests may include:
  1. Complete blood count (CBC) if an elevated white blood cell (WBC) count is concerning
  2. Serum electrolytes, blood urea nitrogen (BUN), and creatinine
  3. Abdominal x-rays or computed tomography (CT) to determine presence of dilation, edema, and inflammation of the intestines

■ NURSING SAFETY PRIORITY: Critical Rescue

A sudden worsening of abdominal pain or a change from localized to generalized abdominal pain may signal a medical emergency. This symptom needs to be communicated, along with vital signs, to the health care provider immediately to avoid patient progression to vascular and respiratory compromise.

Interventions

Nonsurgical Management

- Administer IV fluids and antibiotics.
- Monitor daily weight.
- Record intake and output.
- Keep the patient on NPO status.
- Monitor and record drainage from the nasogastric (NG) tube used for gastric and intestinal decompression.
- Provide pain management with IV analgesics; anticipate use of patient-controlled analgesia (PCA) pump.

- Administer oxygen as prescribed according to the patient's respiratory status.

Surgical Management

- Surgical management may be necessary to identify and repair the underlying cause of the peritonitis.
- Surgery is focused on controlling the contamination, removing foreign material from the peritoneal cavity, and draining fluid collections.
- During surgery, the peritoneum is irrigated with antibiotic solution, and drainage catheters are inserted.
- Provide routine postoperative care as described in Part One, including:
  1. Close monitoring of the patient's cardiovascular stability for early detection of shock (level of consciousness, heart rate, blood pressure, and urine output should remain within normal limits for the patient)
  2. Providing meticulous wound care; irrigating and packing the wound, as prescribed
  3. Assisting the patient to gradually increase his or her activity level

Considerations for Older Adults

The early signs and symptoms of dehydration in the older adult may consist of a subtle decrease in mental status, such as confusion or lethargy. Do not delay in communicating subtle changes in mentation to the prescribing health care provider.

Community-Based Care

- The patient may be discharged home or to a transitional care unit to complete antibiotic therapy and recovery.
- If the patient is discharged home, collaborate with the case manager to determine the need for assistance.
- Provide written and oral postoperative instructions, including:
  1. The necessity to report any redness, swelling, tenderness, or unusual or foul-smelling drainage from the wound
  2. Care of the incision and dressing; ensuring that the patient has the necessary equipment to perform wound care (dressings, solutions, catheter-tipped syringe); and stressing the importance of handwashing
  3. The need to report fever (typically 101° F [38° C]) or abdominal pain to the physician
  4. Administration and monitoring of drugs for pain
  5. Dietary limitations, if necessary
  6. Activity limitations, including limited lifting until healing has occurred

PHEOCHROMOCYTOMA

OVERVIEW

- Pheochromocytoma is a catecholamine-producing tumor that arises in the adrenal medulla.
- These tumors are most often benign, but at least 10% are malignant.
- They produce, store, and release epinephrine and norepinephrine (NE), which stimulate adrenergic receptors and can have wide-ranging adverse effects mimicking the action of the sympathetic division of the autonomic nervous system.

PATIENT-CENTERED COLLABORATIVE CARE

Assessment

- Obtain patient information about intermittent manifestations, including:
  1. Severe headaches
  2. Palpitations
  3. Profuse diaphoresis
  4. Flushing
  5. Apprehension or sense of impending doom
  6. Pain in the chest or abdomen, with nausea and vomiting
- Assess for and document:
  1. Hypertension
  2. Tremors
  3. Weight loss

⬛ NURSING SAFETY PRIORITY: Action Alert

Do not palpate the abdomen, because this action could cause a sudden release of catecholamines and severe hypertension.

- Diagnosis is made on the basis of high urine levels of vanillylmandelic acid (VMA), metanephrine, and catecholamines; the clonidine suppression test; and magnetic resonance imaging (MRI) or computed tomography (CT) scans to precisely locate tumors.

Interventions

- Surgery is performed to remove the tumors and the adrenal gland or glands.
- Provide preoperative care:
  1. Implementing routine preoperative care as discussed in Part One
  2. Monitoring blood pressure regularly; placing the cuff consistently on the same arm, with the patient in lying and standing positions

3. Identifying stressors that may lead to a hypertensive crisis
4. Teaching the patient not to smoke, drink caffeine-containing beverages, or change position suddenly
5. Ensuring adequate hydration
6. Providing a calm, restful environment
7. Administering prescribed drug therapy to stabilize the patient's blood pressure (usually phenoxybenzamine [Dibenzyline])

- Provide postoperative care:
  1. Implementing routine postoperative care discussed in Part One
  2. Closely monitoring for hypertension, hypotension, and hypovolemia
  3. Monitoring for adequate tissue perfusion:
     a. Vital signs with level of consciousness
     b. Fluid intake and output
  4. Checking opioid effects on blood pressure
- If inoperable, tumors are managed with alpha-adrenergic and beta-adrenergic blocking agents and self-measurement of blood pressure with home monitoring equipment.

PHLEBITIS

- Phlebitis is an inflammation of the superficial veins caused by an irritant, commonly IV therapy.
- Phlebitis is manifested as a reddened, warm area radiating up an extremity.
- The patient may experience pain, soreness, and swelling of the extremity.
- Treatment involves application of warm, moist soaks, which dilate the vein and promote circulation. *Do not massage the area.*

PNEUMONIA

OVERVIEW

- Pneumonia is an excess of fluid in the lungs resulting from an inflammatory process.
- It can be caused by many infectious organisms and by inhalation of irritating agents or aspiration of stomach contents.
- Infectious pneumonias are categorized as *community-acquired pneumonia (CAP)* or *hospital-acquired pneumonia (HAP)*; HAP is more likely to be resistant to antibiotics than is CAP.
- *Ventilator-associated pneumonia (VAP)* is an HAP that develops in patients who have an endotracheal tube in place for mechanical ventilation.

- The inflammation and multiplication of organisms result in local capillary leak, edema, and exudate that reduce gas exchange and lead to hypoxemia, interfering with oxygenation and tissue perfusion and possibly leading to death.
- Risk factors for CAP:
  1. Older adult
  2. Never received the pneumococcal vaccination or had received it more than 6 years ago
  3. Not having received the influenza vaccine in the previous year
  4. Presence of a chronic health problem or other coexisting condition
  5. Recent exposure to respiratory viral or influenza infections
  6. Use of tobacco or alcohol
- Risk factors for HAP:
  1. Older adult
  2. Presence of a chronic lung disease
  3. Gram-negative colonization of the mouth, throat, and stomach
  4. Decreased level of consciousness
  5. Recent aspiration event
  6. Presence of endotracheal, tracheostomy, or nasogastric (NG) tube
  7. Poor nutritional status
  8. Immunocompromised status (from disease or drug therapy)
  9. Drugs that increase gastric pH
  10. Mechanical ventilation

PATIENT-CENTERED COLLABORATIVE CARE
Assessment
- Obtain patient information about:
  1. Age
  2. Living, work, and school environments
  3. Diet, exercise, and sleep routines
  4. Swallowing problems
  5. Presence of a nasogastric (NG) tube
  6. Tobacco and alcohol use
  7. Past and current use of drugs, including drug addiction or injection drug use
  8. Past respiratory illnesses
  9. Recent exposure to influenza, pneumonia, or other viral infection
  10. Recent skin rashes, insect bites, or exposure to animals
  11. Chronic respiratory problems
  12. Home respiratory equipment use and cleaning
  13. Date of last influenza or pneumococcal vaccine

- Assess for and document:
  1. General appearance
  2. Breathing pattern; use of accessory muscles
  3. Chest or pleuritic pain or discomfort
  4. Chills and fever
  5. Cough
  6. Tachycardia
  7. Dyspnea and tachypnea
  8. Sputum production
  9. Oxygen saturation
  10. Crackles or wheezes
  11. Hypotension
  12. Mental status changes (especially in an older adult)
  13. Fatigue
  14. Anxiety

Considerations for Older Adults
- Fever and cough may be absent, but hypoxemia is usually present.
- The most common manifestation of pneumonia in the older adult patient is confusion from hypoxia rather than fever or cough.
- Diagnosis is based on manifestations, sputum Gram stain or culture, elevated white blood cell (WBC) count, chest x-ray, peripheral oxygenation (Spo_2) and arterial blood gas (ABG) levels.

Planning and Implementation
- Priority nursing problems are:
  1. Hypoxemia related to decreased diffusion at the alveolar-capillary membrane and potential for airway obstruction related to excessive tracheobronchial secretions, fatigue, chest discomfort, muscle weakness:
     a. Monitor rate, rhythm, depth, and effort of ventilation.
     b. Assess pulse oxymetry and administer oxygen by nasal cannula or mask as prescribed.
     c. Instruct the patient on the correct use of incentive spirometry (sustained maximal inspiration) and encourage him or her to perform 5 to 10 breaths per session every hour while awake.
     d. Assess the patient's ability to cough effectively.
     e. Encourage coughing and deep breathing at least every 2 hours.
     f. Monitor fluid intake and encourage the alert patient to maintain sufficient intake to provide a dilute urine output.

    g. Administer prescribed bronchodilators and corticosteroids by aerosol nebulizer or by metered dose inhaler.

    h. Monitor for complications such as hypoxemia, ventilatory failure, atelectasis, pleural effusion, and pleurisy.

2. Potential for Sepsis related to the presence of microorganisms in a very vascular area:

    a. Administer prescribed anti-infective therapy, based on organism sensitivity.

    b. For pneumonia resulting from aspiration of food or stomach contents, steroids and NSAIDs are used with antibiotics to reduce the inflammatory response.

Community-Based Care

- Teach the patient about:
  1. The importance of completing the full course of antibiotic therapy
  2. Notifying the health care provider if chills, fever, persistent cough, dyspnea, wheezing, hemoptysis, increased sputum production, chest discomfort, or increasing fatigue recurs or if symptoms fail to resolve
  3. The importance of getting plenty of rest and gradually increasing exercise
  4. Preventing upper respiratory tract infections and viruses by:
     a. Avoiding crowds
     b. Avoiding people who have a cold or flu
     c. Avoiding exposure to irritants such as smoke
     d. Obtaining an annual influenza vaccination
     e. Obtaining the pneumococcal vaccination
  5. The importance of eating a balanced diet with adequate fluid intake
- Encourage the patient to quit smoking, and provide information on smoking cessation classes through the American Lung Association (ALA) and American Cancer Society.

✔NATIONAL PATIENT SAFETY GOAL

Three care actions, known as a *ventilator bundle*, have been shown to reduce the incidence of VAP: hand hygiene, oral care, and elevation of the head of the bed.

- Implement these practices for the ventilated patient to reduce VAP:
  1. If possible, use a disinfecting oral rinse immediately *before* the intubation.
  2. Wash hands before and after contact with the patient.
  3. Provide oral care at least every 4 to 6 hours.

4. Remove subglottic secretions; this can be done continuously if the endotracheal tube has a separate lumen that opens directly above the tube cuff.
5. Keep the head of the bed elevated 30 to 45 degrees unless another health problem is a contraindication for this position; avoid supine positioning.
6. Use best practices to promote weaning from the mechanical ventilator.

PNEUMOTHORAX

- Pneumothorax, also called a *collapsed lung*, is an accumulation of air in the pleural space. The lung collapses with the subsequent rise in chest pressure; there is a concurrent reduction in vital capacity.
- Any injury that allows air to enter the pleural space, including blunt chest trauma, can cause a pneumothorax. Injury may also cause some degree of hemothorax. Pneumothorax also may occur spontaneously.
- Assess for and document:
  1. Reduced breath sounds on auscultation
  2. Hyperresonance on percussion
  3. Prominence of the involved side of the chest, which moves poorly with respirations
  4. Deviation of the trachea away from (closed) or toward (open) the affected side
  5. Pleuritic chest pain
  6. Tachypnea
  7. Subcutaneous emphysema (air under the skin in the subcutaneous tissues)
- An ultrasound examination or a chest x-ray is used for diagnosis.
- Chest tubes may be needed to allow the air to escape and the lung to reinflate.

PNEUMOTHORAX, TENSION

- Tension pneumothorax is a rapidly developing and life-threatening complication of large amounts of air entering the pleural space from an air leak in the lung or chest wall.
- Air that enters the pleural space during inspiration does not exit during expiration, allowing air to continue to collect under pressure, collapsing the lung, compressing blood vessels, limiting venous return, and reducing cardiac output.

- Causes include blunt chest trauma, mechanical ventilation with positive end-expiratory pressure (PEEP), closed-chest drainage (chest tubes), burst alveoli blebs, and insertion of central venous access catheters.

∎NURSING SAFETY PRIORITY: Critical Rescue
If not promptly detected and treated, tension pneumothorax is quickly fatal.

- Assess for and document:
  1. Asymmetry of the thorax
  2. Tracheal movement away from midline to the unaffected side
  3. Respiratory distress
  4. Absence of breath sounds on one side
  5. Distended neck veins
  6. Cyanosis
  7. Hypertympanic sound on percussion over the affected side
- Initial management includes insertion of a large-bore needle into the second intercostal space in the midclavicular line of the affected side.
- Chest tube placement into the fourth intercostal space then follows, with water seal drainage until the lung reinflates.

POLIO AND POSTPOLIO SYNDROME

- Poliomyelitis (polio) is an acute viral disease characterized by destruction of the motor cells of the anterior horn of the spinal cord, the brainstem, and the motor strip of the frontal lobe. The disease is rare in North America, because immunization during childhood is prevalent. Treatment is symptomatic.
- Postpolio syndrome is a new onset of weakness, pain, and fatigue in people who had poliomyelitis 30 or more years previously. Physical and emotional stressors are contributing factors. Treatment is symptomatic and includes lifestyle modifications and adaptive devices to preserve energy and function.

POLYNEUROPATHY

OVERVIEW
- The terms *polyneuritis, polyneuropathy,* and *peripheral neuropathy* may be used interchangeably.

  The disorders are characterized by muscle weakness with or without atrophy; pain that is described as stabbing, cutting, or searing; paresthesia or loss of sensation; impaired reflexes; autonomic manifestations; or a combination of these symptoms.

- The most common type is a symmetric polyneuropathy in which the patient experiences decreased sensation along with a feeling that the extremity is asleep. Tingling, burning, tightness, or aching sensations usually start in the feet and progress to the level of the knee before affecting the hands ("glove and stocking" neuropathy).
- The disorders can result from inflammatory or noninflammatory processes; both can damage cranial and peripheral nerves.
- Factors associated with polyneuropathy include diabetes; kidney or hepatic failure; alcoholism; vascular disease; vitamin B_1, B_6, and B_{12} deficiencies; and exposure to heavy metals or industrial solvents.

PATIENT-CENTERED COLLABORATIVE CARE

- Assess for and document:
  1. Light touch sensation and pain in the distal extremities
  2. Position sense and kinesthetic sensation
  3. Any signs of injury
  4. Indications of autonomic dysfunction, such as orthostatic hypotension, abnormal sweating, and miosis
- Treatment consists of elimination or treatment of the underlying cause and symptomatic therapy.
  1. Treat the underlying cause.
  2. Supplement the patient's diet with vitamins.
  3. Provide pain management as needed.
  4. Provide health teaching, including the importance of foot care and of inspecting the extremities for injuries.
  5. Stress the importance of wearing shoes at all times and of purchasing well-fitting shoes.
  6. Teach the patient how to recognize potential hazards, such as exposure to extremes of environmental temperature.
  7. Discourage smoking.
  8. Promote glycemic control.

POLYPS, GASTROINTESTINAL

- GI tract polyps are small growths covered with mucosa that are attached to the intestinal surface; polyps have the potential to become malignant.
- Two forms of inherited GI polyps are particularly concerning to the health care provider: (1) familial adenomatous polyposis

(FAP) and (2) hereditary nonpolyposis colorectal cancer (HNPCC). Both are genetic syndromes characterized by the progressive development of colorectal adenomas. If these conditions are left untreated, colorectal cancer will occur.

- Pedunculated polyps are stalklike, with a thin stem attaching them to the intestinal wall.
- Polyps are usually asymptomatic but can cause rectal bleeding, intestinal obstruction, and intussusception.
- Polyps can usually be removed by polypectomy with an electrocautery snare that fits through a colonoscope, eliminating the need for abdominal surgery.
- After the procedure, monitor for:
  1. Abdominal distention and pain
  2. Rectal bleeding
  3. Mucopurulent rectal drainage
  4. Fever
- Teach the patient about the need for regular, routine monitoring if there is a family history of polyps or a finding of polyps with a screening colonoscopy. The specific follow-up time frame varies but generally occurs with 3 years.

PRESSURE ULCERS

OVERVIEW

- A pressure ulcer is tissue damage that occurs when the skin and the underlying soft tissue are compressed between a bony prominence and an external surface for an extended period.
- They form most commonly over the sacrum, hips, and ankles but can occur on any body surface.
- The major pathologic mechanism is tissue compression from pressure that restricts blood flow to the skin, resulting in reduced tissue perfusion and oxygenation and leading to cell death.
- The forces that lead to pressure ulcer formation include:
  1. *Pressure*: A mechanical force occurring as a result of gravity, compressing blood vessels at the point of contact and leading to ischemia, inflammation, and tissue necrosis
  2. *Friction*: A mechanical force occurring when surfaces rub the skin and irritate or directly pull off epithelial tissue (as when the patient is dragged or pulled across bed linen)
  3. *Shear* or *shearing forces*: Mechanical forces occurring when the skin itself is stationary and the tissues below the skin (e.g., fat, muscle) shift or move, reducing the blood supply to the skin.

Considerations for Older Adults

- Older adults are at particular risk for pressure ulcers because of the presence of age-related skin changes such as epidermal thinning, reduced strength and elasticity, and increased fragility of capillaries in the dermal layer.
- They are exposed to mechanical shearing forces, such as removal of tape or friction from tightly applied restraints.
- Skin moisture and irritation resulting from incontinence and friction over bony prominences can lead to partial-thickness skin destruction and early pressure ulcer formation.

- Once formed, these chronic wounds are slow to heal, resulting in increased morbidity and health care costs.
- Complications include sepsis, kidney failure, infectious arthritis, and osteomyelitis.
- Pressure ulcers are categorized using the following descriptors:
  1. *Stage I*: The skin is intact and red and does not blanch with external pressure.
  2. *Stage II*: The skin is not intact, and there is a partial-thickness skin loss of the epidermis or dermis. It may appear as an abrasion, a blister (open or fluid-filled), or a shallow crater, and bruising is not present.
  3. *Stage III*: Skin loss is full-thickness and subcutaneous tissues may be damaged or necrotic. Bone, tendon, and muscle are not exposed, but the fat may show a deep, crater-like appearance. Undermining and tunneling may or may not be present.
  4. *Stage IV*: Skin loss is full-thickness with exposed or palpable muscle, tendon, or bone. Undermining, tunneling, and sinus tracts may be present. Slough and eschar are often present on at least part of the wound.
  5. *Unstageable*: Skin loss is full-thickness, and the base is completely covered with slough or eschar, obscuring the true depth of the wound.
  6. *Suspected deep tissue injury*: The intact skin area appears purple or maroon and blood-filled blisters may be present. Other changes that may have preceded the discoloration include that the area may have felt more firm, boggy, mushy, warmer, or cooler than the surrounding tissue.
- Health promotion and maintenance:
  1. Intervene early when risk is present to prevent pressure ulcers.
  2. Identify patients at risk for pressure ulcer formation, commonly with a valid and reliable tool such as the Braden Scale. Risk factors include:

    a. Mental status changes
    b. Decreased sensory perception
    c. Impaired mobility
    d. Poor nutritional status
    e. Incontinence

- Implement prevention interventions:
  1. Performing proper positioning by:
     a. Padding contact surfaces with pressure-relieving devices
     b. Repositioning an immobile patient at least every 2 hours
     c. Using a designated slide board or a mechanical lift when moving an immobile patient from a bed to another surface
     d. Keeping the patient's heels off the bed surface with the use of a bed pillow under the ankles
  2. Ensuring adequate nutrition by:
     a. Providing sufficient fluid intake to maintain urine output of 0.5-1 mL/kg/hr.
     b. Helping the patient maintain an adequate intake of protein and calories
  3. Providing skin care, including:
     a. Performing a daily inspection of the patient's entire skin
     b. Documenting and reporting any manifestations of skin infection
     c. Using moisturizers daily on dry skin, and applying them when skin is damp
     d. Keeping moisture from prolonged contact with skin
     e. Using a wicking cloth where two moist skin surfaces touch or where perspiration collects
     f. Using moisture barriers on skin areas where wound drainage or incontinence occurs

❗NURSING SAFETY PRIORITY: Action Alert

Do not massage bony prominences.

  4. Ensuring appropriate skin cleaning by:
     a. Cleaning the skin as soon as possible after soiling occurs and at routine intervals
     b. Using a mild, heavily fatted soap or gentle commercial cleanser for incontinence
     c. Using tepid rather than hot water
     d. Using a disposable cleaning cloth that contains a skin barrier agent when cleaning the perineal area
     e. Using the minimal scrubbing force necessary to remove soil
     f. Patting gently rather than rubbing the skin dry

    g. Avoiding the use of powders or talcs directly on the perineum

    h. Applying a commercial skin barrier after cleansing to those areas in frequent contact with urine or feces

5. Using appropriate pressure-relieving and pressure-reducing devices:

    a. Pressure-relieving devices consistently reduce pressure to less than the capillary closing pressure.

    b. Pressure-reducing devices lower pressure to less than that of a standard hospital mattress or chair surface but do not consistently reduce pressure to less than the capillary closing pressure.

🛑 NURSING SAFETY PRIORITY: Action Alert

These devices are not effective for preventing pressure ulcers when used alone. They must be used together with a turning schedule and other skin care measures. For splints or other pressure-relieving devices, ensure correct fit and sufficient time in place to be therapeutic.

PATIENT-CENTERED COLLABORATIVE CARE
Assessment

- Obtain patient information about:
  1. The cause and specific circumstances of skin loss
  2. Whether any contributing factors are present, such as prolonged bedrest, immobility, incontinence, diabetes mellitus, inadequate nutrition or hydration, Altered Mental Status (decreased sensory perception), or peripheral vascular disease
- Assess for and document:
  1. The entire body for areas of skin injury or pressure
  2. General appearance for body weight and the proportion of weight to height
  3. Overall cleanliness of the skin, hair, and nails
  4. Any loss of mobility or range of joint motion
- Assess existing wounds daily for:
  1. Location, size, color, extent of tissue involvement, using a clock face approach to the wound, with 12 o'clock in the direction of the patient's head and 6 o'clock in the direction of the patient's feet:
     a. Length
     b. Width
     c. Depth
  2. Exudate
  3. Condition of surrounding tissue

4. Presence of foreign bodies
5. Whether reddened areas blanch with pressure
6. Texture of the wound
7. Presence of undermining and tunneling
8. Comparison of existing wound features with those documented previously to determine the current state of healing or deterioration
9. Presence of wound infection:
   a. Inflammation
   b. Induration
   c. Redness
   d. Foul odor
   e. Moderate to heavy exudate
   f. Cellulitis
   g. Progressive increase in ulcer size or depth
   h. Fever (systemic infection)
   i. Elevated white blood cell (WBC) count (systemic infection)
- Assess for psychosocial issues, including:
  1. Altered Body Image
  2. Coping patterns
  3. Changes in lifestyle and ADLs
  4. Financial resources
  5. Patient's and family's willingness and skill in cleaning the wound and applying a dressing
- Assess laboratory data for:
  1. Wound contamination, which is the presence of organisms without any manifestation of infection
  2. Wound infection, which is contamination with pathogenic organisms to the degree that growth and spread cannot be controlled by the body's immune defenses
  3. Systemic infection with bacteremia and sepsis

Planning and Implementation
IMPAIRED SKIN INTEGRITY
  Nonsurgical Management
- Dressing and wound care are the basis for pressure ulcer management. A properly designed dressing can speed healing by removing unwanted debris from the ulcer surface, protecting exposed healthy tissues and creating a barrier between the body and the environment until the ulcer is closed:
  1. *Hydrophobic* (nonabsorbent, waterproof) dressing materials are used when the wound is relatively free of drainage. They protect the ulcer from external contamination.
  2. *Hydrophilic* (absorbent) materials draw excessive drainage away from the ulcer surface, preventing maceration.

- The frequency of dressing changes depends on the amount of necrotic material or exudate:
  1. Dry gauze dressings are changed when "strike-through" occurs or when the outer layer of the dressing first becomes saturated with exudate.
  2. Gauze dressings used for débridement, such as those that are wetted and placed on a wound, allowed to become damp, and then removed, are changed often enough to take off any loose debris or exudate, usually every 4 to 6 hours.
  3. Synthetic dressings are changed when exudate causes the adhesive seal to break and leakage to occur.
- Before reapplying any dressing, gently clean the ulcer surface with saline or a nontoxic wound cleanser as prescribed.
- Drug therapy with topical antibacterial agents is often needed to control bacterial growth.
- Nutrition therapy requires adequate nutritional intake of calories, protein, vitamins, minerals, and water:
  1. Perform a nutritional assessment at least weekly.
  2. Coordinate with the dietitian to encourage the patient to eat a well-balanced diet, emphasizing protein, vegetables, fruit, whole grain breads and cereals, and vitamins.
- New technologies may be useful for chronic ulcers that remain open for months.
  1. *Electrical stimulation* is the application of a low-voltage current to a wound area to increase blood vessel growth and promote granulation.
  2. *Vacuum-assisted wound closure (VAC)* is the use of a suction tube that is covered by a special sponge and sealed in place for 48 hours. During that time, continuous low-level negative pressure is applied through the suction tube.
  3. *Hyperbaric oxygen (HBO)* therapy is the administration of oxygen under high pressure, which raises the tissue oxygen concentration.
  4. *Topical growth factors* are biologically active substances that stimulate cell movement and growth and are applied to the wound.
  5. *Skin substitutes* are engineered products that aid in the temporary or permanent closure of various types of wounds.

Surgical Management
- Surgical management includes removal of necrotic tissue (surgical débridement) and skin grafting or use of muscle flaps to close wounds that cannot heal by epithelialization and contraction.
- Provide preoperative care:
  1. Implementing routine preoperative care as described in Part One

2. Monitoring potential donor sites
3. Maintaining the integrity of the donor skin
4. Avoiding minor injuries that may result in infection and graft loss

- Provide postoperative care, including:
  1. Implementing routine postoperative care as described in Part One
  2. Elevating and resting the grafted area to allow revascularization
  3. Maintaining graft site immobilization with bulky cotton pressure dressings for 3 to 5 days
  4. After dressings are removed, monitoring the graft for indications of failure to vascularize, nonadherence to the wound, or graft necrosis:
     a. A pale flap with delayed capillary filling when blanched
     b. A dusky color or sharp line of color change
  5. Caring for donor sites:
     a. Protecting the area from injury and infection
     b. Positioning the patient to avoid pressure on the site
     c. Using an overbed cradle to tent the sheets
     d. Trimming the separating gauze (when gauze dressings are used) close to the skin surface reduces the chance of accidentally moving the still adherent gauze before healing is complete
     e. Administering analgesics as prescribed
     f. Using special low-pressure or air-fluidized mattresses when grafts or donor sites are on posterior body surface

RISK FOR INFECTION AND WOUND EXTENSION

- Priority nursing interventions focus on preventing wound infections and on identifying wound infections early to prevent complications:
  1. Monitoring the ulcer's appearance using objective criteria
  2. Re-evaluating the treatment plan if an ulcer shows no progress toward healing within 7 to 10 days or worsens
  3. Checking for manifestations of wound infection:
     a. Increased redness at the wound margins
     b. Edema
     c. Purulent and malodorous drainage
     d. Tenderness of the wound margins
     e. Increase in the size or depth of the lesion
     f. Changes in the color or texture of the granulation tissue
  4. Maintaining a safe environment by:
     a. Performing meticulous wound care
     b. Teaching all personnel to use standard precautions
     c. Disposing properly of soiled dressings and linens

Community-Based Care

- Teach the patient and family how to modify the home and obtain supplies to manage wound care.
- Ensure that the patient or the person who will be performing the wound care demonstrates facility in removing the dressing, cleaning the wound, and applying the dressing.
- Explain the manifestations of wound infection, and remind the patient and family to report these to the health care provider or wound care clinic.
- Stress the need for those with pressure ulcers on the legs to rest frequently, with the leg elevated, to avoid or reduce edema.
- Assist the family of an immobile patient in making arrangements for around-the-clock repositioning, as often as every 2 to 4 hours, to prevent further breakdown.
- Work with the social worker or case manager to obtain special beds or mattress overlays for the home.
- Encourage the patient to eat a balanced diet with frequent high-protein snacks.
- Emphasize the need to keep the skin of an incontinent patient clean and dry.
- Make referrals for home care nursing visits, if needed, to monitor wound progress.

PROLAPSE, MITRAL VALVE

- Mitral valve prolapse occurs when the heart valve leaflets prolapse into the left atrium during systole.
- Mitral valve prolapse is usually benign (asymptomatic) but may progress to pronounced mitral regurgitation.
- Assess for and document:
  1. Atypical chest pain; sharp pain localized in the left side of the chest
  2. Palpitations, dizziness or syncope
  3. Family history of mitral valve disease
  4. Midsystolic click or a late systolic murmur that may be audible at the apex
- Valve replacement surgery is indicated for symptomatic mitral prolapse.

PROLAPSE, PELVIC ORGAN

- The pelvic organs are supported by a sling of muscles and tendons, which sometimes become weak and no longer able to hold an organ in place.

- *Uterine prolapse* is the downward displacement of the uterus. It can be caused by neuromuscular damage of childbirth; increased intra-abdominal pressure related to pregnancy, obesity, or physical exertion; or weakening of pelvic support due to decreased estrogen.
- A *cystocele* is a protrusion of the bladder through the vaginal wall (urinary bladder prolapse), which can lead to stress urinary incontinence (SUI) and urinary tract infections (UTIs).
- A *rectocele* is a protrusion of the rectum through a weakened vaginal wall (rectal prolapse).
- Assessment findings include:
  1. Patient's report of feeling as if "something is falling out"
  2. Dyspareunia
  3. Backache
  4. Feeling of heaviness or pressure in the pelvis
  5. Protrusion of the cervix when the woman is asked to bear down
  6. Bowel or bladder problems, such as urinary incontinence, constipation, hemorrhoids, or fecal impaction
- Interventions are based on the degree of prolapse:
  1. Nonsurgical management may include:
     a. Teaching women to improve pelvic support and tone by pelvic floor muscle exercises (PFME, also called *Kegel exercises*)
     b. Using of space-filling devices such as pessaries or spheres worn intravaginally to elevate the uterine prolapse
     c. Administering intravaginal estrogen therapy
     d. Promoting bladder training and attention to complete emptying
     e. Promoting of bowel elimination
  2. Surgical management, usually with a vaginal approach, may be recommended for severe symptoms:
     a. Anterior colporrhaphy (anterior repair) tightens the pelvic muscles for better bladder support.
     b. Posterior colporrhaphy (posterior repair) reduces rectal bulging.
     c. If both a cystocele and a rectocele are present, an anterior and posterior colporrhaphy (A&P repair) is performed.
  3. Nursing care is similar to that for a woman undergoing a vaginal hysterectomy (see *Surgical Management* under *Leiomyomas, Uterine*):
     a. Warn the patient to avoid lifting anything heavier than 5 pounds, strenuous exercises, and sexual intercourse for 6 weeks.
     b. Instruct her to notify her surgeon if she has signs of infection, such as fever, persistent pain, or purulent, foul-smelling discharge.

PROSTATIC HYPERPLASIA, BENIGN

OVERVIEW

- The exact cause of benign prostatic hyperplasia (BPH) is unclear. It is likely the result of a combination of aging and the influence of androgens that are present in prostate tissue, such as dihydrotestosterone (DHT). With aging, the glandular units in the prostate undergo nodular hyperplasia (an increase in the number of cells), resulting in prostatic hypertrophy (enlargement).
- The enlarged prostate extends upward into the bladder and inward, causing bladder outlet obstruction.
- The patient has an increased residual urine (stasis) or acute or chronic urinary retention.
- Increased residual urine causes overflow urinary incontinence in which the urine "leaks" around the enlarged prostate, causing dribbling.
- Urinary stasis can result in urinary tract infections and bladder calculi (stones).

PATIENT-CENTERED COLLABORATIVE CARE

Assessment

- Use a standardized tool to determine the severity of lower urinary tract symptoms such as the International Prostate Symptom Score (I-PSS).
- Assess for and document:
  1. Current urinary patterns such as frequency, straining to begin urination, number of nocturnal voids (nocturia), hesitancy, force and size of urinary stream, sensation of bladder fullness after voiding, and dribbling or leaking post void
  2. Bladder distention (by palpation or bedside ultrasound)
  3. Prostate for size and consistency (by the health care provider or advanced practice nurse): uniform, elastic, and nontender enlargement
  4. Laboratory findings:
     a. Evidence of urinary tract infection and hematuria (white blood cells [WBCs] and red blood cells [RBCs] in the urine)
     b. Prostate-specific antigen (PSA) and a serum acid phosphatase level to rule out prostate cancer

Interventions

Nonsurgical Management

- "Watchful waiting" observation period with yearly examination
- Drug therapy

1. Drugs to lower dihydrotestosterone (DHT) levels:
   a. Finasteride (Proscar)
   b. Dutasteride (Avodart)
2. Alpha-blocking agents that reduce urethral pressure and improve flow:
   a. Tamsulosin (Flomax) (over-the-counter)
   b. Alfuzosin (UroXatral)
   c. Doxazosin (Cardura)
   d. Terazosin (Hytrin)
   e. Silodosin (Rapaflo)

■ NURSING SAFETY PRIORITY: Drug Alert

If giving alpha blockers in an inpatient setting, assess for orthostatic (postural) hypotension, tachycardia, and syncope ("blackout"), especially after the first dose is given to older men. If the patient is taking the drug at home, teach him to be careful when changing position and report any weakness, light-headedness, or dizziness to the health care provider immediately. Bedtime dosing may decrease the risk for problems related to hypotension. Drugs used to treat erection problems (e.g., Viagra) can worsen these side effects. Teach patients taking a 5-alpha-reductase inhibitor (5-ARI) or alpha-blocking drug to keep all appointments for follow-up laboratory testing, because both drug classes can cause liver dysfunction.

- Prostatic fluid can be released and obstructive symptoms reduced with frequent sexual intercourse.
- Teach the patient about ways to prevent bladder distention, such as:
  1. Avoiding drinking large amounts of fluid in a short period
  2. Avoiding alcohol, diuretics, and caffeine
  3. Voiding as soon as the urge is felt
  4. Avoiding drugs that can cause urinary retention, especially anticholinergics, antihistamines, and decongestants
- Minimally invasive techniques to reduce prostate tissue:
  1. *Transurethral needle ablation (TUNA)*, in which low radio-frequency energy shrinks the prostate
  2. *Transurethral microwave therapy (TUMT)*, in which high temperatures heat and destroy excess tissue
  3. *Interstitial laser coagulation (ILC)*, also called *contact laser prostatectomy (CLP)*, in which laser energy coagulates excess tissue
  4. *Electrovaporization of the prostate*, in which high-frequency electrical current cuts and vaporizes excess tissue

5. *Prostatic stents*, which may be placed into the urethra to maintain permanent patency after a procedure for destroying or removing prostatic tissue

Surgical Management

- The most common surgery for BPH is a *transurethral resection of the prostate (TURP)*, in which the enlarged portion of the prostate is cut into pieces and removed through the urethra by an endoscopic instrument. A similar procedure is the *transurethral incision of the prostate (TIUP)*, in which small cuts are made into the prostate to relieve pressure on the urethra.
- Another alternative is an open prostatectomy, although it is rarely performed.
- Newer surgical technologies include *holmium laser enucleation of the prostate (HoLEP)* and *transurethral ultrasound-guided laser incision of the prostate (TULIP)*.
- Provide preoperative care:
  1. Implementing routine preoperative care as described in Part One
  2. Assessing the patient's anxiety
  3. Correcting any misconceptions about the surgery
  4. Informing the patient that he will have an indwelling bladder catheter for at least 24 hours and may have traction on the catheter
  5. Explaining that while the catheter is in place, he will feel the urge to void
  6. Reassuring him that it is normal for the urine to be blood-tinged after surgery
- Provide postoperative care:
  1. Implementing routine postoperative care as described in Part One
  2. Monitoring the patient's urine output every 2 hours and vital signs every 4 hours

∎ NURSING SAFETY PRIORITY: Critical Rescue

If arterial bleeding occurs, notify the surgeon immediately, and increase the continuous bladder irrigation (CBI) rate or intermittently irrigate the catheter with normal saline solution according to physician or hospital protocol.

3. Monitoring for severe bleeding, including serum hemoglobin and hematocrit levels, presence of hematuria, and signs of hypovolemia from blood loss in the first 24 postoperative hours
4. Administering antispasmodic drugs as prescribed
5. Keeping the catheter free of obstruction and kinks; monitoring for clots and sudden cessation of urine output

6. Instructing the patient to increase fluid intake to keep the urine clear
7. Observing for other possible complications of TURP, such as infection or incontinence
8. Teaching the patient that sexual function should not be affected after TURP, but that retrograde ejaculation is possible
9. Reassuring the patient that loss of urine control or dribbling is almost always temporary and will resolve
10. Assisting the patient and his family in finding ways to keep his clothing dry until sphincter control returns

PROSTATITIS

OVERVIEW
- Prostatitis is an inflammation of the prostate gland.
- There are four types: acute bacterial prostatitis (ABP), chronic bacterial prostatitis (CBP), nonbacterial prostatitis (NBP) or chronic pelvic pain syndrome (CPPS), and asymptomatic inflammatory prostatitis.
- ABP often occurs with urethritis or an infection of the lower urinary tract.
- Common organisms are *Escherichia coli*, *Enterobacter*, *Proteus*, and group D streptococci.
- Manifestations of ABP may include:
  1. Fever and chills
  2. Dysuria (painful urination)
  3. Urethral discharge
  4. Boggy, tender prostate
  5. Urinary tract infections
  6. White blood cells (WBCs) in prostatic secretions
- Manifestations of CBP may include:
  1. Hesitancy, urgency, dysuria
  2. Difficulty initiating and terminating the flow of urine
  3. Decreased strength and volume of urine
  4. Discomfort in the perineum, scrotum, and penis
  5. Backache
  6. Hematuria
- Complications include epididymitis and cystitis.

PATIENT-CENTERED COLLABORATIVE CARE
- Treatment includes:
  1. Drug therapy with antimicrobials, which may last from weeks to many months because of poor penetration of antibiotics into prostatic tissue

2. Comfort measures, such as sitz baths, muscle relaxants, and NSAIDs
3. Stool softeners to prevent straining and rectal irritation of the prostate during a bowel movement
4. Drug therapy with alpha blockers such as tamsulosin (Flomax) to promote voiding

- Teach patients about:
  1. Avoiding alcohol, coffee, tea, and spicy foods that irritate symptoms
  2. Avoiding cold preparations containing decongestants or antihistamines that may cause urinary retention
  3. The importance of increasing fluid intake
  4. Activities that drain the prostate:
     a. Sexual intercourse
     b. Masturbation
  5. The fact that prostatitis is not contagious
  6. The importance of adhering to long-term antibiotic therapy for CBP

PSEUDOCYSTS, PANCREATIC

- Pancreatic pseudocysts develop as a complication of acute or chronic pancreatitis or abdominal trauma.
- These "false cysts" do not have an epithelial lining and are encapsulated, saclike structures that form on or surround the pancreas.
- The pancreatic wall is inflamed, vascular, and fibrotic and contains large amounts of straw-colored or dark brown viscous fluid (enzyme exudate from the pancreas).
- The pseudocyst may be palpated as an epigastric mass.
- The primary symptoms are epigastric pain radiating to the back, abdominal fullness, nausea, vomiting, and jaundice. Serum amylase and lipase levels may be elevated.
- Complications include rupture; hemorrhage; infection; obstruction of the bowel, biliary tract, or splenic vein; abscess or fistula formation; and pancreatic ascites.
- A pseudocyst may spontaneously resolve.
- Surgical intervention with internal drainage is accomplished by creating an ostomy between the pseudocyst and the stomach, jejunum, or duodenum; external drainage is provided by insertion of a sump drainage tube to remove pancreatic exudate and secretions.

PSORIASIS

OVERVIEW

- Psoriasis is a lifelong scaling skin disorder with underlying dermal inflammation that has exacerbations and remissions. Normally, cells at the basement membrane of the epidermis take about 28 days to reach the outermost layer where they are shed. In a person with psoriasis, the rate of cell division is speeded up so that cells are shed every 4 to 5 days.
- It appears to be an autoimmune reaction resulting from overstimulation of the immune system that leads to increased keratinocyte cell division and plaque formation.

Genetic/Genomic Considerations

A strong genetic predisposition has been recognized in at least 30% of cases, and several genes appear to be involved in expression of the disease; always ask about a family history when assessing a patient with psoriasis.

- Environmental factors influence whether the disease occurs, its severity, and its response to various treatments.
- Environmental factors that lead to outbreaks and influence the severity of clinical symptoms include skin trauma, surgery, sunburn, and excoriation.
- Treatments include topical agents to reduce inflammation and cell division, ultraviolet light therapy and systemic drugs for immunomodulation in the presence of moderate-to-severe plaque formation, including the use of immunosuppressants and biologic agents (e.g., adalimumab [Humira], alefacept [Amevive], infliximab [Remicade], ustekinumab [Stelara], and etanercept [Enbrel]).
- Some patients with psoriasis also develop a debilitating arthritis.

PATIENT-CENTERED COLLABORATIVE CARE

Assessment

- Obtain patient information about:
  1. Any family history of psoriasis:
     a. Age at onset
     b. Description of the disease progression
     c. Pattern of recurrences
  2. Description of the current flare-up of psoriasis, including:
     a. Whether the onset was gradual or sudden

    b. Where the lesions first appeared
    c. Whether there have been any changes in severity over time
    d. Whether fever and itching are present
  3. Possible precipitating factors, including:
    a. Recent skin trauma
    b. Upper respiratory tract infection
    c. Recent surgeries
    d. Menopause status
    e. Past and current use of drugs
    f. Recent stress
    g. Previous interventions and their effectiveness

- Assess for and document the appearance of psoriasis and its course:
  1. *Psoriasis vulgaris* is the most common type of psoriasis:
     a. Thick, reddened papules or plaques covered by silvery white scales
     b. Sharply defined borders between the lesions and normal skin
     c. Lesions are usually present in the same areas on both sides of the body.
     d. Common lesion sites are the scalp, elbows, trunk, knees, sacrum, and outside surfaces of the limbs.
  2. *Exfoliative psoriasis* (erythrodermic psoriasis) has generalized erythema and scaling that do not form obvious lesions.

Interventions

- Teach the patient about the disease and its treatment, and provide emotional support for the changes in body image often experienced with psoriasis.
- Topical therapy:
  1. Corticosteroids applied to skin lesions, followed by warm, moist dressings to increase absorption
  2. Tar preparations applied to the skin lesions as solutions, ointments, lotions, gels, and shampoos
  3. Anthralin (Anthraforte ✦, Drithocreme, Lasan) application alone or in combination with coal tar baths and ultraviolet (UV) light
  4. Calcipotriene (Dovonex), a synthetic form of vitamin D that regulates skin cell division
  5. Tazarotene (Tazorac), which can cause birth defects even when used topically
- Ultraviolet (UV) radiation therapy decreases dermal growth rates:
  1. Ultraviolet B (UV-B) light
  2. Ultraviolet A (UV-A) light

   3. Psoralen and UV-A (PUVA) treatments involve the ingestion
      of a photosensitizing agent (psoralen) 2 hours before expo-
      sure to UV-A light.
- Systemic therapy:
   1. Examples of biologic agents include:
      a. Alefacept (Amevive)
      b. Etanercept (Enbrel)
   2. Low-dose methotrexate (Folex, Mexate)
   3. Immunosuppressive agents
      a. Cyclosporine (Sandimmune)
      b. Azathioprine (Imuran)
- Often the patient's self-esteem suffers because of the presence of skin lesions and the unpleasantness of some of the
  treatments.
   1. Encourage the patient and family members to express their
      feelings about having an incurable skin problem that can al-
      ter appearance.
   2. Urge patients to contact other people with the disorder.
   3. Use touch without gloves during social interactions to com-
      municate acceptance of the person and the skin problem.
- Teach women of childbearing age who are taking biologic
  agents, methotrexate, or immunosuppressive drugs to use a reliable method of contraception, because these agents can cause
  birth defects when taken during pregnancy.

PULMONARY CONTUSION

- Pulmonary contusion most often follows injuries caused by
  rapid deceleration during vehicular accidents. Hemorrhage
  and edema occur in and between the alveoli, decreasing lung
  movement and reducing the area for gas exchange.
- Respiratory failure often develops over time rather than immediately after the trauma.
- Manifestations include:
   1. Dyspnea
   2. Hypoxemia
   3. Bloody sputum
   4. Decreased breath sounds
   5. Crackles and wheezes
   6. Hazy opacity on chest x-ray in the lobes or parenchyma
- Management is aimed at maintenance of ventilation and
  oxygenation:
   1. Use central venous pressure (CVP) to monitor response to
      fluid therapy and limit overhydration.

2. Provide oxygen therapy and mechanical ventilation with positive end-expiratory pressure (PEEP) to maintain open alveoli.
3. Monitor work of breathing and maintain vigilance for early detection of onset acute respiratory distress syndrome (ARDS), a relatively common complication of extensive lung contusion.

PULMONARY EMBOLISM

OVERVIEW

- Pulmonary embolism (PE) is a collection of particulate matter (solids, liquids, or air), most commonly a blood clot, that enters venous circulation and lodges in the pulmonary vessels.
- Large emboli obstruct pulmonary blood flow, leading to reduced oxygenation of the whole body, pulmonary tissue hypoxia, and, potentially, death.
- The local response includes collection of platelets on the embolus, which triggers the release of substances that cause blood vessel constriction. Widespread pulmonary vessel constriction and pulmonary hypertension impair gas exchange. Deoxygenated blood is moved into the arterial circulation, causing hypoxemia.
- Major risk factors for venothromboembolism (VTE), leading to PE:
  1. Prolonged immobility
  2. Central venous catheters
  3. Surgery (especially pelvic or leg surgery)
  4. Obesity
  5. Advancing age
  6. Conditions that increase blood clotting
  7. History of thromboembolism
- Smoking, pregnancy, estrogen therapy, heart failure, stroke, cancer (particularly lung or prostate), and trauma increase the risk for VTE and PE.

PATIENT-CENTERED COLLABORATIVE CARE
Assessment

- Obtain patient information about:
  1. Sudden onset of breathing difficulty
  2. Risk factors for VTE and PE
- Assess for manifestations:
  1. Pulmonary manifestations:
     a. Dyspnea
     b. Pleuritic chest pain (sharp, stabbing pain on inspiration)

    c. Crackles

    d. Dry cough

    e. Hemoptysis (bloody sputum)

  2. Cardiac manifestations:

    a. Rapid heart rate

    b. Distended neck veins

    c. Syncope (fainting or loss of consciousness)

    d. Cyanosis

    e. Hypotension

█ NURSING SAFETY PRIORITY: Critical Rescue

Assess patients at risk for PE for the symptom cluster of distended neck veins, syncope, cyanosis, and hypotension. If this cluster is present, notify the Rapid Response Team.

    f. Abnormal heart sounds, such as an S_3 or S_4

    g. Electrocardiographic (ECG) abnormalities (nonspecific and transient)

  3. Miscellaneous manifestations:

    a. Low-grade fever

    b. Petechiae on the skin over the chest and in the axillae

    c. Nausea, vomiting, and general malaise

    d. Low $Paco_2$ (early)

    e. Low Pao_2 (late)

    f. High $Paco_2$ (late)

    g. Low arterial pH (late)

  4. Psychosocial manifestations:

    a. Anxiety and fear

    b. Sense of impending doom

    c. Restlessness

- Diagnosis is most commonly made with chest computed tomography (CT) scan.

█ NURSING SAFETY PRIORITY: Critical Rescue

If a patient has sudden onset of dyspnea and chest pain, immediately notify the Rapid Response Team. Reassure the patient, assist him or her to a position of comfort with the head of the bed elevated, and consider applying oxygen therapy.

Planning and Implementation
HYPOXEMIA

- Related to mismatch of lung perfusion and alveolar oxygenation
- Goals of management for PE are to increase gas exchange, improve lung perfusion, reduce the risk for further clot formation, and prevent complications.

Nonsurgical Management
- Oxygen therapy:
  1. Apply oxygen by nasal cannula or by mask in less severe cases.
  2. Institution of mechanical ventilation for the severely hypoxemic patient
  3. Monitor:
     a. Oxygen saturation continually
     b. Vital signs, lung sounds, and cardiac status hourly
  4. Assess for and document increasing or decreasing:
     a. Dyspnea
     b. Dysrhythmias
     c. Distended neck veins
     d. Pedal or sacral edema
     e. Abnormal lung sounds
     f. Cyanosis of lips, conjunctiva, oral mucosa, nail beds
- Drug therapy:
  1. Anticoagulants keep the embolus from enlarging and prevent the formation of new clots:
     a. Heparin
     b. Fibrinolytic drugs (later to break up the existing clot)
     c. Warfarin (Coumadin, Warfilone ♣) starting on the third day of heparin use
  2. Review the patient's partial thromboplastin time (PTT) before therapy is started, every 4 hours after therapy begins, and daily thereafter. Therapeutic PTT values usually range between 1.5 and 2.5 times the control value.
  3. Therapy with both heparin and warfarin continues until the patient has an international normalized ratio (INR) of 2 to 3.

◼ NURSING SAFETY PRIORITY: Drug Alert

Keep antidotes to anticoagulant drugs on the unit for patients undergoing this therapy. The antidote for heparin is protamine sulfate; the antidote for warfarin is injectable phytonadione (vitamin K_1, AquaMEPHYTON, Mephyton). Send a type and screen or type and cross sample to blood bank if implementing antifibrinolytic therapy; antidotes for fibrinolytic therapy include clotting factors, and fresh-frozen plasma. Aminocaproic acid (Amicar) may also be used.

Surgical Management
- *Embolectomy* is the surgical removal of the embolus from pulmonary blood vessels using special thrombectomy catheters that can mechanically break up clots (e.g., AngioJet).

- *Inferior vena cava interruption* with placement of a vena cava filter is a lifesaving measure that prevents further embolus formation for some patients.

HYPOTENSION

- Hypotension is related to inadequate circulation to the left ventricle and or reduced circulation from bleeding due to anticoagulant or antifibrinolytic therapy.
- IV fluid therapy involves giving crystalloid solutions to restore plasma volume and prevent shock:
    1. Continuously monitor:
        a. ECG
        b. Pulmonary artery pressure
        c. Central venous or right atrial pressure
    2. Assess for signs of right-sided heart failure:
        a. Hypoxemia
        b. Dependent edema
- Drug therapy with agents that increase myocardial contractility may be used:
    1. Milrinone (Primacor)
    2. Dobutamine (Dobutrex)
- Drug therapy with vasodilators, such as nitroprusside (Nipride, Nitropress), may be used to decrease pulmonary artery pressure (if it is impeding cardiac contractility)
- Monitor patient response to anticoagulant and antifibrinolytic therapy so as to detect bleeding early.

ANXIETY

- Anxiety is related to hypoxemia and life-threatening illness.
- The patient with PE is anxious and fearful for many reasons.
- Communication:
    1. Acknowledge the anxiety and the patient's perception of a life-threatening situation.
    2. Stay with the patient and speak calmly and clearly, providing reassurance that appropriate measures are being taken.
    3. Explain the rationale and share information with the patient regarding any procedure, assessment, or intervention.
- Drug therapy with an antianxiety drug may be prescribed if the patient's anxiety increases or prevents adequate rest.

RISK FOR BLEEDING

- Assess at least every 2 hours for evidence of bleeding in the form of oozing, bruises that cluster, petechiae, or purpura.
- Examine all stools, urine, drainage, and vomitus visually for gross blood and test for occult blood.
- Measure any blood loss as accurately as possible.

- Measure the patient's abdominal girth every 8 hours.
- Implement best practices for bleeding prevention:
  1. Handling the patient gently
  2. Using and teaching unlicensed assistive personnel (UAP) to use a lift sheet when moving and positioning the patient in bed
  3. Avoiding IM injections and venipunctures
  4. If injections or venipunctures are necessary, using the smallest gauge needle for the task
  5. Applying firm pressure to the needle stick site for 10 minutes or until the site no longer oozes blood
  6. Applying ice to areas of trauma
  7. Testing all urine, vomitus, and stool for the presence of occult blood
  8. Observing IV sites every 4 hours for bleeding
  9. Instructing patients to notify nursing personnel immediately if any trauma occurs or if bleeding or bruising is noticed
  10. Avoiding trauma to rectal tissues by:
      a. Instructing UAP not to take temperatures rectally
      b. Not administering enemas
      c. If suppositories are prescribed, lubricating liberally and administering with caution
  11. Instructing the patient and UAP to use an electric shaver rather than a razor
  12. When providing mouth care or supervising others in providing mouth care:
      a. Using a soft-bristled toothbrush or tooth sponges
      b. Not using floss
      c. Checking to make certain that dentures fit and do not rub
  13. Instructing the patient not to blow the nose forcefully or insert objects into the nose
  14. Instructing UAP and the patient to wear shoes with firm soles whenever he or she is ambulating
  15. Ensuring that antidotes to anticoagulation therapy are on the unit
- Monitor laboratory values daily.
  1. Hematocrit and hemoglobin
  2. Platelet count
  3. Prothrombin time (PT), activated PTT (aPTT), INR

Community-Based Care

- The patient with PE is discharged after hypoxemia and hemodynamic instability have been resolved and adequate anticoagulation has been achieved.

- Anticoagulation therapy usually continues after discharge.
- Teach the patient and family about:
  1. Bleeding precautions
  2. Activities to reduce the risk for VTE
  3. Complications
  4. Need for follow-up care

PULMONARY EMPYEMA

OVERVIEW

- Pulmonary empyema is a collection of pus in the pleural space; the fluid is thick, opaque, exudative, and foul smelling.
- The most common cause is pulmonary infection (pneumonia), lung abscess, or infected pleural effusion that can spread across the pleura, obstructing lymph nodes and leading to a retrograde (backward) flood of infected lymph into the pleural space.
- Other causes include liver or abdominal abscesses that spread infection through the lymphatic system into the lung area, thoracic surgery, and chest trauma.

PATIENT-CENTERED COLLABORATIVE CARE

Assessment

- Obtain patient information about:
  1. Recent febrile illness (including pneumonia)
  2. Chest pain
  3. Dyspnea
  4. Cough
  5. Chest trauma
  6. Fever, chills, night sweats
- Assess for and document:
  1. Character of the sputum
  2. Reduced chest wall motion
  3. Decreased or absent fremitus
  4. Decreased or abnormal breath sounds
  5. Dyspnea, labored breathing, or tachypnea
  6. Weight loss
  7. Hypotension
  8. Displacement of the cardiac point of maximal impulse (PMI)
  9. Hypoxia, decreased SpO_2
- Diagnosis is made by chest x-ray and analysis of pleural fluid obtained by thoracentesis.

Interventions

- Therapy for empyema is focused on emptying the empyema cavity, re-expanding the lung, and controlling the infection.

- Antibiotics appropriate for the identified organism are prescribed.
- Closed-chest drainage is used to promote lung expansion.
- Open thoracotomy and removal of a portion of the pleura may be needed for thick pus or marked pleural thickening.
- Nursing care is the same as for patients with a pleural effusion, pneumothorax, or infection.

PULMONARY HYPERTENSION

OVERVIEW

- Primary pulmonary arterial hypertension (PAH) is a problem of the pulmonary blood vessels in which blood vessel constriction with increasing vascular resistance occurs in the lungs.
- Pulmonary blood pressure rises and blood flow decreases, leading to poor perfusion and hypoxemia. Eventually, the right side of the heart fails (*cor pulmonale*) as a result of the continuous workload of pumping against the high pulmonary pressures.
- Primary PAH is also considered to be idiopathic, because the causes of this life-threatening disorder are unclear.
- Secondary PAH can occur as a complication of other lung disorders.
- Primary PAH is rare and occurs mostly in women between the ages of 20 and 40 years.
- Without treatment for PAH, death usually occurs within 2 years after diagnosis.

Genetic/Genomic Considerations

- About 50% of patients with primary PAH have a genetic mutation in the *BMPR2* gene, which codes for a growth factor receptor. Excessive activation of this receptor allows increased growth of arterial smooth muscle in the lungs, making these arteries thicker.
- Because many more people have mutations in this gene than have PAH, it is thought that the mutations increase susceptibility to PAH when other, often unknown, environmental factors also are present.
- Teach women who have a first-degree relative (parent or sibling) with PAH to have regular health checkups and to consult a health care provider whenever pulmonary problems are present.

PATIENT-CENTERED COLLABORATIVE CARE
Assessment

- Assess for and document:
  1. Dyspnea and fatigue in an otherwise healthy adult
  2. Angina-like chest pain

- Diagnosis is made from the results of right-sided heart catheterization showing elevated pulmonary pressures.

Interventions

- Drug therapy can reduce pulmonary pressures and slow the development of *cor pulmonale* by dilating pulmonary vessels and preventing clot formation:
  1. Natural and synthetic prostacyclin agents provide the best specific dilation of pulmonary blood vessels. These agents are given continuously intravenously or in other parenteral formulations (e.g., epoprostenol [Flolan] or treprostinil [Remodulin])

⊞ NURSING SAFETY PRIORITY: Critical Rescue

Although prostacyclin therapy is very effective, deaths have been reported if intravenous drug delivery is interrupted for even a few minutes. Teach the patient to always have backup drug cassettes and battery packs. If these are not available or the line is disrupted, the patient should go to the emergency department immediately.

  2. Endothelin-receptor antagonists, bosentan (Tracleer)
  3. Warfarin (Coumadin), low-molecular-weight heparin and antiplatelet drugs
  4. Calcium channel blockers, such as nifedipine (Procardia) and diltiazem (Cardizem)
  5. Sildenafil (Revatio, Viagra) administered orally or intravenously with prostacyclins therapy

- Secondary pulmonary hypertension is usually treated by treating the underlying lung pathology. When lung pathology is terminal or untreatable, then management of symptoms or palliative care, becomes the focus of care.
- Teaching patients about the need to:
  1. Use strict aseptic technique in all aspects of manipulating the drug delivery system.
  2. Notify the pulmonologist at the first sign of any respiratory or systemic infection.
- Surgical management of PAH involves single-lung or whole-lung transplantation.
- If *cor pulmonale* also is present, the patient may need combined heart-lung transplantation.

PULMONARY SARCOIDOSIS

- Sarcoidosis is a granulomatous disorder of unknown cause that can affect any organ, especially the lung.

- It develops over time as an autoimmune disorder in which the normally protective T-lymphocytes increase and cause damaging actions in lung tissue.
- Alveolar inflammation (alveolitis) results from the presence of immune cells in the alveoli and the chronic inflammation causes fibrosis that reduces lung compliance (elasticity) and the ability to exchange gases.
- *Cor pulmonale* (right-sided cardiac failure) is often present, because the heart can no longer pump effectively against the stiff, fibrotic lung.
- The disease usually affects young adults.
- Manifestations include enlarged lymph nodes in the hilar area of the lungs, lung infiltrate on chest x-ray, skin lesions, eye lesions, cough, dyspnea, hemoptysis, and chest discomfort.
- The disease may resolve permanently or may lead to progressive pulmonary fibrosis and severe systemic disease.
- The goal of therapy is to lessen symptoms and prevent fibrosis and includes immunomodulating drugs such as corticosteroids and cytokine mediators.

PYELONEPHRITIS

OVERVIEW

- Pyelonephritis is an infection of the kidney and renal pelvis.
- Microorganisms enter the renal pelvis and activate the inflammatory response, which results in mobilization of white blood cells (WBCs) and local edema.
- Pyelonephritis's is generally classified as acute or chronic. Acute pyelonephritis is the active bacterial infection, whereas chronic pyelonephritis results from repeated or continued upper urinary tract infections or the effects of such infections.
- Complications include abscess formation and septicemia.
- Pregnancy, diabetes mellitus, and chronic renal calculi increase the risk for pyelonephritis.
- Structural deformities or obstruction with reflux caused by stones, obstruction, and neurogenic impairment involving the voiding mechanism often lead to chronic pyelonephritis.

PATIENT-CENTERED COLLABORATIVE CARE

Assessment

- Obtain patient information about:
  1. History of urinary tract and kidney infections
  2. History of diabetes mellitus or other conditions and treatment associated with immunocompromise.

3. History of stone disease or other structural or functional abnormalities of the genitourinary tract
- Assess for:
  1. Pregnancy, because pyelonephritis is associated with early onset of labor, compromising fetal health
  2. Flank or abdominal discomfort
  3. Hematuria, cloudy urine
  4. Signs of infection: general malaise, fever, chills
  5. Asymmetry, edema, or erythema at the costovertebral angle
  6. Presence of leukoesterase, nitrogen, WBCs, or bacteria in the urine
- Diagnostic testing may include:
  1. Urinalysis and urine for culture and sensitivity
  2. WBC count with differential; basic metabolic panel for kidney function
  3. X-ray, computed tomography (CT), or urography scans to diagnose stones or obstruction. *Ensure that the patient is not pregnant before any imaging study is performed.*

◼ NURSING SAFETY PRIORITY: Action Alert

A decrease in urine output by more than 0.5 mL/kg of patient weight per hour or an increase of serum creatinine of more than 1.5 times over baseline indicates worsening kidney function and should be communicated to the physician in a timely manner. Early detection of acute kidney injury can prevent progression to kidney failure.

Interventions

- Administer antibiotics. Drug therapy initially includes broad-spectrum antibiotics. With urine and blood culture sensitivity results, a single antibiotic may be ordered.
- Encourage sufficient calories and protein intake to maintain health; consult with dietitian.
- Surgical procedures include:
  1. Pyelolithotomy (removal of a stone from the renal pelvis)
  2. Nephrectomy (removal of a kidney)
  3. Ureteral diversion or reimplantation of the ureter to restore the bladder drainage mechanism
- Maintain sufficient perfusion to the kidneys to prevent acute (hypotensive) or chronic (hypertensive) kidney injury.
- Maintain sufficient fluid intake to promote urine output greater than 1 mL/kg/hr.
- Assess for signs of acute kidney injury, such as increasing blood urea nitrogen (BUN) or creatinine level or decreased urinary output.

Community-Based Care
- Health teaching includes:
  1. Drug administration, including effects, side effects, and importance of following the prescribed duration of therapy
  2. Planning and implementing healthy choices for nutrition and fluid intake
  3. Routine postoperative care
  4. Manifestations of disease recurrence, such as urgency, frequency, or incontinence

RAYNAUD'S PHENOMENON AND RAYNAUD'S DISEASE

- *Raynaud's phenomenon* is caused by vasospasm of the arterioles and arteries of the upper and lower extremities, usually unilaterally.
- *Raynaud's disease* occurs bilaterally. It is more common in women and occurs between the ages of 17 and 50 years.
- The pathophysiology is the same for both entities: vasospasm of the arterioles and arteries of the upper and lower extremities.
- Cutaneous vessels are constricted, causing blanching of the extremities, followed by cyanosis.
- When the vasospasm is relieved, the tissue becomes reddened or hyperemic.
- Patients often have an associated systemic connective tissue disease such as systemic lupus erythematosus (SLE) or progressive systemic sclerosis.
- Assess for:
  1. Color changes in the extremity or digits, ranging from blanched to reddened to cyanotic
  2. Numbness of the extremity or digits
  3. Coldness of the extremity or digits
  4. Pain
  5. Swelling
  6. Ulcerations
  7. Aggravation of symptoms by cold or stress
  8. Gangrene of digits in severe cases
- Interventions include:
  1. Drug therapy to prevent vasoconstriction, including calcium channel blockers
  2. Lumbar sympathectomy to relieve severe symptoms in the feet
  3. Sympathetic ganglionectomy to relieve severe symptoms in the upper extremities

- Health teaching emphasizes methods to minimize vasoconstriction:
    1. Smoking cessation and caffeine reduction
    2. Minimizing exposure to cold by wearing warm clothes, socks, and gloves and maintaining a warm indoor ambient temperature
    3. Stress management

REGURGITATION, AORTIC

- In aortic regurgitation (insufficiency), the aortic valve leaflets do not close properly during diastole, and the annulus may become dilated, loose, or deformed.
- Regurgitation of blood from the aorta into the left ventricle occurs during diastole; the left ventricle dilates to accommodate the greater blood volume and hypertrophies.
- Causes include infective endocarditis, congenital anatomic aortic valvular abnormalities, hypertension, and Marfan syndrome (a generalized, systemic connective tissue disease).
- Patients with aortic insufficiency remain asymptomatic for many years because of the compensatory mechanisms of the left ventricle.
- Signs and symptoms include:
    1. Palpitations (severe disease)
    2. Dyspnea on exertion
    3. Orthopnea
    4. Paroxysmal nocturnal dyspnea
    5. Nocturnal angina with diaphoresis
    6. Bounding arterial pulse
    7. Widened pulse pressure
    8. High-pitched, blowing, decrescendo diastolic murmur
- Nonsurgical therapy focuses on drug therapy and rest. Prophylactic antibiotic therapy is recommended for invasive procedures or surgery.
- Surgical treatment is performed after symptoms of left ventricular failure have developed but before irreversible dysfunction occurs.
- Aortic valve repair or replacement surgery is performed to improve cardiac function in symptomatic patients.
- Repair procedures include valvuloplasty, commissurotomy, and annuloplasty (reconstruction).
- Replacement means that the aortic valve is excised during cardiopulmonary bypass surgery and is replaced with a prosthetic (synthetic) valve or biologic (xenographic or tissue) valve.

- The postoperative patient requires lifetime anticoagulation therapy to prevent thrombus formation on the valve.
- For preoperative and postoperative care, see *Surgical Management* under *Coronary Artery Disease*.

REGURGITATION, MITRAL

- Mitral regurgitation (insufficiency) results from fibrotic and calcific changes that prevent the mitral valve from closing completely during systole, allowing backflow of blood into the left atrium when the left ventricle contracts.
- During diastole, regurgitant output again flows from the left atrium to the left ventricle along with normal blood flow, increasing the volume of blood to be ejected during the next systole.
- To compensate for the increased volume and pressure, the left atrium and ventricle dilate and hypertrophy.
- Degeneration (age-related damage) followed by infective endocarditis are the most common causes of mitral regurgitation. When the causes is rheumatic carditis, regurgitation often co-exists with mitral stenosis.
- Signs and symptoms include:
  1. Right heart failure with neck vein distention, liver enlargement (hepatomegaly) and peripheral edema
  2. Fatigue and weakness
  3. Dyspnea, orthopnea
  4. Anxiety
  5. Atypical chest pains and palpitations
  6. Atrial fibrillation
  7. High-pitched, systolic murmur
- Drug therapy is instituted to maintain normal cardiac output.
- The reparative surgical procedure is mitral annuloplasty, which is performed during cardiopulmonary bypass surgery. Mitral valve leaflets and annuli are reconstructed to narrow the valve orifice.
- The postoperative patient requires lifetime anticoagulation therapy to prevent thrombus formation on the valve.
- For preoperative and postoperative care, see care of the patient undergoing a coronary artery bypass grafting procedure (see *Coronary Artery Disease*).
- Discharge planning includes providing health teaching information:
  1. Drug therapy effects, side effects, and monitoring for anticoagulation
  2. The importance of evaluation the need for antibiotics before any procedure (e.g., dental work, surgery)

RESPIRATORY FAILURE, ACUTE

OVERVIEW

- Acute respiratory failure is classified by blood gas abnormalities: pH less than 7.30, Pao_2 less than 60 mm Hg, Sao_2 less than 90%, and $Paco_2$ greater than 50 mm Hg.
- Acute respiratory failure can be defined in three ways, based on the underlying problem:
  1. *Ventilatory failure* is a problem of oxygen intake (ventilation) and blood delivery (perfusion) that causes a ventilation-perfusion mismatch in which perfusion is normal but ventilation is inadequate. It is often the result of a physical problem of the lungs or chest wall, a defect in the respiratory control center in the brain, or poor function of the respiratory muscles, especially the diaphragm. The $Paco_2$ level is greater than 45 mm Hg in patients who have otherwise healthy lungs.
  2. *Oxygenation failure* is a problem in which chest pressure changes are normal and air moves in and out without difficulty but does not oxygenate the pulmonary blood sufficiently. It occurs in the type of $\dot{V}/\dot{Q}$ mismatch in which air movement and oxygen intake (ventilation or *V*) are normal but lung blood flow (perfusion or *Q*) is decreased. Problems leading to this type of failure include impaired diffusion of oxygen at the alveolar level, right-to-left shunting of blood in the pulmonary vessels, mismatch, breathing air with a low partial pressure of oxygen (a rare problem), and abnormal hemoglobin that fails to bind oxygen.
  3. *Combined ventilatory and oxygenation failure* involves hypoventilation and impairment of oxygenation at the alveolar-capillary membrane. This type of respiratory failure leads to a more profound hypoxemia than either ventilatory failure or oxygenation failure alone. It is seen in patients who have abnormal lungs (chronic bronchitis, emphysema, or during asthma attacks) and in patients who have cardiac failure along with respiratory failure.
- Regardless of the underlying cause, the patient in acute respiratory failure is always hypoxemic.

PATIENT-CENTERED COLLABORATIVE CARE

Assessment

- Assess for and document:
  1. Dyspnea (the hallmark of respiratory failure)
  2. Orthopnea

3. Changes in the respiratory rate or pattern
4. Changes in lung sounds
5. Manifestations of hypoxemia:
   a. Pallor
   b. Cyanosis
   c. Increased heart rate
   d. Restlessness
   e. Confusion
6. Hypercarbia (high arterial blood levels of carbon dioxide)

Interventions

- Management of acute respiratory failure of any origin includes:
  1. Applying oxygen therapy to keep the partial pressure of arterial oxygen (Pao_2) greater than 60 mm Hg
  2. Implementing invasive or noninvasive mechanical ventilation if other measures do not increase oxygenation or reduce hypercarbia
  3. Assisting the patient to find a position of comfort that allows easier breathing, usually a more upright position
  4. Assisting the patient to use relaxation, diversion, and guided imagery to reduce anxiety
  5. Instituting energy-conserving measures of minimal self-care and no unnecessary procedures
  6. Administering drug therapy given systemically or by metered dose inhaler (MDI) to resolve dyspnea
  7. Encouraging deep breathing and techniques to increase oxygen intake or reduce carbon dioxide retention

RETINAL HOLES, TEARS, AND DETACHMENTS

OVERVIEW

- A *retinal hole* is a break in the retina, usually caused by trauma or aging.
- A *retinal tear* is a more jagged and irregularly shaped break, often caused by traction on the retina.
- A *retinal detachment* is the separation of the retina from the epithelium. Detachments are classified by the nature of their development.
  1. *Rhegmatogenous detachments* occur after a hole or tear in the retina is caused by mechanical force, creating an opening for the vitreous to move under the retina, pushing the retina away from its attachment.
  2. *Traction detachments* occur when the retina is pulled away from the support tissue by bands of fibrous tissue in the vitreous.
  3. *Exudative detachments* are caused by fluid collecting under the retina.

PATIENT-CENTERED COLLABORATIVE CARE
Assessment
- Subjective manifestations:
  1. Bright flashes of light (*photopsia*) or floating dark spots in the affected eye
  2. The sensation of a curtain being pulled over part of the visual field
  3. No pain
- Ophthalmoscopic manifestations:
  1. Gray bulges or folds in the retina that quiver
  2. Possibly a hole or tear at the edge of the detachment

Interventions
- For an actual detachment, surgical repair is needed to place the retina in contact with the underlying structures. A common repair procedure is scleral buckling.
- Preoperative care:
  1. Reassuring the patient to allay fears of permanent vision loss
  2. Teaching the patient to restrict activity and head movement before surgery to prevent further tearing or detachment and to promote drainage of any fluid under the retina
  3. Applying an eye patch over the affected eye to reduce eye movement
  4. Applying prescribed topical drugs to inhibit pupil constriction and accommodation
- Postoperative care:
  1. Applying an eye patch and shield
  2. Monitoring the patient's vital signs and checking the eye patch and shield for any drainage
  3. Positioning the patient as prescribed to allow the agent being used to promote reattachment to press the retina against the interior surface of the eye
  4. Administering analgesics and antiemetics as prescribed
  5. Instructing the patient to report any sudden increase in pain or pain occurring with nausea, which may indicate development of complications
  6. Reminding the patient to avoid activities that increase intraocular pressure (IOP)
  7. Teaching the patient to avoid reading, writing, and close work, such as sewing, during the first week after surgery, because these activities cause rapid eye movements and promote detachment
  8. Teaching the patient the manifestations of infection and detachment (sudden reduced visual acuity, eye pain, pupil that does not respond to light by constricting)
  9. Instructing the patient to notify the surgeon immediately if these manifestations occur

R

ROTATOR CUFF INJURIES

- The function of the rotator cuff is to stabilize the head of the humerus in the glenoid cavity during shoulder abduction.
- It may be injured by substantial trauma and also undergoes degenerative changes with aging.
- Older adults tend to have small tears related to aging, repetitive motions, or falls.
- Younger adults sustain tears by trauma, including falling, throwing a ball, or lifting heavy objects.
- Manifestations include shoulder pain and the inability to achieve or maintain abduction of the arm at the shoulder.
- Conservative management involves the use of NSAIDs, physical therapy, sling or immobilizer support, and ice or heat applications while the tear heals.
- Surgical cuff repair may be needed for patients who do not respond to conservative treatment or for those who have a complete tear.

SCABIES

- Scabies is a contagious skin disease that is caused by mite infestations and transmitted by close and prolonged contact with an infested companion or infested bedding.
- It is manifested by curved or linear ridges in the skin, especially between the fingers and on the palms and inner aspects of the wrists, and intense itching.
- Hypersensitivity reactions result in excoriated erythematous papules, pustules, and crusted lesions on the elbows, nipples, lower abdomen, buttocks, thighs, and penis and in the axillary folds.
- Infestation is confirmed by the presence of mites and eggs on microscopic examination of lesion scrapings.
- Treatment involves the use of scabicides, such as permethrin (Acticin), lindane (Kwell, Kildane, Scabene), malathion (Ovide), or benzyl benzoate (Ascabiol).
- Clothing and personal items must be cleaned with hot water and detergent.
- Social contacts should also be treated.

SCLERODERMA (SYSTEMIC SCLEROSIS)

OVERVIEW

- Systemic sclerosis (SSc), also called *scleroderma,* is a chronic, inflammatory, autoimmune connective tissue disease that usually first manifests with hardening of the skin.

- The disease is often confused with systemic lupus erythematosus (SLE) but is less common and has a higher mortality rate.
- The manifestations vary widely from person to person.
- The etiology is unclear, but SSc is thought to be an autoimmune disorder.
- It is classified as:
  1. *Diffuse cutaneous SSc,* with skin thickening on the trunk, face, and proximal and distal extremities (over most of the body). The first symptom is hand and forearm edema, which may exist with bilateral carpal tunnel syndrome.
  2. *Limited cutaneous SSc,* with thick skin limited to sites distal to the elbow and knee but also involving the face and neck. Patients have the *CREST syndrome:*
     a. *C*alcinosis (calcium deposits)
     b. *R*aynaud's phenomenon
     c. *E*sophageal dysmotility
     d. *S*clerodactyly (scleroderma of the digits)
     e. *T*elangiectasia (spider-like hemangiomas)
- Women are affected more often than men and usually are between 25 and 65 years old.

PATIENT-CENTERED COLLABORATIVE CARE
Assessment

- SSc manifests with joint pain and stiffness; painless, symmetric, pitting edema of the hands and fingers that may progress to include the entire upper and lower extremities and face; and taut, shiny skin that is free of wrinkles.
- When scleroderma progresses, swelling is replaced by tightening, hardening, and thickening of skin tissue with loss of elasticity and greatly decreased range of motion (ROM).
- Ulcerations and joint contractures may develop, and the patient may be unable to perform ADLs.
- Major organ involvement is manifested by:
  1. GI tract changes, especially in the esophagus, with dysphagia and esophageal reflux (GERD). A small, sliding hiatal hernia may be present. Intestinal peristalsis is diminished, leading to partial bowel obstruction and malabsorption.
  2. Cardiovascular system changes, especially Raynaud's phenomenon with digit necrosis, excruciating pain, and autoamputation of the distal digits. Myocardial fibrosis may be present with cardiac dysrhythmias and chest pain.
  3. Lung changes include fibrosis of the alveoli and interstitial tissues, and pulmonary hypertension may develop.
  4. Involvement of renal vasculature contributes to chronic kidney disease and may cause malignant hypertension and death.

Interventions
- The focus of medical management is to induce disease remission and slow disease progression.
- Systemic steroids and immunosuppressants are used in large doses and often in combination.
- Nursing management includes:
  1. Local skin protective measures:
     a. Teaching the patient to use mild soap and lotions and gentle cleaning techniques
     b. Inspecting the skin for further changes or open lesions
     c. Caring for skin ulcers according to their type and location
     d. Using bed cradles and foot boards
     e. Adjusting room temperature to prevent chilling
  2. Implementing and teaching about drug therapy
  3. Teaching patients to avoid or minimize cigarette smoking with associated vasoconstriction
  4. Promoting nutrition:
     a. Providing small, frequent meals
     b. Instructing the patient to avoid foods that may exacerbate GERD (e.g., spicy foods, caffeine, alcohol)
     c. Teaching the patient to keep the head elevated for 1 to 2 hours after a meal
  5. Reducing pain and maintaining joint mobility using interventions similar to those for rheumatoid arthritis
  6. Referring patients and families to community resources

SEIZURE DISORDERS

OVERVIEW
- A seizure is an abnormal, sudden, excessive, uncontrolled electrical discharge of neurons within the brain that may result in alterations in consciousness, motor or sensory ability, or behavior.
- Epilepsy is a chronic disorder characterized by two or more seizures.
- Three major categories:
  1. Generalized seizures that involve both cerebral hemispheres:
     a. *Tonic-clonic seizure* (formerly called a *grand mal seizure*) is characterized by stiffening or rigidity of the muscles, followed by rhythmic jerking of the extremities. Immediate unconsciousness occurs, and the patient may be incontinent of urine or feces and may bite his or her tongue.

    b. *Tonic seizures* are characterized by an abrupt increase in muscle tone, loss of consciousness, and loss of autonomic signs lasting from 30 seconds to several minutes.

    c. *Clonic seizures* last several minutes and are characterized by muscle contraction and relaxation.

    d. *Absence seizure* (formerly called *petit mal seizure*) consists of a brief (often seconds) period of loss of consciousness and blank staring, as if the patient were daydreaming.

    e. *Myoclonic seizure* is a brief, generalized jerking or stiffening of the extremities and may occur singly or in groups.

    f. *Atonic seizures* (formerly called *drop attacks*) are characterized by sudden loss of muscle tone, which in most cases causes the patient to fall.

  2. Partial (focal) seizures that begin in one cerebral hemisphere:

    a. *Complex seizure* (often called a *psychomotor seizure* or a *temporal lobe seizure*) causes the patient to lose consciousness or black out for 1 to 3 minutes. Characteristic behavior, known as automatism, may occur (e.g., lip smacking, patting, picking at clothes).

    b. *Simple seizure* consists of an aura or unusual sensation (déjà vu phenomenon, perception of an offensive smell, or sudden onset of pain) before the seizure takes place. It may be followed by unilateral movement of an extremity or autonomic or psychic symptoms. Simple seizures do not fit well into the generalized or partial classification.

  3. Unclassified or idiopathic seizures that occur for no known reason and account for nearly half of all seizure diagnoses

- *Status epilepticus* is a seizure that lasts longer than 10 minutes or repeated seizures over the course of 30 minutes. It is a neurologic emergency and must be treated promptly, or brain damage and possibly death from anoxia, cardiac dysrhythmias, or lactic acidosis may occur.
- Status epilepticus is usually caused by:
  1. Sudden withdrawal from anticonvulsant drugs
  2. Acute alcohol withdrawal
  3. Head trauma
  4. Cerebral edema
  5. Metabolic disturbances
- Primary seizures are not associated with any identifiable brain lesions, are usually inherited, and are often age-related.
- Secondary seizures often result from underlying brain pathology, such as a head injury, vascular disease, brain tumor, aneurysm, opportunistic infection from acquired immunodeficiency syndrome (AIDS), or meningitis. They may also occur in the presence of metabolic or electrolyte disorders, drug withdrawal,

S

acute alcohol intoxication, water intoxication, or kidney or liver failure. Seizures resulting from these disorders are not considered epilepsy.

Considerations for Older Adults

Complex partial seizures are the most common seizure disorder among older adults. Symptoms appear similar to dementia, psychosis, or Alzheimer's disease (AD), especially in the post-ictal stage (after the seizure). New-onset seizures in older adults are typically associated with conditions such as hypertension, cardiac disease, diabetes mellitus, stroke, or AD.

PATIENT-CENTERED COLLABORATIVE CARE
Assessment

- Obtain patient information about:
  1. Frequency, duration, and pattern of occurrence for seizure activity
  2. Description of pre-ictal symptoms and post-ictal activity (aura, motor activity, sequence of progression, eye signs, consciousness, respiratory patterns) and events surrounding the seizure
  3. Current drugs, including dosage, frequency of administration, and the time at which the drug was last taken
  4. Compliance with the drug schedule and reasons for non-compliance, if appropriate
- Note whether an observed seizure is new (first occurrence) or acute. Seizures occurring in greater intensity, number, or length than the patient's usual seizures are considered *acute.* They may also appear in clusters that are different from the patient's typical seizure pattern.

Interventions
Nonsurgical Management

- Administration of anti-epileptic drugs and monitoring patient response with serum levels for effectiveness. Anticipate multiple drug-drug interactions with anti-epileptic drugs and other medications.
- Care of the patient during a tonic-clonic or complete partial seizure:
  1. Protect the patient from injury.
  2. Do not force anything into the patient's mouth.
  3. Turn the patient to the side.
  4. Loosen any restrictive clothing.
  5. Maintain the airway, and suction as needed.
  6. Do not restrain the patient; rather, guide the patient's movements.

7. At the completion of the seizure:
   a. Take vital signs.
   b. Perform neurologic assessment.
   c. Allow the patient to rest.
   d. Document the seizure.
- Nursing observations and documentation of a seizure include:
   1. Onset and cessation of seizure activity: date, time, and duration
   2. Sequence and type of movement and whether more than one activity occurs
   3. Observations during the seizure:
      a. Changes in pupil size and any eye deviation
      b. Level of consciousness (LOC)
      c. Presence of apnea, cyanosis, salivation
      d. Incontinence of bowel or bladder
      e. Eye fluttering
      f. Movement and progression of motor activity
      g. Lip smacking or other automatism
      h. Tongue or lip biting
   4. How long the seizure lasted
   5. Presence and description of aura or precipitating events
   6. Post-ictal status
   7. Length of time before the patient returns to pre-seizure status
- Drug therapy is the major component of management; the health care provider introduces one anticonvulsant at a time to achieve seizure control.
- Serum drug levels are monitored for the first 3 days after the start of anticonvulsants and thereafter as needed.
- Follow agency policy for the implementation of Seizure Precautions:
   1. Keep oxygen, suctioning equipment, and an airway available at the bedside.
   2. Maintain IV access (a saline lock) for patients at risk for tonic-clonic seizures.
   3. Padded tongue blades do not belong at the bedside; nothing should be inserted into the patient's mouth after a seizure begins.
   4. Keep the bed in the low position. Use of padded siderails is controversial; siderails are rarely the source of significant injury, and the use of padded siderails may embarrass the patient and family.
- Convulsive status epilepticus is a neurologic emergency and must be treated promptly and aggressively. Notify the health care provider immediately. Immediate treatment of status epilepticus includes:
   1. Establishing an airway (intubation may be necessary)

2. Monitoring the patient's respiratory status carefully
3. Administering oxygen
4. Establishing an IV line and starting 0.9% saline infusion
5. Drawing blood for arterial blood gas analysis and identifying metabolic, toxic, and other causes of uncontrolled seizures
6. Administering drugs such as IV lorazepam (Ativan, Apo-Lorazepam ✦) or possibly diazepam (Valium) to stop motor movement, followed by phenytoin (Dilantin) or fosphenytoin (Cerebyx) to prevent recurrence. General anesthesia may be used as a last resort to stop the seizure activity.
7. Monitoring vital signs every 15 minutes or more frequently until the patient's condition stabilizes

⬛ NURSING SAFETY PRIORITY: Critical Rescue

Ensure that oxygen and suction are available at the bedside of any patient who is at risk for seizure activity. Maintaining the airway and supporting ventilation can prevent brain injury during a seizure.

Surgical Management
- Several procedures may be performed when traditional methods fail to maintain seizure control.
  1. Vagal nerve stimulation involves surgically implanting a vagal nerve-stimulating device below the left clavicle to control partial seizures.
  2. Corpus callostomy involves severing the corpus callosum to prevent neuronal discharges from passing through the two hemispheres of the brain. It is used to treat tonic-clonic or atonic seizures.
  3. Other procedures, including anterior temporal lobe resection for complex partial seizures of temporal origin, cortical resection, and removal of part or all of a cerebral hemisphere may be performed.
- Perioperative care is as outlined in Part One, with the addition of assessing neurologic status with vital signs postoperatively.

Community-Based Care
- Health teaching includes:
  1. The importance of taking all drugs consistently as prescribed and monitoring for effects and side effects. Dosage or effectiveness may change over time or with the occurrence of comorbid conditions.
  2. The importance of not taking any herbal remedies or over-the-counter (OTC) drugs without notifying the health care

provider. Anti-seizure medications have multiple and serious drug-drug and drug-herb interactions.
  3. Components of a balanced diet and the effects of alcohol (Alcohol should be avoided.)
  4. The role of rest, time management, and stress management in health promotion
  5. The utility of keeping a seizure diary to determine whether there are factors that tend to be associated with seizure activity
  6. Restrictions (if any), such as driving or operating dangerous equipment and participating in certain physical activities or sports
  7. The importance of follow-up visits with the health care provider
  8. The value of wearing a medical alert bracelet or necklace
- Inform the patient that state laws prohibit discrimination against people who have epilepsy.
- Refer the patient to the state Vocational Rehabilitative Services, Epilepsy Foundation of America, National Epilepsy League, or National Association to Control Epilepsy and to local support groups.

SEVERE ACUTE RESPIRATORY SYNDROME

OVERVIEW
- Severe acute respiratory syndrome (SARS) is an atypical pneumonia with a high mortality rate caused by a new coronavirus known as *SARS Co-V*, which is highly contagious.
- The virus infects cells of the respiratory tract, triggering an inflammatory response.
- It is easily spread by airborne droplets from infected people through sneezing, coughing, and talking and from contaminated surfaces and objects.
- People at greatest risk for SARS are those in close direct contact with an infected person. The portals of entry for infection with the virus are the mucous membranes of the eyes, nose, and mouth.

PATIENT-CENTERED COLLABORATIVE CARE
Assessment
- The manifestations of SARS are the same as those of any respiratory infection:
  1. Fever higher than 100.4° F (38° C)
  2. Headache and general body aches

3. Cold symptoms of a runny nose, sore throat, and watery eyes
4. A dry cough and dyspnea developing within 2 to 7 days
5. Late symptoms: hypoxia with cyanosis, low oxygen saturation

- Diagnosis is made by the manifestations and the use of a rapid SARS test, the reverse transcriptase-polymerase chain reaction (RT-PCR) assay that detects SARS-CoV RNA in the blood within 2 days after symptoms begin.

Interventions for Patient Care
- There is no completely effective treatment at this time.
- Interventions are supportive to allow the patient's own immune system to fight the infection:
  1. Oxygen therapy
  2. Bronchodilators
  3. Intubation and mechanical ventilation
  4. Antibiotics if bacterial pneumonia occurs with SARS

Interventions for Prevention of Infection Spread
- Isolating the person with SARS and adhering to strict Isolation Precautions are effective measures for containing the infection and preventing an epidemic:
  1. Performing frequent handwashing
  2. Using Airborne and Contact Precautions if SARS is suspected
  3. Using gowns and eye protection when coming into direct contact with the patient
  4. Ensuring that the patient wears a mask and protective clothing when he or she is out of the isolation environment (the patient can contaminate surfaces with the virus)
  5. Wearing a disposable particulate mask respirator (e.g., N-95, N-99, N-100) and protective eyewear when performing procedures that normally induce coughing or promote aerosolization of particles (e.g., suctioning, using a positive-pressure face mask, obtaining a sputum culture, giving aerosolized treatments)
  6. Keeping the door to the patient's room closed
  7. Avoiding touching your face with contaminated gloves

SHOCK

OVERVIEW
- Shock is a widespread abnormal cellular metabolism that occurs when oxygenation and tissue perfusion are not sufficient to maintain cell function.

- All body organs are affected by shock, and they work harder to adapt and compensate for reduced oxygenation or fail to function because of hypoxia.
- Shock is a syndrome, because the cellular, tissue, and organ events that occur in response to its presence happen in a predictable sequence.
- Any problem that impairs oxygen delivery to tissues and organs can start the syndrome of shock and lead to a life-threatening emergency.
- Shock is classified as one of four types, and more than one type may be present:
  1. *Hypovolemic shock* occurs when too little circulating blood volume causes a decrease in mean arterial pressure (MAP) so that the body's total need for oxygen is not met. Common problems leading to hypovolemic shock are hemorrhage (external or internal) and dehydration.
  2. *Cardiogenic shock* occurs when the heart muscle is unhealthy and pumping is impaired. Heart failure from myocardial infarction (MI) is the most common cause of cardiogenic shock.
  3. *Distributive shock* occurs when blood volume is not lost from the body but is distributed to the interstitial tissues, where it cannot circulate and deliver oxygen. It has several origins:
     a. Neural-induced distributive shock, in which a loss of MAP occurs because sympathetic nerve impulses controlling blood vessel smooth muscle decrease and the smooth muscles of blood vessels relax, causing widespread vasodilation
     b. Chemical-induced distributive shock, which occurs when certain chemicals or foreign substances within the blood and blood vessels initiate widespread changes in blood vessel walls. Common conditions leading to this type of shock include:
        (1) Anaphylaxis after exposure to a specific allergen in a susceptible person, which results in widespread loss of blood vessel tone and decreased cardiac output
        (2) Sepsis resulting from widespread infection, which triggers a whole-body inflammatory response when pathologic microorganisms are present in the blood (also called *septic shock*)
        (3) Capillary leak syndrome, which is the response of capillaries to the presence of biologic chemicals (mediators) that change blood vessel integrity and allow fluid to leak from the blood in the vascular space into the interstitial tissues. Once in the interstitial tissue, these fluids are stagnant and not able

to deliver oxygen or remove tissue waste products. Problems causing fluid shifts include severe burns, liver disorders, ascites, peritonitis, paralytic ileus, severe malnutrition, large wounds, hyperglycemia, kidney disease, hypoproteinemia, and trauma.

4. *Obstructive shock* occurs when the normal heart muscle is prevented from pumping effectively. The heart itself remains normal, but conditions outside the heart prevent adequate filling of the heart or adequate contraction of the healthy heart muscle. Common causes of obstructive shock are pericarditis and cardiac tamponade.

- Although the causes and initial manifestations associated with the different types of shock vary, eventually the effects of hypotension and anaerobic cellular metabolism result in the common key features:
  1. Cardiovascular manifestations:
     a. Decreased cardiac output
     b. Pulse rate increased, quality decreased
     c. Decreased systolic blood pressure
     d. Narrowed pulse pressure
     e. Postural hypotension
     f. Flat neck and hand veins in dependent positions
     g. Slow capillary refill in nail beds
     h. Diminished peripheral pulses
  2. Respiratory manifestations:
     a. Increased respiratory rate
     b. Shallow depth of respirations
     c. Increased $Paco_2$; decreased Pao_2
     d. Cyanosis, especially around lips and nail beds
  3. Neuromuscular manifestations:
     a. Early:
        (1) Anxiety and restlessness
        (2) Increased thirst
     b. Late:
        (1) Lethargy to coma
        (2) Generalized muscle weakness
        (3) Diminished or absent deep tendon reflexes
        (4) Sluggish pupillary response to light
  4. Kidney manifestations:
     a. Decreased urine output
     b. Increased specific gravity
  5. Skin and mucous membrane manifestations:
     a. Cool to cold
     b. Pale to mottled to cyanotic
     c. Moist, clammy

- Hypovolemic shock:
  1. The basic problem of hypovolemic shock is a loss of blood volume from the vascular space, which results in a decreased MAP and decreased oxygen-carrying capacity from the loss of circulating red blood cells (RBCs).
  2. These problems decrease tissue perfusion and oxygenation, leading to anaerobic cellular metabolism.
  3. The most common problems leading to hypovolemic shock are hemorrhage (external or internal) and dehydration.
  4. Uncorrected hypovolemic shock progresses in four stages as poor cellular oxygenation continues:
     a. *Initial stage of shock (early shock)* occurs when the patient's baseline MAP is decreased by less than 10 mm Hg. Adaptive (compensatory) mechanisms are effective at returning MAP to normal levels, and oxygenated blood flow to all vital organs is maintained. Heart and respiratory rates are increased from the patient's baseline level, or a slight increase in diastolic blood pressure may be the only objective manifestation.
     b. *Nonprogressive stage (compensatory stage)* occurs when MAP decreases by 10 to 15 mm Hg from baseline. Kidney and hormonal adaptive (compensatory) mechanisms are activated, because cardiovascular adjustments alone are not enough to maintain MAP and supply needed oxygen to the vital organs. Tissue hypoxia occurs in the skin, GI tract, and kidney but is not great enough to cause permanent damage. The cellular effects of this stage are reversible if the problem is recognized and appropriate interventions are started.
     c. *Progressive stage of shock (intermediate stage)* occurs when there is a sustained decrease in MAP of more than 20 mm Hg from baseline. Adaptive (compensatory) mechanisms are functioning but can no longer deliver sufficient oxygen, even to vital organs. As a result of poor oxygenation and a buildup of toxic metabolites, some tissues have severe cell damage and die.
     d. *Refractory stage of shock (irreversible stage)* occurs when too much cell death and tissue damage results from too little oxygen reaching the tissues. Vital organs have overwhelming damage, the body can no longer respond effectively to interventions, and shock continues. Widespread release of toxic metabolites and destructive enzymes causes cell damage in vital organs to continue despite aggressive interventions, and multiple organ dysfunction syndrome (MODS) leads to death.

PATIENT-CENTERED COLLABORATIVE CARE
Assessment
- Obtain patient information about:
  1. Recent illness, trauma, procedures, or chronic health problems:
     a. GI ulcers
     b. General surgery
     c. Hemophilia
     d. Liver disorders
     e. Prolonged vomiting or diarrhea
  2. Drug use, especially aspirin, diuretics, and antacids
  3. Fluid intake and output during the previous 24 hours
- Assess for and document:
  1. Bleeding of gums, wounds, and sites of dressings, drains, and vascular accesses
  2. Swelling or skin discoloration that may indicate an internal hemorrhage
  3. Cardiovascular changes:
     a. Increased heart rate and decreased pulse quality
     b. Decreased peripheral pulses

▮NURSING SAFETY PRIORITY: Action Alert
Changes in systolic blood pressure are not always present in the initial stage of shock and should not be used as the main indicator of shock presence or progression.

     c. Trends of decreasing systolic pressure and narrowing pulse pressure
     d. Decreasing oxygen saturation
  4. Respiratory changes:
     a. Increased rate
     b. Decreased depth
  5. Kidney and urinary changes:
     a. Decreased urine output
     b. Increased urine specific gravity
  6. Skin changes:
     a. Cool temperature
     b. Pallor or cyanosis, especially oral mucous membranes
     c. Clammy or moist skin
     d. Slow or sluggish capillary refill
  7. Central nervous system (CNS) changes:
     a. Thirst
     b. Decreasing alertness and level of consciousness (LOC)
  8. Psychosocial changes:
     a. Restlessness and sense of "impending doom"

    b. Decreasing orientation
    c. Decreased cognition
 9. Laboratory changes:
    a. Decreased hematocrit and hemoglobin levels if shock is caused by hemorrhage
    b. Increased hematocrit and hemoglobin levels if shock is caused by dehydration or a fluid shift

Interventions

Nonsurgical Management

- Oxygen therapy is useful whenever shock is present. It can be delivered by mask, hood, nasal cannula, nasopharyngeal tube, endotracheal tube, or tracheostomy tube.
- IV therapy (fluid resuscitation) is initiated as prescribed.
  1. Crystalloid solutions contain nonprotein substances and include normal saline and Ringer's lactate.

■ NURSING SAFETY PRIORITY: Drug Alert

Do not infuse Ringer's lactate with blood or blood products, because the calcium induces clotting of the infusing blood.

S

  2. Colloid solutions contain large molecules (usually proteins or starches) to help restore osmotic pressure and fluid volume. These fluids include whole blood, packed RBCs, plasma, plasma fractions, and synthetic plasma expanders.
  3. Drug therapy is initiated as prescribed when the volume deficit is severe and the patient does not respond sufficiently to the replacement of fluid volume and blood products:
     a. Vasoconstricting agents:
        (1) Dopamine (Intropin, Revimine ♣)
        (2) Norepinephrine (Levophed)
     b. Inotropic agents
        (1) Dobutamine (Dobutrex)
        (2) Milrinone (Primacor)
     c. Drugs that enhance myocardial perfusion, such as sodium nitroprusside (Nitropress, Nipride ♣)
- Additional nursing interventions include assessing the patient's response to therapy.
  1. Monitor every 30 to 60 minutes until shock is controlled:
     a. Pulse pressure and mean MAP
     b. Skin and mucosal color
     c. Urine output
     d. LOC
     e. Vital signs, including heart rate, blood pressure, respiratory rate, and peripheral oxygenation (SpO_2)

Surgical Management

- After a cause has been established, surgical intervention may be needed to correct the cause of shock. Such procedures include vascular repair or revision, surgical hemostasis of major wounds, closure of bleeding ulcers, and chemical scarring (chemosclerosis) of varicosities.
- Sepsis and septic shock are a complex type of distributive shock that usually begins as a bacterial or fungal infection and progresses to a dangerous condition over a period of days.

INFECTION

- When infection is confined to a local area, it does not lead to sepsis and shock. The invasion first sets off a helpful, nonspecific series of local responses to confine and eliminate the organism and to prevent the infection from becoming worse or widespread.
- The white blood cells (WBCs) in the area of invasion secrete cytokines to trigger a local inflammatory response and bring more phagocytic WBCs to the area to fight and kill the invading organisms. The results of this local response constrict the small veins and dilate the arterioles in the area of injury. These blood vessel changes cause redness and warmth of the locally infected tissues and increase blood flow to the area to deliver more nutrients.
- Blood flow to the area increases, and edema forms at the site of injury or invasion. Capillary leak also occurs, allowing blood plasma to leak into the tissues. This response causes swelling and pain. The duration of these responses depends on the size and severity of the infection, but usually they subside within a few days, when the infection has been managed by these responses.
- An important feature of the benefit of these responses is that they are limited only to the area of infection and stop as soon as they are no longer needed. The patient does not have fever, tachycardia, decreased oxygen saturation, or reduced urine output.

Sepsis and SIRS

- Sepsis is a widespread infection coupled with a more general inflammatory response, known as *systemic inflammatory response syndrome (SIRS)*, which is triggered when an infection escapes local control.
- With the organisms and their toxins or endotoxins in the bloodstream and entering other body areas, the inflammatory responses become an enemy, leading to extensive tissue and vascular changes that further impair oxygenation and tissue perfusion.

- The WBCs are producing many pro-inflammatory cytokines, leading to widespread vasodilation and pooling of blood in some tissues.
- The patient has a low-grade fever, mild hypotension, a urine output that is lower than expected for fluid intake, and an increased respiratory rate. These actions result in a hypodynamic state with decreased cardiac output.
- Microthrombi begin to form within the capillaries of some organs, causing some cell hypoxia and reducing organ function. The microthrombi increase the number of cells that are operating under anaerobic conditions, which results in the generation of more toxic metabolites. These cause more cell damage and increase the production of pro-inflammatory cytokines, intensifying or amplifying the SIRS and leading to a vicious repeating cycle of poor oxygenation and tissue perfusion.
- These subtle manifestations indicate early sepsis and usually progress unless intervention occurs at this time:
  1. If early sepsis is identified and treated aggressively, the cycle of progression is stopped and the outcome is good.
  2. If early sepsis is not identified and treated at this stage, it almost always progresses to severe sepsis, which is much harder to control.

Severe Sepsis

- Severe sepsis is the progression of sepsis with an amplified inflammatory response. All tissues are involved, and all have some degree of hypoxia.
- Microthrombi formation is widespread and consumes much of the available platelets and clotting factors, a condition known as *disseminated intravascular coagulation (DIC)*.
- The amplified SIRS and cytokine release increase capillary leakiness, injure cells (especially endothelial cells of blood vessels), and increase cell metabolism.
- Damage to endothelial cells reduces anticlotting actions and triggers the formation of even more small clots, allowing anaerobic metabolism to continue.
- The continued stress response triggers continued release of glucose from the liver, causing hyperglycemia. The more severe the response, the higher the blood glucose level.
- At this time, cardiac function is hyperdynamic, because the pooling of blood and widespread capillary leak stimulate the heart. Heart rate is rapid, and systolic blood pressure is elevated. The patient's extremities may feel warm, and there is little or no cyanosis.

S

- Additional manifestations at this stage are lower oxygen saturation, rapid respiratory rate, decreased to absent urine output, and a change in the patient's cognition and affect.
  Septic Shock
- Septic shock is the stage of sepsis and SIRS in which multiple organ failure is evident and uncontrolled bleeding occurs. *Even with appropriate intervention, the death rate is very high.*
- Severe hypovolemic shock is present with hypodynamic cardiac function. The clinical manifestations resemble the late stage of hypovolemic shock.
  Interventions to Prevent Sepsis and Septic Shock
- Evaluate all patients for their risk for sepsis.
- Use aseptic technique during invasive procedures and when working with nonintact skin and mucous membranes in immunocompromised patients.
- Remove indwelling urinary catheters and IV access lines as soon as they are no longer needed.
- Assess vital signs often (at least twice per shift) for changes from baseline levels.
- Review laboratory data for changes in serum lactate levels, in total WBC count, and in the differential. The hallmark of sepsis is a left shift, an increasing serum lactate level, a normal or low total WBC count, and a decreasing segmented neutrophil level with a rising band neutrophil level.
- Assess other laboratory indicators of sepsis and septic shock, especially a low blood level of activated protein C, rising plasma D-dimer levels, rising interleukin-6 (IL-6), and normal or decreasing levels of IL-10.
  Management of Sepsis and Septic Shock
- The health care team implements the Sepsis Resuscitation Bundle:
  1. Measuring serum lactate levels
  2. Obtaining blood cultures before administering antibiotics unless this intervention delays antibiotic administration
  3. Administering broad-spectrum antibiotic therapy within 1 to 3 hours of suspected diagnosis
  4. If hypotension or a serum lactate level greater than 4 mmol/L (36 mg/dL) is present:
     a. Institute IV delivery of 20 mL/kg of crystalloid fluids (or the colloid equivalent).
     b. If hypotension does not respond to initial fluid resuscitation by increasing MAP to at least 65 mm Hg, start IV vasopressor therapy.
  5. If hypotension persists despite fluid resuscitation and vasopressor therapy, and septic shock is present or the serum

lactate level remains greater than 4 mmol/L (36 mg/dL), use the following parameters to monitor therapy effectiveness:

    a. Central venous pressure (CVP) of at least 8 mm Hg

    b. Central venous oxygen saturation ($Scvo_2$) of at least 70% or a mixed venous oxygen saturation (Svo_2) of at least 65%

6. Obtain procalcitonin (PCT) serum level. PCT shows a rapid elevation at early stages of bloodstream infection and decreases nearly as rapidly as bloodstream infections clear

- The health care team implements the Sepsis Management Bundle:

    1. When septic shock is present, administer low-dose steroids (200 to 300 mg hydrocortisone IV daily in divided doses) in accordance with intensive care unit (ICU) protocol.

    2. Administer drotrecogin alfa (activated) for patients meeting ICU and drotrecogin criteria.

    3. Administer insulin to maintain blood glucose levels at least lower than 150 mg/dL.

    4. Use mechanical ventilation to maintain inspiratory plateau pressures less than 30 cm H_2O to prevent lung injury.

- Blood replacement therapy is used when septic shock progresses to hemorrhage:

    1. Clotting factors (cryoprecipitate)

    2. Fresh-frozen plasma (FFP)

    3. Whole blood

    4. Packed RBCs

S

SICKLE CELL DISEASE AND TRAIT

OVERVIEW

- Sickle cell disease (SCD), which used to be called *sickle cell anemia,* is a genetic disorder that results in chronic anemia, pain, disability, organ damage, increased risk for infection, and early death.
- In SCD, inheritance of two alleles (autosomal recessive trait) results in at least 40% (and often much more) of the total hemoglobin composed of abnormal beta chains, known as *hemoglobin S (HbS).*
- In *sickle cell trait,* one normal gene allele and one abnormal gene allele for hemoglobin are inherited, so that only half of the hemoglobin chains produced are abnormal
- When red blood cells (RBCs) having large amounts of HbS are exposed to decreased oxygen conditions, the abnormal beta chains contract and pile together within the cell, distorting the shape of the RBC, resulting in a sickle-shaped RBC. The

distorted RBC is rigid and becomes "sticky" and fragile, forming a clump that blocks blood flow.

- Episodes of vascular occlusion from clumped, sickled RBCs causes ischemia, leading to potential organ damage from anoxia and infarction. Episodes of severe sickling are called *crisis.*
- Conditions that cause sickling include hypoxia, dehydration, infections, venous stasis, pregnancy, alcohol consumption, high altitudes, low environmental or body temperatures, acidosis, strenuous exercise, and anesthesia.

PATIENT-CENTERED COLLABORATIVE CARE
Assessment
- Family history
- Previous crises, what led to the crises, severity, and usual treatments
- Onset of pain, and events leading to current symptoms
- Potential organ damage (e.g., chronic kidney disease or acute kidney injury, heart failure, lung damage, cirrhosis/liver damage, joint swelling, bone necrosis muscle damage, and open sores from poor skin perfusion and stroke or seizure) from occlusive events

Interventions
- Evaluate presence of HbS in a newly diagnosed patient.
- Manage pain from ischemia; severe pain can cause/prolong crisis. Opioids are used during crisis.
- Administer hydroxyurea (Droxia) to reduce sickling episodes and pain.
- Provide hydration by the oral or IV route to reduce the duration of pain episodes.
- Use oxygen therapy and optimize perfusion to prevent or minimize multi-organ dysfunction as a result of occlusion and ischemia during sickling episodes.
- Reduce risk for infection, because splanchnic injury can result in immunocompromise; consider reverse isolation precautions during crisis. Monitor vital signs, temperature, and other symptoms of infection regularly to detect early signs of sepsis and avoid septic shock.

SJÖGREN'S SYNDROME

- Sjögren's syndrome (SS) is a group of problems that often appear with other autoimmune disorders, typically rheumatoid arthritis or fibromyalgia. Inflammation and autoimmune responses obstruct certain secretory ducts and glands.

- Problems include dry eyes (sicca syndrome), dry mucous membranes of the nose and mouth (xerostomia), and vaginal dryness.
  1. Insufficient tears cause inflammation and ulceration of the cornea. Other manifestations include blurred vision, burning and itching of the eyes, and thick mattering in the conjunctiva.
  2. Insufficient saliva decreases digestion of carbohydrates, promotes tooth decay, and increases the incidence of oral and nasal infections. Difficulty swallowing food, changes in taste sensation, nosebleeds, and frequent upper respiratory infections may also occur.
  3. Vaginal dryness increases the incidence of infection and may cause pain during sexual intercourse.
- There is no cure, and management focuses on slowing the intensity and the progression of the disorder by suppressing immune and inflammatory responses.
- Drug therapy may include:
  1. Immunomodulators (e.g., methotrexate [Rheumatrex]; cyclophosphamide [Cytoxan]; cyclosporine [Neoral, Sandimmune])
  2. Corticosteroids
  3. Hydroxychloroquine (Plaquenil)
- Dry eye and dry mouth symptoms may be managed with a variety of artificial tears and artificial saliva.
- Use of water-soluble vaginal lubricants and moisturizers can increase patient comfort and reduce the incidence of vaginitis.
- Use humidifiers/humidified air or oxygen to decrease airway dryness.

SKIN INFECTIONS

OVERVIEW

- Skin infections can be bacterial, viral, or fungal, but most are bacterial, caused by *Staphylococcus* or *Streptococcus* microorganisms.
- *Folliculitis* is a superficial infection involving only the upper portion of the follicle. It usually manifests as a raised, red rash with small pustules.
- *Furuncles* (boils) are deeper follicle infections with a large, sore-looking, raised bump that may or may not have a pustular "head" at its point.
- *Cellulitis* is a generalized infection and involves the deeper connective tissue.
- The major cause of bacterial skin infection is minor skin trauma.

- An increasingly common skin problem is infection with methicillin-resistant *Staphylococcus aureus* (MRSA). This highly contagious specific infection is described elsewhere (see *Methicillin-Resistant* Staphylococcus aureus).
- Viral skin infections are commonly caused by the herpes simplex virus (HSV) and include type I infections (common cold sore), type II infections (genital herpes), and herpes zoster (shingles) (see *Herpes, Genital*). Viral infections differ from bacterial infections in two ways:
  1. After the first infection, the virus remains in the body in a dormant state in the nerve ganglia, and the patient has no symptoms.
  2. Reactivation stimulates the virus to travel the pathways of sensory nerves to the skin, where lesions reappear.
- Many fungal infections also affect the skin:
  1. Superficial dermatophyte infections include:
     a. Tinea pedis ("athlete's foot")
     b. Tinea manus (hands)
     c. Tinea cruris (groin, "jock itch")
     d. Tinea capitis (head)
     e. Tinea corporis (ringworm)
  2. *Candida albicans*, also known as yeast *infection*, is another common superficial fungal infection of skin and mucous membranes:
     a. Risk factors include immunosuppression, long-term antibiotic therapy, diabetes mellitus, and obesity.
     b. The incidence is higher in hot, humid climates.
     c. Infected skin (most often of the mouth, perineum, vagina, axillae, and under the breasts) has a moist, red, irritated appearance, usually with itching and burning.
- Prevention of skin infections, especially bacterial and fungal infections, involves avoiding the offending organism and good personal hygiene to remove the organism before infection can occur.

⬛ NURSING SAFETY PRIORITY: Critical Rescue

Handwashing and not sharing personal items with others are the best ways to avoid contact with some of the most easily transmitted organisms, including MRSA.

PATIENT-CENTERED COLLABORATIVE CARE
Assessment

- Obtain patient information about:
  1. Recent history of skin trauma
  2. Past or current staphylococcal or streptococcal infections

3. Living conditions, home sanitation, personal hygiene habits, and leisure or sport activities
4. Whether fever and malaise are also present
5. Lesions locations, especially lips, mouth, or genital region
6. History of similar lesions in the same location
7. Presence of burning, tingling, or pain
8. Recent stress factors
9. Recent contact with an infected person
10. Whether the patient has had ever chickenpox or shingles
11. Whether the patient has received the shingles prevention vaccine, Zostavax
12. Social and environmental factors:
    a. Direct contact with an infected person
    b. Personal hygiene practices
    c. Frequent contact with animals
    d. Type and frequency of athletic activities

- Assess for and document the condition of the skin, including local or general:
1. Redness
2. Warmth
3. Edema
4. Tenderness
5. Pain
6. Itching
7. Stinging
8. Location of areas of inflammation, rash, or infection
9. Presence of:
    a. Blisters or vesicles
    b. Pustules
    c. Papules
    d. Scaling
    e. Single or multiple lesions

Interventions

- Most skin infections heal well with nonsurgical management, but surgery may be required if an infectious agent is present in deep tissue layers.
- Nursing interventions include:
1. Skin care instructions:
    a. Bathing daily with an antibacterial soap. Chlorhexidine showers or dilute bleach baths can reduce bacterial load, especially in the presence of MRSA.
    b. Not squeezing any pustules or crusts but removing them gently
    c. Applying warm compresses twice a day to furuncles or areas of cellulitis

    d. Avoiding constricting garments that might rub the lesions
    e. Keeping the skin dry between treatments
    f. Positioning for optimal air circulation to the area
  2. Prevention of transmission:
    a. Using handwashing and antimicrobial hand solutions to prevent cross-contamination
    b. Isolating the patient if infections are colonized with *Staphylococcus* that is resistant to antibiotic therapy
    c. Teaching patients to avoid sharing personal items such as hairbrushes, articles of clothing, or footwear
    d. Teaching patients to avoid sexual contact when recurrent herpes lesions are present

- Drug therapy includes:
  1. Topical agents for superficial infections and mild bacterial infections
  2. Systemic antibiotic therapy for extensive infections, especially if fever or lymphadenopathy is present
     a. Antiviral agents such as acyclovir (Zovirax), valacyclovir (Valtrex), or famciclovir (Famvir)
     b. Antifungal agents such as ketoconazole (Nizoral)

SPINAL CORD INJURY

OVERVIEW

- An injury to the vertebral column and spinal cord may be caused by motor vehicle accidents, falls, sports such as diving and football, and penetrating trauma from violence.
- As a result of spinal cord injury (SCI), losses of or decreases in motor function, sensation, reflex activity, and bowel and bladder function may occur.
- The extent of the injury can be classified as:
  1. *Complete* if the spinal cord is severed or damaged in a way that eliminates all innervation below the level of injury, and total motor and sensory loss occurs
  2. *Incomplete* (more common) if there is preservation of a mixed pattern of motor, sensory, and reflex function
- Cervical SCIs may result in specific syndromes:
  1. Anterior cord injury is characterized by loss of motor function, pain, and temperature sensation below the level of the injury; sensations of touch, position, and vibration remain intact.
  2. Posterior cord injury is characterized by intact motor function and loss of vibratory sense, crude touch, and position sense.

3. Central cord injury is characterized by loss of motor function that is more pronounced in the upper extremities than in the lower extremities.
- Complications of SCI include pressure ulcers, contractures, and deep vein thrombosis (DVT) or pulmonary emboli. Muscle spasticity and bone loss can occur over time.

PATIENT-CENTERED COLLABORATIVE CARE
Assessment
- Obtain information about:
  1. How the injury occurred and the probable mechanism of injury
  2. Position immediately after the injury
  3. Symptoms that occurred after the injury and what changes have occurred since
  4. Prehospital rescue personnel are questioned about:
     a. Problems encountered during the extrication and transport
     b. Type of immobilization devices used
     c. Medical treatment given at the scene
  5. Medical history, with particular attention to a history of arthritis of the spine, congenital deformities, osteoarthritis or osteomyelitis, cancer, previous back or spinal cord injury, and respiratory problems
- Assess for and document:
  1. Adequacy of airway, breathing, and circulation
  2. Vital signs and indication of hemorrhage or bleeding around the fracture sites or in the abdomen
  3. Indications of a head injury, such as a change in level of consciousness (LOC), abnormal pupil size and reaction to light, and change in behavior or ability to respond to directions
  4. Spinal shock is characterized by complete, but temporary loss, of motor, sensory, reflex, and autonomic function that often lasts less than 48 hours but may continue for several weeks:
     a. Evaluate motor strength, comparing bilateral movement; the ability to shrug the shoulders, flex and extend the arms, elevate the arms and legs off the bed, extend the wrist, wiggle the toes, and flex and extend the feet and legs; and deep tendon reflexes.
     b. Evaluate sensation, comparing bilaterally and documenting decreased or absent tactile sensation.
     c. Evaluate cardiovascular dysfunction, such as bradycardia, hypotension, and cardiac dysrhythmias.

S

5. Change in thermoregulatory capacity, with the patient's body tending to assume the temperature of the environment (hypothermia)

6. Evaluate breathing problems resulting from an interruption of spinal innervation to the respiratory muscles, assessing for atelectasis and/or pneumonia symptoms. *Patients with injuries at or above T6 are especially at risk for respiratory complications and pulmonary embolus during the first 5 days after injury.*

7. Evaluate the patient's abdomen for manifestations of internal bleeding, distention, or paralytic ileus. Paralytic ileus is manifested by decreased or absent bowel sounds and distended abdomen, usually 72 hours or longer after injury.

8. Autonomic dysfunction initially causes an areflexic (neurogenic) bladder (no reflex ability for bladder contraction), which later leads to urinary retention. The patient is at risk for urinary tract infection from an indwelling urinary catheter; intermittent catheterizations; or bladder distention, stasis, and/or overflow.

9. Coping strategies used in the past to deal with illness, difficult situations, or disappointments; initial hospitalization after SCI lasts for 3 or more months to include rehabilitation.

Planning and Implementation

- The patient may have difficulty breathing related to upper motor neuron injury.
- Monitor airway and breathing closely. Document effort, SpO_2 and secretions.
- Maintain suction at the bedside.
- Use a cough assist technique with cervical injury.
- Implement incentive spirometry.

⊟ NURSING SAFETY PRIORITY: Critical Rescue

Assess breath sounds every 2 to 4 hours during the first few days after injury, and document and report any adventitious or diminished sounds. Monitor vital signs carefully, and watch for changes in respiratory pattern, effort and secretions. Note also tachycardia, bradycardia, and changes in level of consciousness with respiratory evaluation.

- Potential for neurogenic shock is related to loss of interruption of sympathetic innervation in patients with SCIs above T6:
  1. Maintain adequate hydration with IV and oral fluids.
  2. Relate vital signs to patient condition.

⬛ NURSING SAFETY PRIORITY: Critical Rescue

Monitor the patient at least hourly for:

- Severe bradycardia
- Warm, dry skin
- Severe hypotension

Notify the physician immediately if these symptoms occur, because this problem is an emergency! Neurogenic shock is treated symptomatically by restoring fluids to the circulating blood volume and providing supportive care to stabilize the patient.

- There is a potential for further spinal cord injury related to swelling and/or fractures:
  1. Immobilize the fracture to prevent further damage to the spinal cord from bone fragments. Skeletal traction (e.g., halo fixator) may be used.
  2. Log roll the patient to avoid an inbed position that bends the spine. Use reverse Trendelenburg position to elevate the head rather than pillows or backrest elevation.
  3. Anticipate surgery to reduce or repair vertebral fractures.
- The patient may experience Impaired Physical Mobility and/or Self-Care Deficit (the level depends on the extent and level of the injury) related to decreased or absent muscle control:
  1. The patient with an SCI is especially at risk for pressure ulcers, contractures, venous thromboembolism (deep vein thrombosis and/or pulmonary embolus), and fractures related to osteoporosis. Patients with high SCIs are also at risk for orthostatic hypotension.
  2. Provide safe, effective positioning and repositioning
  3. Use pressure-relieving devices, implementing pressure ulcer prevention strategies at all times.
  4. Assist with slow transitions to upright posture, especially after a period of supine positioning.
- The patient may have spastic or flaccid bladder and bowel related to direct neurologic damage or disruption in nerve impulses.
- The type of bladder emptying program depends on the usual elimination pattern and whether the injury involved upper motor neurons (UMNs) or lower motor neurons (LMNs).
- Use a bedside bladder ultrasound device to measure bladder residual and determine effectiveness of bladder-emptying strategies.
- Teach the patient that the essential elements of a bowel program include stool softeners, increased fluid intake (unless medically contraindicated), high-fiber diet, and a consistent time for elimination.

S

- Evaluate for urinary tract infection (UTI), particularly foul-smelling urine; the SCI patient may not develop flank pain, urgency, frequency, or other signs of UTI.

◼ NURSING SAFETY PRIORITY: Critical Rescue

Observe the patient with an upper SCI (above the level of T6) for signs of autonomic dysreflexia (hyperreflexia). Although it does not occur often, autonomic dysreflexia is an excessive, uncontrolled sympathetic output. It is characterized by severe hypertension, bradycardia, severe headache, nasal stuffiness, and flushing. The cause of this syndrome is a noxious stimulus, usually a distended bladder or constipation. *This is a neurologic emergency and must be promptly treated to prevent a hypertensive stroke.*

- Treatment of autonomic dysreflexia includes:
  1. Raising the head of the bed to a high Fowler's position
  2. Loosening tight clothing
  3. Checking the Foley catheter tubing (if present) for kinks or obstruction
  4. If a Foley catheter is not in place, checking for bladder distention and catheterizing immediately
  5. Checking the patient for fecal impaction and, if present, disimpacting immediately using anesthetic ointment
  6. Checking the room temperature to ensure that it is not too cool or drafty
  7. Monitoring blood pressure every 15 minutes; hypertension may be treated with nitrates or hydralazine
- The patient may experience impaired adjustment related to disability requiring need for life change:
  1. Help to set and reinforce realistic goals for managing self-care while promoting independence and decision making daily.
  2. Provide opportunities for emotional and spiritual support.
  3. Collaborate with the case manager or discharge planner for a review of the patient's insurance and financial status.
- Drug therapy during the acute phase may include:
  1. Methylprednisolone (Solu-Medrol) may be given after the initial injury in a very high loading dose and then as a continuous drip for 24 hours.
  2. IV fluids and vasopressors may be used to maintain perfusion to the spinal cord, typically to maintain a mean arterial pressure (MAP) >70 mm Hg.
  3. Atropine sulfate is used to treat bradycardia with neurogenic shock.

- Drug therapy for chronic SCI may include treatments to manage the effects of prolonged immobility and denervation of the motor system:
  1. Dantrolene (Dantrium) or baclofen (Lioresal) to treat spasticity
  2. Drugs to prevent osteoporosis and abnormal bony overgrowth
  3. Drugs to prevent venothromboembolism (VTE)
  4. Drugs to promote regular bowel evacuation

Community-Based Care

- Discharge planning: most patients are discharged to a rehabilitation setting, where they learn more about self-care, mobility skills, and bladder and bowel retraining:
  1. Psychosocial adaptation is a crucial factor in determining the success of rehabilitation:
     a. Assist the patient to verbalize feelings and fears about body image, self-concept, role performance, and self-esteem.
     b. Talk to the patient about the expected reactions of those outside the hospital environment.
- To prepare for discharge to home or for a weekend home visit:
  1. Collaborate with the patient, family, case manager, and rehabilitation professionals to assess the home environment to ensure that it is free from hazards and can accommodate the patient's special needs.
  2. Ensure that the patient can correctly use all adaptive devices ordered for home use.
  3. Ensure that adaptive equipment is installed in the home before discharge.
- Teach the patient and family, in collaboration with other health care team members:
  1. ADL skills
  2. Bowel and bladder program
  3. Drug regimen
  4. Pressure ulcer prevention strategies
  5. Sexual functioning
  6. Mobility skills
- Refer the patient to local, state, and national support groups.

STENOSIS, AORTIC

OVERVIEW

- The most common cause of aortic stenosis (AS) is age ("wear and tear").
- In AS, the aortic valve orifice narrows, obstructing left ventricular outflow during systole. As afterload increases, the left ventricle hypertrophies.

- As stenosis progresses, cardiac output becomes fixed and unable to meet the demands of the body during exertion and symptoms develop.
- Over time, left ventricular failure (heart failure [HF]) develops, volume backs up in the left atrium, and the pulmonary system becomes congested. Right-sided HF can occur late in the disease.

Considerations for Older Adults

Atherosclerosis and degenerative calcification of the aortic valve are the predominant causative factors in people older than 70 years. Aortic stenosis has become the most common valvular disorder in countries with an aging population.

PATIENT-CENTERED COLLABORATIVE CARE

- Assess for and document:
  1. Dyspnea, angina, and syncope on exertion
  2. Systolic crescendo-decrescendo murmur
  3. Signs of left heart failure: fatigue and pulmonary edema
- Aortic valve surgery is the treatment of choice when the patient is symptomatic with AS:
  1. Balloon valvuloplasty may be performed to repair the valve. A balloon catheter is inserted through the femoral artery and advanced to the aortic valve, where the balloon is inflated, enlarging the orifice of the valve.
  2. In aortic valve replacement surgery, the valve is excised during cardiopulmonary bypass surgery and then replaced with a prosthetic (synthetic) or biologic (tissue) valve.
- The postoperative patient requires lifetime anticoagulation therapy to prevent thrombus formation on the valve.
- For preoperative and postoperative care, see *Perioperative Care* (Part One) and *Surgical Management* under *Coronary Artery Disease*.

STENOSIS, MITRAL

OVERVIEW

- Mitral stenosis is most commonly caused by rheumatic carditis and congenital cardiac anomalies.
- Valve leaflets fuse together, becoming stiff; the chordae tendineae contract and shorten; the valve opening narrows, preventing normal blood flow from the left atrium to the left ventricle; and as a result, the left atrial pressure rises, the left ventricle dilates, pulmonary artery pressures increase, and the right ventricle hypertrophies.

- Pulmonary congestion and right-sided heart failure occur; later, preload is decreased and cardiac output declines.

PATIENT-CENTERED COLLABORATIVE CARE
Assessment
- Assess for and document:
  1. Changes in respiratory patterns: orthopnea, dyspnea with exertion, paroxysmal nocturnal dyspnea, cough
  2. Symptoms of right ventricular failure: hepatomegaly, neck vein distention, peripheral pitting edema that occur initially in disease progression
  3. Symptoms of left ventricular failure: pulmonary edema, S_3 heart sound, crackles in lungs, frothy sputum that occur later in disease progression
  4. Atrial fibrillation resulting from right atrial hypertrophy
  5. Rumbling, apical diastolic murmur
  6. A history of rheumatic fever

Interventions
- Mitral valve repair or replacement surgery is the treatment of choice for symptomatic mitral valve stenosis:
  1. Balloon valvuloplasty, an invasive nonsurgical procedure, involves passing a balloon catheter from the femoral vein, through the atrial septum, to the mitral valve. The balloon is inflated to enlarge the mitral orifice.
  2. Mitral commissurotomy is performed during cardiopulmonary bypass surgery. The surgeon removes thrombi from the atria, incises the fused commissures (leaflets), and débrides calcium from the leaflets, thus widening the orifice.
  3. Mitral valve replacement is indicated if the leaflets are calcified and immobile. The valve is excised during cardiopulmonary bypass surgery, and a new valve is sutured into place.
- The postoperative patient requires lifetime anticoagulant therapy to prevent the formation of a thrombus on the valve.
- Perioperative care:
  1. For care of the patient undergoing coronary artery bypass grafting, see *Coronary Artery Disease.*
  2. After the procedure, observe the patient for bleeding from the catheter insertion site and institute postangiography precautions.
  3. Observe for signs of a regurgitant valve by closely monitoring for change in quality of a murmuring heart sound, cardiac output, and heart rhythm.

    4. Observe for signs of vascular occlusion (reduced peripheral pulses, stroke, and acute coronary syndrome) from emboli while establishing anticoagulation therapy.

Community-Based Care

- Provide health teaching information regarding:
  1. Drugs, especially anticoagulant therapy
  2. Plan of work, activity, and rest to conserve energy
  3. The potential need for an antibiotic before invasive procedures (e.g., dental work, surgery)
- Refer the patient to community resources, such as the American Heart Association.

🔲 NURSING SAFETY PRIORITY: Drug Alert

Heparin and warfarin (Coumadin) are two drugs commonly associated with significant errors in the hospital setting. Be especially vigilant in verifying the correct patient, dosage, route, time of administration, and drug (including concentration) when giving these powerful drugs.

STENOSIS, RENAL ARTERY

- Renal artery stenosis involves pathologic processes affecting the renal arteries that result in severe narrowing of the lumen and reduced blood flow to the kidney tissues.
- Uncorrected stenosis leads to ischemia and atrophy of kidneys.
- Renal artery stenosis is suspected when a sudden onset of hypertension occurs. Reduced renal blood flow from stenosis results in neurohormonal changes (such as activation of the renin-angiotensin-aldosterone system) that elevate blood pressure in a compensatory response to improve renal blood flow.
- Pathology may be fibrotic, atherosclerotic, or both. Fibromuscular changes of the vessel wall occur throughout the length of the renal artery from the aortic junction to the point of branching into the renal segmental arteries. Atherosclerotic changes in the renal artery are associated with similar plaque formation in other major vessels.
- The location of the defect, the overall condition of the patient, and the size of the atrophied kidney influence the decision for therapeutic intervention.
- Treatment includes:
  1. Antihypertensive drugs
  2. Percutaneous transluminal balloon angioplasty or stent placement
  3. Renal artery bypass surgery

STOMATITIS

- Stomatitis is a broad term that refers to inflammation within the oral cavity and may manifest as painful single or multiple ulcerations of the oral mucosa, impairing the protective lining of the mouth.
- Primary stomatitis includes herpes simplex infection and traumatic insults.
- Secondary stomatitis results from infection by opportunistic viruses, fungi, or bacteria or as a result of chemotherapy for cancer.
- A common type of secondary stomatitis is caused by *Candida albicans*. Candidiasis is common in patients undergoing long-term antibiotic therapy and in those undergoing immunosuppressive therapy, such as chemotherapy, radiation, and steroids.
- The patient is instructed to:
  1. Use a soft-bristled brush to gently clean teeth, gums, and the oral cavity.
  2. Rinse the mouth often with sodium bicarbonate solution, warm saline, or hydrogen peroxide solution. Avoid alcohol-based commercial mouthwashes.
  3. Take drugs (antimicrobials, immune modulators, and symptomatic topical agents) as prescribed.

STROKE (BRAIN ATTACK)

OVERVIEW

- Stroke is caused by a change in the blood supply to the brain. The National Stroke Association now uses the term *brain attack* to describe a stroke.
- A stroke is a medical emergency that strikes suddenly, and it should be treated immediately to prevent neurologic deficit and permanent disability.
- Strokes may be classified as:
  1. *Acute ischemic stroke*, which is caused by the occlusion of a cerebral artery:
     a. Types of ischemic strokes include:
        (1) A *thrombotic stroke* is commonly associated with the development of atherosclerosis of the blood vessel wall. Rupture of one or more atherosclerotic plaque exposes foam cells to clot-promoting elements in the blood. The end result is clot formation. The artery becomes occluded, and blood flow to the area is markedly diminished, causing transient ischemia

and then complete ischemia and infarction of brain tissue. Signs and symptoms occur over minutes to hours.

(2) A *lacunar stroke* is a type of thrombotic stroke that causes a soft area or cavity to develop in the white matter or deep gray matter of the brain.

(3) An *embolic stroke* is caused by a thrombus or group of thrombi that travel to the cerebral arteries through the carotid artery and block the artery, resulting in ischemia. Sudden and rapid development of focal neurologic deficits occurs. Cerebral hemorrhage may result if the vessel wall is damaged. Embolic strokes are associated with atrial fibrillation, coronary disease, and heart valve disease or repair.

b. Ischemic stroke may be preceded by warning signs, including:

(1) *Transient ischemic attack (TIA),* a transient focal neurologic deficit such as vertigo or blurred vision that lasts a few minutes to fewer than 24 hours

(2) *Reversible ischemic neurologic deficit (RIND),* which is characterized by neurologic symptoms that last longer than 24 hours but less than 1 week

2. *Hemorrhagic stroke,* in which the integrity of the vessel wall is interrupted and bleeding occurs into the brain tissue (intracerebral) or spaces surrounding the brain (ventricular, subdural, subarachnoid). Causes include hypertension, ruptured aneurysm, and arteriovenous malformation (AVM):

a. An *aneurysm* is an abnormal ballooning or blister on the involved artery that may become stretched or thinned and rupture.

b. *AVM* is a tangled or spaghetti-like mass of malformed, thin-walled, dilated vessels that form an abnormal communication between the arterial and venous systems.

c. *Vasospasm,* a sudden and periodic constriction of a cerebral artery, often results from a cerebral hemorrhage caused by aneurysm rupture. Blood flow to distal areas of the brain supplied by the artery is markedly diminished, leading to cerebral ischemia and infarction and further neurologic dysfunction.

PATIENT-CENTERED COLLABORATIVE CARE
Assessment
- Obtain patient information about:
  1. Activity at onset of the stroke

2. Progression and severity of symptoms, including the presence of a previous TIA or RIND
3. Level of consciousness (LOC), orientation, and other measures of cognitive function
4. Motor status: gait, balance, reading and writing abilities
5. Sensory status: speech, hearing, vision
6. Medical history
7. Social history, with attention to identifying risk factors such as smoking, diet, and exercise
8. Current drugs and nonprescribed drugs, especially anticoagulants, aspirin, vasodilators, and illegal drugs

- Assess for and document:
  1. Neurologic function using a standard stroke screening tool such as the National Institutes of Health (NIH) Stroke Scale, including:
     a. LOC
     b. Orientation
     c. Motor ability
     d. Pupil size and reaction to light, extraocular movement, visual field deficits, ptosis (drooping eyelid)
     e. Speech and language
  2. Vital signs
  3. Blood glucose
  4. Additional assessment includes:
     a. Cognition, memory, judgment, and problem-solving and decision-making abilities
     b. Ability to concentrate and attend to tasks
     c. Range of motion (ROM), proprioception, head and trunk control, balance, gait, coordination, bowel and bladder control
     d. Sensory status (response to touch and painful stimuli; ability to distinguish between two tactile stimuli presented simultaneously; ability to read, write, and follow verbal directions; and ability to name objects and use them correctly)
     e. Speech pattern (rhythm, clarity, aphasia)
     f. Visual system (homonymous hemianopsia, bitemporal hemianopsia, amaurosis fugax)
     g. Cranial nerve function
     h. Cardiac system (dysrhythmias and murmurs)
     i. Coping mechanisms or personality changes
  5. Emotional lability and screen for depression
  6. Nutritional status
  7. Social support, financial status, and occupation

S

- Diagnostic tests:
  1. Computed tomography (CT) scan of the head without contrast is performed within 30 minutes after arrival at the emergency department. This study is essential to determine patient eligibility for fibrinolytic therapy.
  2. Magnetic resonance imaging (MRI) and related multimodal imaging demonstrates ischemia earlier than CT scan and is used to identify the presence of hemorrhage or a cerebral aneurysm. Results also help differentiate stroke from other pathologic changes that mimic a stroke.
  3. Complete blood count (CBC), serum electrolytes, and coagulation factors
  4. Carotid ultrasound
  5. Electrocardiogram and echocardiography to determine whether cardiac disease or dysrhythmia is a contributing factor to stroke

Planning and Implementation
INEFFECTIVE CEREBRAL TISSUE PERFUSION
  Nonsurgical Management
- Management includes either fibrinolytic therapy or endovascular procedures.
- Monitor for neurologic changes or complications before, during and after medical interventions:
  1. Perform a neurologic assessment at least every 2 to 4 hours, checking:
     a. Verbal ability, orientation
     b. Eye opening, pupil size, and reaction to light
     c. Motor response
  2. Monitor vital signs with neurologic checks:
     a. Ask the physician for acceptable limits for blood pressure.

◼ NURSING SAFETY PRIORITY: Critical Rescue
Be alert for symptoms of increased intracranial pressure (ICP) and report any deterioration in the patient's neurologic status to the health care provider immediately! The first sign of increased ICP is a declining LOC.

  3. Perform a cardiac assessment:
     a. Monitor the patient for dysrhythmias; palpate peripheral pulses to help identify new irregularities in heart rhythm in the absence of a cardiac monitor.
  4. Position the backrest to promote cerebral perfusion. In the presence of ischemic stroke, a flat backrest initially may be preferred.

5. Avoid activities that may increase ICP:
   a. Maintain the patient's head in a midline neutral position.
   b. Position the patient to avoid extreme hip or neck flexion.
   c. Avoid clustering of nursing procedures.
   d. Provide a quiet environment; room lights should be low.
   e. Assess the need for suctioning; hyperoxygenate the patient before suctioning.
- Drug therapy:
  1. Fibrinolytic therapy may be used for an acute ischemic stroke:
     a. Recombinant tissue plasminogen activator (rtPA) may be given IV within 3 to 4.5 hours after the onset of symptoms:
        (1) Patients who have had a stroke or serious head trauma in the past 3 months, a hemorrhagic stroke, recent myocardial infarction (MI), increased partial thromboplastin time (PTT), anticoagulant therapy, or who are pregnant are not candidates for this therapy.
     b. Catheter-directed fibrinolytic therapy may be performed as an alternative treatment for up to 6 hours after initial symptoms.
  2. Anticoagulant therapy and antiplatelet therapy may be prescribed depending on the health care provider's preference.
     a. Obtain a baseline prothrombin time (for oral anticoagulation therapy) and PTT (for heparin [Hepalean] therapy) before initiating therapy, 6 to 8 hours after the start of the drug, and every morning thereafter. International normalized ratio (INR) is used to monitor warfarin (Coumadin) therapy and signs of bruising and bleeding.
     b. Aspirin or other antiplatelet drugs may be used to prevent progression or future thrombotic and embolic strokes.
  3. Other drugs used to treat symptoms associated with stroke include:
     a. Phenytoin (Dilantin) or gabapentin (Neurontin), which may be used to prevent seizures
     b. Calcium channel blockers (nimodipine [Nimotop]), which may be administered to treat vasospasm or chronic spasm of the vessel that inhibits blood flow to the area
     c. Stool softeners, analgesics for pain, and antianxiety drugs
     d. Antihypertensives to maintain cerebral perfusion within prescribed limits

S

- Monitor the patient for complications such as:
  1. Vasospasm, or narrowing of the cerebral arteries, which leads to cerebral ischemia and infarction and is manifested by a decreased LOC, motor and reflex changes, and increased neurologic deficits (cranial nerve deficits, aphasia)
  2. Bleeding following fibrinolytic therapy or rebleeding with hemorrhagic stroke
  3. Bleeding caused by thrombolytic, anticoagulant, or anti-platelet therapy. Observe for blood in the urine and stool, epistaxis (nosebleed), bleeding gums, and easy bruising.
  4. Hydrocephalus-enlarged ventricles manifested by a change in the LOC, gait disturbances, and behavior changes
- Carotid artery angioplasty is a nonsurgical intervention used to treat certain types of ischemic stroke. A distal protection device may be placed beyond the stenosis to catch any debris that breaks off during the angioplasty or stenting procedure.

Surgical Management
- Two surgical procedures that may be used for ischemic stroke are:
  1. Carotid endarterectomy to remove atherosclerotic plaque from the inner lining of the carotid artery
  2. Extracranial-intracranial bypass to bypass the occluded area and re-establish blood flow to the affected area
- Surgical procedures to treat AVM include:
  1. Injecting an embolic agent such as a liquid agent that hardens
  2. Surgically removing involved vessels through gamma knife or conventional approaches
- Surgical procedures to treat aneurysm include:
  1. Placing a clip or clamp at the base or neck of the aneurysm
  2. Wrapping the aneurysm with muscle, muslin, or plastic coating
- The nursing care for these procedures is similar to that discussed in *Perioperative Care* (Part One) including neurologic assessment with vital signs.

IMPAIRED SWALLOWING
- Nursing interventions include:
  1. Initiating aspirations precautions
  2. Before feeding, assessing the patient's ability to swallow using an evidence-based tool. Observe for facial drooping, drooling, impaired voluntary cough, hoarseness, incomplete mouth closure, or cranial nerve palsies. A runny nose may also indicate impaired swallowing with saliva discharged through the nasal passages. Next check the gag and cough reflex.

    3. Positioning the patient to facilitate swallowing:
       a. Place the patient in a chair or sitting straight up in bed.
       b. Position the patient's head and neck slightly forward and flexed.
    4. Providing soft or semisoft foods and thickened fluids (e.g., mechanical soft, dental diet; custards, scrambled eggs)
    5. Maintaining a quiet room with few distractions while the patient is eating
    6. Providing nutritional supplementation if needed
    7. Encouraging family members to participate in mealtimes and feeding
    8. Weighing the patient twice a week
    9. Consultation with speech pathology specialist for additional evaluation

IMPAIRED PHYSICAL MOBILITY; SELF-CARE DEFICIT
- Treatment includes:
    1. Performing ROM exercises and progressing to chair and ambulation
    2. Consulting with physical therapist and occupational therapist to evaluate strength and ability, promote mobility, and evaluate for discharge placement
    3. Carefully positioning the patient in proper body alignment, using splint or brace if needed
    4. Using sequential compression devices or pneumatic compression boots to prevent venothromboembolism (VTE) when limited mobility is present
    5. Monitoring the patient for signs of VTE and iatrogenic pneumonia
    6. Supporting nutritional intake

APHASIA OR DYSARTHRIA
- Interventions to help the patient with impaired speech to develop communication strategies include:
    1. Present one idea or thought in a sentence (e.g., "I am going to help you get into the chair").
    2. Use simple one-step commands rather than ask patients to do multiple tasks.
    3. Speak slowly but not loudly; use cues or gestures as needed.
    4. Avoid "yes" and "no" questions for patients with expressive aphasia, because they often give automatic responses that may be incorrect.
    5. Use alternative forms of communication if needed, such as a computer, communication board, or flash cards (often with pictures).
    6. Collaborating with the speech language pathologist or therapist

BOWEL AND BLADDER INCONTINENCE
- Interventions to help the patient become continent include:
  1. Establishing the type (bowel or bladder) and cause of the problem:
     a. Altered LOC
     b. Impaired innervation
     c. Inability to communicate the need to urinate or defecate
  2. Determining the patient's usual voiding or bowel movement pattern
  3. Implementing an individualized bladder training program (see *Incontinence*)
     a. Place the patient on a bedpan or commode every 2 hours; encourage fluid intake to 2000 mL daily unless contraindicated.
     b. Use an intermittent catheterization program if retraining is not feasible.
  4. Implementing an individualized bowel training program:
     a. Determine the normal time or routine for bowel elimination.
     b. Place the patient on a bedpan or commode at the same time each day; use a suppository or stool softener, if needed.
     c. Provide a diet high in bulk or fiber (may require consultation with a nutritionist).

SENSORY CHANGES
- Nursing interventions include:
  1. Providing frequent verbal and tactile cues to help the patient perform ADLs
  2. Breaking down tasks into small steps when cueing
  3. Approaching the patient from the nonaffected side
  4. Placing objects within the patient's field of vision
  5. Placing a patch over the affected eye if diplopia is present
  6. Removing clutter from the room
  7. Orienting the patient to time, place, and event with each encounter
  8. Providing a structured, repetitious, and consistent routine or schedule
  9. Presenting information in a clear, simple, concise manner
  10. Using a step-by-step approach
  11. Placing pictures and other familiar objects in the room

UNILATERAL NEGLECT
- Interventions include:
  1. Teaching the patient to use both sides of the body
  2. Teaching the patient to scan with the eyes and turn the head from side to side

Community-Based Care

- Provide a detailed plan of care at the time of discharge for patients to be transferred to a rehabilitation center or long-term care facility.
- If possible, a case manager should be assigned to help coordinate plans for the patient discharged to the home setting. The case manager should collaborate with the home health agency and with physical and occupational therapists to:
  1. Identify and suggest corrections of hazards in the home before discharge.
  2. Ensure that the patient and family can correctly use all adaptive devices ordered for home use.
  3. Arrange follow-up appointments, as needed.
- Discharge teaching includes:
  1. Providing drug information as needed
  2. Reinforcing mobility skills (in collaboration with other therapists):
     a. How to safely climb stairs, transfer from bed to chair, and get into and out of a car
     b. How to use adaptive equipment
  3. Teaching the family that depression and emotional lability may occur:
     a. Depression is usually self-limited; antidepressants may be needed.
     b. Advise the family to avoid being overprotective.
     c. Assist the family and patient to develop realistic and achievable goals.
- Depending on the location of the lesion, the patient may be anxious, slow, cautious, hesitant, or impulsive; may lack initiative; or may be seemingly unaware of the deficit.
- Refer the family to a social worker for further support and counseling. Family members may need a referral for respite care.
- Provide the family with a variety of publications available from the American Heart Association and National Stroke Association.

⚠ NURSING SAFETY PRIORITY: Action Alert

Hand-off errors lead to patient harm. Be sure that clear, consistent communication and complete documentation are available when the patient transfers between in-hospital care units or procedural suites or to rehabilitative or home care.

SUBCLAVIAN STEAL

- Subclavian steal occurs in the upper extremities from a subclavian artery occlusion or stenosis and results in altered blood flow and ischemia in the arm.

- The disorder can occur at any age but is more common when the patient also has risk factors for atherosclerosis.
- Assess for:
  1. Paresthesias
  2. Light-headedness
  3. Dizziness
  4. Pain and discomfort when the arms are elevated
  5. Difference in blood pressure between arms
  6. Subclavian bruit or decreased pulse on the occluded side
  7. Edema, redness or cyanosis, and delayed capillary refill of the affected arm
- Surgical intervention involves one of three procedures:
  1. Endarterectomy of the subclavian artery
  2. Carotid-subclavian bypass
  3. Dilation of the subclavian artery

SYNDROME OF INAPPROPRIATE ANTIDIURETIC HORMONE

OVERVIEW

- Syndrome of inappropriate antidiuretic hormone (SIADH) occurs when vasopressin (antidiuretic hormone [ADH]) is secreted even though plasma osmolarity is low or normal.
- Water is retained, which results in dilutional hyponatremia (a decreased serum sodium level) and expansion of the extracellular fluid volume.
- SIADH occurs with many pathologic conditions and some drugs, including:
  1. Malignancies (associated with small cell lung cancer; pancreatic, duodenal, and genitourinary carcinomas; thymoma; Hodgkin's lymphoma and non-Hodgkin's lymphoma)
  2. Pulmonary disorders (such as pneumonia, lung abscesses, active tuberculosis, pneumothorax, chronic lung diseases)
  3. Central nervous system (CNS) disorders (typically trauma, infection, tumors, and strokes)
  4. Drugs:
     a. Exogenous ADH
     b. Chlorpropamide
     c. Chemotherapy drugs (vincristine, cyclophosphamide)
     d. Carbamazepine
     e. Opioids
     f. Tricyclic antidepressants
     g. Selective serotonin reuptake inhibitors (SSRIs)
     h. General anesthetics

PATIENT-CENTERED COLLABORATIVE CARE
Assessment
- Obtain patient information about:
  1. Recent head trauma
  2. Cerebrovascular disease
  3. Tuberculosis or other pulmonary disease
  4. Cancer
  5. All past and current drug use
  6. Loss of appetite
  7. Nausea and vomiting
  8. Recent weight gain
- Assess for and document:
  1. Lethargy and headaches
  2. Change in level of consciousness (LOC)
  3. Decreased deep tendon reflexes
  4. Decreased responsiveness, seizures, and coma
  5. Tachycardia
  6. Hyponatremia
  7. Hypo-osmolarity of the blood
  8. Decreased urine output with high specific gravity

Interventions
- Fluid restriction:
  1. Intake may be kept as low as 500 to 600 mL/24 hr.
  2. Use saline to irrigate and dilute medications when using an enteral or gastric tube.
- Assess degree of fluid retention and therapy effectiveness.
  1. Measure intake and output.
  2. Weigh the patient daily.
- Promote comfort by offering frequent oral rinsing.
- Drug therapy may include:
  1. Diuretics if heart failure results from fluid overload
  2. Hypertonic saline (i.e., 3% sodium chloride [3% NaCl]) infusions
  3. Administering ADH antagonists:
     a. Tolvaptan (oral) (Samsca) or conivaptan (IV) (Vaprisol). These drugs promote water loss without urinary sodium excretion.

> **■ NURSING SAFETY PRIORITY: Drug Alert Only**
>
> Administer tolvaptan or conivaptan only in the hospital setting, so serum sodium levels can be monitored closely for the development of hypernatremia.

     b. Demeclocycline (Declomycin), an antibiotic with ADH antagonist properties

- Assess for fluid overload, electrolyte derangements, pulmonary edema, and heart failure:
  1. Monitor for indicators of increased fluid overload at least every 2 hours:
     a. Increased pulse quality
     b. Increasing neck vein distention
     c. Presence of crackles in lungs
     d. Increasing peripheral edema
     e. Altered serum sodium, potassium, calcium, phosphate, and magnesium levels
     f. Reduced and concentrated urine output

◼ NURSING SAFETY PRIORITY: Critical Rescue

Pulmonary edema can occur very quickly and can lead to death. Notify the health care provider about any change that indicates the fluid overload from SIADH is not responding to therapy or is becoming worse.

- Provide a safe environment:
  1. Monitor the patient's neurologic status for:
     a. Muscle twitching
     b. Orientation to time, place, and person
  2. Reduce environmental noise and lighting to prevent over-stimulation.

SYPHILIS

OVERVIEW

- Syphilis is a complex sexually transmitted disease (STD) that can become systemic and can cause serious complications, including death.
- The causative organism is a spirochete called *Treponema pallidum*.
- Syphilis progresses through four stages: primary, secondary, latent, and tertiary.
  1. In *primary syphilis*, a chancre develops at the site of entry (inoculation) of the organism, within 3 weeks on average. Without treatment, the chancre disappears within 6 weeks; however, the organism spreads throughout the body, and the patient is still infectious.
  2. *Secondary* syphilis develops 6 weeks to 6 months after the on-set of primary syphilis. Manifestations are typical of systemic infections: fever, malaise, and generalized aches with a rash, often manifested on palms and soles, that progress to pustules.

3. *Latent syphilis* is a later stage of the disease and has two phases:
   a. *Early latent syphilis* occurs during the first year after infection, and infectious lesions can recur.
   b. *Late latent syphilis* is a disease occurring more than 1 year after infection. It is not infectious except to the fetus of a pregnant woman.
4. *Tertiary syphilis*, or *late syphilis*, occurs after a highly variable period, from 4 to 20 years in untreated cases. Any organ system can be affected, and manifestations vary widely. Manifestations include benign lesions (gummas) of the skin, mucous membranes, and bones; aortic valvular disease and aortic aneurysms; and neurosyphilis with central nervous system (CNS) problems (e.g., meningitis, hearing loss, generalized paresis).

PATIENT-CENTERED COLLABORATIVE CARE

- Diagnosis of primary or secondary syphilis is confirmed by a finding of *T. pallidum* on microscopic examination, by a positive Venereal Disease Research Laboratory (VDRL) serum test, or by a positive rapid plasma reagin (RPR) test result. Latent and tertiary syphilis may be confirmed by the fluorescent treponemal antibody absorption (FTA-ABS) test or the microhemagglutination assay for *T. pallidum* (MHA-TP).

Interventions

- Antibiotic therapy is the treatment for primary, secondary, and early latent syphilis. A course of antibiotics for the late latent stage may require intravenous administration and a prolonged therapeutic course over weeks or months.

❗ NURSING SAFETY PRIORITY: Drug Alert

Discuss with the patient the importance of partner notification and treatment, including the risk for re-infection if the partner goes untreated. All sexual partners must be prophylactically treated as soon as possible, preferably within 90 days of the syphilis diagnosis.

- Provide education about safe sex practices.
- It is essential to teach patient follow-up at 6, 12, and 24 months after initial treatment.
- Inform the patient that the disease will be reported to the local health authority and that all information will be held in strict confidence.

S

- Encourage the patient to provide accurate information for this follow-up to ensure that all at-risk partners are treated appropriately.
- Provide a setting that offers privacy and encourages open discussion.

SYSTEMIC LUPUS ERYTHEMATOSUS

OVERVIEW
- Systemic lupus erythematosus (SLE) is a chronic, progressive, inflammatory connective tissue disease that can cause major body organs and systems to fail.
- The main mechanism of organ damage is the formation of immune complexes that form in organ tissues and in blood vessels, which deprive the organ of essential oxygen.
- It is classified as an autoimmune disease and has periods of spontaneous remissions and exacerbations (flares) with a wide variation in symptoms. However, most patients with SLE have kidney involvement, because the immune complexes tend to aggregate in that system.
- *Discoid lupus erythematosus (DLE)* affects only the skin and is not as common as SLE.
- Lupus mainly affects 10 times more women than men.
- The cause is unknown, although like many autoimmune disorders, a genetic predisposition with environmental interactions is likely.

PATIENT-CENTERED COLLABORATIVE CARE
Assessment
- Assess for and document:
  1. Dry, scaly, raised rash on the face (butterfly rash) or upper body
  2. Individual round lesions (scarring lesions of discoid lupus)
  3. Joint involvement:
     a. Initial changes are similar to rheumatoid arthritis.
     b. Later changes may include joint deformity.
  4. Muscle aches and atrophy
  5. Fever
  6. Various degrees of weakness, fatigue, anorexia, and weight loss
  7. Kidney insufficiency characterized by reduced urine output, proteinuria, hematuria, and fluid retention
  8. Pulmonary effusions or pneumonia
  9. Pericarditis (the most common cardiovascular change):
     a. Tachycardia

      b. Chest pain

      c. Myocardial ischemia

  10. Neurologic changes:

      a. Psychoses

      b. Seizures

      c. Paresis

      d. Migraine headaches

      e. Cranial nerve palsies

  11. Raynaud's phenomenon or other manifestations of vasculitis

  12. Abdominal pain from peritoneal and blood vessel inflammation

  13. Liver enlargement

  14. Osteonecrosis

  15. Body image changes

  16. Social isolation

  17. Fear, anxiety

- Diagnostic tests include:
  1. Skin biopsy
  2. Positive blood tests for:
     a. Rheumatoid factor
     b. Antinuclear antibodies
     c. Erythrocyte sedimentation rate
     d. Anti-SS-A (Ro), anti-SS-B (La), anti-Smith (anti-SM), anti-DNA, extractable nuclear antigens (ENA)
  3. Serum protein electrophoresis
  4. CBC showing pancytopenia
  5. Electrolyte levels
  6. Renal function tests, cardiac and liver enzymes

Interventions

- Drug therapy may include:
  1. Topical steroid preparations
  2. Hydroxychloroquine (Plaquenil) to reduce inflammatory responses
  3. Chronic oral steroid therapy
  4. Immunosuppressive agents, such as methotrexate (Rheumatrex) or azathioprine (Imuran) for renal or central nervous system (CNS) lupus
  5. Antineoplastic drugs, such as cyclophosphamide (Cytoxan, Procytox ✦)

◼ NURSING SAFETY PRIORITY: Action Alert

Stress the importance of avoiding large crowds and people who are ill. Teach them to report any early sign of infection to their health care provider. Observe for side effects and toxic effects of these drugs, and report their occurrence immediately.

- Teach the patient how to protect the skin by:
  1. Minimizing exposure to sunlight and other forms of ultra-violet light:
     a. Wearing long sleeves and wide-brimmed hats
     b. Using sun-blocking agents with a sun protective factor of at least 30
  2. Cleaning the skin with a mild soap and avoiding harsh, perfumed products
  3. Using cosmetics with moisturizers and sun protectants
  4. Using mild protein shampoo and avoiding hair bleaching agents, permanents, and dyes
- Reinforce measures for joint protection and energy conservation (see *Arthritis, Rheumatoid*).
- Help the patient identify coping strategies and support systems that can help him or her deal with the unpredictable nature of the exacerbations.
- Teach the patient about:
  1. The importance of monitoring for fever (the first sign of exacerbation)
  2. The importance of joint protection and energy conservation
  3. Sexual counseling for risk of pregnancy and for contraception options
  4. Resources such as the Lupus Foundation and the Arthritis Foundation
  5. Drug therapy information for scheduling, side effects, and any precautions

TETANUS

- Tetanus, also known as *lockjaw,* is caused by *Clostridium tetani.*
- Tetanus vaccination is initiated in childhood and re-administered every 10 years ("booster") to provide protection against this infection. A booster dose may be given at 5 to 7 years if an injury with a high risk for tetanus infection is present. In addition, tetanus vaccination is given with trauma injuries, burns, and animal/spider bites to prevent secondary infection. Tetanus is preventable with vaccination.
- Tetanus is characterized by muscle rigidity, opisthotonos (abnormal posturing that includes arching the back), cramps, muscle spasms, stiffness, and headache.
- When infection occurs, treatment includes prompt (within 72 hours) IM administration of antitoxin: human tetanus immune globulin or hyperimmune equine or bovine serum.

- Sedation, antianxiety agents, and muscle relaxants to decrease muscle spasms and increase comfort are provided.
- Beta blockers or another antidysrhythmic agent may be given to treat cardiac irregularities, and the patient may need aggressive respiratory support.

THORACIC OUTLET SYNDROME

- Thoracic outlet syndrome is a compression of the subclavian artery at the thoracic outlet by anatomic structures, such as a rib or muscle.
- Damage to the arterial wall can produce thrombosis or embolization in distal arteries of the arm.
- The common sites of compression of the thoracic outlet are the costoclavicular space (most common), the interscalene triangle and between the coracoid process of the scapula, and the pectoralis minor tendon,
- Assess for:
  1. Neck, shoulder, and arm pain or numbness that increases when the arm is extended or held above the shoulder
  2. Moderate edema of the extremity
- Conservative treatment includes:
  1. Physical therapy
  2. Avoidance of aggravating positions
- Surgical treatment involves resection of the anatomic structures that are compressing the artery.

THROMBOCYTOPENIA PURPURA, AUTOIMMUNE

OVERVIEW

- In autoimmune thrombocytopenic purpura, also called *idiopathic thrombocytopenic purpura (ITP)*, there is a greatly reduced number of circulating platelets, increasing the patient's risk for hemorrhage and death.
- In this type of thrombocytopenia, platelet production in the bone marrow is normal, but an antiplatelet antibody is made, causing macrophages in the spleen to increase the rate of platelet destruction.
- When the rate of platelet destruction exceeds the rate of platelet production, the number of circulating platelets decreases and blood clotting slows.
- The problem is most common among women between the ages of 20 and 40 years and among people who have other autoimmune disorders.

PATIENT-CENTERED COLLABORATIVE CARE
- Assess for and document:
  1. Large bruises
  2. Presence of blood in body fluids
  3. Petechial rash on the arms, legs, upper chest, and neck
  4. Mucosal bleeding
  5. Anemia
  6. Neurologic impairment as a result of an intracranial bleed-induced stroke
  7. Laboratory findings: decreased platelet count, large numbers of megakaryocytes in the bone marrow, presence of antiplatelet antibodies in the blood, low hematocrit, and low hemoglobin levels
- Interventions include:
  1. Drug therapy to suppress immune function:
     a. Corticosteroids
     b. Azathioprine (Imuran)
  2. Administration of IV immunoglobulin and IV anti-Rho to prevent the destruction of antibody-coated platelets
  3. Platelet transfusions (when platelet counts are less than $20,000/mm^3$)
  4. Maintaining safety:
     a. Injury prevention
     b. Infection prevention
  5. A possible splenectomy if there is no response to drug therapy

TONSILLITIS

- Tonsillitis is an inflammation and infection of the tonsils and lymphatic tissues located on each side of the throat.
- It is a contagious airborne infection.
- The acute form usually lasts 7 to 10 days and often is caused by bacteria, such as *Streptococcus, Staphylococcus aureus, Haemophilus influenzae,* or *Pneumococcus,* or by viruses.
- Manifestations of acute tonsillitis include the sudden onset of:
  1. Mild to severe sore throat
  2. Fever, muscle aches, chills
  3. Dysphagia, odynophagia (painful swallowing of food)
  4. Pain in the ears
  5. Headache, anorexia, malaise
  6. "Hot potato" voice (thickened voice of poor quality)
  7. Tonsils visually swollen and red with white or yellow exudate
  8. Edematous or inflamed uvula
  9. Enlarged cervical lymph nodes

- Treatment includes:
  1. Oral antibiotics for 7 to 10 days
  2. Teaching the patient about:
     a. Supportive care (rest, increasing fluid intake, humidifying the air, analgesics for pain, gargling several times daily with warm saline, throat lozenges containing mild anesthetics)
     b. The importance of completing antibiotic therapy
- Surgical intervention may be needed for recurrent acute infections (especially group A beta-hemolytic streptococcal infections), chronic infections that have not responded to antibiotic therapy, a peritonsillar abscess, or enlarged tonsils or adenoids that obstruct the airway.
- Procedures may include:
  1. Traditional tonsillectomy and adenoidectomy
  2. Laser tonsillectomy
  3. Radiothermal ablation tonsillectomy
  4. Tonsillar "shaving"

TOXIC SHOCK SYNDROME

- Toxic shock syndrome (TSS) is a form of septic shock caused by *Staphylococcus aureus* or *Streptococcus* infection and is related to menstruation and tampon use.
- Other conditions associated with TSS include internal contraceptive devices, surgical wound infection, nonsurgical infections, and gynecologic surgeries.
- In menstrual-related infection, menstrual blood provides a growth medium for the bacteria, which produces endotoxins that cross the vaginal mucosa to the bloodstream. Tampon insertion or prolonged use can cause vaginal dryness and microabrasions that provide an entry for the microorganisms.
- Assess for:
  1. Abrupt onset of a high fever
  2. Headache and flu-like symptoms
  3. Severe hypotension
  4. Sunburn-like rash with broken capillaries in the eyes and on the skin
- Management includes:
  1. Removal of the infection source
  2. Management of fluids and electrolyte imbalances; avoiding hypotension
  3. IV antibiotics and other measures included in the management of sepsis and septic shock

T

- Patient education focuses on prevention by teaching all women about the proper use of tampons, internal contraceptive devices such as vaginal sponges and diaphragms, and prompt treatment of gynecologic infections.

TRACHOMA

- Trachoma is a chronic, bilateral scarring form of conjunctivitis caused by *Chlamydia trachomatis*. It is the chief cause of preventable blindness in the world.
- Manifestations include tears, photophobia, edema of the eyelids and conjunctiva, and follicles on the upper eyelid conjunctiva. With disease progression, the eyelid scars and turns inward, causing the eyelashes to damage the cornea.
- Drug therapy management involves a 4-week course of oral or topical tetracycline (Achromycin, Apo-Tetra ✦) or erythromycin (Apo-Erythro-EC ✦, E-Mycin, E.E.S.). Azithromycin (Zithromax) may be used once weekly for 1 to 3 weeks.
- Prevention through infection control is effective. Teach patients to:
  1. Wash the hands before and after touching the eyes.
  2. Keep washcloths separate from those of unaffected people, and launder them separately.
  3. Complete the entire course of antibiotics.

TRAUMA, ABDOMINAL

OVERVIEW

- Abdominal trauma is an injury to the structures located between the diaphragm and the pelvis that occurs when the abdomen is subjected to blunt or penetrating force.
- Organs that may be injured include the large and small bowel, liver, spleen, duodenum, pancreas, kidneys, and urinary bladder.
- Two broad categories are:
  1. Blunt trauma, which commonly results from automobile accidents but is also caused by falls, assaults, and contact sports
  2. Penetrating trauma, most often caused by gunshot wounds and stab wounds

PATIENT-CENTERED COLLABORATIVE CARE

Assessment

- Assess for airway, breathing, and circulation (ABCs).
- The focus of the assessment is on the risk of hemorrhage, shock, and peritonitis. The spleen is vulnerable to blunt trauma and contributes to significant blood loss.

- The key assessment factors related to early shock detection are decreased mental status, altered vital signs (e.g., hypotension, tachycardia, tachypnea and decreased SpO_2), and skin perfusion (see *Shock* for discussions of hemorrhagic and hypovolemic forms):
  1. In mild shock, the skin is pale, cool, and moist.
  2. In moderate shock, diaphoresis is marked and urine output decreased.
  3. In severe shock, changes in mental status are manifested by agitation, disorientation, and recent memory loss.
- Assess for and document:
  1. Mental status, vital signs (HR, BP, RR, and SpO_2), bowel sounds, urinary output, and changes in clinical findings every 15 to 30 minutes until stable, then hourly. Report any deterioration immediately to the physician.
  2. The patient's report about the presence, location, and quality of pain, including referred pain (e.g., right shoulder) and nausea
  3. Inspection of the abdomen, back, flanks, genitalia, and rectum for contusions, abrasions, lacerations, ecchymoses, penetrating injuries, and symmetry. Ecchymosis around the umbilicus (Cullen's sign) and ecchymosis in either flank (Turner's sign) may indicate retroperitoneal bleeding into the abdominal wall. Be aware that a large volume of blood can accumulate in the abdominal cavity before there is a change in the size or color during inspection.
  4. Auscultation of the abdomen for absent or diminished bowel sounds and bruits
  5. Percussion for abnormal sounds, such as resonance over the liver or dullness over the stomach or intestines (Ballance's sign)
  6. Results from light palpation of the abdomen to identify areas of tenderness, guarding, rigidity, and spasm
  7. Kehr's sign, indicating splenic injury, which is left shoulder pain resulting from diaphragmatic irritation
  8. Blood in peritoneal lavage, nasogastric tube output, or emesis

Interventions

Nonsurgical Management
- Interventions include:
  1. Placing two large-bore IV catheters to provide rapid fluid resuscitation
  2. Infusing IV fluids at a rapid rate, as ordered, and monitoring patient responses
  3. Obtaining blood samples for analysis
  4. Inserting an indwelling Foley catheter and monitoring urine output hourly for at least 24 hours

5. Inserting a nasogastric (NG) tube to prevent vomiting and reduce intra-abdominal pressure
6. Monitoring intra-abdominal pressure (in some facilities) to detect compartment syndrome, which is compression of structures in the abdominal cavity (see *Compartment Syndrome*)

- Diagnostic studies may include:
  1. Abdominal ultrasound in the presence of blunt trauma
  2. Peritoneal lavage
  3. Abdominal flat plate x-ray
  4. Abdominal computed tomography (CT) scan
  5. Chest x-ray
  6. Electrocardiogram (ECG) and ongoing ECG monitoring
  7. Serum analyses: complete blood count (CBC), basic metabolic panel, coagulation factors, tests for liver function and blood typing with antibody screening for possible transfusion
  8. Continuous intra-abdominal pressure monitoring
- Analgesics for pain, with careful attention to maintaining airway and breathing

Surgical Management

- For patients with severe abdominal trauma, an exploratory laparotomy with repair of abdominal injuries is performed.
- Most patients with gunshot or stab wounds require an exploratory laparotomy to assess for internal damage.
- Perioperative care is performed as outlined in Part One.
- A colostomy, either temporary or permanent, may be required (see *Surgical Management* under *Cancer, Colorectal*).

✓ NATIONAL PATIENT SAFETY GOAL

Before administering medications or implementing procedures, ensure that the right patient is receiving interventions by using at least two identifiers. This process is challenging to implement in the emergency department, where the fast pace of admissions and rapidly changing condition of the patient may not prioritize "routine" admission activities such a placing a name band. Nonetheless, accurate identification is essential for risk reduction and avoidance of adverse errors.

TRAUMA, BLADDER

- Bladder trauma occurs as a result of blunt or penetrating injury to the lower abdomen.
- The most common cause is a fractured pelvis (bone fragments puncture the bladder).

- Assess for:
  1. Anuria
  2. Hematuria
  3. Bloody urinary meatus
  4. Results of cystogram and voiding cystourethrogram
- Patients with bladder trauma other than a simple contusion require surgical intervention, including closure repair of the bladder wall and peritoneal membrane.
- Recovery may include prolonged use (more than 2 weeks) of a Foley or suprapubic catheter while the repaired bladder heals.

TRAUMA, BRAIN (ACUTE BRAIN INJURY WITH OR WITHOUT SKULL FRACTURE)

OVERVIEW

- A head injury occurs as the result of blow or jolt to the head or penetration of the head by a bullet or other foreign object. As a result, the normal functioning of the brain is disrupted. Traumatic brain injury (TBI) may produce a diminished state of consciousness and changes in cognitive abilities, physical functioning, or behavioral and emotional functioning. These changes may be immediate or delayed and may resolve or persist long after the original injury.
- Direct brain injury is the result of primary forces applied to the head. The primary injury occurs at the point of injury, with potential for additional primary injury from contrecoup forces when the intracranial tissue "bounces" against the skull opposite the site of direct injury. Indirect brain injury results from forces applied to another body part with a rebound effect to the brain.
- Brain damage from trauma most often involves the frontal or temporal lobes.
- Damage to brain tissue depends on the location, degree, and mechanism of injury:
  1. Brain injury can be classified as mild, moderate, or severe, depending on the initial Glasgow Coma Scale (GCS) score, which has implications for both treatment and prognosis.
  2. It may be also described by the degree of apparent damage to the brain:
     a. A *concussion* is a shaking of the brain and may be associated with a brief loss of consciousness and no damage visible by computed tomography (CT).
     b. A *contusion* causes bruising of the brain tissue.
     c. A *laceration* causes tearing of the cortical surface vessels and may lead to secondary hemorrhage.

    d. Neuronal injury, ischemia, and infarct
    e. Damage to supporting structures and cells, including blood vessels, the dura, and glial and microglial cells that secrete repair and growth factors, releases substances that can extend the area of injury or interfere with normal repair.

- Brain injury can also be from physiologic, vascular, and biochemical events that are an extension of the primary injury and involve cellular changes that contribute to tissue injury. The most common responses are hypotension, hypoxia, ischemia, and cerebral edema. Prevention of secondary injury is a major focus of acute care.
- A closed head injury is caused by blunt trauma. The integrity of the skull is not violated. One severe form of closed head injury is diffuse axonal injury, in which neuronal axons are damaged as a result of the rotating and high-velocity force of the primary injury.
- An open head injury occurs when the skull is fractured or penetrated by an object (e.g., bullet, projectile, knife), violating the integrity of brain and dura and exposing brain tissue to extracranial contaminants.
- Brain injury may be accompanied by skull fracture, which increases the risk of central nervous system (CNS) infection and additional brain damage. Types of skull fractures include:
  1. *Linear,* a simple, clean break
  2. *Depressed,* in which bone is pressed inward into brain tissue
  3. *Open,* in which the scalp is lacerated along with the skull fracture
  4. *Comminuted,* in which the skull is fragmented and bone is depressed into the brain tissue
  5. *Basilar,* which occurs at the base of the skull, usually along the paranasal sinus and which may result in a cerebrospinal fluid (CSF) leak from the nose or ear and potential damage to cranial nerves I, II, VII, and VIII

PATIENT-CENTERED COLLABORATIVE CARE
Assessment
- Obtain patient information about:
  1. When, where, and how the injury occurred
  2. The patient's level of consciousness (LOC) immediately after the injury and on admission to the hospital or unit and whether there have been any changes or fluctuations
  3. Presence of seizure activity
  4. Age, gender, and race

5. Medical and social history, especially presence of alcohol or drug use
6. Hand dominance
7. Allergies to drugs and foods, especially seafood (patients allergic to seafood are often allergic to the medium used in diagnostic testing)

- Assess for:
  1. Impaired airway or breathing pattern: respiratory rate, depth, and quality with peripheral oxygenation (SpO_2)
  2. Signs and symptoms of hypovolemic shock or hemorrhage, which may indicate additional traumatic injuries, such as abdominal bleeding or bleeding into soft tissue around major fractures
  3. Cardiac dysrhythmias from chest trauma, bruising of the heart, or interference with the autonomic nervous system
  4. Heart rate, blood pressure, peripheral pulses, and core temperature
  5. Baseline and ongoing neurologic status with a standard assessment tool such as the GCS:
     a. Decreased or garbled verbal response to auditory or tactile stimulus; new aphasia
     b. Inability to follow commands; confusion
     c. Pupils that are large, pinpoint, or ovoid, and nonreactive to light (indicates cranial nerve dysfunction, especially III, IV, and VII; may indicate brainstem dysfunction)
     d. Decreased or absent motor strength in the extremities; hemiparesis or hemiplegia
     e. Complaints of severe headache, nausea, or vomiting
     f. Seizure activity
     g. Drainage of CSF from the ear or nose ("halo sign")
  6. Indications of post-traumatic sequelae in the patient who experienced a minor head injury (symptoms may persist for weeks or months):
     a. Persistent headache
     b. Weakness
     c. Dizziness
     d. Loss of memory
     e. Personality and behavioral changes
     f. Problems with perception, reasoning abilities, and concept formation
  7. Changes in personality, behavior, and abilities, such as:
     a. Increased incidence of temper outbursts, risk-taking behavior, depression, and denial of disability
     b. Becoming more talkative and developing a very outgoing personality

T

   c. Decreased ability to learn new information, to concen-
      trate, and to plan
   d. Impaired memory, especially recent or short-term
      memory; this should not be confused with problems
      of aphasia
- Assess family dynamics. Family members may be angry with the
  patient for being injured, especially if the patient's behavior
  resulted in an injury that could have been prevented, or they
  may feel guilty that they could not prevent the injury.
- Diagnostic studies may include:
   1. Complete blood count (CBC), basic metabolic panel, coag-
      ulation studies, arterial blood gases (ABGs), and toxicology
      screen
   2. CT scan
   3. Chest x-ray and abdominal x-ray to evaluate for the presence
      of additional injuries

◼ NURSING SAFETY PRIORITY: Critical Rescue

LOC is the most sensitive and specific indicator of neurologic
deterioration. Immediately inform the physician about changes
in mentation, orientation, or behavior. A decrease in GCS score
of 2 points or more should be reported immediately.

Interventions
Nonsurgical Management
- Assess vital signs with a standard neurologic assessment every 1
  to 2 hours to detect early signs of decreased levels of consciousness, poor perfusion, hypovolemia, and dangerous elevations of
  blood pressure that may cause further brain damage. Cardiac
  monitoring to detect cardiac dysrhythmias may be implemented. Report derangements immediately.
- The patient may be placed in systemic or local (cranial) hypothermia devices (blanket, helmet) to slow brain metabolism
  during the acute phase.
- Maintain normothermia; fever may extend the area of brain
  damage during the acute phase.
- Position the patient to avoid extreme flexion or extension of
  the neck, which interferes with CSF outflow. Maintain the
  head in a midline, central position; log roll the patient and
  elevate the backrest 30 degrees unless contraindicated; use reverse Trendelenburg position if spinal cord injury is still being
  evaluated.
- The patient on a ventilator may receive settings to maintain
  the $Paco_2$ at 35 to 38 mm Hg during the first 2 to 24 hours
  to promote cerebral vasoconstriction and reduce intercranial
  hypertension.

- Maintain the Pao_2 at 85 to 100 mm Hg and Spo_2 at greater than 92% to maintain sufficient oxygen to brain cells, preventing secondary brain injury.
- Monitor intracranial pressure (ICP) with a specialized device in the intensive care unit (ICU) if the patient presents with coma; manage ICP and cerebral perfusion pressure to maintain adequate blood flow to brain tissue. Maintain infection control/prevention processes specific to the use of ICP monitoring devices to prevent secondary brain injury from infection.
- Monitor brain tissue oxygenation with jugular venous oxygen apparatus (Sjo_2).
- Drug therapy:
  1. Osmotic diuretics (mannitol) are given through, or drawn up through, a needle with a filter to eliminate microscopic crystals. These drugs are used to pull fluid out of the intracranial space and into the vasculature for excretion. Osmotics are most effective when given as a bolus rather than a continuous infusion.
  2. Opioids may be used if the patient is mechanically ventilated to control restlessness and agitation if activity is causing increased ICP.
  3. Antiepileptic drugs may be used to treat actual or risk for seizure activity.
  4. Barbiturate coma (with severe injury and use of mechanical ventilation) may be induced to reduce the oxygen demands of the brain during acute injury and subsequent increases in intracranial pressure.
- Pulmonary management includes:
  1. Encouraging the conscious patient to breathe deeply every hour while awake; avoid coughing, which can increase ICP
  2. Turning and repositioning the patient at least once every 2 hours; consider the use of continuous lateral rotational therapy if the patient is comatose, hypoxic, and mechanically ventilated
- Fluid and electrolyte management includes:
  1. Monitoring electrolytes and serum and urine osmolarity to maintain/replace a normal range of values, particularly during diuretic/osmotic treatment
  2. Measuring intake and output every hour to avoid overhydration and subsequent increased intracranial pressure or dehydration and subsequent poor perfusion
  3. Measuring urine osmolality, sodium, and specific gravity when there is a significant increase in urine output (greater than 300 mL/hr for 2 hours) to evaluate for syndrome of inappropriate antidiuretic hormone (SIADH)

T

4. Using a Foley catheter to monitor hourly output if acute moderate or severe brain injury is diagnosed
5. Monitoring daily weight
6. Instituting institutional specific seizure precautions
- Sensory, cognitive, and behavioral management includes:
  1. Providing a balance between sensory stimulation and quiet rest to promote brain recovery
  2. Monitoring the patient for nutritional deficits that may occur secondary to loss of smell and loss of ability to taste, swallow, or feel food in the oral cavity
     a. Ensure that mealtime is a pleasant experience.
     b. Check the temperature of food and beverages on the tray before serving.
     c. Position the patient to maximize swallowing ability.
     d. Collaborate with the speech-language pathologist to develop and implement a swallowing program for the patient, as needed.
  3. Providing a safe environment with frequent monitoring, use of a sitter, or if needed, use of restraints following institutional policy
  4. Initiating a sensory stimulation program, such as audio-tapes used for no longer than 10 to 15 minutes for patients in coma; awake or alert patients may enjoy longer tapes
  5. Orienting the patient to environment, time, place, and the reason for hospitalization with each encounter if short-term memory loss or coma is present
  6. Reassuring the patient realistically about concerns, visitation, and plan for care at least once per shift
  7. Providing simple, short explanations of procedures and activities immediately before any interventions
  8. Collaborating with physical and occupational therapists to plan exercise and ADL programs
  9. Maintaining the patient on a normal sleep-wake cycle for mild brain injury, and providing periods of rest for patients with moderate or severe injury
  10. Asking the family to bring in familiar objects, such as pictures or music
  11. Monitoring the patient's reaction to television or radio (the brain-injured patient is often unable to differentiate programs from what is happening within his or her own environment)
  12. Keeping the bed in the low position if the patient is awake
  13. Observing and documenting behavior; providing constant supervision if the patient is unable to consistently follow directions or is unsafe due to short-term memory failure

- Nutrition management includes:
  1. Beginning nutritional support as soon as possible with hyperalimentation, tube feedings (nasal or gastrostomy), or oral feedings
  2. Monitoring the patient's weight and serum albumin, prealbumin, and transferrin levels to ensure adequate protein intake

Surgical Management
- A craniotomy may be indicated to:
  1. Evacuate a subdural or epidural hematoma
  2. Treat uncontrolled increased ICP; remove ischemic tissue or tips of temporal lobe
  3. Treat hydrocephalus
- Bedside surgical insertion of an ICP-monitoring device is often performed. Types of devices include:
  1. Intraventricular catheter
  2. Epidural catheter or sensor
  3. Subarachnoid bolt or screw
  4. Fiberoptic transducer-tipped sensor

Community-Based Care
- Respite care may be needed to help the family cope with feelings of isolation, increased responsibility, financial or emotional stress, or role reversal; refer them to support groups.
- The patient may experience a sense of isolation and loneliness, because personality and behavior changes make it difficult to resume or maintain pre-injury social contacts.
- Discharge planning often involves a case manager and includes:
  1. Providing a detailed plan of care at the time of transfer to a rehabilitation or long-term care facility:
     a. Drugs, including dosage and possible side effects
     b. Current patient activity
     c. Techniques used to motivate or calm the patient
     d. Successful coping strategies identified by the patient or family
  2. Referring the patient to follow-up and home care to promote adjustment
  3. Informing the patient and family about resources such as the National Head Injury Foundation or a local head injury support group
- Health teaching includes:
  1. Reviewing seizure precautions
  2. Strategies to adapt to sensory dysfunction and to cope with the personality or behavior problems that may arise
  3. Explaining the purpose, dosage, schedule, and route of administration of drugs

4. Encouraging the patient to participate in activities as tolerated
5. Teaching the patient and family measures to treat sensory dysfunctions:
   a. The home should have functioning smoke detectors (the patient may have loss of the sense of smell).
   b. Objects and furniture should be kept in consistent locations.
   c. The measures described for sensory and perceptual management also are relevant here.
   d. Help the family and patient develop a home routine that is structured, repetitious, and consistent.
6. For minor head injury, discuss symptoms of post-traumatic stress disorder and mild cognitive deficit disorder. Inform the patient that these symptoms are common and refer the patient and family to a specialist in brain injury or cognitive therapy and a support group if symptoms persist. Symptoms include:
   a. Personality changes
   b. Irritability
   c. Headaches
   d. Dizziness
   e. Restlessness
   f. Nervousness
   g. Insomnia
   h. Memory loss
   i. Depression

TRAUMA, ESOPHAGEAL

- Trauma to the esophagus can result from blunt injuries, chemical burns, surgery or endoscopy, or the stress of protracted severe vomiting.
- Trauma may affect the esophagus directly, impairing swallowing and nutrition, or it may create problems and complications in related structures such as the lungs or mediastinum.
- Assess for and document:
  1. Airway patency, breathing
  2. Chest pain
  3. Dysphagia
  4. Vomiting
  5. Bleeding
  6. Results of x-ray examination, computed tomography (CT), and endoscopy

- Treatment includes:
  1. Maintaining the patient on NPO status to prevent further leakage of esophageal secretions
  2. Maintaining nasogastric (NG) or gastrostomy tube drainage to rest the patient's esophagus
  3. Administering total parenteral nutrition (TPN) during esophageal rest (usually for at least 10 days)
  4. Administering broad-spectrum antibiotics, corticosteroids, and analgesics
- Surgery may be needed to remove the tissue. A resection or replacement of the damaged esophageal segment with small bowel tissue may be required.

TRAUMA, FACIAL

OVERVIEW
- Facial trauma is defined by the specific bones (mandibular, maxillary, orbital, or nasal fractures) and the side of the face involved.
- Mandibular (lower jaw) fractures can occur at any point on the mandible and are the most common facial fractures.
- The rich blood supply of the face leads to extensive bleeding and bruising with facial trauma.

PATIENT-CENTERED COLLABORATIVE CARE
Assessment
- The first action to take for a patient with facial trauma is airway assessment.
- Assess for:
  1. Manifestations of airway obstruction:
     a. Stridor
     b. Shortness of breath
     c. Anxiety and restlessness
     d. Hypoxia and hypercarbia
  2. Soft tissue trauma
     a. Edema
     b. Facial asymmetry
     c. Pain
     d. Leakage of spinal fluid through the ears or nose
     e. Vision and eye movement
     f. Bruising behind the ears in the mastoid area ("battle sign")
Interventions
- The priority action is to establish and maintain a patent airway.

- Other interventions include:
  1. Anticipating the need for emergency intubation, tracheotomy, or cricothyroidotomy
  2. Controlling hemorrhage
  3. Assessing for the extent of injury
  4. Establishing IV access and initiating fluid resuscitation
  5. Assisting in the stabilization of fractures
  6. Administering prescribed antibiotics
  7. For mandibular fixation with plates, teaching the patient about:
     a. Oral care with an irrigating device
     b. Soft diet or dental liquid diet restrictions
     c. How to cut the wires if emesis occurs

⚠ NURSING SAFETY PRIORITY: Critical Rescue
Instruct the patient to keep wire cutters with him or her at all times in case this emergency arises.

TRAUMA, KIDNEY

- Kidney (renal) trauma is injury to one or both kidneys. Injury can be blunt or penetrating.
- Injuries:
  1. Minor injuries (contusion, small lacerations, tearing of the parenchyma and the calyx) are likely to follow falls, contact sports, and blows to the back or torso.
  2. Major injuries (lacerations to the cortex, medulla, or one of the branches of the renal artery or vein) are likely to follow penetrating abdominal, flank, or back wounds.
  3. Pedicle injuries (laceration or disruption of the renal artery or vein) result in rapid and extensive hemorrhage and death unless diagnosis and intervention are prompt.
- Obtain patient information about:
  1. History of events surrounding the trauma
  2. History of kidney or urologic disease, including previous surgical intervention
  3. History of diabetes, hypertension, or atherosclerosis
- Assess for and document:
  1. Vital signs, particularly derangements in HR, BP, and RR indicating poor perfusion or reduced ventilation. Use SpO_2 to monitor oxygenation; maintain values greater than 92%. Fever contributes to brain injury and must be treated early and aggressively.
  2. Abdominal or flank pain
  3. Penetrating injuries of the lower thorax, back, or abdomen

4. Abdominal or flank bruising
5. Abdominal distention or flank asymmetry
6. Urine output hourly and abnormal urine, especially blood in the urine
7. Decreased serum hemoglobin and hematocrit values
- Treatment includes drugs for vascular support, fluids to restore volume, and surgery when indicated.
  1. Administer fluids, such as crystalloids or packed red blood cells, to restore circulatory blood volume; plasma volume expanders may also be given.
  2. Assess the need for clotting factors such as vitamin K and platelets.
- Depending on the extent of the injury, nephrectomy (surgical removal of the kidney) may be required.
- For major vascular tearing, the kidney may be surgically removed, repaired through revascularization techniques, and then surgically reimplanted.

TRAUMA, KNEE

- There are two semilunar cartilaginous structures (menisci) in the knee joint, the medial meniscus and the lateral meniscus, which act as shock absorbers.
- Meniscus injuries are usually tears and occur more often in the medial meniscus, usually causing the knee to lock.
- Manifestations include pain, swelling, tenderness in the knee, and a clicking or snapping sound when the knee is moved.
- A common diagnostic technique is the McMurray test. The examiner flexes and rotates the knee and then presses on the medial aspect while slowly extending the leg. The test result is positive if clicking is palpated or heard, but a negative finding does not rule out a tear.
- Management of a locked knee is manipulation followed by splinting or casting for 3 to 6 weeks.
- A partial or total meniscectomy may be required and is performed either as an open procedure (rare) or as a closed procedure by arthroscopy.
- Postoperative care includes:
  1. Monitoring the surgical dressing for bleeding and drainage
  2. Monitoring vital signs for sings of hypovolemia, poor perfusion, and impaired oxygenation
  3. Performing neurovascular checks:
     a. Skin temperature and color
     b. Movement and sensation
     c. Distal pulses

      d. Capillary refill

      e. Pain

  4. Teaching the patient to perform exercises (e.g., quadriceps setting, straight-leg raises)

  5. Teaching the patient to use a knee immobilizer

  6. Elevating the knee and applying ice

- Ligament injuries result in sprains and tears.
- Manifestations of an anterior cruciate ligament (ACL) tear include feeling a snap and the knee giving way, swelling and stiffness, and pain.
- Management may be nonsurgical (exercises, bracing, activity limitation) or surgical, depending on the severity of the injury and the anticipated activity of the patient.
- For a rupture of the patellar tendon, management includes surgical repair and casting for 6 to 8 weeks, or tendon transplantation. See *Fracture* for care of the patient in a cast.

TRAUMA, LARYNGEAL

- Laryngeal trauma is the result of a crushing or direct blow, fracture, or an injury such as that induced by prolonged endotracheal intubation.
- Manifestations include dyspnea, aphonia, hoarseness, subcutaneous emphysema, and hemoptysis.
- Respiratory assessment includes:
  1. Assessing the airway every 15 to 30 minutes
  2. Monitoring vital signs and pulse oximetry every 15 to 30 minutes to evaluate perfusion and oxygenation
  3. Applying oxygen and humidification as prescribed
  4. Assessing for increased respiratory difficulty:
     a. Increasing tachypnea
     b. Nasal flaring
     c. Anxiety
     d. Sternal retraction
     e. Dyspnea
     f. Restlessness
     g. Decreased oxygen saturation
     h. Decreased level of consciousness
     i. Stridor

◼ NURSING SAFETY PRIORITY: Critical Rescue

If the patient has respiratory difficulty, stay with him or her, and instruct other trauma team members or the Rapid Response Team to prepare for an emergency intubation or tracheostomy.

- Surgical intervention is necessary for lacerations of the mucous membranes, cartilage exposure, or paralysis of the cords.
- An artificial airway may be needed.

TRAUMA, LIVER

- The liver is one of the organs most commonly injured in patients with abdominal trauma. Damage or injury should be suspected whenever any upper abdominal or lower chest trauma is sustained.
- Common injuries to the liver include simple lacerations, multiple lacerations, avulsions (tears), and crush injuries.
- Because the liver is a vascular organ, blood loss is massive when trauma occurs (see *Shock* , especially the discussion of hemorrhagic and hypovolemic shock).
- Clinical manifestations of liver trauma include right upper quadrant pain with abdominal tenderness, distention, guarding, rigidity, and abdominal pain that is aggravated by deep breathing and is referred to the right shoulder.
- Exploratory laparotomy is done to determine the source and type of bleeding. Operative procedures may include suture placement, wound packing, and decompression; liver lobe resection may be necessary.
- The patient requires infusion of multiple blood products, packed red blood cells (RBCs), fresh-frozen plasma, and massive volume replacement to maintain hydration. Anticipate perioperative bleeding and prolonged coagulopathy with severe liver injury.

TRAUMA, PERIPHERAL NERVE

- The peripheral nerves are subject to injuries associated with mechanical or vehicular accidents, sports, the injection of particular drugs, military conflicts or wars, and acts of violence (e.g., knife or gunshot wounds).
- Specific mechanisms of injury include:
  1. Partial or complete severance of a nerve or nerves
  2. Contusion, stretching, constriction, or compression of a nerve or nerves
  3. Ischemia
  4. Electrical, thermal, or radiation injury
- Most commonly affected are the median, ulnar, and radial nerves of the arms and the peroneal, femoral, and sciatic nerves of the legs.

- Nerve damage is characterized by pain, burning, or other abnormal sensations distal to the trauma; weakness or flaccid paralysis; and change in skin color and temperature (a warm phase and a cold phase).
- Nonsurgical treatment consists of immobilization of the area with a splint, cast, or traction followed by physical and occupational therapy.
- Surgery may include resection and suturing to reapproximate the severed nerve ends, nerve grafting, and nerve and tendon transplantation.
- Regeneration of the damaged nerve and return of sensation may occur several years after the injury; motor movement is less likely to recover long after the event.
- Postoperative nursing care is directed toward frequent skin care and assessment, management of pain, and instructing the patient to protect the involved area from trauma.

TRAUMA, TRACHEOBRONCHIAL

- Most tears of the tracheobronchial tree result from severe blunt trauma or rapid deceleration and primarily involve the mainstem bronchi.
- Injuries to the trachea usually occur at the junction of the trachea and cricoid cartilage.
- Patients with tracheobronchial trauma develop massive air leaks, causing air to enter the mediastinum and leading to extensive subcutaneous emphysema.
- Upper airway obstruction may occur, causing severe respiratory distress and inspiratory stridor.
- Large tracheal tears are managed by cricothyroidotomy or tracheotomy below the level of injury.
- Management includes:
  1. Assessing for hypoxemia
  2. Administering oxygen as needed
  3. Initiating mechanical ventilation
  4. Assessing for subcutaneous emphysema
  5. Assessing oxygenation, ventilation, and work of breathing along with lung sounds.
  6. Providing tracheostomy care if surgical repair was needed

TUBERCULOSIS

OVERVIEW

- Pulmonary tuberculosis (TB) is a highly communicable disease caused by *Mycobacterium tuberculosis* infection.

- The organism is transmitted by aerosolization (airborne route) from an infected person during coughing, laughing, sneezing, whistling, or singing.
- Far more people are infected with the bacillus than actually develop active TB.
- When the bacillus is inhaled into a susceptible site, it multiplies freely, causing an exudative pneumonitis. Only a few people develop active TB from this initial infection.
- Initial infection is seen more often in the middle or lower lobes of the lung, and reactivation occurs more in the upper lobes.
- Progression of infection leads to an inflammatory lump that surrounds the bacilli and is filled with collagen, fibroblasts, and lymphocytes. The lump necroses, causing calcification or liquefaction and leading to destruction of lung tissue with cavity formation.
- *Miliary,* or *hematogenous,* TB is the spread of TB throughout the body when a large number of organisms enter the blood and can then infect the brain, liver, kidney, or bone marrow.
- An infected individual is not infectious to others until manifestations of disease occur.
- People at greatest risk for developing TB are those who have repeated close contact with an infectious person who has not yet been diagnosed with TB. People at risk include:
  1. Those in constant, frequent contact with an untreated individual
  2. Those who have immune dysfunction or HIV infection
  3. Those who live in crowded areas such as long-term care facilities, prisons, and mental health facilities
  4. Older people
  5. Homeless people
  6. Abusers of injection drugs or alcohol
  7. Members of lower socioeconomic groups
  8. Foreign immigrants (especially from Mexico, the Philippines, and Vietnam)

PATIENT-CENTERED COLLABORATIVE CARE
Assessment
- Obtain patient information about:
  1. Persistent cough
  2. Weight loss
  3. Anorexia
  4. Night sweats
  5. Fever or chills
  6. Dyspnea or hemoptysis
  7. Past exposure to TB

  8. Country of origin and travel to foreign countries
  9. History of bacillus Calmette-Guérin (BCG) vaccination
- Assess for and document:
  1. Dullness with percussion over involved the lung fields
  2. Bronchial breath sounds
  3. Crackles, wheezes
  4. Enlarged lymph nodes
- TB is diagnosed on the basis of manifestations, a positive nucleic acid amplification test (NAAT), or a positive sputum smear for acid-fast bacillus. Blood analysis by an enzyme-linked immunosorbent assay using the QuantiFERON-TB Gold (QFT-G) may be used for testing in the acute care setting. A purified protein derivative (PPD) two-step test may be used for screening purposes.

◼ NURSING SAFETY PRIORITY: Action Alert

- Do not assume that a positive PPD reaction means that active disease is present. It only indicates exposure to TB, TB vaccination, or the presence of inactive (dormant) disease.
- A reduced PPD skin reaction or a negative PPD skin test result does not rule out TB disease or infection in the very old or in anyone who is severely immunocompromised.

Interventions

- Combination drug therapy is the most effective method of treating TB and preventing transmission. Current first-line therapy uses four medications:
  1. Isoniazid (INH) for 6 months
  2. Rifampin for 6 months
  3. Pyrazinamide for the first 2 months
  4. Ethambutol for 6 months
- Variations of the first-line drugs along with other drug types are used if the patient does not tolerate the standard first-line therapy.
- Nursing interventions include:
  1. Caring for the hospitalized patient using strict Airborne Precautions
  2. Patient teaching about drug therapy:
     a. Explaining the actions, side effects, dosing, and scheduling of the drugs
     b. Stressing the importance of taking each drug regularly, exactly as prescribed
     c. Presenting drug information in multiple formats, such as pamphlets, videos, and drug-schedule worksheets

    d. Asking the patient to describe the treatment regimen, major side effects, and when to call the health care agency and physician

    e. Explaining that nausea can be prevented by taking the drugs at bedtime

3. Patient teaching about multidrug-resistant strains of TB. Higher doses of some drugs for longer periods and absolute adherence to therapy are required for survival and cure of the disease.

4. Patient teaching about infection control:

    a. Reminding patients that Airborne Precautions are not necessary in the home, because family members have already been exposed

    b. Teaching family members in the household about the need to undergo TB testing

    c. Teaching the patient to cover the mouth and nose with a tissue when coughing or sneezing and to place used tissues in plastic bags

    d. Teaching the patient to wear a mask when in contact with crowds until the drugs suppress infection

5. Patient teaching about health and general care issues:

    a. Fatigue will diminish as the treatment progresses.

    b. Avoid exposure to any inhalation irritants, because they can cause further lung damage.

    c. Eat a well-balanced diet containing adequate amounts of protein and vitamins.

    d. Get adequate rest and sleep.

6. Report the TB infection to the local public health department

Community-Based Care

- Consult with the social service worker in the hospital or the community health nursing agency to ensure that the patient is discharged to the appropriate environment with continued supervision.

- Teach the patient to follow the drug regimen exactly as prescribed and always to have a supply on hand.

- Teach about side effects and ways of reducing them to ensure adherence.

- Remind the patient that the disease is usually no longer contagious after drugs have been taken for 2 to 3 consecutive weeks and clinical improvement is seen; however, he or she *must continue with the drugs for 6 months or longer as prescribed.*

- Determine the need for *directly observed therapy (DOT)*, in which the nurse or other health care provider watches the patient swallow the drugs.

- Remind the patient to receive follow-up care by a health care provider for at least 1 year during active treatment.
- Refer the patient to community resources such as the American Lung Association (ALA).
- Urge smokers to quit, and assist them in finding an appropriate smoking-cessation program.
- Ensure that active cases are reported to the local public health department or agency.

TUMORS, BRAIN

OVERVIEW

- Brain tumors can arise anywhere within the brain structures and are named according to the cell or tissue where they are located.
- *Primary tumors* originate within the central nervous system (CNS).
- *Secondary tumors (metastatic tumors)* spread to the brain from cancers in other body areas, such as the lungs, breast, kidney, and GI tract.
- Regardless of brain tumor type or location, the tumor expands and invades, infiltrates, compresses, and displaces normal brain tissue, leading to one or more problems, including:
  1. Cerebral edema/brain tissue inflammation
  2. Increased intracranial pressure (ICP); intracranial hypertension
  3. Neurologic deficits
  4. Hydrocephalus
  5. Pituitary dysfunction
  6. Seizure activity
- *Supratentorial tumors* are located within the cerebral hemispheres, and *infratentorial tumors* are located in the brainstem structures and cerebellum.
- Some brain tumors are benign (noninvasive), and others are cancerous. Regardless of type, most brain tumors must be treated or death will occur.
- Classification by cell type or tissue type includes tumors arising from:
  1. Neurons, which are responsible for nerve impulse conduction
  2. Neuroglial cells (glial cells), which provide support, nourishment, and protection
     a. Astrocytes (astrocytomas)
     b. Oligodendroglia
     c. Ependymal cells
     d. Microglia (gliomas, which are malignant)

3. Meninges, which are the coverings of the brain (meningiomas)
4. Pituitary (pituitary adenomas)
5. The sheath of Schwann cells in cranial nerve VII (acoustic neuromas)

- Metastatic, or secondary, tumors from other body areas make up about 30% of brain tumors.
- The exact cause of brain tumors is unknown but may be related to genetic changes, heredity, errors in fetal development, ionizing radiation, electromagnetic fields, environmental hazards, diet, viruses, or injury.

PATIENT-CENTERED COLLABORATIVE CARE
Assessment

- Obtain patient information about general symptoms of a brain tumor, including:
  1. Headaches that are usually more severe on awakening in the morning
  2. Nausea and vomiting
  3. Vision changes (blurred or double vision)
  4. Seizures
  5. Changes in mentation or personality
  6. Papilledema (swelling of the optic disc)
  7. Specific neurologic deficits:
     a. Supratentorial (cerebral) tumors usually result in paralysis, seizures, memory loss, cognitive impairment, language impairment, or vision problems.
     b. Infratentorial tumors produce ataxia, autonomic nervous system dysfunction, vomiting, drooling, hearing loss, and vision impairment.

- Diagnosis is based on the history, neurologic assessment, clinical examination, results of neurodiagnostic testing, computed tomography (CT), magnetic resonance imaging (MRI), and skull x-rays. Cerebral angiography, electroencephalography (EEG), lumbar puncture (LP), brain scan, and positron emission tomography (PET) may be also be used to further define the tumor.

Interventions
Nonsurgical Management

- Management depends on tumor size and location, patient symptoms and general condition, and whether the tumor is primary or has recurred.
- Drug therapy for symptom management may include:
  1. Analgesics for headache:
     a. Codeine
     b. Acetaminophen

2. Agents to control cerebral edema:
   a. Dexamethasone (Decadron)
   b. Glucocorticoids
3. Phenytoin (Dilantin) or other antiepileptic drug for seizure activity
4. Agents to prevent stress ulcers, typically proton pump inhibitors (e.g., pantoprazole [Protonix])
5. Institution-specific seizure precautions

- Chemotherapy may be given alone, in combination with radiation therapy and surgery, and with tumor progression. More than one agent may be given orally, IV, intra-arterially, or intrathecally through an Ommaya reservoir placed in a cranial ventricle. Both cytotoxic and targeted therapy agents may be used:
  1. Direct drug delivery to the tumor, using a disk-shaped drug wafer (polifeprosan 20 with carmustine implant [Gliadel]) placed directly into the cavity created during surgical tumor removal (interstitial chemotherapy), is an emerging practice.
  2. General management issues for care of patients undergoing chemotherapy are presented in Part One, under *Cancer Therapy.*

- Radiation therapy may be used alone, after surgery, or in combination with chemotherapy and surgery.
  1. Traditional external beam radiation may be used.
  2. A radioactive monoclonal antibody may be directly injected into the cavity from which the tumor was removed.
  3. General management issues for care of patients undergoing radiation therapy are presented in Part One under *Cancer Therapy.*

- Stereotactic radiosurgery (SRS) is an alternative to traditional surgery. Techniques used may include:
  1. Modified linear accelerator using accelerated x-rays (LINAC)
  2. Particle accelerator using beams of protons (cyclotron)
  3. Isotope seeds implanted in the tumor (brachytherapy)
  4. Gamma knife using a single high dose of ionized radiation to focus 201 beams of gamma radiation produced by the radioisotope cobalt 60
  5. CyberKnife

Surgical Management

- Brain biopsy is done to determine the specific pathology. Then a craniotomy (incision into the cranium) may be performed to improve symptoms related to the lesion or to decrease pressure effect from the tumor. Complete removal is possible with some tumors, which results in a "surgical cure."

1. Minimally invasive surgery (MIS) may involve:
   a. The transnasal approach with endoscopy for pituitary tumors
   b. Stereotactic surgery using burr holes and local anesthesia
   c. Laser surgery
2. In traditional open craniotomy, the patient's head is placed in a skull fixation device, and a piece of bone (bone flap) is removed to expose the tumor area. The tumor is removed, the bone flap is replaced, and a drain or monitoring device may be inserted.

- Provide preoperative care, including:
  1. Implementing routine preoperative care as described in Part One
  2. Allowing the patient to express anxiety and concerns about:
     a. Surgery into the brain
     b. Possibility of neurologic deficits
     c. Changes in appearance and self-image
  3. Teaching the patient and family about what to expect immediately after surgery and throughout the recovery period
  4. Ensuring that the patient has refrained from alcohol, tobacco, anticoagulants, or NSAIDs for at least 5 days before surgery

◼ NURSING SAFETY PRIORITY: Action Alert

The focus of postoperative care is to monitor the patient to detect changes in status and to prevent or minimize complications, especially increased ICP.

- Provide postoperative care, including:
  1. Implementing routine postoperative care as described in Part One
  2. Assessing neurologic (level of consciousness) and vital signs every 15 to 30 minutes for the first 4 to 6 hours after surgery and then every hour
  3. Assessing for:
     a. Decreased level of consciousness (LOC)
     b. Motor weakness or paralysis
     c. Aphasia
     d. Visual changes
     e. Personality changes
  4. Ensuring appropriate positioning:
     a. After supratentorial surgery:
        (1) Elevating the head of the bed 30 degrees
        (2) Avoiding extreme hip or neck flexion
        (3) Maintaining the head in a midline, neutral position
        (4) Placing the patient on the nonoperative side

b. After infratentorial (brainstem) craniotomy
   (1) Keeping the patient flat
   (2) Positioning the patient on either side for 24 to 48 hours
5. Maintaining NPO status for at least the first 24 hours after surgery
6. Administering prescribed drug therapy:
   a. Antiepileptic drugs
   b. Proton pump inhibitors
   c. Corticosteroids
   d. Analgesics
7. Monitoring the dressing every 1 to 2 hours for:
   a. Amount, type, and color of drainage
   b. Suction of drains maintained as prescribed

⚠ NURSING SAFETY PRIORITY: Critical Rescue

Immediately report a saturated head dressing or drainage greater than 50 mL in 8 hours to the surgeon.

8. Applying cold compresses for periorbital edema and ecchymosis of one or both eyes
9. Irrigating the affected eye with warm saline solution or artificial tears
10. Assessing the airway and managing mechanical ventilation:
    a. Keeping $Paco_2$ at about 35 mm Hg
    b. Keeping the arterial oxygen levels higher than 95 mm Hg
    c. Hyperoxygenating the patient carefully before suctioning
11. Assessing the cardiac monitor for dysrhythmias
12. Precisely measuring intake and output to maintain a balance, avoiding overhydration and underhydration
13. Implementing any prescribed fluid restriction
14. Ensuring that range of motion (ROM) exercises are performed with all extremities at least every 2 to 3 hours
15. Ensuring that the patient turns, coughs, and breathes deeply every 2 hours (if permitted)
16. Maintaining VTE prophylaxis until the patient ambulates
17. Monitoring laboratory values for changes and abnormalities:
    a. Complete blood count (CBC)
    b. Serum electrolyte levels and osmolarity
    c. Coagulation studies
    d. Arterial blood gases (ABGs)

18. Assessing for fluid volume overload or syndrome of inappropriate antidiuretic hormone (SIADH):
    a. Irritability
    b. Rapid weight gain
    c. Low serum sodium and potassium values
    d. Low urine output in relation to fluid intake
19. Assessing for diabetes insipidus (DI):
    a. High serum sodium and osmolarity
    b. Muscle weakness and restlessness
    c. Extreme thirst and dry mouth
    d. High output of dilute urine
20. Assessing for cerebral salt wasting (CSW):
    a. Low serum sodium and decreased osmolarity
    b. No dilution of other electrolytes or of hematocrit and hemoglobin
21. Preventing and assessing for other postoperative complications, including:
    a. Increased ICP:
       (1) Severe headache
       (2) Deteriorating LOC
       (3) Restlessness and irritability
       (4) Dilated or pinpoint pupils that are slow to react or nonreactive to light
    b. Subdural and epidural hematomas and intracranial hemorrhage:
       (1) Severe headache
       (2) Rapid change in LOC
       (3) Progressive neurologic deficits
       (4) Sudden cardiovascular and respiratory arrest
    c. Hydrocephalus (increased CSF in the brain)
    d. Respiratory complications:
       (1) Atelectasis
       (2) Pneumonia
       (3) Neurogenic pulmonary edema
    e. Wound infections:
       (1) Reddened and puffy wound appearance
       (2) Area sensitive to touch
       (3) Area warm
    f. Meningitis

Community-Based Care
- Assist the family to make the environment safe for prevention of falls (e.g., remove scatter rugs, install grab bars in the bathroom).

- When needed, work with the case manager or discharge planner to help the family select a facility with experience in providing care for neurologically impaired patients.
- Teach patients and families about:
  1. Seizure precautions and what to do if a seizure occurs
  2. Drug therapy and person to call if adverse drug events occur
  3. Avoiding any over-the-counter (OTC) drugs unless approved by the health care provider
  4. The importance of recommended follow-up health care appointments
  5. The need for adequate caloric intake during radiation therapy or chemotherapy
- Refer the patient and family to support groups and community resources such as the American Brain Tumor Association, the National Brain Tumor Foundation, the American Cancer Society, home care agencies, and hospice services or palliative care services (for those who are terminally ill).

ULCERS, PEPTIC

OVERVIEW

- A peptic ulcer is a mucosal lesion of the stomach or duodenum. The term is used to describe both gastric and duodenal ulcers.
- Peptic ulcer disease (PUD) results when mucosal defenses become impaired and no longer protect the epithelium from the effects of acid and pepsin.
- Peptic ulcer development is primarily associated with bacterial infection with *Helicobacter pylori* and NSAID use. Caffeine, smoking, alcohol, and radiation contribute to PUD.
- Recurrent ulcer can be caused by incomplete vagotomy or persistent *H. pylori* infection.
- Types of peptic ulcers include:
  1. *Gastric ulcer,* which occurs when there is a break in the mucosal barrier and hydrochloric acid injures the epithelium. Gastric emptying is delayed, causing regurgitation of duodenal contents. Gastric ulcers are deep and penetrating, and they usually occur on the lesser curvature of the stomach near the pylorus.
  2. *Duodenal ulcer,* a chronic break in the duodenal mucosa that extends through the muscularis mucosa and leaves a scar after healing. It is characterized by high gastric acid secretion and is the most common type of peptic ulcer.
  3. *Stress ulcer,* which occurs with acute and chronic diseases or major trauma. Bleeding resulting from gastric erosion is the principal manifestation, and multiple lesions occur in the

proximal portion of the stomach, beginning with the area of
ischemia and evolving into erosions.
- Complications of PUD include:
  1. Hemorrhage
  2. Perforation, with the gastroduodenal contents emptying
     through the anterior wall of the stomach or duodenum into
     the peritoneal cavity
  3. Pyloric obstruction
  4. Intractable disease, which is characterized by lack of re-
     sponse to conservative management and with symptoms
     that interfere with ADLs

PATIENT-CENTERED COLLABORATIVE CARE
Assessment
- Obtain patient information about:
  1. Tobacco use
  2. Dietary intake, including alcohol, caffeine, other foods
     known to cause gastric irritation, and patterns of eating
  3. Medical history focusing on GI problems
  4. Prescribed and over-the-counter (OTC) drugs, such as cor-
     ticosteroids and NSAIDs
  5. Recent severe, serious, complex, or traumatic illness
  6. Symptoms, including epigastric discomfort, abdominal ten-
     derness, cramps, indigestion, nausea, or vomiting and their
     onset, duration, location, and frequency, as well as aggravat-
     ing and alleviating factors, including sleep patterns
  7. Presence of chronic disease and recent changes in flares or
     medications
- Assess for and document:
  1. Epigastric pain and tenderness; rigid, boardlike abdomen
     accompanied by rebound tenderness (if perforation
     occurred)
  2. Effect of eating on GI symptoms, because gastric ulcer pain
     may be relieved by food, and duodenal ulcer pain occurs
     90 minutes to 3 hours after eating and often awakens the
     patient at night
  3. Dyspepsia and effects of certain foods that may exacerbate
     GI symptoms
  4. Melena, especially in older adults
  5. Vomiting
  6. Orthostatic vital signs
  7. Deficient fluid volume, including orthostatic hypotension
     and dizziness
  8. Low hemoglobin and hematocrit levels
  9. Results of esophagogastroduodenoscopy (EGD), which
     visualizes the ulcer

U

10. *H. pylori* testing
11. Impact of chronic disease on the patient
- Diagnostic studies may include:
  1. Hemoglobin and hematocrit levels
  2. Testing for *H. pylori*
  3. An upper GI series if no perforation is suspected,
  4. If perforation is suspected, the health care provider usually requests abdominal computed tomography (CT) scan.
  5. The major diagnostic test for PUD is EGD, which is the most accurate means of establishing a diagnosis. Direct visualization of the ulcer crater by EGD allows the health care provider to take specimens for *H. pylori* testing and for biopsy and cytologic studies for ruling out gastric cancer.

Considerations for Older Adults
- The older adult may use OTC remedies to treat symptoms, often delaying appropriate treatment for PUD.
- Ulcer-producing drugs for chronic illnesses are often consumed by older adults.
- The older adult may be at increased risk for bleeding, complications, and death with hemorrhagic PUD.

Planning and Implementation
ACUTE OR CHRONIC PAIN
- Perform a comprehensive pain assessment. Carefully assess changes in the characteristic of location or peptic ulcer pain, because this may indicate the development of complications.
- Drug therapy includes:
  1. Proton pump inhibitors (PPI) or histamine (H_2) receptor blockersto inhibit gastric acid secretion
  2. As an alternative to PPI or H_2 blockers, prostaglandin analogues to inhibit acid secretion and contribute to the mucosal barrier
  3. Antacids as buffering agents to decrease pain (given 2 hours after meals)
  4. Mucosal barrier fortifiers to provide a protective coat, preventing digestive action
  5. *H. pylori* infection treatment with 1 to 2 antibiotics and a drug to reduce gastric acidity, most often a PPI or H_2 blocker. Antibiotics may include metronidazole, amoxicillin, ciprofloxacin, or tetracycline.
- There is no evidence that dietary restrictions reduce gastric acid secretion or promote tissue healing. When diet therapy is used, teach the patient to:
  1. Avoid caffeine-containing coffee, tea, and cola and other foods that cause discomfort.
  2. Avoid alcohol and tobacco.

- Monitor for gastric outflow or pyloric obstruction caused by edema, spasm, or scar tissue. Obstruction may be manifested by abdominal pain, bloating, distention, tenderness, and reduced bowel sounds.

RISK FOR GI BLEEDING
Nonsurgical Management

- The patient is at risk for fluid volume deficit (hypovolemia), hemorrhage, and perforation.
  1. Management of hypovolemia includes:
     a. Monitoring vital signs to detect hypovolemia manifested by tachycardia, hypotension, increased rate and depth of respirations, decreased SpO_2, and reduced level of consciousness
     b. Recording volumes of fluid loss from bleeding or vomiting
     c. Maintaining strict intake and output
     d. Monitoring serum electrolytes and hematocrit and hemoglobin for derangements from a normal range and reporting derangements to the prescribing health care provider in a timely manner
     e. Inserting two peripheral IV catheters (see *Shock*)
     f. Replacing fluids with IV fluids such as normal saline or lactated Ringer's solution
     g. Ordering blood products in the presence of symptomatic anemia or hypoxemia from low hemoglobin
  2. Management of hemorrhage includes:
     a. Monitoring for signs and symptoms indicating GI bleeding and documenting findings:
        (1) Observe secretions (emesis, sputum, stool, urine, and nasogastric drainage) for frank or occult blood.
        (2) Document color, amount, and character of stools.
        (3) Obtain stool to test for occult blood and report positive results to prescribing health care provider.
        (4) Monitor hematocrit, hemoglobin, and coagulation studies for changes from baseline.
     b. Inserting a nasogastric (NG) tube to ascertain the presence of blood in the stomach, assess the rate of bleeding, prevent gastric dilation, and provide lavage; irrigating the NG tube to maintain patency and prevent obstruction with blood
     c. Administering acid-decreasing drugs such as a proton pump inhibitor or H_2 histamine blocker
     d. Treatment measures include:
        (1) EGD to identify and coagulate bleeding sites
        (2) Possible room temperature, sterile water, or saline lavage through the NG tube to remove gastric blood

U

3. Management of perforation includes the immediate replacement of fluid, blood, and electrolytes:
   a. Maintain NG suction to drain gastric secretions.
   b. Keep the patient on NPO status, and monitor intake and output carefully to avoid dehydration and poor perfusion.
   c. Check the patient's vital signs at least once hourly.
   d. Monitor the patient for poor systemic perfusion or symptoms of shock.
   e. Anticipate emergency surgery (see *Perioperative Care* in Part One).

Community-Based Care

- Collaborate with the patient and family to identify gastric irritants
- Instruct the patient about symptoms that should be brought to the attention of the health care provider:
  1. Abdominal pain
  2. Nausea and vomiting
  3. Black, tarry stools
  4. Weakness and dizziness
- Instruct the patient to avoid NSAIDs unless under the care of a health care provider who may prescribe concurrent acid-reducing medication.
- Teach dietary management to the postoperative patient, especially the patient who has had a partial stomach removal:
  1. Eat small volume meals.
  2. Avoid drinking liquids with meals.
  3. Abstain from foods that contribute to discomfort.
  4. Eliminate caffeine and alcohol consumption.
  5. Begin a smoking cessation program.
  6. Receive vitamin B_{12} injections as appropriate.
- Teach the patient and family to recognize symptoms of pyloric obstruction that can occur from edema, spasm, or scar tissue. Symptoms of obstruction related to difficulty in emptying the stomach include feelings of fullness, distention, or nausea after eating, as well as vomiting copious amounts of undigested food.

URETHRITIS

- Urethritis is inflammation of the urethra.
- Symptoms of urethritis are:
  1. Burning, painful urination similar to cystitis/urinary tract infection symptoms
  2. Urgency and frequency
  3. Weak urine stream (men)
  4. Incontinence

5. Discharge from the urethral meatus, especially in men
6. Pyuria (cloudy) or foul-smelling urine
- The most common cause of urethritis in males is sexually transmitted disease (STD).
- In postmenopausal women, urethritis is probably caused by tissue changes related to low estrogen levels, and it is treated with estrogen vaginal cream.
- Noninfectious urethritis may be caused by increased serum urea levels.
- STDs and infectious processes are treated with appropriate antibiotic therapy.

URINARY INCONTINENCE

OVERVIEW
- Urinary incontinence (UI) is the involuntary loss of urine that is severe enough to cause social or hygienic problems. It may be transient or permanent. It is not a normal change associated with aging.
- Common forms of urinary incontinence (UI):
    1. *Stress incontinence* is the loss of small amounts of urine during coughing, sneezing, jogging, or lifting. Patients are unable to tighten the urethra sufficiently to overcome the increased detrusor pressure, and leakage of urine results.
    2. *Urge UI* is the involuntary loss of urine associated with a sudden, strong desire to urinate. Patients are unable to suppress the signal for bladder contractions. It is also known as *overactive bladder*.
    3. *Mixed incontinence* is a combination of stress and urge incontinence.
    4. *Reflex incontinence* occurs when the bladder has reached a specific bladder volume. There is a decreased or absent ability to sense a full bladder, usually from neurologic impairment or bladder damage.
    5. *Functional incontinence* is leakage of urine caused by factors other than pathology of the lower urinary tract, such as impaired cognition, impaired vision, or inability to reach a toilet.
- In adult patients younger than 65 years, incontinence occurs twice as often in women than in men.

PATIENT-CENTERED COLLABORATIVE CARE
Assessment
- Obtain patient information:
    1. Presence and severity of incontinence with effective screening questions. Ask the patient to respond with *always*, *sometimes*, or *never* to the following questions:

   a. Do you ever leak urine when you do not want to?
   b. Do you ever leak urine or water when you cough, laugh, or exercise?
   c. Do you ever leak urine on the way to the bathroom?
   d. Do you ever use pads, tissue, or cloth in your underwear to catch urine?
2. Risk factors for UI
   a. Age
   b. Menopausal status
   c. Conditions that may affect the autonomic nervous system or cognition, such as:
      (1) Parkinson disease
      (2) Dementia
      (3) Multiple sclerosis
      (4) Stroke
      (5) Neurogenic complications from diabetes mellitus
      (6) Spinal cord injury
   d. Childbirth
   e. Urologic procedures
   f. Drugs, especially drugs that affect the autonomic nervous system
   g. Bowel pattern
   h. Stress or anxiety level
3. Limited mobility, reduced ability to ambulate and to transfer to a chair or toilet
4. Communication pattern
5. Barriers to toileting:
   a. Lack of privacy
   b. Restrictive clothing
   c. Access to toilet
6. Presence of urinary tract infection (cystitis). Assess for and document the findings:
   a. Palpate the abdominal area for evidence of bladder fullness.
   b. Percuss the abdomen, and listen for the dull sound of a distended bladder.
   c. Observe for urine leakage while the patient strains by coughing or bearing down in the standing position.
   d. Determine the amount of residual urine by portable ultrasound or by catheterizing the patient immediately after voiding.
   e. Inspect the external genitalia of women to determine urethral or uterine prolapse, cystocele, or rectocele.
   f. Describe any secretions from the genitourinary openings.

   g. Inspect the urinary meatus of men for the presence of discharge or other characteristics.

   h. Query the patient regarding the effects of incontinence on socialization, family relationships, and emotional status.

   i. Monitor the urine for color, odor, and presence of sediment or cloudiness, and report abnormal results of a urinalysis in a timely manner to the prescribing health care provider.

   j. Review the results of the voiding cystourethrogram, which detects the anatomic structure and function of the bladder, as well as the postvoiding residual.

Planning and Implementation
REDUCING STRESS URINARY INCONTINENCE
Nonsurgical Management

- Nonsurgical management of incontinence may include:
  1. Drug therapy to reduce urgency and frequency
     a. Phenylpropanolamine, an alpha-adrenergic agonist
     b. Tricyclic antidepressants: imipramine (Tofranil, Novo-Pramine ♥)
     c. Estrogen for postmenopausal women
     d. Tolterodine, an anticholinergic
  2. Dietary counseling to assist the obese patient with weight loss and to encourage all patients to avoid alcohol and caffeine (bladder irritants)
     a. Collaborate with the nutritionist to promote goals to achieve body weight goals.
  3. Exercise therapy:
     a. Teach women how to do Kegel exercises to strengthen the muscles of the pelvic floor; biofeedback devices may be used to help the patient detect the effectiveness of the exercises.
     b. Instruct the patient in the correct use of vaginal cones:
        (1) The lightest cone is inserted into the vagina with the string to the outside for a 1-minute test period.
        (2) If the patient is able to hold the first cone in place without its slipping out while she walks around, she proceeds to the second cone and repeats the procedure.
        (3) Treatment is begun with the heaviest cone that the patient can hold in her vagina for the 1-minute test period.
        (4) The treatment is for 15 minutes twice daily; when the patient can hold the cone comfortably in her vagina for 15 minutes, proceed to the next heaviest weight.

U

4. Other treatments include behavior modification, psycho-
therapy, and electrical devices for the inhibition of bladder
contraction.
   a. The Reliance insert is a tampon-like device inserted into
   the urethra. The patient inflates the attached balloon,
   which prevents urine flow.

Surgical Management

- Provide preoperative care as described in Part One.
- Operative procedures for women are used to elevate the bladder
  and urethra into a normal intra-abdominal position, increase
  the length of the urethra, and decrease hypermobility of the
  bladder neck:
    1. Anterior vaginal repair (colporrhaphy) to elevate the urethra
       and repair any cystocele
    2. Retropubic suspension to elevate the urethra and provide
       longer-lasting results
    3. Needle bladder neck suspension (Pereyra or Stamey proce-
       dure) to elevate the urethra and provide a longer-lasting
       result without a long operative time
    4. Pubovaginal sling procedure, in which a sling made of syn-
       thetic material is placed under the urethrovesical junction to
       elevate the bladder neck
    5. An artificial sphincter, a mechanical device that opens and
       closes the urethra, placed around the anatomic urethra;
       the procedure is used for men more often than for women.
- Provide postoperative care as described earlier, and take the following steps:
    1. Secure the urethral catheter to prevent unnecessary move-
       ment or traction on the bladder neck.
    2. Monitor the suprapubic catheter, if present, for leakage of
       urine and serosanguineous drainage.

REDUCING URGE URINARY INCONTINENCE

- Interventions for urge UI include drug and behavioral interventions such as bladder and habit training. Surgery is not
  recommended:
    1. Drug therapy includes:
        a. Anticholinergic agents and anticholinergics with smooth
           muscle relaxant properties
        b. Tricyclic antidepressants
    2. Diet therapy includes:
        a. Instructing the patient to avoid foods that have a bladder-
           stimulating effect, such as caffeine and alcohol
        b. Instructing the patient to space fluids throughout the day
           and to limit fluids after dinner

3. Bladder training is an educational program to help patients gain control of their bladder:
   a. A regular schedule of voiding is established.
   b. The patient is instructed to void during the established time frame and to ignore any urge to urinate that occurs between the mandated interval.
   c. After the patient is comfortable with the initial interval, the interval time is increased by 15 to 30 minutes.
4. Habit training is a variation of bladder training that is useful for cognitively impaired patients. The caregiver assists the patient to void every 2 hours.
5. Exercise therapies, such as Kegel exercises and vaginal cone therapy, are also useful.
6. Electrical stimulation with a variety of intravaginal and intrarectal devices has been used to treat both stress and urge UI.

REDUCING REFLEX URINARY INCONTINENCE

- Interventions for reflex incontinence include surgery, drugs, and teaching the patient interventions to empty the bladder. Avoid urine volumes greater than 300 mL to maintain continence in this condition:
  1. Surgery, which includes removal of the prostate and repair of genital prolapse to relieve the obstruction of the bladder outlet
  2. Drug therapy, which includes bethanechol chloride for the short-term management of urinary retention
  3. Interventions can assist with bladder emptying:
     a. Using or teaching the Credé maneuver, Valsalva maneuver, or double-voiding technique to assist in promoting bladder contraction
     b. Teaching intermittent self-catheterization to patients with neurogenic bladder disorders and other long-term problems of incomplete bladder emptying

REDUCING FUNCTIONAL URINARY INCONTINENCE

- The primary focus of the intervention is to treat reversible causes of incontinence. When that is not possible, the goal is to contain the urine and protect the patient's skin. Interventions include:
  1. Altering the environment so the patient can reach the toilet easily
  2. Implementing habit training for the cognitively impaired patient
  3. Using absorbent pads and briefs to collect urine and keep the patient's skin and clothing dry

4. Using an external catheter for men or any patient, inserting a Foley catheter, or implementing intermittent catheterization, especially when perineal skin impairment is present

■ NURSING SAFETY PRIORITY: Critical Rescue

Assessing the patient's risk for incontinence while he or she is hospitalized is an essential step in preventing iatrogenic skin damage and preventing pressure ulcer formation.

Community-Based Care
- Discharge planning includes:
  1. Assessing the home environment for barriers that impede access to the toileting facilities
  2. Considering the personal, physical, emotional, and social resources of the patient
  3. Considering who the primary caretaker will be and what circumstances or factors exist in the environment that will influence the effectiveness of the plan
  4. Assisting the patient to control or manage fears and anxieties related to incontinence while in public
  5. Referring the patient to home care agencies
- Teach the patient and family about:
  1. The causes of incontinence and treatment options available
  2. Prescribed drugs (purpose, dosage, method, route of administration, and expected and potential side effects)
  3. The importance of weight reduction and dietary modification
  4. Options available for external devices or incontinence pads, considering the patient's lifestyle and resources
  5. The technique of self-catheterization, ensuring that a return demonstration is correct

UROLITHIASIS

OVERVIEW
- Urolithiasis is the presence of calculi (stones) in the urinary tract. Stones often do not cause symptoms until they pass into the lower urinary tract, where they can cause excruciating pain. Nephrolithiasis is the formation of stones in the kidney. Formation of stones in the ureter is ureterolithiasis.
- The exact mechanism of formation is not known, but three factors contribute to stone formation through slow urine flow, resulting in supersaturation of the urine with the particular element (e.g., calcium) that first becomes crystallized and later becomes the stone:

1. Damage to the lining of the urinary tract (from crystals)
2. Decreased inhibitor substances in the urine that would otherwise prevent supersaturation and crystal aggregation
3. High urine acidity (as with uric acid and cystine stones), high alkalinity (as with calcium phosphate and struvite stones), and drugs (triamterene, indinavir, and acetazolamide)

- Calculi may be formed from calcium, phosphate, oxalate, uric acid, struvite, and cystine crystals, but most stones contain calcium as one component.

⊕ Cultural Awareness

- There is an increased incidence of urolithiasis in the southeastern United States and a rising incidence in Japan and Western Europe.

- Urolithiasis is more common in men than in women and tends to occur in young adulthood or early middle adulthood.

PATIENT-CENTERED COLLABORATIVE CARE
Assessment
- Obtain patient information about:
  1. History of renal stones
  2. Family history of renal stones
  3. Metabolic disorders and diet history
  4. Previous interventions to eliminate stones
- Assess for and document:
  1. Location and duration of pain, which is often described as severe, unbearable, spasmodic (colic), and in the region of the trunk, back, and thighs ("flank" pain)
  2. Nausea and vomiting
  3. Hematuria, oliguria, or anuria
  4. Increased turbidity and odor of urine
  5. Bladder distention
  6. Diaphoresis
  7. Pale, ashen skin
  8. Presence of red blood cells (RBCs), white blood cells (WBCs), and bacteria in the urine

Planning and Implementation
MANAGE ACUTE PAIN
  Nonsurgical Management
- Drug therapy includes:
  1. Opioid agents, such as hydromorphone or morphine
  2. NSAIDs, such as ketorolac (Toradol)
  3. Spasmolytic agents, such as oxybutynin chloride (Ditropan) and propantheline bromide (Pro-Banthine, Propanthel)
- Assess the patient's response to drug interventions.

- Encourage ambulation and an upright position to drain the renal calyx and pass renal calculi.
- Assist the patient to find a comfortable position and to use relaxation techniques.
- Distraction or relaxation techniques such as hypnosis, imagery, or acupuncture can be used to relieve pain.
- Lithotripsy, or extracorporeal shock wave lithotripsy (ESWL), is the application of ultrasound or dry shock wave energies to fragment the calculus. The patient receives conscious sedation as the lithotriptor and fluoroscope locate and break up the calculus. After lithotripsy, implement routine postoperative care with additional monitoring for urine output (quantity, quality, and presence of sediment or stones).

Surgical Management

- Stone removal procedures include:
  1. *Ureteroscopy,* which is the use of an endoscope through the urethra to visualize stones and to extract stones with a basket, or the use of a laser to fragment stones. Stents may be used to dilate the ureter and create a passageway for the stone.
  2. *Percutaneous ureterolithotomy and nephrolithotomy,* or the use of an endoscope to visualize the stone with a special attachment to extract the calculus through a small flank incision
  3. *Laparoscopic ureterolithotomy,* which is the use of a laparoscope through the ureter to remove the calculus
  4. *Pyelolithotomy,* which is direct visualization of renal pelvis through a large flank incision and removal of stone
  5. *Nephrolithotomy,* which is direct visualization of the kidney through a large flank incision and removal of the stone
  6. *Ureterolithotomy,* which is direct visualization of the ureter through a large flank or lower abdominal incision and removal of the stone
- Preoperative care includes routine care described in Part One and:
  1. Providing individualized instructions, depending on the procedure to be performed
  2. Preparing bowel according to the physician's preference
- Postoperative care includes routine care described in Part One and:
  1. Monitoring the amount and character (color, presence of sediment or clots) of urine output every 1 to 2 hours for 24 hours to prevent urinary obstruction from stone fragments or clots
  2. Straining the patient's urine to capture stones for analysis
  3. Reducing risk for infection including:
     a. Monitoring for signs of infection (fever, chills, altered mental status)

    b. Evaluating the results of serum and urine tests

    c. Administering antibiotics to eliminate existing infections or prevent new ones and monitoring patient responses including serum drug levels

    d. Ensuring adequate nutrition and fluid intake, which may include additional fluid intake to "flush" the kidneys for the first 24 hours after diagnosis.

4. Administering drug therapy to promote elimination of chemicals contributing to stone formation and assessing for adverse effects, including:

    a. Acetohydroxamic acid (Lithostat) and hydroxyurea (Hydrea) for patients with struvite stones; monitoring serum creatinine levels (contraindicated for levels above 2 mg/dL)

    b. Thiazide diuretics to treat hypercalciuria (high levels of calcium in the urine)

    c. Allopurinol (Zyloprim) and vitamin B_6 (pyridoxine) to treat hyperoxaluria (high levels of oxalic acid in the urine) or gout

    d. Alpha-mercaptopropionylglycine (AMPG) and captopril (Capoten) to treat cystinuria (high levels of cystine in the urine)

Community-Based Care

- Inform the patient that:
  1. Extensive bruising may occur after lithotripsy and may take several weeks to resolve.
  2. Urine may be bloody for several days after surgical intervention.

- Instructing the patient about:
  1. The importance of following the prescribed drug regimen
  2. Diet, depending on metabolic evaluation or stone type
  3. The rationale for preventing dehydration, stressing the importance of dilute urine from adequate fluid intake
  4. The importance of reporting symptoms of infection or formation of another stone, such as pain, fever, chills, and difficulty with urination
  5. The importance of keeping follow-up appointments to check on resolution of symptoms or postoperative recovery

UTERINE BLEEDING (DYSFUNCTIONAL)

OVERVIEW

- Dysfunctional uterine bleeding (DUB) is bleeding that is excessive or frequent (more than every 21 days).
- Most cases of DUB are classified into two types: anovulatory DUB (most common) and ovulatory DUB.

- DUB is associated with polycystic ovary disease, stress, extreme weight changes, and long-term use of drugs, including anticholinergics, morphine, and oral contraceptives.

PATIENT-CENTERED COLLABORATIVE CARE
Assessment
- Common risk factors for DUB include:
  1. Extreme weight loss or gain
  2. Age over 40
  3. High stress levels
  4. Polycystic ovary disease
  5. Long-term drug use (e.g., oral contraceptives)
  6. Excessive exercise
  7. Anatomic abnormalities such as leiomyomas (fibroids)

Interventions
Nonsurgical Management
- Hormone therapy with progestin or combined estrogen-progestin therapy.
- Evaluate the patient's knowledge about the effects, dosage, and administration schedule of her prescribed hormone therapy.
- Teach the patient the information she needs to know about her prescribed hormone therapy.

Surgical Management
- Surgical management includes laser endometrial ablation, uterine artery embolization, dilation and curettage, and hysterectomy.
- Nursing care is similar to that for a woman undergoing a vaginal hysterectomy (see *Surgical Management* under *Leiomyomas, Uterine*).

UTERINE FIBROIDS (LEIOMYOMAS)

See *Leiomyomas (Uterine Fibroids)*.

UVEITIS

OVERVIEW
- Uveitis is a general term for inflammation of the eye's uveal tract. It may occur in the anterior or posterior portion of the eye.
- Anterior uveitis:
  1. May be inflammation of the iris, inflammation of the ciliary body, or both
  2. The cause of anterior uveitis is unknown but often follows exposure to allergens, infectious agents, trauma, or systemic disease (rheumatoid arthritis, herpes simplex, herpes zoster). It can follow any local or systemic bacterial infection.

3. Manifestations include aching around the eye; tearing; blurred vision; photophobia; a small, irregular, nonreactive pupil; and a "bloodshot" appearance of the sclera.
- Posterior uveitis:
  1. Posterior uveitis involves inflammation of the retina (retinitis) or inflammation of both the choroid and the retina (chorioretinitis).
  2. Common causes include tuberculosis, syphilis, and toxoplasmosis.
  3. Manifestations include visual impairment in the affected eye; a small, nonreactive, and irregularly shaped pupil; black dots on the optic fundus; and grayish yellow patches on the retinal surface.

PATIENT-CENTERED COLLABORATIVE CARE
- Drug therapies:
  1. Resting the ciliary body with a cycloplegic agent
  2. Administering steroid drops given hourly to reduce the inflammation and to prevent adhesion of the iris to the cornea and lens
- Symptom management:
  1. Applying cool or warm compresses
  2. Darkening the room, having the patient wear dark glasses
- Safety management:
  1. Instructing the patient not to drive or operate machinery
  2. Reviewing the manifestations of eye ulcers and those of increased intraocular pressure (IOP)

VANCOMYCIN-RESISTANT ENTEROCOCCUS

V

OVERVIEW
- Enterococci are bacteria that live in the intestinal tract and are important for digestion. These organisms are tougher than other bacteria, because they must survive pH changes, enzymes, and other environmental dangers. As long as they remain only in the intestinal tract, they pose no health problem.
- When they move to another area of the body, such as during surgery, they can cause an infection, which usually is treatable with the antibiotic vancomycin. However, in recent years, more than one fourth of these bacterial strains have become resistant to the drug, and infection with vancomycin-resistant enterococci (VRE) results.
- Unfortunately, VRE can live on almost any surface (e.g., toilet seats, door handles, other objects) for days or weeks and still be able to cause an infection.

- The most common infections caused by VRE include wound infections, urinary tract infections (UTIs), and bloodstream infections.
- Risk factors for this infection apply to patients who:
  1. Are hospitalized, especially in the ICU, and have received prolonged antibiotic therapy
  2. Have been previously treated with the antibiotic vancomycin or other antibiotics for long periods
  3. Are immunosuppressed (patients receiving cancer chemotherapy, have HIV disease, have received solid organ or bone marrow transplants) or are taking immunosuppressive drugs
  4. Have extensive open wounds or have undergone surgical procedures such as abdominal or chest surgery
  5. Have a long-term internal medical device that opens to the outside, such as urinary catheters, central venous catheters, and peripherally inserted central catheters (PICCs)
- Most VRE infections occur in hospitals.

PATIENT-CENTERED COLLABORATIVE CARE
- Management includes use of contact precautions for patients who are hospitalized with VRE infection, recent infection, or colonization. Also:
  1. People who have intestinal or mucous membrane VRE do not usually need antibiotic treatment if they are colonized.
  2. For patients with indwelling urinary catheters and a VRE UTI, catheter removal usually halts the infection.
  3. VRE infections can be treated with antibiotics other than vancomycin after culture and sensitivity testing to determine which antibiotics are most likely to be effective.
- Prevention:
  1. Performing meticulous hand-washing with soap and water is the best method of preventing VRE spread.
  2. Using special cleaning of rooms and items in contact with patients who have VRE infection

VASCULAR DISEASE, PERIPHERAL

- Peripheral vascular disease (PVD) includes disorders that alter the natural flow of blood through the arteries and veins of the peripheral circulation.
- It affects the lower extremities much more commonly than the upper extremities.
- A diagnosis of PVD usually implies arterial disease rather than venous involvement. Some patients have arterial and venous disease.
- Atherosclerosis is the most common cause of peripheral arterial disease (PAD) (see *Peripheral Arterial Disease, Atherosclerosis*).

VEINS, VARICOSE

- Varicose veins are distended, protruding veins that appear darkened or tortuous.
- The vein walls weaken and dilate. Venous pressure increases, and the valves become incompetent. Incompetent valves enhance vessel dilation, and veins become tortuous and distended.
- Varicose veins occur primarily in patients subjected to prolonged standing. They also occur in pregnant women and in patients with systemic problems, such as heart disease or obesity, and a family history of varicose veins.
- Conservative treatment measures include:
  1. Wearing elastic stockings
  2. Elevating the legs as often as possible
- Outpatient surgery includes routine perioperative care and restrictions to weight-bearing for several days. Procedures include:
  1. Sclerotherapy, in which the physician injects a chemical to sclerose the vein, performed on small or a limited number of varicosities
  2. Laser treatment uses a laser to heat and close the main vessel that is contributing to the varicosity.
  3. Radiofrequency (RF) ablation involves heating the vein from the inside by the RF energy and shrinking the vein. Surgical intervention entails ligation (tying) and stripping (removal) the affected veins with the patient under general anesthesia.
- Collateral veins take over supplying blood to tissues after laser, RF, or surgical interventions.

VENOUS THROMBOEMBOLISM

V

Venous thromboembolism (VTE) includes both thrombus and embolus complications. A thrombus (also called a *thrombosis*) is a blood clot believed to result from an endothelial injury, venous stasis, or hypercoagulability.

VISUAL IMPAIRMENT (REDUCED VISION)

OVERVIEW

- Visual impairment can range from total blindness in both eyes to various degrees and types of partial impairment.
- Patients are legally blind if their best visual acuity with corrective lenses is 20/200 or less in the better eye or if the widest diameter of the visual field in that eye is no greater than 20 degrees.
- Blindness can occur in one or both eyes. When one eye is affected, the field of vision is narrowed, and depth perception is impaired.

- Central vision can be impaired by diseases involving the macula, such as macular edema or macular degeneration.
- Peripheral vision loss affects the patient's ability to drive and awareness of hazards in the periphery.

PATIENT-CENTERED COLLABORATIVE CARE

- Test the visual acuity of both eyes immediately of any person who experiences an eye injury or any sudden change in vision.
- Ask the patient about vision problems in any other members of the family, because some vision problems have a genetic component.
- Urge all patients to wear eye protection when they are performing yard work, working in a woodshop or metal shop, using chemicals, or are in any environment in which drops or particulate matter is airborne.
- Nursing interventions for the patient with reduced sight focus on teaching patients techniques to make better use of existing vision, communication, safety, ambulation, self-care, and support.
  1. To make better use of existing vision, teach the patient:
     a. To move the head slightly up and down to enhance a three-dimensional effect
     b. When shaking hands or pouring water, to line up the object and move toward it
     c. To choose a position that favors the good eye; for example, people with vision in the right eye should position people and items on their right
  2. Instruct the patient about safety:
     a. Teach patients to count the number of footsteps needed to move from one area to another
     b. Stress to hospital staff, family, and friends that changes in item location should not be made without input from the person with reduced vision.
     c. Orient the patient to the immediate environment, including the size of the room. Use one object in the room, such as a chair or hospital bed, as the focal point during your description. Guide the person to the focal point and describe all other objects in relation to the focal point.
     d. Go with the patient to other important areas, such as the bathroom. Highlight landmarks such as the location of the toilet, sink, and toilet paper holder.

■ NURSING SAFETY PRIORITY: Action Alert

Never leave the patient with reduced vision in the center of an unfamiliar room.

    e. Allow the patient to establish the location of important objects, such as the call bell, water pitcher, and clock. Do not move these items after their locations have been fixed.

    f. Set up food trays using imaginary clock placement to orient the patient to the location of specific items.

3. Teach safe ambulation:

    a. Allow the patient to grasp your arm at the elbow while keeping the arm close to your body so that he or she can detect your direction of movement.

    b. Alert the patient when obstacles are in the path ahead.

    c. Assist with the correct use of a cane to detect obstacles (the cane is held in the dominant hand several inches off the floor and sweeps the ground where the patient's foot will be placed next).

4. Promote self-management:

    a. Knock on the door before entering the room and state your name and the reason for visiting when entering the room. Use a normal tone of voice unless there is a hearing problem.

    b. Explain all diagnostic procedures, restrictions, and follow-up care to the patient scheduled for tests.

    c. Encourage the mastery of one task at a time.

    d. Provide positive reinforcement for each success when adapting to visual loss or impairment.

    e. Use local resources that provide adaptive items such as large print books for reduced vision or talking clocks for any impaired vision.

5. Provide emotional support:

    a. Provide opportunities for the patient and family to express their concerns about a possible change in vision status.

    b. Allow the newly blind person a period of grieving for loss of vision.

W

WEST NILE VIRUS

- West Nile virus infection is spread by infected mosquitoes and contaminated substances such as blood products, breast milk, or organ transplantation.
- Although not common in the United States, the Centers for Disease Control tracks exposure and infections for all 50 states annually, with warm weather states reporting the most cases (i.e., Arizona, California, Florida, and Mississippi).

- The infection is generally mild, and the patient usually is asymptomatic or has only flu-like symptoms (e.g., fever, body aches, nausea, vomiting).
- A small percentage of patients develop encephalitis with symptoms that include:
  1. High fever
  2. Severe headache
  3. Decreased level of consciousness
  4. Tremors
  5. Vision loss
  6. Seizures
  7. Muscle weakness or paralysis
- Diagnostic tests include enzyme-linked immunosorbent assay (ELISA) and West Nile virus-specific IgM antibody in serum or cerebrospinal fluid (CSF).
- Management is symptomatic, as for any other type of viral encephalitis.
- For the severe form of the disease, manifestations may last for several weeks, and neurologic deficits may be permanent.
- To prevent West Nile Virus infection, avoid mosquito bites by using an insect repellent containing an Environmental Protection Agency (EPA)-registered active ingredient such as DEET or Picaridin, wearing long sleeves and pants at dusk when mosquitoes abound or consider staying indoors during these hours, making sure you have good screens on your windows and doors to keep mosquitoes out, and getting rid of mosquito breeding sites by emptying standing water from flower pots, buckets, wading pools, and barrels. Do not handle dead birds, because they may have died from West Nile infection.

Guide to Head-to-Toe Physical Assessment of Adults

Guide to Head-to-Toe Physical Assessment of Adults*

Nursing Activity	Typical Finding	Changes Associated with Aging
NEUROLOGIC SYSTEM		
1. Determine level of consciousness.	1. Awake, alert	1. None
2. Test for orientation.	2. States name, place, and time	2. None
SKIN		
1. Inspect skin.	1. Intact, warm, dry, elastic skin without lesions	1a. Excessive dryness; wrinkles; discolorations from ultraviolet exposure ("age spots") and hemangiomas; inelastic, sagging skin
		1b. Ecchymotic areas as a result of increased capillary fragility
HEAD AND FACE		
1. Inspect and palpate the scalp, hair, and skull.	1. No lesions, shiny hair	1. Alopecia, thinning and dullness of hair
2. Inspect the face for symmetry of expression.	2. Symmetric expression	2. None

Continued

Guide to Head-to-Toe Physical Assessment of Adults*—cont'd

Nursing Activity	Typical Finding	Changes Associated with Aging
EYE		
1. Inspect the external eye structures.	1. No structural abnormalities	1. Entropion (inverted eyelid) or ectropion (everted eyelid)
2. Inspect the conjunctivae, sclerae, corneas, and irides.	2. No abnormalities; round irides	2. None
3. Use a penlight to test pupillary response (direct and consensual).	3. Pupils are equal and round and react to light and accommodation.	3. None
4. Test vision by asking the client to read (if able) or interpret an eye chart. NOTE: Be sure that glasses or contact lenses are in place, if used.	4. No vision impairment	4. Presbyopia (farsightedness)
EAR		
1. Inspect the external structure.	1. No structural abnormalities	1. No major change
2. Inspect the auditory meatus for drainage.	2. No drainage; small amount of cerumen may be present	2. None
3. Test hearing by whispering to the client while turning head away. NOTE: Be sure that hearing aid, if used, is in place.	3. No difficulty in hearing	3. Hearing loss, especially high-frequency sounds

Guide to Head-to-Toe Physical Assessment of Adults*—cont'd

Nursing Activity	Typical Finding	Changes Associated with Aging
MOUTH		
1. Use a penlight to inspect mouth, teeth, and gums.	1. No lesions, extensive dental caries, or gum disease	1. None
NECK		
1. Inspect for symmetry, lesions, pulsations, and JVD.	1. Symmetric, without lesions or JVD	1. None
2. Palpate the carotid pulse, one side at a time; check for bruits.	2. No bruits; pulses equal	2. None
3. Palpate the cervical lymph nodes.	3. Unable to palpate	3. None
4. Test ROM.	4. No limitations	4. Possible reduced neck flexion and extension; possible crepitus
CHEST (POSTERIOR, ANTERIOR, AND LATERAL)		
1. Inspect the chest for deformity, symmetry, expansion, and lesions; note pulsations or heaves (lifts).	1. Symmetric; without lesions; anteroposterior-lateral ratio of 1:2; no heaves	1. Slight change in anteroposterior-lateral ratio (1:1.5)
2. Palpate any chest lesions.	2. No lesions	2. None
3. Locate the PMI.	3. PMI at the left MCL, fifth ICS	3. None
4. Palpate each vertebra of the spine.	4. No tenderness or bony spurs	4. Thoracic kyphosis
5. Auscultate breath sounds throughout all lung fields.	5. Unlabored excursion of air; no adventitious sounds	5. Shallow respirations

Continued

Guide to Head-to-Toe Physical Assessment of Adults*—cont'd

Nursing Activity	Typical Finding	Changes Associated with Aging
CHEST (POSTERIOR, ANTERIOR, AND LATERAL)—cont'd		
6. Auscultate apical rate and rhythm; auscultate heart sounds.	6. S_1 and S_2 heart sounds	6. Possible S_4 heart sound
UPPER EXTREMITIES		
1. Inspect and palpate joints for swelling, tenderness, and deformity.	1. No swelling, tenderness, or deformity	1. Tenderness of one or more joints
2. Palpate brachial and radial arteries; assess for pulse deficit.	2. Pulses equal and within normal limits	2. None
3. Test ROM in all joints and sensation.	3. No restriction	3. Slight decrease in ROM; possible crepitus
4. Test muscle strength of arms, hands, and shoulders.	4. Movement against both gravity and resistance (5/5)	4. None or slight decrease (4+/5)
5. Palpate axillary nodes.	5. Nodes not palpable	5. None
ABDOMEN		
1. Inspect for contour, symmetry, lesions, and pulsations.	1. Symmetric; without lesions or pulsations	1. None
2. Auscultate bowel sounds in all four quadrants.	2. 5-15 sounds/min in each quadrant	2. May be slightly decreased (hypoactive)
3. Auscultate over abdominal aorta for bruit.	3. No bruit	3. None
4. Palpate for liver enlargement.	4. Liver not below costal margin	4. None

Guide to Head-to-Toe Physical Assessment of Adults*—cont'd

Nursing Activity	Typical Finding	Changes Associated with Aging
LOWER EXTREMITIES		
1. Inspect and palpate for swelling, tenderness, and deformity.	1. No swelling, tenderness, or deformity	1. Tenderness of one or more joints
2. Test ROM and sensation.	2. No limitation	2. Slight decrease in ROM; possible crepitus
3. Test muscle strength.	3. Movement against gravity and resistance (5/5)	3. None or slight decrease (4+/5)
4. Palpate femoral, popliteal, and pedal pulses.	4. Pulses equal and within normal range	4. Pedal pulses may be weak or not palpable.
5. Palpate inguinal nodes.	5. Nodes not palpable	5. None
GENITALIA		
1. Inspect external genitalia for lesions or drainage.	1. No lesions or drainage	1. None

ICS, intercostal space; *JVD,* jugular venous distension; *MCL,* midclavicular line; *PMI,* point of maximal impulse; *ROM,* range of motion.

*Additional assessments may be needed, depending on the patient's concerns and the medical diagnoses. For more information on physical assessment, see Ignatavicius, D.D., & Workman, M.L. (2013). *Medical-surgical nursing: patient-centered collaborative care* (7th ed.). Philadelphia: Saunders.

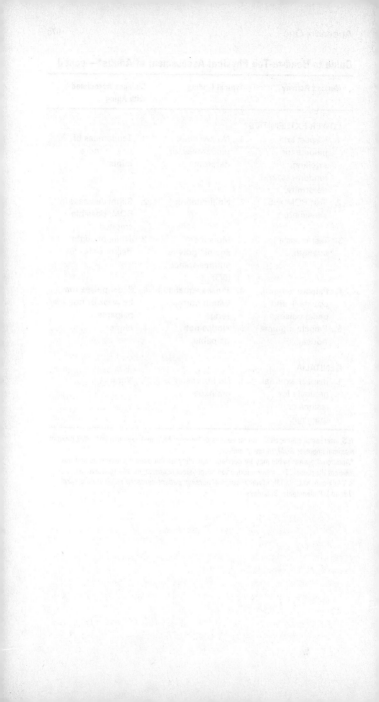

Terminology Associated with Fluid and Electrolyte Balance

active transport Assisted movement of a substance through a permeable membrane between two fluid compartments; occurs against a concentration, electrical, or pressure gradient; requires the expenditure of chemical energy

adenosine triphosphate (ATP) A substance that is generated by the metabolism of glucose or fat within cells and releases chemical energy for physiologic function when a high-energy phosphate bond ($\sim$P) is broken

aldosterone A hormone secreted by the adrenal cortex that stimulates the renal reabsorption of sodium and water and the renal excretion of potassium

anion A molecule (electrolyte) that carries an overall negative charge when dissolved in water

antidiuretic hormone (ADH) A hormone secreted from the posterior pituitary gland that increases the renal reabsorption of pure water and decreases urine output; also known as vasopressin

atrial natriuretic peptide (ANP) A hormone secreted by cardiac atrial cells that increases the renal excretion of sodium and water

Brownian motion Inherent molecular motion

capillary (plasma) hydrostatic pressure The force generated by fluid within a capillary that tends to move fluid out from the capillary and into the interstitial space

capillary (plasma) osmotic pressure The force generated by the concentration of plasma solutes (osmotic and oncotic pressures) that tends to retain fluid within the capillary or move fluid from the interstitial space into the capillary

cation A molecule (electrolyte) that carries an overall positive charge when dissolved in water

cofactor A substance required to enhance the activity of an enzyme or a physiologic reaction

colloidal oncotic pressure The osmotic pressure exerted by the concentration of colloids (proteins) within a solution; also known as *oncotic pressure*

diffusion Unimpeded movement of a substance through a permeable membrane between two fluid compartments; occurs down a concentration gradient; does not require the expenditure of chemical energy

disequilibrium   A state in which two fluid compartments are unequal in at least one characteristic

electrolytes   Substances that carry an electrical charge when dissolved in water

electroneutrality   A state in which a body fluid has an equal number of cations and anions so that the fluid does not express an electrical charge

equilibrium   A state in which two fluid compartments are equal in one or more characteristics

extracellular fluid (ECF)   Body fluid present outside of cells, which includes plasma, interstitial fluid, and transcellular fluid

facilitated diffusion   Assisted movement of a substance through a permeable membrane between two fluid compartments; occurs down a concentration gradient; does not require the expenditure of chemical energy

filtration   The movement of fluid through a biologic membrane as a result of hydrostatic pressure differences on the two sides of the membrane

gradient   A graded difference in some characteristic between two fluid compartments

hydrostatic pressure   The force of pressure exerted by static water in a confined space-"water-pushing" pressure

hypertonic (hyperosmotic)   Any solution with a solute concentration (osmolarity) greater than that of normal body fluids (greater than 310 mOsm/L)

hypotonic (hypo-osmotic)   Any solution with a solute concentration (osmolarity) less than that of normal body fluids (less than 270 mOsm/L)

impermeable membrane   A membrane separating two fluid compartments that does not permit the movement of one or more substances through the membrane (by diffusion) from one compartment to the other

insensible fluid loss   Fluid losses from the skin, gastrointestinal tract, wounds, and pulmonary epithelium

interstitial fluid   Fluid in the spaces between cells

intracellular fluid (ICF)   Fluid found inside cells

isotonic (isosmotic)   Any solution with a solute concentration equal to the osmolarity of normal body fluids or normal saline (0.9% NaCl), or about 300 mOsm/L

obligatory urine output   The minimal amount of urine output necessary to ensure the excretion of metabolic wastes (approximately 400 mL/day); a clinical goal for urine output may be higher.

osmolality   The concentration of solute within a solution as measured by the amount of solute osmoles per kilogram of solvent

osmolarity   The concentration of solute within a solution as measured by the amount of solute osmoles per liter of solution

osmoreceptor   Specialized sensory nerve cells in the thalamus or hypothalamus that are sensitive to changes in the osmolarity of extracellular fluid

osmosis   Diffusion of water (no other substance) through a selectively permeable membrane from an area of lower osmotic pressure to an area of greater osmotic pressure

osmotic pressure   The pressure exerted by a solution that contains a relatively high concentration of solute; this pressure draws water from areas or compartments with lower concentrations of solute into the areas or compartments with higher concentrations of solute-"water-pulling" pressure

permeable membrane   A membrane separating two fluid compartments that permits the movement of one or more substances through the membrane (by diffusion) from one compartment to the other

solubility   The degree to which any given solute completely dissolves (dissociates) in water

solute   The solid particles dissolved in a solution

solvent   The fluid (water) portion of a solution

tissue hydrostatic pressure (THP)   The force generated by fluid within the interstitial spaces that tends to move fluid into the capillary from the interstitial space

tissue osmotic pressure (TOP)   The force generated by the concentration of interstitial fluid solutes that tend to retain fluid in the interstitial space or move fluid from the capillary into the interstitial space

transcellular fluid   Extracellular fluid confined to a specific area or region of the body (cerebrospinal fluid, pericardial fluid, visceral fluid, aqueous humor, peritoneal fluid, and pleural fluid)

viscosity   Gumminess or thickness of the molecules in a solution, causing friction within that solution

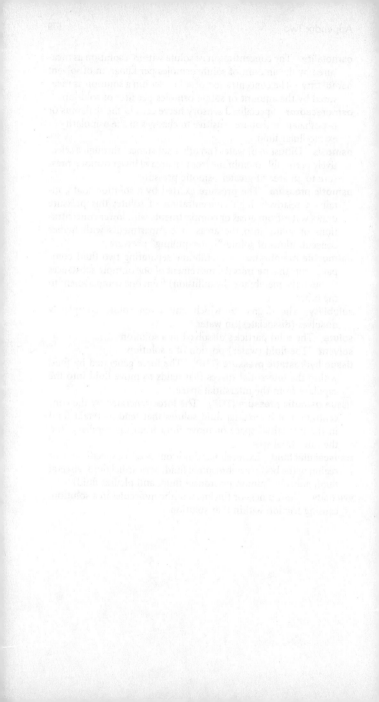

Laboratory Values

Major Serum Electrolyte Concentrations, Chemistries, and Functions

Electrolyte	Reference Range	International Recommended Units	Functions
Sodium (Na⁺)	136-145 mEq/L	136-145 mmol/L	Maintains plasma and interstitial osmolarity Generates action potentials; maintains resting cell-membrane electrical potential Contributes to acid-base balance Maintains electroneutrality
Potassium (K⁺)	3.5-5 mEq/L	3.5-5 mmol/L	Maintains plasma and cellular osmolarity Contributes to action potential; maintains resting cell membrane electrical potential Maintenance of plasma acid-base balance
Calcium (Ca²⁺)	9-10.5 mg/dL	2.25-2.75 mmol/L	Acts as a cofactor in blood-clotting cascade Provides plateau phase in action potential Contributes to neurotransmitter release Adds strength and density to bones and teeth Essential component of contractile processes in cardiac, skeletal, and smooth muscle

Chloride (Cl⁻)	98-106 mEq/L	98-106 mmol/L	Maintains plasma acid-base balance Maintains plasma electroneutrality Forms hydrochloric acid in specialized gastrointestinal cells

Chloride (Cl⁻)	98-106 mEq/L	98-106 mmol/L	Maintains plasma acid-base balance Maintains plasma electroneutrality Forms hydrochloric acid in specialized gastrointestinal cells
Magnesium (Mg^{2+})	1.3-2.1 mEq/L	0.65-1.05 mmol/L	Stabilizes excitable cell membranes Contributes to cardiac, skeletal, and smooth muscle contraction Acts as a cofactor in blood-clotting cascade Acts as a cofactor in DNA and protein synthesis
Phosphorus (P_i)	3-4.5 mg/dL	0.97-1.45 mmol/L	Activates B-complex vitamins Forms adenosine triphosphate and other high-energy substances Acts as a cofactor in carbohydrate, protein, and lipid metabolism
Blood urea nitrogen (BUN)	10-20 mg/dL	3.6-7.1 mmol/L	The amount of nitrogen in the blood in the form of urea. Measures renal function
Creatinine	Female: 0.5-1.1 mg/dL Male: 0.6-1.2 mg/dL	Female: 44-97 µmol/L Male: 53-106 µmol/L	A waster product of muscle metabolism Measures renal function

Continued

Major Serum Electrolyte Concentrations, Chemistries, and Functions—cont'd

Electrolyte	Reference Range	International Recommended Units	Functions
Hemoglobin A1C (concentration of glucose) HgbA1C	Female: 12-16 g/dL Male: 14-18 g/dL	Female: 8.7-11.2 mmol/L Male: 7.4-9.9 mmol/L	Measures the amount of hemoglobin bound to glucose Reflects how much glucose has been in the blood during the past 2-4 months
B-type natriuretic peptide (BNP)	<100 pg/mL	<100 ng/L	A hormone stored mainly in the cardiac ventricular myocardium Contributes to diuresis when cardiac tissue is "stretched" Blood levels of BNP are elevated in hypervolemic states, such as congestive heart failure
Cholesterol (Total)	<200 mg/dL	<5.20 mmol/L	A sterol compound found in most body tissues and important in metabolism Elevated plasma concentrations are thought to promote atherosclerosis Measures low-, high- and other densities of cholesterol circulating in the blood
Low-density lipoprotein (LDL)	<130 mg/dL		A form of cholesterol associated with atherosclerotic plaque

| High-density lipoprotein (HDL) | Female: >55 mg/dL Male: >45 mg/dL | Female: >0.91 mmol/L Male: >0.75 mmol/L | A form of cholesterol associated with scavenging large molecules of cholesterol, like LDL, and returning the molecules to the liver for further metabolism, reducing the risk for atherosclerotic pathology |
| Albumin | 3.5-5 g/dL | 35-50 g/L | A major plasma protein Provides oncotic or colloidal pressure for fluid balance and serves as a transport protein for large organic anions Indicates protein nutritional status |

Data from Pagana, K. & Pagana, T. (2009). *Mosby's manual of diagnostic and laboratory tests* (4th ed.). St. Louis: Mosby.

Cells and Indices from a Complete Blood Count (CBC) and Their Functions

Cell/Component	Reference	International Units	Functions
Red blood cell (RBC)/ erythrocyte	Men: 4.7-6.1 million RBCs per microliter Women: 4.2-5.4 million RBCs per microliter	$4.7\text{-}6.1 \times 10^{12}$ per liter $4.7\text{-}6.1 \times 10^{12}$ per liter	RBCs carry oxygen from lungs to tissues and carry some carbon dioxide from tissues to lungs.
Hemoglobin (Hgb)	Men: 14-18 g/dL Women: 12-16 g/dL	8.7-11.2 mmol/L 7.4-9.9 mmol/L	Hemoglobin is the protein in the RBC that binds to oxygen.
Hematocrit (Hct)	Men: 42%-52% Women: 37%-47%	0.42-0.52 volume fraction 0.37-0.47 volume fraction	This test measures the amount of volume RBCs use in the blood.
Indices			
Mean corpuscular volume (MCV)	82-98 fL		These values refer to the size of RBCs (MCV), the amount of hemoglobin in a single cell (MCH), and the averaged hemoglobin in the sample (MCHC).
Mean corpuscular hemoglobin (MCH)	26-34 pg		

Mean corpuscular hemoglobin concentration (MCHC)	31-38 g/dL or 31%-38%		
Platelets	150,000-400,000 per mm³	150-400 × 10⁹ per liter	Platelets provide an initial response to blood vessel injury and hemorrhage by forming a stick plug and activating the clotting cascade.
White blood cells (WBC)/leukocytes (men and nonpregnant women)	4,500-11,000 per mcL³	4.5-11 × 10⁹ per liter	WBCs protect the body against infection and produce signals for inflammation.
WBC Differential			Each of these WBCs provides a range of activities to protect the body against invading pathogens, repair injury, and remove malignant cells. The differential provides important information about the immune system and the presence of injury, infection, or inflammation.
Neutrophils	50%-62%		
Band Neutrophils	3%-6%		
Lymphocytes	25%-40%		
Monocytes	3%-7%		
Eosinophils	0-3%		
Basophils	0-1%		

fL, Femtoliter; *pg*, picogram.
Data from Pagana, K. & Pagana, T. (2009). *Mosby's manual of diagnostic and laboratory tests* (4th ed.). St. Louis: Mosby.

Major Urine Electrolytes, Osmolarity, and Specific Gravity

Electrolytes and Characteristics	Normal Value*	Significance of Abnormal Value†
Calcium	2.5-7.5 mmol/day	Increased: malignancy, thyrotoxicosis, hyperparathyroidism, osteoporosis, vitamin D intoxication
Chloride	110-250 mEq/day 110-250 mmol/day	Increased: increased salt intake, drug-induced diuresis, adrenocortical insufficiency Decreased: reduced salt intake, water retention, vomiting, cerebral edema, adrenocortical hyperfunction
Magnesium	3-5 mmol/day	Increased: alcohol intake, diuretics, corticosteroid therapy, cisplatin therapy Decreased: dietary insufficiency
Phosphorus	12.9-42 mmol/day	Increased: hyperparathyroidism, renal tubular damage, immobility, nonrenal acidosis Decreased: hypoparathyroidism
Potassium	25-100 mmol/day (varies with diet)	Increased: early starvation, hyperaldosteronism, metabolic acidosis Decreased: Addison's disease, renal disease
Sodium	40-220 mEq/day 40-220 mmol/day	Increased: increased dietary intake, adrenal failure, diuretic therapy Decreased: low sodium intake, sodium and water retention, adrenocortical hyperfunction, excessive diaphoresis, diarrhea

| Osmolarity (osmolality), random | 50-1200 mOsm/kg water | Increased: dehydration, SIADH
Decreased: diabetes insipidus, primary polydipsia |
| Specific gravity | 1.015-1.025 | Increased: dehydration, SIADH, diabetes mellitus, toxemia of pregnancy
Decreased: chronic renal insufficiency, diabetes insipidus, lithium toxicity, early renal disease |

Data from Pagana, K., & Pagana, T. (2009). *Mosby's manual of diagnostic and laboratory tests* (4th ed.). St. Louis: Mosby.

SIADH, syndrome of inappropriate antidiuretic hormone.

*Based on a 24-hour total volume urine sample.

†Common conditions associated with abnormal values.

Interventions for Common Environmental Emergencies

Interventions for Common Environmental Emergencies

	Clinical Manifestations	Collaborative Management
HEAT-RELATED ILLNESS		

Heat exhaustion	Patient complains of flu-like symptoms:
	  Headache
	  Fatigue
	  Anorexia
	  Nausea
	  Vomiting
	  Hypotension
	  Tachycardia
	May have normal temperature
		Home care:
		Move to cool environment.
		Remove constrictive clothing.
		Provide an oral rehydrating solution such as water, a sports drink or IV fluids (9% saline solution).
		Place cool or cold packs on neck, chest, abdomen, and groin.
		Place in cool water.
		Fan while spraying water on the skin.
		Hospital care (if necessary):
		Monitor vital signs.
		Rehydrate with oral or IV fluids.

Heat stroke:
elevated temperature
(> 105° F or 40.5° C)
	Hot, dry skin
	Mental status changes
	Anxiety
	Confusion
	Bizarre behavior
	Loss of coordination
	Hallucinations
		Prehospital care:
		Call for emergency help.
		Provide ABCs of emergency care (airway, breathing, circulation).
		Initiate rapid cooling:
		  Remove clothes.
		  Place ice packs on neck, axillae, chest, and groin.

Agitation
Seizures
Coma
Hypotension
Tachycardia
Tachypnea

Immerse in cold water.
Wet the body with tepid water and fan rapidly to aid
   in cooling by evaporation.
Hospital care:
Maintain and monitor ABCs
Oxygen
IV fluids with 9% saline solution
Aggressive methods to decrease temperature
   (continuously monitor temperature)
Cooling blanket
Iced lavage
Peritoneal lavage
Monitor neurologic status
Seizure precautions

COLD-RELATED INJURIES

Hypothermia: core body temperature below 95° F (35° C)

Mild: 32-35° C

Mild:
Shivering
Dysarthria
Tachycardia

Mild:
Shelter from cold environment
Remove wet clothes and apply warm clothes or
   blankets; warm room.

Continued

Interventions for Common Environmental Emergencies—cont'd

Clinical Manifestations	Collaborative Management
Mild: 32-35° C—cont'd Muscular incoordination, impaired cognitive abilities, and diuresis Increased respiratory rate	Provide warm, high-carbonate liquids that do not contain alcohol or caffeine.
Moderate: 28-32° C *Moderate:* Obvious motor impairment such as stumbling, falling Weakness Confusion, apathy Irrational, incoherent Stupor and coma Shivering stops Patient may perceive warmth and undress Bradycardia and hypotension Decreased respiratory rate and cardiac output Dysrhythmias Coagulopathy Thrombocytopenia	*Moderate and severe:* Hospital care required Do not use external rewarming methods, which promote "after drop," a continued decrease in core body temperature after the victim is removed from the cold environment. Applying external heat may produce peripheral vasodilation, which stimulates return of cold blood from periphery to warmer core. Standard resuscitation measures, if needed. Handle gently to prevent ventricular irritability. Place patient in horizontal position. Core rewarming methods include administration of warm IV fluids, heated oxygen, and inspired gas.

| Severe: <28° C | **Severe:**
Absent neurologic reflexes; no response to pain
Hypotension
Acid-base abnormalities
Ventricular fibrillation, asystole
Coagulopathy
Thrombocytopenia | **Severe:**
Extracorporeal rewarming methods used for severe hypothermia such as cardiopulmonary bypass, hemodialysis, or continuous arteriovenous rewarming
Administer medications cautiously: Metabolism is unpredictable, and a drug can accumulate without obvious therapeutic effect while the patient is cold, but it will become active and may lead to drug toxicity as effective rewarming is underway. |
| Frostbite | **Frostnip:**
Pain, numbness, pallor of affected area (white or waxy appearance)

First-degree frostbite:
Hyperemia and edema
Second-degree frostbite:
Large, fluid-filled blisters with partial-thickness skin necrosis
Third-degree frostbite:
Small blisters that contain dark fluid
Full-thickness and subcutaneous necrosis | **Frostnip:**
Use body heat to warm affected area. For example, place warm hands over cold ears or cold hands under axillary region.
Frostbite:
Hospital care required
Rapid rewarming in a water bath at temperature of 38° C (41° C)
Premedicate for pain before rewarming.
Do not apply dry heat or rub affected area.
After rewarming, elevate an involved extremity above the heart to decrease tissue edema. |

Continued

Interventions for Common Environmental Emergencies—cont'd

	Clinical Manifestations	Collaborative Management
Frostbite—cont'd	Affected area cool, numb, blue, or red that does not blanch *Fourth-degree frostbite:* No blisters or edema Affected area is numb, cold, and bloodless. Full-thickness necrosis extends into muscle and bone.	Administer tetanus prophylaxis, if needed. Surgical management for deep wounds Amputation may be necessary.
SNAKE BITES North American pit viper: Rattlesnake Copperhead Water moccasin (cottonmouth)	One or more puncture wounds Severe pain Swelling Redness or ecchymosis Later: vesicles or hemorrhagic bullae Minty, rubbery, or metallic taste in mouth Tingling or paresthesias of scalp, face, and lips Muscle fasciculations and weakness Nausea, vomiting Hypotension Seizures Coagulopathy Disseminated intravascular coagulation	*Prehospital care:* Move patient to safe location. Encourage patient to rest to decrease venom circulation. Remove constrictive clothing and jewelry. If extremity is affected, immobilize and keep below level of heart. Keep patient warm. Provide reassurance. If hospital care and definitive treatment will be delayed, a constricting band may be applied proximal to an extremity wound to impede venom circulation through lymphatic flow but not tight enough to impair venous drainage or arterial

flow. Loosen band if peripheral edema contributes to undue tightening/loss of pulse, edema.

Hospital care:

ABCs

Assess distal circulation frequently.

Insert two 16-18 gauge (large-bore) IV catheters and begin fluids.

Continuous cardiac and blood pressure monitoring

Pain management

Tetanus prophylaxis

Broad-spectrum antibiotic to reduce risk of infection

Laboratory studies:

CBC, electrolytes

Coagulation studies

Creatinine kinase

Type and crossmatch

Urinalysis

Electrocardiogram

Measure and record circumference of bite site every 15-30 minutes, if possible.

Continued

Interventions for Common Environmental Emergencies—cont'd

	Clinical Manifestations	Collaborative Management
North American pit viper—cont'd		Monitor for bleeding because of potential of coagulopathy. Contact the poison control center. Administer antivenom if ordered and monitor for adverse reactions and anaphylaxis.
Coral snake	Pain may be only mild and transient. Fang marks difficult to visualize Coagulopathy does not occur. Toxic effect may be delayed 12-13 hours. Nausea, vomiting Headache Pallor Abdominal pain Neurologic manifestations Paresthesias Numbness Mental status changes Cranial and peripheral nerve involvement Later may see total flaccid paralysis Difficulty speaking, swallowing, and breathing Cardiovascular collapse	Continuous cardiac, blood pressure, and pulse oximetry monitoring. Aggressive airway management Monitor and initiate interventions to prevent aspiration. Contact the poison control center. Administer antivenom, if ordered, and monitor for side effects.

Continued

ARTHROPOD (SPIDER) BITES

Brown recluse spider

Bite is painless, stinging, sharp, or painful.

Intense local aching and pruritus

Central bite site appears as a bleb or vesicle surrounded by edema and erythema, which may expand.

Over 1-3 days, central lesion becomes dark and necrotic; eschar forms.

When the eschar sloughs, an open wound or ulcer can remain for weeks to months.

Surgical intervention may be needed.

Systemic toxicity manifested by:

Fever, chills

Nausea and vomiting

Malaise, joint pain

Petechiae

Hemolytic reactions, renal failure, and death may occur.

Home care:

Call primary care provider.

Cold compresses—never use heat.

Rest, elevate affected extremity.

Hospital care:

Wound care includes oral or topical antibiotics, antiseptic cream, and a sterile dressing to cover the bite area.

Surgical evaluation to determine the need for debridement and skin grafting

Black widow spider

Little to severe pain

Tiny papule or small, red punctuate mark

Systemic signs and symptoms:

Severe abdominal pain

Muscle rigidity/spasm

Hypertension

Home care:

Call primary care provider

Apply ice pack.

Hospital care:

Monitor ABCs.

Pain medication

Interventions for Common Environmental Emergencies—cont'd

	Clinical Manifestations	Collaborative Management

Black widow spider—cont'd	Nausea and vomiting
	Facial edema
	Ptosis
	Diaphoresis
	Weakness
	Increased salivation
	Priapism
	Respiratory difficulty
	Increased respiratory secretions
	Fasciculations
	Paresthesias
		Muscle relaxants
		Calcium gluconate may be used for muscle spasms, rigidity, and pain.
		Institute seizure precautions.
		Medications include:
		  Tetanus prophylaxis
		  Antihypertensive agents
		Monitor for pulmonary edema and shock.
		Hospital admission is recommended for pregnant women and patients with hypertension.

Tarantula	Pain at bite site Swelling Redness Numbness Lymphangitis	Call primary care provider Supportive management Analgesics Elevate and immobilize an extremity if affected.
Scorpions	Pain and inflammation Mild systemic symptoms	Call primary care provider Analgesics, supportive management Clean wound and apply most dressing for 24 hours.
Bark scorpion	Severe pain Systemic manifestations Respiratory failure Pancreatitis	Transport to hospital; call primary care provider Monitor vital signs Continuous cardiac monitoring Monitor for respiratory failure.

Musculoskeletal dysfunction | IV fluids
Cranial nerve dysfunction | Analgesics
| Tetanus prophylaxis
| Atropine is used if hypersalivation occurs.
| Antivenom if ordered

LIGHTNING INJURIES Cardiovascular

Asystole or ventricular fibrillation | Initiate basic life support; monitor ABCs.
Mottled skin | Follow advanced life support guidelines.
Absent peripheral pulses | Cardiac monitoring
Respiratory arrest, hypoxia | Immobilize for spinal cord injury.

Central nervous system | Monitor vital signs.

Temporary paralysis lasting from minutes to hours | Note entrance and exit site injuries to evaluate internal pathway damage; burn care if needed
Loss of consciousness | Laboratory studies for muscle damage such as creatinine kinase (CK)
Amnesia | Tetanus prophylaxis if needed
Confusion, disorientation | Monitor for rhabdomyolysis and kidney injury with serial serum and urine laboratory analyses of BUN, creatinine, CK, anion gap and hourly urine output.
Photophobia |
Seizures |
Hemorrhage |
Cerebellar dysfunction |
Spinal cord injury |

Integumentary

Burns (superficial to full thickness)

Continued

Interventions for Common Environmental Emergencies—cont'd

	Clinical Manifestations	Collaborative Management
ALTITUDE-RELATED ILLNESSES		
High altitude is an elevation above 5000 feet.		
Acute mountain sickness (AMS)	Throbbing headache Anorexia Nausea and vomiting Irritability, apathy Variable vital signs Dyspnea on exertion, at rest	Rest and allow time to acclimate to altitude. Remove to lower altitude. Administer oxygen if available. Medications Acetazolamide (Diamox) to prevent and treat AMS Dexamethasone (Decadron) may be given while patient moves to lower altitude.
High altitude cerebral edema (HACE)	Unable to perform activities of daily living Extreme apathy Confusion, lack of judgment Cranial nerve dysfunction Seizures Stupor, coma, death	Rapid descent to lower altitude Supplemental oxygen Keep patient warm. Medications, if available, during descent Dexamethasone (Decadron) Loop diuretics Hospital care required Monitor ABCs. Symptom management
High altitude pulmonary edema (HAPE)	Poor exercise tolerance Dyspnea on exertion Dry cough Cyanosis of nails and lips Tachycardia, tachypnea Rales, pink frothy sputum	As above

ABCs Airway, breathing, circulation.

Chemical and Biological Agents of Terrorism

The Centers for Disease Control and Prevention list the following indications of intentional release of a biological agent:

1. An unusual clustering of illness (e.g., persons who attended the same public event or gathering) or patients experiencing clinical signs and symptoms that suggest an infectious disease outbreak

2. An unusual age distribution for common diseases (e.g., increase in what appears to be a chickenpox-like illness among adult patients but that may be smallpox)

3. A large number of cases of acute flaccid paralysis with prominent bulbar palsies manifested by cranial nerve paralysis (e.g., facial weakness, dysphagia, or dysarthria), suggesting a release of botulinum toxin

Information for this Appendix is taken from the Centers for Disease Control and Prevention website (www.bt.cdc.gov).

Chemical and Biological Agents of Terrorism

Agent	Clinical Manifestations	Mode of Transmission	Collaborative Management
Anthrax, cutaneous A bacterial infection caused by the gram-positive, rod-shaped organism, *Bacillus anthracis*, which lives as a spore in contaminated soil	Raised vesicle may itch and resemble an insect bite. Center of the vesicle becomes hemorrhagic and sinks inward. An area of necrosis and ulceration begins; the tissue around the wound swells and becomes edematous. It is distinguished from insect bites or other skin lesions in that it is painless and that eschar forms regardless of treatment.	Incubation period of 3-5 days after exposure Direct contact	Treatment includes ciprofloxacin or doxycycline. Prevention: vaccine is given in 5 divided doses over 18 months and requires annual boosters.
Anthrax, inhalation	*Prodromal stage (early):* Fever Fatigue Mild chest pain Dry cough No manifestations of upper respiratory infection of rhinitis, headache, watery eyes, or sore throat	Incubation period of 1 day to 6 weeks Spread through direct contact Not spread by person-to-person contact	Treatment with ciprofloxacin or doxycycline, and amoxicillin These drugs are used individually in oral form for prophylaxis when people have been exposed to inhalation anthrax.

		Fulminant stage (late):	Death can occur within 24-36 hours after the onset of breathlessness, even if antibiotic is started at this stage
		Sudden onset of breathlessness, progressing to severe respiratory distress	
		Diaphoresis	
		Stridor on inhalation and exhalation	
		Hypoxia	
		High fever	
		Mediastinitis and pleural effusion	
		Hypotension	
		Septic shock, meningitis	
Botulism	A muscle-paralyzing disease caused by a toxin made by the bacterium *Clostridium botulinum*	*Foodborne botulism:*	Incubation period is 12-72 hours. Antitoxin can prevent symptoms from worsening if given early. Supportive therapy, including intravenous fluids and mechanical ventilation
		Abdominal cramps	Airborne or foodborne illness
		Nausea, vomiting, diarrhea	
		Drooping eyelids	
		Blurred or double vision	
		Dysphagia	
		Dry mouth	
		Slurred speech	
		Descending muscle weakness	
		Inhalation botulism (includes all of the above except the GI symptoms plus):	
		Dyspnea	

Continued

Chemical and Biological Agents of Terrorism—cont'd

Agent	Clinical Manifestations	Mode of Transmission	Collaborative Management
	Decreasing respirations that may lead to apnea and respiratory arrest		
Smallpox An acute, contagious, and sometimes fatal disease caused by the variola virus	*Initial symptoms:* Fever (usually high), malaise, vomiting Head and body aches Small, red spots on the tongue and in the mouth Rash that starts on the face and legs, hands, and feet *After 3 days:* Rash becomes raised bumps, which fill with a thick, opaque fluid and often have a depression in the center that looks like a bellybutton (a major distinguishing characteristic of smallpox). Bumps become pustules. Pustules begin to form a crust and then scab.	Incubation period of 7-17 days Prolonged face-to-face contact with someone who has smallpox (usually someone who already has a smallpox rash) Direct contact with infected bodily fluids or an object such as bedding or clothing that has a virus on it Exposure to an aerosol release of smallpox Infected person is contagious to others until all of the scabs have fallen off.	No proven treatment Intravenous fluids Medication to control fever, pain and support/increase blood pressure may be used Routine smallpox vaccination ended in 1972.

Plague Disease caused by *Yersinia pestis*, a bacterium found in rodents and their fleas	*By the end of the second week:* After the rash appears, most of the sores have scabbed over. Fever, weakness Rapidly developing pneumonia Dyspnea, chest pain Cough, bloody or watery sputum Nausea, vomiting, and abdominal pain May lead to respiratory failure, shock, and rapid death	Incubation period of 2-4 days Respiratory droplets Intentional aerosol release	Streptomycin, gentamicin, doxycycline, or ciprofloxacin may be used
Tularemia Inhalational *Francisella tularensis*	Resembles the flu Fever, fatigue Swollen glands Sore throat Pneumonia	Incubation period of 3-7 days	Streptomycin, gentamicin, doxycycline, ciprofloxacin, and tetracycline may be used.
Hemorrhagic fever Caused by Ebola, Marburg, Lassa, and Crimean-Congo hemorrhagic fever viruses and resulting in multisystem organ failure syndrome	Specific signs and symptoms vary by the type of viral hemorrhagic fever (VHF). Marked fever, fatigue Dizziness Muscle aches Loss of strength Bleeding under the skin, in internal organs, or from body orifices such as the mouth, eyes, and ears	Carried by rodents, mosquitoes, and tics Incubation period of 5-10 days May spread from one person to another after an initial person has become infected Secondary transmission of the virus can occur directly through close contact with infected people or their body fluids.	Supportive therapy; no other treatment or established cure for VHFs Ribavirin, an antiviral drug, has been effective in treating some individuals with Lassa fever. Treatment with convalescent-phase plasma has been used with success in some

Continued

Chemical and Biological Agents of Terrorism—cont'd

Agent	Clinical Manifestations	Mode of Transmission	Collaborative Management
	Signs of shock Nervous system malfunction, coma, delirium, and seizures Renal failure	It can also occur indirectly through contact with objects contaminated with infected body fluids.	patients with Argentine hemorrhagic fever.
Ricin A toxic protein made from castor beans. The poison can be extracted from the beans, purified, and treated to form a powder that can be inhaled.	*Inhalation:* Respiratory distress (difficulty breathing), tightness in the chest Fever, cough, nausea Heavy sweating Pulmonary edema Hypotension and respiratory failure, leading to death *Ingestion:* Vomiting and diarrhea that may be bloody and result in severe dehydration Hypotension Hallucinations Seizures Blood in the urine Skin and eye exposure: Redness and pain of the skin and the eyes	Symptoms within 8 hours of inhalation	No antidote exists. Supportive care, including intravenous fluid, vasopressors, gastric lavage, and mechanical ventilation can be used. Death may take place within 36-72 hours of exposure, depending on the route of exposure and the dose received. If death has not occurred in 3-5 days, the victim usually recovers.

Agent	Signs and symptoms	Exposure/incubation	Treatment
Sarin (GB) and soman (GD) Both are human-made chemical warfare agents classified as nerve agents, which can evaporate into a vapor (gas) and spread into the environment.	Runny nose Watery eyes Small, pinpoint pupils Eye pain Blurred vision Drooling and excessive sweating Cough Chest tightness Rapid breathing Diarrhea Increased urination Confusion Drowsiness Weakness Headache Nausea, vomiting, abdominal pain Slow or fast heart rate Low or high blood pressure Loss of consciousness Convulsions Paralysis Respiratory failure possibly leading to death	Incubation is a few minutes to several hours. Clothing can give off vapors for up to 30 minutes after exposure. The patient can be exposed through skin or eye contact; breathing air that contains the agents; touching or drinking contaminated water, eating contaminated food, or touching contaminated clothes	First responders should wear full protective gear to prevent nerve damage. Remove patient's clothing to reduce symptomatic damage. Rapidly wash the patient's entire body with soap and water. Give antidote, as ordered. Provide airway, breathing, and circulatory support. Provide supportive care based on patient's signs and symptoms.
Tabun The manmade chemical warfare agent is	Same as sarin and soman	Tabun is an immediate but short-lived threat and does not last a long time in the environment.	Give antidote, as ordered. Provide airway, breathing, and circulatory support.

Continued

Chemical and Biological Agents of Terrorism—cont'd

Agent	Clinical Manifestations	Mode of Transmission	Collaborative Management
classified as a nerve agent.		Tabun is more volatile than VX, and it remains on exposed surfaces for a shorter period than VX. Tabun is less volatile than sarin, and it remains on exposed surfaces for a longer period than sarin.	Supportive care based on patient's signs and symptoms
VX The human-made chemical warfare agent is classified as a nerve agent. It is the most potent of all nerve agents and affects breathing function.	Same as sarin and soman	Symptoms appear within a few seconds after exposure to the vapor form of VX and within a few minutes to up to 18 hours after exposure to the liquid form. Under average weather conditions, VX can last for days on objects that it has come in contact with. Under very cold conditions, VX can last for months. It evaporates slowly and can be a long-term threat as well as a short-term threat. Surfaces contaminated with VX should be considered a long-term hazard.	Recovery from VX exposure is possible with treatment, but the antidote must be used quickly to be effective.

Discharge Planning

- Discharge planning begins on admission.
- Information to ask the patient to assist with discharge planning:
  1. Where do you live?
  2. How will you get home?
  3. Can you describe your home?
  4. How many stairs must you climb to get into your house?
  5. Are your bedroom, bathroom, laundry, and kitchen on the same floor, or will you need to use steps?
  6. Do you live alone, or does someone live with you?
     a. Who lives with you? Will they need help with caregiving?
     b. Will the person be able to help you after your discharge?
     c. Is there a neighbor or church member who can help you after you are discharged?
     d. Is anyone available to help you with grocery shopping, laundry, or driving to doctors' appointments?
- Collaborate with physician(s), physical therapist, occupational therapist, speech therapist, dietitian, pharmacist, stoma/skin care specialist, diabetic educator, social worker, case manager, or discharge planner to identify the patient's needs related to care after hospitalization, including education, meal preparation, support to complete activities of daily living and personal hygiene, wound care, acquisition of durable medical goods, supplies, and prescriptive drugs.
- Provide written and verbal information about referrals for housing, finances, insurance, legal services, funeral arrangements, and spiritual counseling if they are part of the discharge plan.

▼ NATIONAL PATIENT SAFETY GOAL

Accurately and completely reconcile drugs that the patient take at home. Ensure new drug and established drug regimens are clear and emphasize the importance of prescribed drugs and regimens. Provide an up-to-date list of medications and document communication of this list to the patient or family. Ensure that this list is accessible to the health care provider(s) who will provide follow-up care. Remind the patient or family members to call the primary care provider to report side effects or challenges to drug adherence.

- Provide patient and family education:
  1. Provide verbal and written information about the disease process, how to recognize complications (if appropriate), and how to manage the disease at home.
  2. Provide verbal and written information to reinforce need to contact primary care provider for ongoing care, to schedule and attend follow-up care. Include contact information (e.g., phone number for appointments, clinic name, and specialty provider name).
  3. Teach the patient about drugs:
     a. Names of drugs
     b. Purpose of drugs
     c. Dosage
     d. Side effects
     e. Interactions, if any, with foods or other drugs
     f. Importance of taking drugs as prescribed
     g. Schedule follow-up labs and ensure skills and supplies are in place for checking blood sugar as prescribed at home. Inform patient to reporting abnormal values and trends to primary care provider.
     h. Provide and help patient evaluate reliable sources of information and to avoid altering or stopping prescribed treatment without informing primary care provider.
  4. Teach the patient about the use of supplies or equipment prescribed for use after discharge, such as dressing changes, suctioning, tube feeding, or other special care that may be required at home.
  5. Explain signs and symptoms that should be reported to the health care provider. Focus on information that must be reported immediately.
- Use established guidelines and teaching tools from reliable sources to reinforce teaching.
- Use institutional forms and policies to document discharge instructions and obtain the patient's or a family member's signature to acknowledge receipt of written instructions for the patient record.

Electrocardiographic Complexes, Segments, Intervals

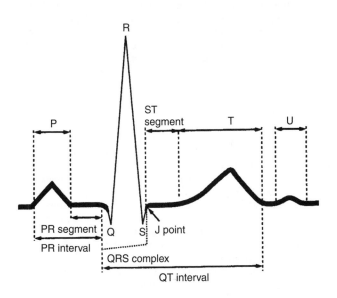

The electrocardiogram (ECG) is the graphic record of electrical activity of the heart. The spread of electrical current in the heart is detected by surface electrodes, and the amplified electrical signals are recorded on calibrated paper.

The first step in reading an ECG is to analyze the rhythm and rate. Determine whether the rhythm is regular or irregular, then calculate the heart rate by counting the number of PP or RR intervals that occur in 6 seconds, and multiply that number by 10. A normal rate is 60-100 beats per minute.

The second step is to systematically examine the waveforms, intervals, and segments:

P wave represents atrial depolarization.

PR segment represents the time required for the impulse to travel through the atrioventricular (AV) node (where the impulse is delayed).

PR interval represents the time required for atrial depolarization and impulse travel through the AV node, inclusive of the P wave and PR segment. It is measured from the beginning of the P wave to the end of the PR segment, and a normal time in adults is 0.12 to 0.2 second.

QRS complex represents depolarization of both ventricles and is measured from the point at which the complex first leaves the baseline to the end of the last appearing wave (from the end of the PR interval to the J point). This is normally 0.04 to 0.1 second. A wide (i.e., >0.12 seconds) QRS complex indicates a delay in the conduction time in the ventricles. Delay in ventricular depolarization(i.e., a wide QRS) can be the result of myocardial ischemia, injury, or infarct; it may also result from ventricular hypertrophy or electrolytes imbalances.

J point represents the junction where the QRS complex ends and the ST segment begin.

ST segment represents early ventricular repolarization. It is measured from the J point to the beginning of the T wave.

T wave represents ventricular repolarization.

U wave represents late ventricular repolarization. It is not normally seen in all leads.

QT interval represents the total time required for ventricular depolarization and repolarization. It is measured from the beginning of the QRS complex to the end of the T wave. It varies with age, gender, and heart rate. It must be corrected to a heart rate of 60 after measurement (QTc). The upper limit of normal QTc is less than 0.43 second in men and less than 0.45 second in women with a normal rate of 60-100 beats/min.

The third and final step is to interpret the recording. Rhythm strips in this appendix illustrate common and clinically important ECG patterns.

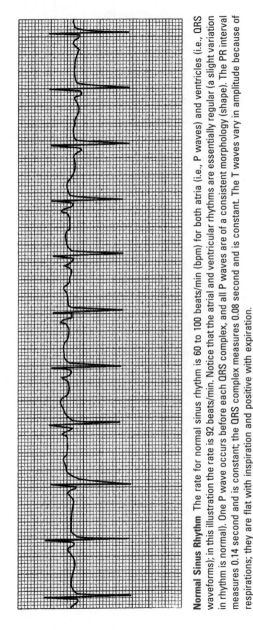

Normal Sinus Rhythm The rate for normal sinus rhythm is 60 to 100 beats/min (bpm) for both atria (i.e., P waves) and ventricles (i.e., QRS waveforms); in this illustration the rate is 92 beats/min. Notice that the atrial and ventricular rhythms are essentially regular (a slight variation in rhythm is normal). One P wave occurs before each QRS complex, and all P waves are of a consistent morphology (shape). The PR interval measures 0.14 second and is constant; the QRS complex measures 0.08 second and is constant. The T waves vary in amplitude because of respirations; they are flat with inspiration and positive with expiration.

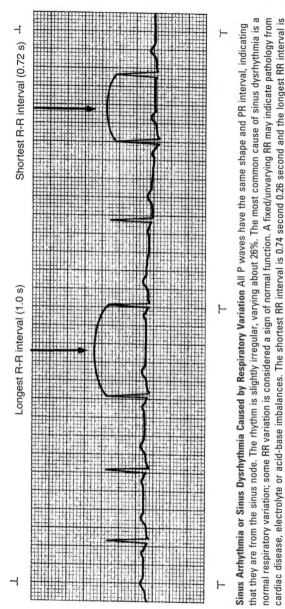

Sinus Arrhythmia or Sinus Dysrhythmia Caused by Respiratory Variation All P waves have the same shape and PR interval, indicating that they are from the sinus node. The rhythm is slightly irregular, varying about 26%. The most common cause of sinus dysrhythmia is a normal respiratory variation; some RR variation is considered a sign of normal function. A fixed/unvarying RR may indicate pathology from cardiac disease, electrolyte or acid-base imbalances. The shortest RR interval is 0.74 second 0.26 second and the longest RR interval is 1 second.

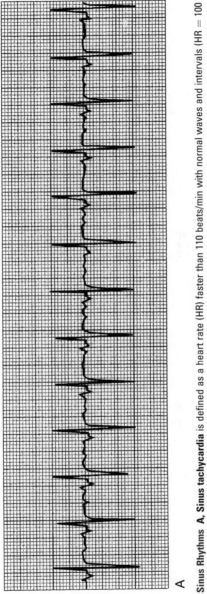

Sinus Rhythms A, Sinus tachycardia is defined as a heart rate (HR) faster than 110 beats/min with normal waves and intervals (HR = 100 beats/min, PR = 0.12 second, QRS = 0.08 second).

Continued

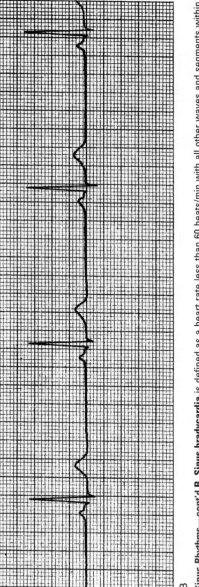

Sinus Rhythms—cont'd B, Sinus bradycardia is defined as a heart rate less than 60 beats/min with all other waves and segments within normal values (HR = 35 beats/min, PR = 0.16 second, QRS = 0.10 second).

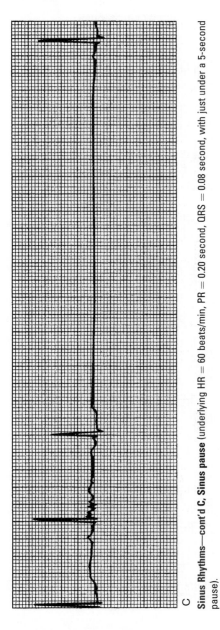

Sinus Rhythms—cont'd C, Sinus pause (underlying HR = 60 beats/min, PR = 0.20 second, QRS = 0.08 second, with just under a 5-second pause).

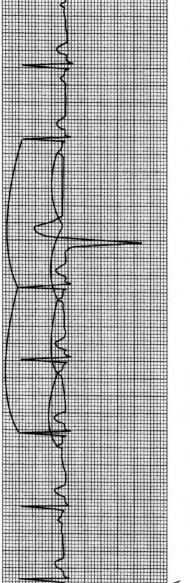

A

Normal Sinus Rhythm with a Premature Contraction A, Normal sinus rhythm with a premature ventricular contraction (PVC). A complete compensatory pause follows the PVC, indicated by the fact that the sinus P wave after the pause comes exactly when it was due to occur.

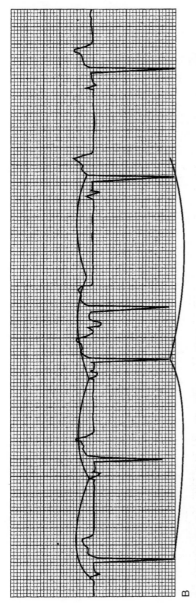

Normal Sinus Rhythm with a Premature Contraction—cont'd B, Normal sinus rhythm with a premature atrial contraction (PAC). An incomplete or noncompensatory pause follows the PAC, indicated by the sinus P wave after the pause coming before it was originally due to occur. The QRS complex also comes before it was due.

B

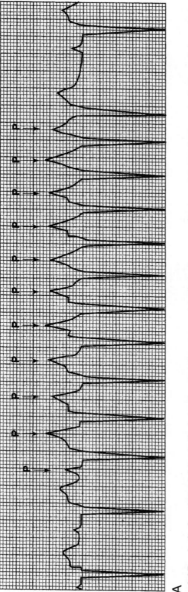

A

Atrial Dysrhythmias An atrial dysrhythmia implies that the source of the irregular rate or rhythm originates in the atria. **A,** Normal sinus rhythm with an 11-beat run of paroxysmal atrial tachycardia (PAT) with 1:1 conduction.

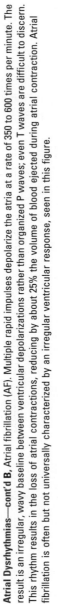

Atrial Dysrhythmias—cont'd B, Atrial fibrillation (AF). Multiple rapid impulses depolarize the atria at a rate of 350 to 600 times per minute. The result is an irregular, wavy baseline between ventricular depolarizations rather than organized P waves; even T waves are difficult to discern. This rhythm results in the loss of atrial contractions, reducing by about 25% the volume of blood ejected during atrial contraction. Atrial fibrillation is often but not universally characterized by an irregular ventricular response, seen in this figure.

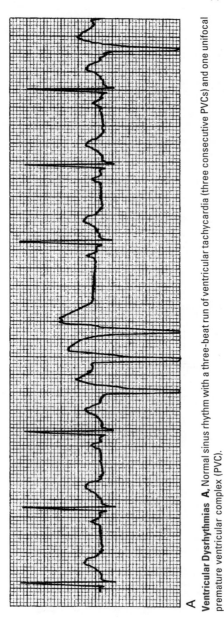

Ventricular Dysrhythmias A, Normal sinus rhythm with a three-beat run of ventricular tachycardia (three consecutive PVCs) and one unifocal premature ventricular complex (PVC).

A

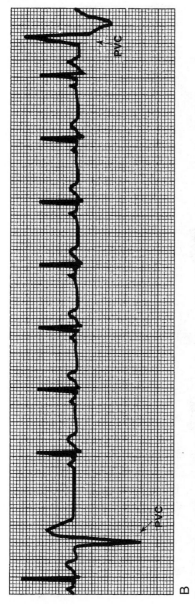

Ventricular Dysrhythmias—cont'd B, Normal sinus rhythm with multifocal PVCs (one negative and the other positive).

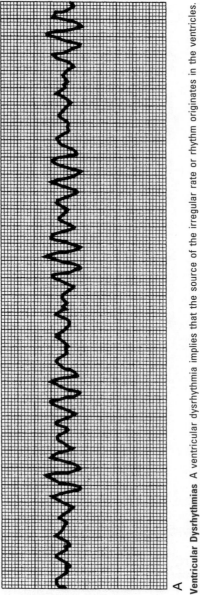

Ventricular Dysrhythmias A ventricular dysrhythmia implies that the source of the irregular rate or rhythm originates in the ventricles. **A,** Coarse ventricular fibrillation.

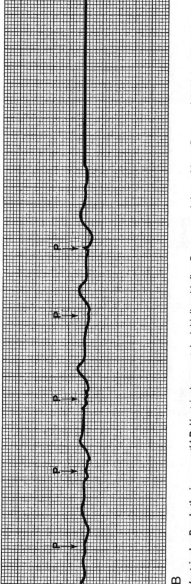

Ventricular Dysrhythmias—cont'd B, Ventricular asystole, initially with five P waves and then with no P waves (arterial and ventricular standstill).

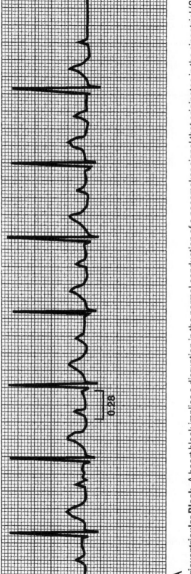

Atrioventricular Block A heart block implies a disruption in the normal conduction of a pacemaker signal that originates in the sinoatrial (SA) node. **A,** Normal sinus rhythm with a first-degree AV block (PR interval = 0.28 second). First- and second-degree heart block imply a delay at the AV node.

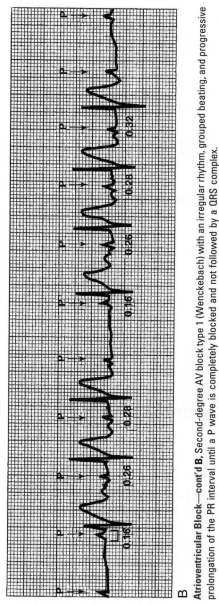

Atrioventricular Block—cont'd B, Second-degree AV block type 1 (Wenckebach) with an irregular rhythm, grouped beating, and progressive prolongation of the PR interval until a P wave is completely blocked and not followed by a QRS complex.

Continued

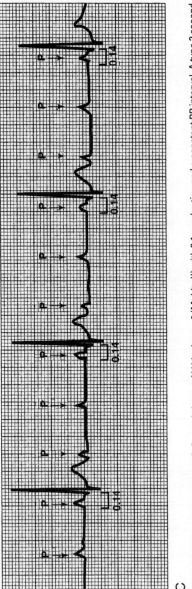

Atrioventricular Block—cont'd C, Second-degree AV block type 2 (Mobitz II) with 3:1 conduction and a constant PR interval. A type 2 second-degree block is more serious and indicates the need for more urgent intervention, such as placing a transcutaneous pacemaker and anticipating the placement of a permanent placement.

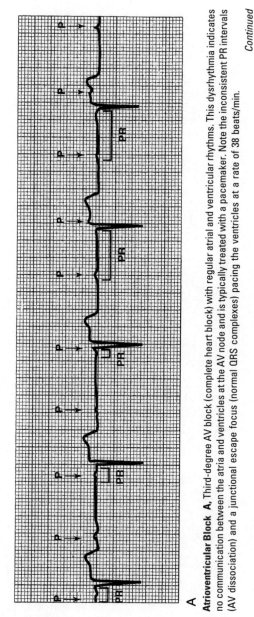

Atrioventricular Block A, Third-degree AV block (complete heart block) with regular atrial and ventricular rhythms. This dysrhythmia indicates no communication between the atria and ventricles at the AV node and is typically treated with a pacemaker. Note the inconsistent PR intervals (AV dissociation) and a junctional escape focus (normal QRS complexes) pacing the ventricles at a rate of 38 beats/min.

Continued

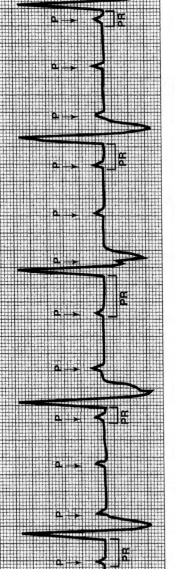

Atrioventricular Block—cont'd B, Third-degree AV block with regular atrial and ventricular rhythms, inconsistent PR intervals (AV dissociation), and ventricular escape focus pacing the ventricles at a rate of 35 beats/min, with wide QRS complexes. Third-degree heart block implies a more serious condition and a delay low in the AV node or along the bundle of His. New onset of this rhythm should be communicated to the physician immediately and a transcutaneous pacemaker should be placed until the patient can be fully evaluated for possible permanent pacemaker placement.

The Patient Requiring Intubation and Ventilation

OVERVIEW

- Mechanical ventilation is usually a temporary life-support technique, although it may be lifelong for those with severe, restrictive lung disease such as fibrotic pneumonitis and for those with chronic, progressive neuromuscular diseases such as amyotrophic lateral sclerosis that reduce effective ventilation.
- It is most often used for patients with hypoxemia and progressive alveolar hypoventilation with respiratory acidosis.
- Mechanical ventilation requires intubation to establish an artificial airway.
- The purposes of intubation are to maintain a patent airway, to provide a means to remove secretions, and to provide ventilation and oxygen.
- The most common type of airway for a short-term basis is the endotracheal (ET) tube.

PATIENT-CENTERED COLLABORATIVE CARE

- Endotracheal intubation
  1. Most often, the long, polyvinyl chloride ET tube is passed through the mouth into the trachea, usually by an anesthesiologist, nurse anesthetist, pulmonologist, or advanced practice nurse. The nasal route is reserved for pre-existing facial anomalies, new facial or oral traumas, and surgeries when oral intubation is not possible.
  2. When properly positioned, the tip of the ET tube rests about 2 cm above the carina.
  3. The main parts of the ET tube are:
     a. The shaft, with a radiopaque line running its length
     b. The cuff at the distal end, which is inflated after placement to create a seal between the trachea and the cuff
     c. The pilot balloon, which is a one-way valve, allows air to be inserted into the cuff, and prevents air from escaping
     d. The adaptor, which connects the ET tube to ventilator tubing or to other types of oxygen delivery systems

4. Prepare for emergency intubation by:
   a. Summoning intubation personnel in the facility to the bedside in an emergency situation
   b. Explaining the procedure to the patient as clearly as possible
   c. Ensuring that the code ("crash") cart, airway equipment box, and suction equipment (often already on the code cart) are at the bedside
   d. Maintaining a patent airway through positioning and inserting an oral or nasopharyngeal airway until the patient is intubated
   e. During the intubation, continuously monitoring for changes in vital signs, signs of hypoxia or hypoxemia, dysrhythmias, and aspiration
   f. Ensuring that each intubation attempt lasts no longer than 30 seconds, preferably fewer than 15 seconds, and after 30 seconds, providing oxygen by means of a mask and manual resuscitation bag to prevent hypoxia and cardiac arrest
   g. Suctioning, as necessary
   h. Verifying tube placement by assessing for:
      (1) End-tidal carbon dioxide levels
      (2) Bilateral breath sounds
      (3) Symmetrical chest movement
      (4) Air emerging from the ET tube
      (5) Concurrence with the documented insertion landmark with ET centimeter mark (e.g.,"23 cm at the lips" or "22 cm at the teeth") after chest x-ray confirms correct placement.
   i. Stabilizing ET tube at the mouth or nose and marking the tube where it touches the lip, incisor tooth, or naris
   j. Inserting an oral airway to keep the patient from biting the ET tube
5. Providing nursing care, including:
   a. Regularly assessing tube placement via chest x-ray and landmark (e.g.,"23 cm at the lips"), minimal cuff leak, breath sounds, and chest wall movement
   b. Preventing pulling or tugging on the tube by the patient to prevent dislodgment or "slipping" of the tube
      (1) Ensuring proper positioning
      (2) Ensuring adequate sedation
      (3) Providing constant supervision, often with the help of family members
      (4) Applying soft wrist restraints as a last resort

      c. Checking the pilot balloon to ensure that the cuff is inflated

      d. Assessing and changing the device or tape that secures the ET tube

         (1) If using adhesive tape, always taping the tube to the upper lip, never the lower lip

         (2) Inspecting the device or tape at least every shift for signs of loosening or skin irritation or breakdown

         (3) Checking anchoring each shift if swelling in the face and neck occurs or if there is an increase in fluid retention

         (4) Applying skin protectants to the areas under the tape or device

         (5) Keeping the ET tube from touching the corners of the mouth

- Mechanical ventilation
  1. The purposes of mechanical ventilation are to improve gas exchange and to decrease the work needed for an effective breathing pattern.
  2. Mechanical ventilation does not cure diseased lungs; it provides ventilation until the patient is able to resume the process of breathing.
  3. Positive-pressure ventilators generate pressure that pushes air into the lungs and expands the chest. There are four types:
     a. *Pressure-cycled ventilators* (bi-level positive airway pressure [BIPAP], positive end-expiratory pressure [PEEP]) push air into the lungs until a preset airway pressure is reached.
     b. *Time-cycled ventilators* push air into the lungs until a preset time has elapsed.
     c. *Volume-cycled ventilators* push air into the lungs until a preset volume is delivered.
     d. *Microprocessor ventilators* are computer-managed, positive-pressure ventilators that often have the components of volume-, time-, and pressure-cycled ventilators.
  4. Modes of ventilation are the way in which the patient receives breaths from the ventilator:
     a. *Assist-control ventilation* (ACV), in which the ventilator takes over the work of breathing for the patient. The tidal volume and ventilatory rate are preset to establish a minimal ventilatory pattern if the patient does not trigger spontaneous breaths.

b. *Synchronized intermittent mandatory ventilation* (SIMV), in which the tidal volume and ventilatory rate are preset to establish a minimal ventilatory pattern when the patient does not trigger breaths, but it also allows spontaneous breathing at the patient's own rate and tidal volume between the ventilator breaths.

c. *BIPAP* provides noninvasive pressure support ventilation by nasal mask or facemask.

d. Additional, less commonly used modes include:
    (1) Pressure support
    (2) Continuous flow (flow-by)
    (3) Maximum mandatory ventilation (MMV)
    (4) Inverse inspiration-expiration (I/E) ratio
    (5) Permissive hypercarbia
    (6) Airway pressure-release ventilation
    (7) Proportional assist ventilation
    (8) High-frequency ventilation
    (9) High-frequency oscillation

5. Common ventilator controls and settings include:

a. *Tidal volume* (V_T): The volume of air the patient receives with each breath ranges between 74 and 10 mL/kg of body weight. In the presence of acute lung injury (ALI) or acute respiratory distress syndrome (ARDS), a reduced tidal volume of 5 to 6 mL/kg is used to prevent additional lung injury.

b. *Rate*: The number of ventilator breaths delivered per minute is usually between 10 and 14 breaths/min.

c. *Fraction of inspired oxygen* (Fio_2): The oxygen level delivered to the patient can range between 21% and 100% oxygen.

d. *Peak airway (inspiratory) pressure* (PIP): This is the pressure needed by the ventilator to deliver a set tidal volume at a given lung compliance.

e. *Continuous positive airway pressure* (CPAP): Positive airway pressure is applied throughout the entire respiratory cycle for patients who are breathing spontaneously. It keeps the alveoli open during inspiration and prevents alveolar collapse during expiration. Normal levels of CPAP are 5 to 15 cm H_2O.

f. *PEEP*: Positive pressure is exerted during the expiratory phase of ventilation to improve oxygenation by enhancing gas exchange and preventing atelectasis. The amount of PEEP is usually 5 to 15 cm H_2O.

g. *Flow*: This rate is how fast each breath is delivered, and it is usually set at 40 L/min.

⚠ NURSING SAFETY PRIORITY: Critical Rescue

If a patient is agitated or restless, has a widely fluctuating pressure reading on inspiration, or has other signs of air hunger, the flow may be set too low. Increasing the flow and investigating oxygenation status (either peripheral oxygenation [SpO_2] or arterial [P_aO_2] values) should be tried before using chemical restraints.

6. Three nursing priorities in caring for the patient during mechanical ventilation are monitoring and evaluating patient responses, managing the ventilator system safely, and preventing complications.
7. Provide nursing care, including:
   a. Assessing respiratory status, including auscultating lung sounds, assessing respiratory rate and quality, indicating presence/absence of air leak, evaluating SpO_2, characteristics of the artificial airway, secretions, and patient comfort with mechanical ventilation settings.
   b. Assessing the patient's baseline respiratory status every 4 hours when hemodynamically stable, as well as his or her response to interventions
      (1) Taking vital signs with each respiratory assessment
      (2) Observing the patient's color (especially lips and nail beds)
      (3) Observing the patient's chest for bilateral expansion
      (4) Assessing the placement of the nasotracheal or endotracheal tube via chest x-ray and documented landmarks such as centimeter (cm) mark at lips or teeth.
      (5) Measuring oxygen saturation
      (6) Evaluating arterial blood gases (ABGs), as indicated
      (7) Maintaining head of the bed higher than 30 degrees to prevent microaspiration and ventilator-associated pneumonia
      (8) Noting the peak and plateau inspiratory pressures from the ventilator, because increasing pressure may indicate a need for suctioning or worsening lung disease
   c. Explaining all procedures and treatments, providing access to a call bell, and visiting the patient often
   d. Providing a light touch or blow-by call light. A magic slate, letter/picture board, or pencil and paper for communication is also essential
   e. Documenting pertinent observations in the patient's medical record (chart)

f. Checking at least every 4 to 8 hours to be sure the ventilator settings are set as prescribed

g. Checking to be sure alarms are set (especially low-pressure and low-exhaled volume)

⚠ NURSING SAFETY PRIORITY: Critical Rescue

Alarm systems must be activated and functional at all times. If the cause of the alarm cannot be determined, ventilate the patient manually with a resuscitation bag until the problem is corrected by another health care professional.

h. If the patient is on PEEP, observing the peak airway pressure dial to determine the proper level of PEEP

i. Observing the exhaled volume digital display to be sure the patient is receiving the prescribed tidal volume

j. Monitoring for water collected in ventilator tubing and removing/draining collected water

⚠ NURSING SAFETY PRIORITY: Critical Rescue

Never empty fluid in the tubing back into the ventilator or humidification reservoir.

k. Ensuring humidity by keeping delivered air temperature maintained at body temperature

l. Ensuring the airway cuff (is adequately inflated to provide adequate tidal volume

m. Auscultating the lungs for crackles, wheezes, equal breath sounds, and decreased or absent breath sounds

n. Observing the patient's need for tracheal, oral, or nasal suctioning every 2 hours

o. Performing suctioning, as needed

p. Inspecting the patient's mouth for internal and external pressure ulcers, especially at the point of contact with the ET tube.

q. Performing mouth care every 2 hours. Include cleaning gums, tongue, and teeth to decrease the oral bioburden and subsequent airway infection.

r. Changing the airway anchor (e.g., tape or commercial device) per institutional policy, whenever airway device is not secure and as needed for hygiene

s. Carefully move the oral ET tube to the opposite side of the mouth once daily to prevent ulcers.

t. Assessing patients for GI distress (diarrhea, constipation, tarry stools)

    u. Maintaining accurate intake and output records to monitor fluid balance

    v. Turning the patient at least every 2 hours to promote lung expansion. Consider continuous lateral rotation therapy if the patient is comatose or at high risk for or experiences acute lung injury or adult respiratory distress syndrome.

    w. Altering treatments and nursing care with intervals for rest

    x. Monitoring for the effectiveness of mechanical ventilation in terms the patient's physiologic and psychological status

    y. Monitoring for adverse effects of mechanical ventilation: infection, barotrauma, and reduced cardiac output

    z. Positioning the patient to facilitate ventilation-perfusion matching ("good lung down"), as appropriate

    aa. Administering prescribed muscle-paralyzing agents, sedatives, and narcotic analgesics. Anticipate a sedation holiday for at least 20 minutes daily when sedatives are given continuously as IV. Analgesics may also be stopped when given continuously IV during the holiday. This period is used to assess patient neurologic status, evaluate for the presence of delirium, and measure spontaneous breathing parameters with the respiratory therapist.

8. Preventing these complications (most are caused by the positive pressure from the ventilator)

    a. Cardiac problems include hypotension and fluid retention.

       (1) Teach the patient to avoid a Valsalva maneuver (bearing down while holding the breath).

       (2) Prevent constipation.

       (3) Monitor the patient's fluid intake and output, weight, hydration, and signs of hypovolemia.

    b. Lung problems include barotrauma (damage to the lungs by positive pressure), volutrauma (damage to the lung by excess volume delivered to one lung over the other), and acid-base imbalance.

    c. GI and nutritional problems result from the stress of mechanical ventilation.

       (1) Administer prescribed drug therapy (antacids, sucralfate [Carafate, Sulcrate <can>], histamine blockers such as ranitidine [Zantac], or proton-pump inhibitors such as esomeprazole [Nexium]).

       (2) Consult with a nutritionist to provide balanced nutrition through the diet, enteral feedings, or parenteral feedings.

(3) Closely monitor potassium, calcium, magnesium, and phosphate levels, and replenish deficits as prescribed.

(4) Monitor sodium, renal function (i.e., BUN, creatinine, urine output, peripheral edema), because fluid overload and dehydration can impair optimal respiratory function

(5) Monitor for anemia in patients with chronic ventilation. Reduced oxygen-carrying capacity in anemia can contribute to delayed weaning from mechanical ventilation.

d. Monitor for infection, especially ventilator-associated pneumonia (VAP), and implement these practices for the ventilator bundle:

(1) If possible, perform oral care with a disinfecting oral rinse *immediately before* the intubation.

(2) Do not wear hand jewelry, especially rings, when providing care to ventilator patients.

(3) Wash hands before and after contact with the patient.

(4) Provide oral care per institutional policy, typically every 2 to 4 hours.

(5) Remove subglottic secretions frequently (at least every 2 hours) or continuously (when the ET tube has a separate lumen that opens directly above the tube cuff).

(6) Keep the head of the bed elevated to at least 30 degrees unless another health problem is a contraindication for this position.

(7) Verify that an initial x-ray has been obtained to confirm the placement of any nasogastric tube before instilling drugs, fluids, or feedings into the tube.

(8) Work with the patient and health care team to assist in the weaning process as soon as possible.

(9) When weaning is delayed beyond 7 to 21 days or is unlikely to be successful because of the patient's condition, anticipate a surgical tracheostomy with subsequent placement of a tracheostomy tube.

i.   Maintain a clean surgical site, following institutional policy for new tracheostomy site care.

ii. Inform surgeon of bright red or copious or recurrent bleeding immediately and about the presence of persistent blood at the site or in endotracheal secretions beyond 3 to 4 days after surgery.

iii. Provide tracheostomy tube management per institutional policy.

    iv. If using inline suction equipment, use tracheostomy-compatible equipment. It is shorter, reflecting the decreased length of the airway.

    v. In some cases, a patient may progress to a permanent tracheotomy without tubing to mechanical ventilation. A tracheotomy may close over time if it is not needed to maintain an airway.

  e. Muscle deconditioning and weakness are caused by immobility.

    (1) Get the patient out of bed as soon as possible.

    (2) Ambulate the patient with assistance.

    (3) Encourage the patient to perform active range-of-motion (ROM) exercises; provide passive ROM to maintain joint mobility in patients who are not able to assist with or complete independent ROM.

    (4) Premedicate with analgesics before initiating activity if pain interferes with mobility.

    (5) Consult with physical and occupational therapists to provide assistive devices, positioning devices, and splints to maintain function in weak or comatose patients.

9. Perform extubation (ET tube removal).

  a. Explain the procedure to the patient.

  b. Set up the prescribed oxygen delivery system.

  c. Have the equipment for emergency reintubation at the bedside.

  d. Hyperoxygenate the patient.

  e. Thoroughly suction the ET tube and the oral cavity.

  f. Rapidly deflate the cuff of the ET tube, and remove the tube at peak inspiration.

  g. Immediately instruct the patient to cough.

  h. Give oxygen by facemask or nasal cannula.

  i. Assess the patient's responses, ability to maintain adequate gas exchange, and the possible need for reintubation.

🛑 NURSING SAFETY PRIORITY: Critical Rescue

Monitor vital signs every 5 minutes at first, and assess ventilatory pattern for manifestations of respiratory distress (dyspnea, coughing, and the inability to expectorate secretions). Notify the physician or Rapid Response Team at the onset of these problems.

🛑 NURSING SAFETY PRIORITY: Critical Rescue

If stridor (high-pitched, crowing noise during inspiration) develops at any time, immediately call the Rapid Response Team.

The Patient Requiring Chest Tubes

OVERVIEW

- A chest tube is a drain placed in the pleural space to restore intrapleural pressure and allow re-expansion of the lung through the use of gravity and pressure.
- The drainage system consists of one or more chest tubes or drains, a collection container placed below the chest level, and a water seal to keep air from entering the chest.
- The tip of the tube used to drain air is placed near the front lung's apex and usually sutured in place. The tube that drains liquid is placed on the side near the base of the lung. The sites are covered with airtight dressings.
- The chest tube is connected to about 6 feet (2 meters) of tubing that leads to a collection device placed several feet below the chest.
- Standard stationary chest-tube drainage systems usually have three chambers connected to each other:
  1. Chamber 1 is the drainage collection container with the tube (s) from the patient connected to it, penetrating shallowly and never having the tip touch the fluid collection.
  2. Chamber 2 is the water seal that prevents air from entering the patient's pleural space. Air from the pleural space also enters chamber 1 but moves immediately to chamber 2 through the connecting tube. This tube must always be under the water level in chamber 2 to prevent air from returning to the patient. The tube acts as a one-way valve, allowing air to move into the water and preventing air in this chamber from re-entering the tube. As long as the tip of the tube from the first chamber is under water in the water seal chamber, air that has escaped from the patient's chest tube cannot re-enter the patient.
     a. Bubbling of the fluid in this chamber indicates air drainage from the patient and is usually seen when the patient exhales, coughs, or sneezes.
     b. When the air in the pleural space has been removed and the pleural space re-seals, bubbling stops. A blocked or kinked chest tube also can cause bubbling to stop.

    3. Chamber 3 is the suction control of the system. The health care provider prescribes the amount of suction (typical about −20 mm Hg) to be maintained in this chamber.

PATIENT-CENTERED COLLABORATIVE CARE

- Initial care includes:
  1. Checking hourly to ensure the sterility and patency of any chest drainage system
  2. Taping tubing junctions to prevent accidental disconnections
  3. Keeping an occlusive dressing at the chest-tube insertion site
  4. Keeping sterile gauze at the bedside to cover the insertion site immediately if the chest tube becomes dislodged
  5. Keeping padded clamps at the bedside for use if the drainage system is interrupted
  6. Positioning the drainage tubing to prevent kinks and large loops of tubing that can block drainage and prevent lung re-expansion
- Specific nursing care includes:
  1. Assessing for difficulty breathing
  2. Assessing breathing effectiveness by pulse oximetry
  3. Checking alignment of the trachea
  4. Ensuring that the dressing on the chest around the tube is tight and intact
  5. Reinforcing or changing loose dressings according to agency policy and surgeon preference
  6. Checking the tube insertion site for condition of the skin and palpating the area for puffiness or crackling that may indicate subcutaneous emphysema
  7. Inspecting the site for signs of infection (redness, purulent drainage) or excessive bleeding
  8. Assessing the depth of tube placement
  9. Listening to breath sounds in each lung
  10. Assessing for pain and its location and intensity, and administering prescribed drugs for pain as prescribed
  11. Assisting the patient to deep breathe, cough, perform maximal sustained inhalations, and use incentive spirometry
  12. Repositioning the patient who reports a "burning" pain in the chest
- Manage the drainage system by:
  1. Not "stripping" the chest tube
  2. Keeping the drainage system lower than the level of the patient's chest
  3. Keeping the chest tube as straight as possible, avoiding kinks and dependent loops

4. Ensuring the chest tube is securely taped to the connector and that the connector is taped to the tubing going into the collection chamber

5. Assessing the water-seal chamber, which, in some systems, gentle bubbles during the patient's exhalation, forceful cough, or position changes. If the system is "dry," then assess fluctuation of the sealed chamber.

6. Assessing for normal "tidaling" (water in the long tube of the second chamber rises and falls 2 to 4 inches during inhalation and exhalation)

7. Checking that the prescribed suction pressure is maintained

8. Checking and documenting the amount, color, and characteristics of fluid in the collection chamber as often as needed according to the patient's condition and agency policy

9. Changing the system if the collection chamber becomes more than 75% full

10. Obtaining drainage samples (when prescribed) using institutional or manufacturer practice guidelines

11. Immediately notifying the physician or Rapid Response Team about:
    a. Tracheal deviation
    b. Sudden onset or increased intensity of dyspnea
    c. Oxygen saturation less than 90%
    d. Drainage greater than 70 mL/hr for 2 or more hours
    e. Visible eyelets on the chest tube or the chest tube falling out of the patient's chest. Cover the area with dry, sterile gauze
    f. Chest tube disconnecting from the drainage system (first put the end of tube in a container of sterile water and keep it below the level of the patient's chest)
    g. Drainage in the tube stopping in the first 24 hours

Communication Quick Reference for Spanish-Speaking Patients

THE BODY • EL CUERPO (ehl koo-EHR-poh)

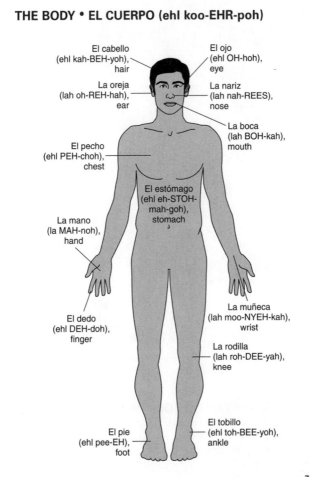

El cabello
(ehl kah-BEH-yoh),
hair

El ojo
(ehl OH-hoh),
eye

La oreja
(lah oh-REH-hah),
ear

La nariz
(lah nah-REES),
nose

La boca
(lah BOH-kah),
mouth

El pecho
(ehl PEH-choh),
chest

El estómago
(ehl eh-STOH-mah-goh),
stomach

La mano
(la MAH-noh),
hand

La muñeca
(lah moo-NYEH-kah),
wrist

El dedo
(ehl DEH-doh),
finger

La rodilla
(lah roh-DEE-yah),
knee

El tobillo
(ehl toh-BEE-yoh),
ankle

El pie
(ehl pee-EH),
foot

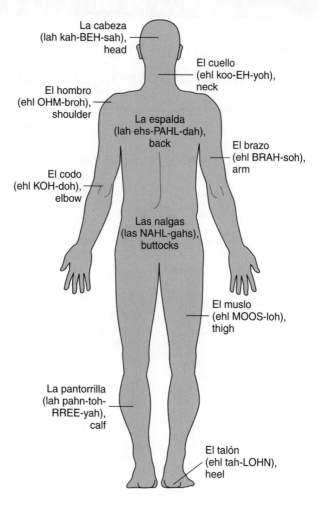

La cabeza
(lah kah-BEH-sah),
head

El cuello
(ehl koo-EH-yoh),
neck

El hombro
(ehl OHM-broh),
shoulder

La espalda
(lah ehs-PAHL-dah),
back

El brazo
(ehl BRAH-soh),
arm

El codo
(ehl KOH-doh),
elbow

Las nalgas
(las NAHL-gahs),
buttocks

El muslo
(ehl MOOS-loh),
thigh

La pantorrilla
(lah pahn-toh-
RREE-yah),
calf

El talón
(ehl tah-LOHN),
heel

COMMON TERMS FOR BODY PARTS

Move the, Mueva (mooh-EH-bah)
Touch the, Toque (TOH-keh)
Point to the, Señale (seh-NYAH-leh)

MORE PARTS OF THE BODY
Armpit, la axila (lah ahk-SEE-lah)
Breasts, los senos (lohs SEH-nohs)
Collarbone, la clavícula (lah klah-BEE-koo-lah)
Diaphragm, el diafragma (ehl dee-ah-FRAHG-mah)
Forearm, el antebrazo (ehl ahn-teh-BRAH-soh)
Groin, la ingle (lah EEN-gleh)
Hip, la cadera (lah kah-DEH-rah)
Kneecap, la rótula (lah ROH-too-lah)
Nail, la uña (lah OO-nyah)
Pelvis, la pelvis (lah PEHL-bees)
Rectum, el recto (ehl REHK-toh)
Rib, la costilla (lah kohs-TEE-yah)
Spine, la espina dorsal (lah ehs-PEE-nah DOHR-sahl)
Throat, la garganta (lah gahr-GAHN-tah)
Tongue, le lengua (lah LEHN-goo-ah)

ORGANS
Appendix, el apéndice (ehl ah-PEHN-dee-seh)
Bladder, la vejiga (lah beh-HEE-gah)
Brain, el cerebro (ehl seh-REH-broh)
Colon, el colon (ehl KOH-lohn)
Esophagus, el esófago (ehl eh-SOH-fah-goh)
Gallbladder, la vesícula biliar (lah beh-SEE-koo-lah bee-lee-AHR)
Genitals, los genitales (lohs heh-nee-TAH-lehs)
Heart, el corazón (ehl koh-rah-SOHN)
Kidney, el riñón (ehl ree-NYOHN)
Large intestine, el intestino grueso (ehl een-tehs-TEE-noh groo-EH-soh)
Liver, el hígado (ehl EE-gah-doh)
Lungs, los pulmones (lohs pool-MOH-nehs)
Pancreas, el páncreas (ehl PAHN-kreh-ahs)
Small intestine, el intestino delgado (ehl een-tehs-TEE-noh dehl-GAH-doh)
Spleen, el bazo (ehl BAH-soh)
Thyroid gland, la tiroides (lah tee-ROH-ee-dehs)
Tonsils, las amígdalas (lahs ah-MEEG-dah-lahs)
Uterus, el útero (ehl OO-teh-roh)

ESSENTIAL PHRASES

Good morning.	*Buenos días.*	Boo-EH-nohs DEE-ahs.
Good afternoon.	*Buenas tardes.*	Boo-EH-nahs TAHR-dehs.
Good night.	*Buenas noches.*	Boo-EH-nahs NOH-chehs.
Hello.	*Hola.*	OH-lah.
How are you?	*¿Cómo está?*	¿Koh-moh ehs-TAH?
Good (fine).	*Bien.*	Bee-EHN.
Bad, Better, Worse	*Mal, Mejor, Peor*	Mahl, Meh-OHR, peh-OHR
The same	*Igual*	Ee-GOO-ahl
Do you speak English?	*¿Habla Inglés?*	¿Ah-blah een-GLEHS?
I don't understand.	*No comprendo.*	Noh kom-PREHN-doh.
Excuse me.	*Discúlpeme.*	Dees-KOOL-peh-meh.
Please speak slowly.	*Por favor, hable más lento*	Pohr fah-VOHR, AH-bleh mahs LEHN-toh
Are you in pain?	*¿Está adolorido(a)?*	¿Ehs-TAH ah-doh-loh-REE-doh(dah)?
Yes, No	*Sí, No*	SEE, Noh
Tell me where it hurts.	*Digame donde le duele.*	DEE-gah-meh DOHN-deh leh doo-EH-leh.
Here, there	*Aquí, ahi*	Ah-KEE, ah-EE

DESCRIPTION OF PAIN

Is your pain ...	*Tiene un dolor ...*	Tee-EH-neh oon doh-LOHR ...
burning?	*¿que arde?*	¿keh AHR-deh?
constant?	*¿constante?*	¿kohns-TAHN-teh?
dull?	*¿amortiguado?*	¿ah-MOHR-tee-goo-AH-doh?
intermittent?	*¿intermitente?*	¿een-tehr-mee-TEHN-teh?
mild?	*¿moderado?*	¿moh-deh-RAH-doh?
severe?	*¿muy fuerte?*	¿MOO-ee foo-EHR-teh?
sharp?	*¿agudo?*	¿ah-GOO-doh?
throbbing?	*¿pulsante?*	¿pool-SAHN-teh?
worse?	*¿peor?*	¿peh-OHR?

Are you allergic to any medication?	*¿Es usted alérgico (a) a algun medicamento?*	¿Ehs oos-TEHD ah-LEHR-hee-koh(kah) ah ahl-GOON meh-dee-kah-MEHN-toh?
I'm here to help you.	*Estoy aquí para ayudarle.*	Ehs-TOH-ee ah-KEE pah-rah ah-yoo-DAHR-leh.
Calm down.	*Cálmese.*	KAHL-meh-seh.
Please.	*Por favor.*	Pohr fah-VOHR.
Thank you.	*Gracias.*	GRAH-see-ahs.
You're welcome.	*De nada.*	Deh NAH-dah
May I?	*¿Puedo?*	¿Poo-EH-doh?
Who, What, When, Where?	*¿Quién, Qué, Cuándo, Dónde?*	¿Kee-ehn, Keh, Koo-AHN-doh, DOHN-deh?
Zero, one, two, three, four	*Cero, uno, dos, tres, cuatro*	SEH-roh, OO-noh, dohs, trehs, koo-AH-troh
Five, six, seven, eight, nine, ten	*Cinco, seis, siete, ocho, nueve, diez*	SEEN-koh, SEH-ees, see-EH-teh, OH-choh, noo-EH-beh, dee-EHS

PRELIMINARY EXAMINATION

My name is _____, and I am your nurse.	*Me llamo _____, y soy su enfermera (o).*	Meh YAH-moh ___, ee SOH-ee soo ehn-fehr-MEH-rah(roh).
I'm going to ...	*Le voy a ...*	Leh VOH-ee ah ...
take your vital signs.	*tomar los signos vitales.*	toh-MAHR lohs SEEG-nohs vee-TAH-lehs.
weigh you.	*pesar.*	peh-SAHR.
take your blood pressure.	*tomar la presión.*	toh-MAHR lah preh-see-OHN.
Extend your arm and relax.	*Extienda su brazo y descánselo.*	Ehks-tee-EHN-dah soo BRAH-soh ee dehs-KAHN-seh-loh.
I'm going to take your ...	*Le voy a tomar ...*	Leh voy ah toh-MAHR...
pulse.	*el pulso.*	ehl POOL-soh.
temperature.	*su temperatura.*	soo tehm-peh-rah-TOO-rah.
I'm going to count your respirations.	*Voy a contar sus respiraciones.*	VOH-ee ah kohn-TAHR soos rehs-pee-rah-see-OH-nehs.

OBTAINING A BLOOD SAMPLE

I need to draw a blood sample.	*Necesito tomar una muestra de la sangre.*	Neh-seh-SEE-toh toh-MAHR OO-nah MOO-ehs-trah deh lah SAHN-greh.
Please give me your arm.	*Por favor, déme el brazo.*	Pohr fah-VOHR, DEH-meh ehl BRAH-soh.
It may cause a little discomfort.	*Le puede causar alguna molestia.*	Leh-poo-EH-deh kah-OO-sahr ahl-GOO-nah moh-LEHS-tee-ah.
I am going to put a tourniquet around your arm.	*Le voy a poner una liga alrededor del brazo.*	Leh VOH-ee ah poh-NEHR OO-nah LEE-gah ahl-reh-deh-DOHR dehl BRAH-soh.
I am going to draw blood from this vein.	*Voy a sacar la sangre de esta vena.*	Voy ah sah-KAHR lah SAHN-greh deh EHS-tah VEH-nah.

OBTAINING BLOOD FROM A FINGER STICK

I need to take a few drops of blood from your finger.	*Necesito sacar unas gotas de sangre de uno de sus dedos.*	Neh-seh-SEE-toh sah-KAHR OO-nahs GOH-tahs deh SAHN-greh deh OO-noh dehsoos DEH-dohs.

OBTAINING A URINE SAMPLE

We also need a urine sample.	*También necesitamos una muestra de la orina.*	Tahm-bee-EHN neh-seh-see-TAH-mohs OO-nah moo-EHS trah deh lah oh-REE-nah.
It has to be from the middle of the stream.	*Tiene que ser de la mitad del chorro.*	Tee-EH-neh keh sehr deh lah mee-TAHD dehl CHOH-rroh.
Put the urine in this cup.	*Ponga la orina en esta tasa.*	POHN-gah lah oh-REE-nah ehn EHS-tah TAH-sah.

OBTAINING A STOOL SPECIMEN

I need a sample of your stool.	*Necesito una muestra de su excremento.*	Neh-seh-SEE-toh OO-nah moo- EHS-trah deh soo ehks-kreh-MEN-toh.
Please put a small amount in this cup.	*Por favor ponga un poco en esta tasa.*	Pohr fah-VOHR POHN-gah oon POH-koh ehn EHS-tah TAH-sah.

OBTAINING A SPUTUM SPECIMEN

I need a sample of your sputum.	*Necesito una muestra de su esputo.*	Neh-seh-SEE-toh OO-nah MOO-ehs-trah deh soo ehs-POO-toh.
Please spit in this cup.	*Por favor, escupa en este vaso.*	Pohr fah-VOHR, ehs-KOO-pah ehn EHS-tah VAH-soh.

ORDERS

You need . . .	*Necesita . . .*	Neh-seh-SEE-tah . . .
a bandage.	*un vendaje.*	oon behn-DAH-heh.
a blood transfusion.	*una transfusión de sangre.*	OO-nah trahns-foo-see-OHN deh SAHN-greh.
a cast.	*un molde de yeso.*	oon MOHL-deh deh YEH-soh.
gauze.	*la gasa.*	lah GAH-sah.
intensive care.	*cuidado intensivo.*	koo-ee-DAH-doh een-tehn-SEE-boh.
intravenous fluids.	*líquidos intravenosos.*	LEE-kee-dohs een-trah-beh-NOH-sohs.
an operation.	*una operación.*	OO-nah oh-peh-rah-see-OHN.
physical therapy.	*terapia física.*	teh-RAH-pee-ah FEE-see-kah.
a shot.	*una inyección.*	OO-nah een-yehk-see-OHN.
x-rays.	*rayos equis.*	RAH-yohs EH-kees.
We're going to . . .	*Vamos a . . .*	VAH-mohs ah . . .
change the bandage.	*cambiarle el vendaje.*	kahm-bee-AHR-leh ehl behn-DAH-heh.
give you a bath.	*darle un baño.*	DAHR-leh oon BAH-nyoh.
take out the IV.	*sacarle el tubo intravenoso.*	sah-KAHR-leh ehl TOO-boh een-trah-beh-NOH-soh.

DESCRIPTION OF TUBES

The tube in your ...	*El tubo en su* ...	Ehl TOO-boh ehn soo ...
arm is for IV fluids.	*brazo es para líquidos intravenosos.*	BRAH-soh ehs PAH-rah LEE-kee-dohs een-trah-beh-NOH-sohs.
bladder is for urinating.	*vejiga es para orinar.*	beh-HEE-gah ehs PAH-rah oh-ree-NAHR.
stomach is for the food.	*estómago es para los alimentos.*	ehs-TOH-mah-goh ehs PAH-rah lohs ah-lee-MEN-tohs.
throat is for breathing.	*garganta es para respirar.*	gahr-GAHN-tah ehs PAH-rah rehs-pee-RAHR.

Index

Note: Page numbers followed by *b* indicate boxes and *t* indicate tables.

NOTES

NOTES

NOTES

NOTES